CHECK for CD on
ISSUE and
RETURN

ER010

Geriatric Rehabilitation

A Clinical Approach

Third Edition

Carole B. Lewis, PT, DPT, GCS, GTC, MSG, MPA, PhD, FAPTA
President
Premier Physical Therapy Services of Washington
Adjunct Professor
George Washington University
College of Medicine
School of Health Care Sciences
Washington, DC

Jennifer M. Bottomley, PT, MS, PhD
Geriatric Rehabilitation Program Consultant
Wayland, MA

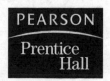

PEARSON

Prentice
Hall

Upper Saddle River, New Jersey 07458

Publisher: Julie Levin Alexander
Executive Assistant: Regina Bruno
Executive Editor: Mark Cohen
Associate Editor: Melissa Kerian
Editorial Assistant: Nicole Ragonese
Managing Editor for Production: Patrick Walsh
Production Liaison: Yagnesh Jani
Manufacturing Manager: Ilene Sanford
Manufacturing Buyer: Pat Brown
Cover Design Coordinator: Maria Guglielmo-Walsh
Formatting: Pine Tree Composition
Marketing Manager: Harper Coles
Marketing Coordinator: Michael Sirinides
Marketing Assistant: Wayne Celia
Printer/Binder: Von Hoffman/Owensville
Copy Editor: Nancy Marcello
Cover Design: Gary Sella
Cover Printer: Phoenix Color
Media Product Manager: John Jordon
Media Project Manager: Steve Hartner

Notice: The authors and the publisher of this volume have taken care to make certain that the doses of drugs and schedules of treatment are correct and compatible with the standards generally accepted at the time of publication. Nevertheless, as new information becomes available, changes in treatment and the use of drugs become necessary. The reader is advised to carefully consult the instruction and information material included in the package insert of each drug or therapeutic agent before administration. This advice is especially important when using new or infrequently used drugs. The publisher disclaims any liability, loss, injury, or damage incurred as a consequence, directly or indirectly, of the use and application of any of the contents of this volume.

■

This book is dedicated to the memory of Art Buchwald. He brought joy to many and enriched our lives.

Carole and Jennifer

Pearson Prentice Hall™ is a trademark of Pearson Education, Inc.
Pearson® is a registered trademark of Pearson plc
Prentice Hall® is a registered trademark of Pearson Education, Inc.

Pearson Education Ltd., *London*
Pearson Education Australia Pty. Limited, *Sydney*
Pearson Education Singapore, Pte. Ltd.
Pearson Education North Asia Ltd., *Hong Kong*
Pearson Education Canada, Ltd., *Toronto*
Pearson Educación de Mexico, S.A. de C.V.
Pearson Education—Japan, *Tokyo*
Pearson Education Malaysia, Pte. Ltd.
Pearson Education, Upper Saddle River, New Jersey

10 9 8 7 6 5 4 3 2

ISBN 0-13-170826-0
9780131708266

Table of Contents

NOTE: This book was in press when the latest statistics from the 2006 Federal Interagency Forum on Aging Related Statisics: 2006 was released. To ensure that the reader receive the latest statistics we are enclosing this entire report on the Student CD. Thanks to the Federal Interagency Forum on Aging-Related Satistics. Older Americans Update 2006: Key Indicators of Well-Being. Federal Interagency Forum on Aging-Related Statistics.Washington, DC: U.S. government Printing Office. May 2006

Preface to the Third Edition

I remember when I was six years old and I accidentally knocked a robin's nest from a tall bush in our backyard. The nest came hurling to the ground with all the newly hatched robins still very much alive. I could see the mouths of the tiny hungry creatures open and ready and even demanding of food. What stands out my memory is when the mother bird returned to the nest and supplied the food. The baby birds devoured the food with such fervor and then they were satiated.

I see today's therapists in the field of geriatrics as these hungry birds, wanting, and demanding usable information. These therapists have their minds open to new ideas and solutions to the care of this wonderful aging population. It is my hope for this new edition, that it will be just the right amount of usable information for the hungry therapist in geriatrics. I am excited to present this new information in a way that will make them want to devour all this book has to offer.

So how is this edition different form the previous editions? There are many changes:

- *Evidence-Based Medicine* The most exciting change to the 3rd edition is the inclusion of Evidence Based Medicine (EBM) interventions throughout. EBM treatment suggestions are given for a myriad of diagnoses. These EBM treatment ideas are boxed in so they are easy to locate. Each EBM suggestion provides the complete reference as it would appear in medical literature searches for further reading if more detail of the study is needed. When you see boxed in prose it is an EBM treatment suggestion.

- *Enhanced images courtesy of VHI* Visual Health Information (VHI), the maker of the popular exercise cards and software, has given us rights to use a number of their outstanding exercises.

- *CD-ROM included* Long tables, forms, and worksheets from prior editions, along with additional resources have been moved to the CD-ROM. This provides readers with an electronic tools and documents library and allows for a more manageable printed text. Throughout the book, whenever you see this symbol ● you can go to the CD ROM for a printable version. Additionally, the CD-ROM contains a fully functional demonstration version of the VHI exercise software.

- *Pearls* We've retained this popular feature, providing readers with the essence of what's most important, however the Pearls have been streamlined and moved to the beginning of each chapter.

- *Enhanced readability* In an effort to make the book more inviting and understandable, we have trimmed down the text, and added subheadings, introductions, and conclusions to each chapter.

- *Critical-evaluation questions* I hope the readers of this text will have a satisfying experience as they feed their hunger to answer many perplexing issues in the exciting care of older persons. Jennifer and I share an enthusiasm for this field and we hope that our passion explodes through the pages in our new exciting format.

Enjoy devouring as much as we enjoy creating and doing.

Carole B. Lewis

Acknowledgments

If there were an academy award for supporting people writing a book, it would go hands down to my family. Gratitude is not a large enough word to encompass my appreciation. They showed me constant patience, understanding, and a sense of humor during this somewhat grueling process. They stood by me and still loved me while I went through the numerous re-writes and frustrations to get this book to its current state. Your love and support through the years it took in researching, re-writing, editing and creating a virtually new text was deeply treasured by me. Barry, Madison and Gerald consider this your Oscar from me with all my heart. Thank you.

I would also like to thank Yagnesh Jani and Mark Cohen for being saints and putting up with my whining and assisting me in every step of the process. It is great to get that kind of support from a publisher. Thank you.

Carole B. Lewis

Reviewers

Evan Prost, PT, GCS
Clinical Instructor
Department of Physical Therapy
University of Missouri-Columbia
Columbia, Missouri

Joseph A. Lucca, PT, DPT, PhD, GCS
Associate Professor
Department of Physical Therapy
University of Delaware
Newark, Delaware

David Village, MSPT, D.H.Sc.
Associate Professor
Department of Physical Therapy
Andrews University
Berrien Springs, Michigan

Larry J. Nosse, MAPT, Ph.D.
Associate Professor
Department of Physical Therapy
Marquette University
Milwaukee, Wisconsin

Chad Cook, PT, PhD, MBA, OCS
Assistant Clinical Professor
Physical Therapy Program
Duke University Medical Center
Durham, North Carolina

Lynda Jack, MS, PT
Assistant Professor
Department of Physical Therapy
Florida Gulf University
Fort Myers, Florida

Lisa R. Dehner, PhD, PT
Assistant Professor
Health Sciences Department
College of Mount Saint Joseph
Cincinnati, Ohio

William H. Staples, PT, DPT, GCS
Assistant Professor
Krannert School of Physical Therapy
University of Indianapolis
Indianapolis, Indiana

Lynne Tierney, B.A., M.P.T.
Associate Professor
Department of Physical Therapy
Chapman University
Orange, California

PART I

Applied Gerontological Concepts

1

Demographics of Aging

Pearls

- Change in population size depends on the rates of birth, immigration, death, and emigration. Growth in the total population is most sensitive to a decline in mortality rates, whereas growth in the older population is due to a decline in fertility rates.
- The elderly made up 12.6% of the US population in 1990, and this figure is expected to climb to 20% by 2030.
- The US birthrate will stay below 3.7 million per year or decline, and the death rate will steadily decrease.
- The current ratio of elderly women to elderly men is three to two, and it is five to two for those over age 85. These ratios are expected gradually to increase through the 21st century.

- Viewed as a homogeneous group, the majority of elderly are free of disability until extreme old age.
- It is estimated that the number of minority elderly will grow at a more rapid rate than the number of white elderly over the next 60 years.
- In approximately 30 years, there will be 850 million elderly worldwide.

INTRODUCTION

Demography is the scientific study of the population. The demography of aging as a subfield of general demography has become increasingly important as it relates to the concerns of social gerontologists.[1] The study of the demography of aging is currently focused on determining: the state of the older population; changes in the numbers, proportionate size, and composition of this subpopulation; the component forces of fertility, mortality, morbidity, migration, and immigration; and the impact of these demographic changes on issues related to the social, economic, and health status of the elderly in an aging society.[1,2]

Distinct subgroups within the older population, somewhat ignored in the past, have also been receiving increased demographic emphasis in the past few years.[3] This development appears to reflect societal concerns about the policy challenges of meeting the welfare and health needs of all components of an aging society.[4]

Gilford[5] has determined that there are serious data gaps in existing demographic information. One such data gap has been identified in the area of the subgroup termed the "oldest-old" (also called the "frail elderly" or the "ex-

tremely old"). Because of the special concerns regarding the relatively high rates of illness and disability, and the concomitant implications for health care and social service provisions in this age group, the oldest-old have been presented by demographers as a geriatric imperative for future research.[6]

AN HISTORICAL PERSPECTIVE OF THE STUDY OF POPULATION AGING

The study of population aging has a relatively long history. Attention to population aging emerged in France at the close of the nineteenth century, when the proportion of persons aged 65 years of age and over exceeded 5%. By the 1900s, this had increased to 8%.[7] Sweden also experienced considerable population aging in the nineteenth century.[8] Sundbarg[8] was the first to place emphasis on the relative proportions of aged individuals in a society, and the first demographer to note systematic differences in age composition among countries. By implication, he hypothesized that there would be a demographic shift over time toward an aging population structure in all countries.[9]

For most western countries, the aging of the population has been a distinctly twentieth-century phenomenon. In the United States, concerted demographic attention to the aging process can be found as early as the 1920s,[10] and increasing concern was expressed in the 1930s when the declining fertility of the Depression led demographers to project rapid changes in the age structure of the United States.[11–13] Today, there is an increasing awareness that population aging will be an important issue in developing countries currently experiencing social and economic growth.[14] Population aging is now recognized as a worldwide phenomenon that commands immediate attention if effective societal responses are to be made to changing demographic realities.[1] As a result, many issues have emerged, such as the degree to which countries are able to make commitments to social welfare and health care policies in light of other priorities they face in the allocation of social and economic resources.[15,16]

DEMOGRAPHIC PROCESSES AND POPULATION AGE STRUCTURE

Change in the size of a population over time depends on the rate persons join the population through birth or immigration and the rate they leave the population through death or emigration. Persons born in a common year (i.e., classified by common age) are often grouped together as a birth cohort.[17] Such cohorts can be followed to reconstruct population history and to project future population change.

Traditionally, demographers have used the age of 65 for delineating old age. This facilitates standardized analyses and is grounded in social practices (e.g., retirement, Social Security provisions). In addition, because slightly more males than females are born in human populations and the mortality experiences of men and women differ, demographers typically distinguish the sex of persons in constructing models of population change.[3]

The number of persons who survive to any given age depends on the number of persons born into that cohort, the rate at which they survive, and the extent to which their numbers have changed because of cumulative differences between immigrants and emigrants. For example, the number of persons reaching the age of 65 in 1990 depended on the number of persons born in 1925; the cumulative probability that they survived each of the next sixty-five years; and the relative balance between the movement of persons from that age cohort into the United States or out of the United States from 1925 to 1990. The number of persons aged 65 and older in 1990 increased compared to the number of the elderly in 1989 because of the addition of this new cohort to the population of older persons was greater than the subtraction of persons who died in all cohorts aged 65 and older during that year.[3] The population of older persons can thus grow either because the size of the entering birth cohort is much larger than that of previous cohorts or because improvements in survivorship have reduced the number of deaths that might otherwise have occurred among the elderly. Demographers utilize the aging pyramid to graphically depict cohort distribution from year to year. Figure 1.1 shows the age structure of the US population in 1910.[18] Contrast this pyramid with the age structure of the US population in 1980 depicted in Figure 1.2 when the 1900–1910 birth cohort reached the 70 years of age and older category.[18] Figures 1.3, 1.4, and 1.5 demonstrate the significant shift in the aged population that occurred in the year 2000 (Figure 1.3) and the anticipated increase in the elderly population projected for 2025 (Figure 1.4) and 2050 (Figure 1.5). A distinction is drawn between "aging at the apex" (i.e., when the proportion of older persons in a population increases) and "aging from the base" (i.e., when the proportion of younger persons in a population decreases).

Historically, fertility is the most important determinant of population growth and the age structure of the population. Demographers view fertility as the critical process of renewal. When the fertility rate is high, the cohort born each year has more members than the cohorts that preceded it. At moderate to low levels of mortality, then, the number of newborns added to the population exceeds the number of older persons who die; the proportion of the population that is young increases, and its median age declines. When the birthrate is low, the proportion of the population that is old increases, and its median age rises.

The effect of a decline in mortality from high to moderate levels, which occurred in the United States in the late nineteenth century and early twentieth century as infectious diseases were brought under control, paradoxically caused the population to become younger.[19] The reason for this relationship between mortality and age structure is that the most important improvements in survivorship during this period occurred in the age groups of infants and children. Recent advances in the prevention and treatment of cardiovascular disease, however, have increased the survivorship of older persons. Since 1940, the major reason for the increase in the number of the oldest-old, those aged 85 years and older, has been the improved survivorship of the old.[20] About two-thirds of the 1980 to 1985 increase in the proportion of older persons in the population was caused by the mortality decline.[21] The tremendous increase in the projected number of elderly during the next fifty years results from the large cohorts born during the post–World War II baby boom reaching old age and the improved survivorship at all ages, especially the oldest-old.[19]

The growth of the total population is particularly sensitive to declining mortality rates, whereas the growth of the older population, especially in its proportionate size relative to the total population, occurs when the fertility rate declines.[22] In fact, declines in mortality focused at younger ages that are not accompanied by decreases in the fertility rate can lead to an overall younger population. The

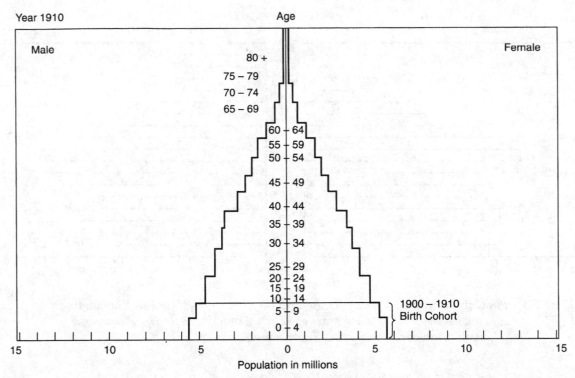

Figure 1.1   Population Pyramid Summary of Age Structure of the US Population: 1910 Census. (Adapted from the US Bureau of the Census, 1970 Census of Population: United States Summary, General Population Characteristics, PC(1):81, Washington, DC: US Government Printing Office; 1972. Reproduced with permission from Soldo, B.J. America's elderly in 1980's. *Pop Bull.* 1980; 35[1]:1–48.)

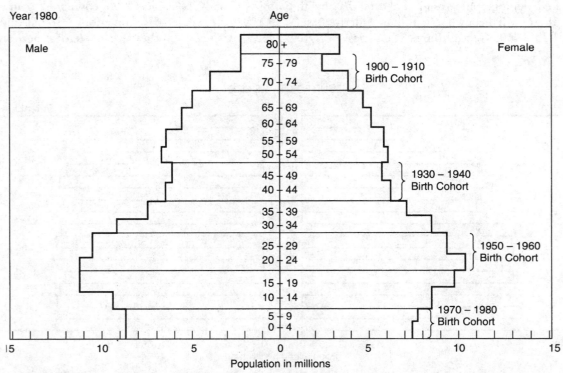

Figure 1.2   Population Pyramid Summary of Age Structure of the US Population: 1980 Census. (Adapted from Bouvier, L.F. America's baby boom generation: The fateful bulge. *Pop Bull.* Vol. 35:1. Washington, DC: Population Reference Bureau; 1980; 35[1]:1–48.)

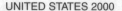
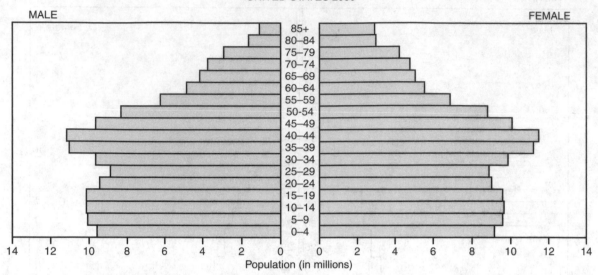

Figure 1.3   Population Pyramid US Population in 2000. (Source: U.S. Census Bureau, International Data Base. US Census Bureau. Accessed online at: http://www.census.gov/population/projections/nation/summary/np-t3-a.txt.)

sustained decrease in mortality that extends into older ages is the main reason for current population aging.[21]

PROJECTED POPULATION TRENDS IN AN AGING SOCIETY

The projected demographic trends indicate that by the year 2030 there will be over 69 million elderly Americans.[19,23,24] In 1960, Census Bureau statistics indicated that there were 16.7 million persons aged 65 and over In 1998, 34.4 million people were aged 65 years or older,[24] reflecting major changes in the population structure of the United States in this century. Figure 1.6 represents the growth of elderly individuals in the United States since 1900 and anticipated growth to the year 2030.

The number of older Americans has increased by 3.2 million, or 10.1%, since 1990, compared to an increase of 8.1% for the under-65 population.[25] To put things in perspective, since 1900 the percentage of Americans aged 65

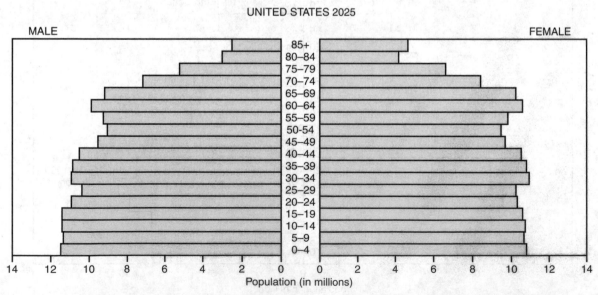

Figure 1.4   Population Pyramid Projected US Population: 2025. (Source: U.S. Census Bureau, International Data Base. US Census Bureau. Accessed online at: http://www.census.gov/population/projections/nation/summary/np-t3-a.txt.)

UNITED STATES 2050

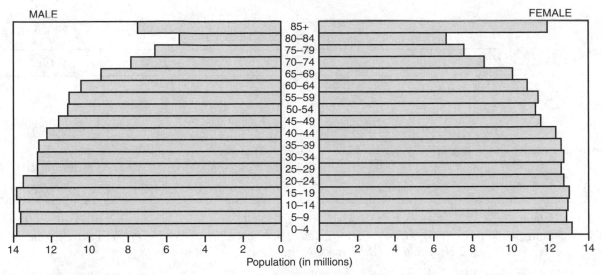

Figure 1.5   Population Pyramid Projected US Population: 2050. (Source: U.S. Census Bureau, International Data Base. US Census Bureau. Accessed online at: http://www.census.gov/population/projections/nation/summary/np-t3-a.txt.)

or older has more than tripled (4.1% in 1900 to 12.7% in 1998) and the number has increased eleven times (3.1 million to 34.4 million). If Census Bureau projections are accurate, it is anticipated that these proportions will climb to 17.7% in 2020, to 20% by the year 2030 when the children of the postwar baby boom will be well into old age, and to 22.9% by 2050.[25]

Between the years 1960 and 1990 there was a 2% annual growth in the overall elderly population. This trend is actually expected to decrease to about 1% by the year 2010 as a result of the smaller Depression era and World War II age cohorts that will be reaching the age of 65. However, after 2010, the annual rate of growth will exceed 2% as the baby-boom cohort reaches the age of 65 years. This trend is anticipated to persist until 2030. Between 2030 and 2050, it is projected that the population of elderly Americans will stabilize to a 1% level of growth annually.[19]

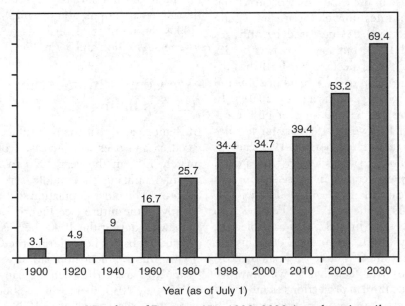

Figure 1.6   Number of Persons 65+, 1900–2030 (numbers in millions). Data for this section compiled primarily from Internet releases of the U.S. Bureau of the Census and the National Center for Health Statistics.

TABLE 1.1   Life Expectancy of us Population at Birth, by Race and Gender: 1900, 1940, 1950, 1960, 1970, 1980, 1990, 1994, 1997

Race and Gender	Life Expectancy at Birth								
	1900	*1940*	*1950*	*1960*	*1970*	*1980*	*1990*	*1994*	*1997*
White									
Men	47	62.1	66.5	67.4	68	70.7	72.7	73.3	73.6
Women	49	66.6	72.2	74.1	75.6	78.1	79.4	79.6	80.5
Nonwhite									
Men	33	51.5	59.1	61.1	61.3	65.3	67	67.6	68.2
Women	34	54.9	62.9	66.3	69.4	73.6	75.2	75.7	76.3

Compiled from data in Singh, G.K., Kochanek, K.D., MacDorman, M.F. Advance report of final mortality statistics, 1994. Monthly Vital Statistics Report. 45(3), suppl.:19. Hyattsville, MD: National Center for Health Statistics 1996 and Monthly Vital Statistics Report. 46(12):2 Hyattsville, MD: National Center for Health Statistics 1998.

Projected demographic trends reflect an assumption that there will be a sharply declining fertility rate accompanied by a decreasing mortality rate until the year 2050.[19] These forecasted changes indicate that there will be a reduction in the growth of the total population to a level of 1% annually.[1] However, even at a level of 1% annual growth, it is anticipated that the total population will double over the next sixty years.[19]

Table 1.1 shows how dramatically life expectancy of the US population has increased from the early 1900s to the projected life expectancy of the year 2050.[18,25] The major part of the current increase in life expectancy occurred because of reduced death rates for children and young adults. Life expectancy at age 65 increased by only 2.4 years between 1900 and 1960, but has increased by 3.3 years since 1960. In fact, life expectancy at birth has increased from 74.3 years in 1982 to 76.7 years in 2000 and is projected to increase to 81 years of age by 2050.[19] In 1997, Americans reaching age 65 had an average life expectancy of an additional 17.6 years (19 years for females and 15.8 years for males).[25] A child born in 1997 can expect to live 76.5 years, about 29 years longer than a child born in 1900.[25] Male life expectancy increased from 70.6 years in 1982 to 72.9 years in the year 2000 and is expected to rise to 76.7 years by the year 2050. Females who could expect to live 78.1 years in 1982, and as projected, attained a life expectancy of 80.5 years in 2000. This life expectancy is anticipated to increase to 85.2 years by 2050 for women. Some researchers feel that it will improve even more than the Census Bureau projections assume.[26–28] Life expectancy is expected to gain an additional 12.8 years if the current demographic trends persist over the next fifty years.

PROJECTED COMPONENTS OF CHANGE IN AN AGING POPULATION

Fertility Patterns

In the middle series for the overall US population, the number of births is expected to remain above the present level of 3.7 million throughout the early 2000s. The peak number of births (3.9 million) may actually have already occurred in the late 1980s.[19] After the early 1990s, the birthrate did not surpass 3.7 million because of a decline in the female population of childbearing age. In the early 2000s the number of births is projected to fluctuate between 3.4 million and 3.7 million.

Age Composition of the Aging US Population

It is anticipated that the percentage of the total population aged 65 and over will increase from the level of approximately 13% in the year 2000 to 21.2% by 2030 (nearly double) utilizing the middle series Census Bureau estimates.[24] The older population will continue to grow significantly in the future (see Figure 1.6). This growth slowed somewhat during the 1990s because of the relatively small number of babies born during the Great Depression of the 1930s. But the older population will burgeon between the years 2010 and 2030 when the baby boomers reach the age of 65.[25] By 2030, there will be about 70 million older persons, twice their numbers in 1998.

The older population itself is getting older. The 85 years of age and over population will grow at a more rapid rate than the entire 65 and over population, assuming that the extremely old will benefit from the improvements in future mortality rates. In 1998, the 65- to 74-year-old age group (18.4 million) was eight times larger than in 1900, but the 75- to 84-year-old group (12.0 million) was sixteen times larger, and the over-85 group (4.0 million) was thirty-three times larger.[25] According to population studies, there are currently more than 4 million Americans aged 85 and over. This number is projected to increase during the beginning of the twenty-first century to approximately 4.9 million, and reach 8.6 million persons over the age of 85 by 2030.[19,25] Currently, about 1% of the population is aged 85 years and older. By 2050, 5.2% of the population will be that old. Within the present population of 65 years of age and older, this comprises 9.1% aged 85 and above.[23] Projections indicate that by the year 2050, those 85 years of age and older will make up one-quarter of the entire elderly population.[25,27]

For the population of those aged 100 years and over, a substantial growth in the overall numbers is also anticipated. According to the 1990 Census Bureau report,[23] there were about 32,000 centenarians in the population. By the year 2000, this number grew to 108,000 and is expected to reach an estimated 492,000 persons over the age of 100 by the year 2030. Currently, about ninety elderly persons turn 100 every day, and by the year 2030, two hundred eighty persons each day are expected to be passing their first century of life.[25]

Gender Composition of the Aging US Population

Accompanying the aging of the population is an increasing proportion of females compared to males as age increases. Elderly women outnumbered men by three to two as a result of sex differentials in mortality that favor females at all ages over 65. For those 85 years of age and older, women outnumbered men five to two in 1990,[29] which increased to a ratio of seven to one by 1998.[30,31] In other words, higher proportions of females than males survive to old age. These ratios are expected to sharply increase through the middle of the twenty-first century as large entry cohorts, in which the sex ratios are higher, enter the 65 years of age and older population.[1]

Geographical Distribution of the Aging US Population

Elderly individuals tend to concentrate in specific regions of the country. In 1998, about half (52%) of persons over 65 lived in nine states. California had more than 3.5 million, Florida had 2.7 million, and New York 2.4 million, Texas and Pennsylvania had almost 2 million, and Ohio, Illinois, Michigan, and New Jersey each had over 1 million individuals 65 years of age and older.[25,31]

Marital Status of the Aging US Population

Another demographic characteristic that warrants examination is the marital status of older persons. The importance of this characteristic is its meaning for the elderly individual and its impact on family status, living arrangements, and available support systems.[32] The composition of the aged population with respect to marital status is influenced by complex patterns of family formation and dissolution that vary cross-culturally as well as by the important constraints imposed by differential mortality rates of males and females.[33] In 1998, older men were much more likely to be married than older women—75% of men and 43% of women (see Figure 1–7). The reduced mortality that distinguishes the demographic transitions reportedly occurring, lengthens the duration of marriage as the joint survival of both men and women is extended. However, with the widening gap in survival between the sexes, widowhood becomes more common for women at older ages. For males over 65 years of age, over 15% were widowed in 1998, but, for females, over 45% are widowed, as depicted in Figure 1.7.[24,25] There were four times as many widows (8.4 million) as widowers (2.0 million).[25]

Projections of marital status in the United States indicate that there will be a slight reduction in the proportions of older males married and widowed as the century progresses, and that there will be proportionately fewer females who are widowed.[34] It is anticipated, however, that cohorts reaching the older ages after 2000 will be more likely to be divorced or separated as a result of the substantially higher proportions of divorced and separated persons in younger cohorts.

Living Arrangements of the Aging US Population

Associated with these marital changes have been pronounced changes in the living arrangements of the elderly. The most notable of these have been the sharp increase in the proportion of women living alone and the sharp decline in the proportion of women living with other family members.[25,32] There has been relatively little change in the proportion of elderly men living alone or with other family members. The majority (67%) of older noninstitutionalized persons lived in a family setting. Elderly men are much more likely to be living with a wife than to be widowed or living with other family members.[25,38,39] About 13% of older persons over the age of 85 (7% of men, 17% of women) were not living with a spouse but were living with children, siblings, or other relatives in 1998. An additional 3% of men and 2% of women, or 718,000 older persons, lived with nonrelatives.[25]

Living alone correlates with advanced age. Among women aged 85 and over, for example, three of every five

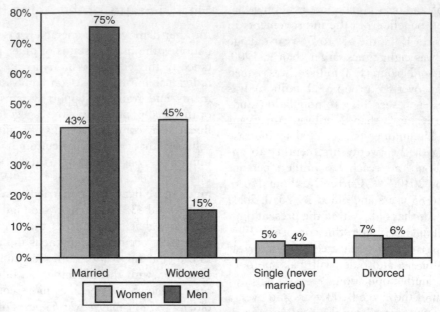

Figure 1.7   Marital Status of Persons 65+, 1998. (Based on data from the U.S. Bureau of the Census. Marital Status and Living Arrangements: March 1998 [Update], Current Population Reports, PPL-100.)

lived outside a family setting.[25] The increased tendency of older women, including extremely aged women, to live alone, is likely to continue. It is expected that by 2005, over 70% of women 75 years of age and over will be living alone. The proportion of aged men living alone is not expected to change much. The trend toward independent living has come about partly as a result of improvements in the economic and health status of the elderly, partly from a desire not to be dependent on others and partly, for some, from a simple lack of an alternative.[36]

There is an unfortunate and growing trend for homelessness among the elderly population.[37,38] In the United States, according to the 1990 Population Census *S-Night* (shelter and street count), there were 400,000 homeless elderly people on the streets and in shelters, and 6,000 to 9,000 in temporary accommodations, such as hotels, prisons, and staying with friends.[39] A recent assessment is that anywhere between 60,000 and 400,000 older persons are homeless, and that although the absolute number has recently increased, the proportion of elderly among the total homeless population has declined.[40] Other estimates of the national total are, however, highly variable, as are the reported proportions of homeless aged 50 years and over (2% to 27% in studies of homeless people).[41–42]

While a comparatively small number (1.43 million) and percentage (4.2%) of the over-65 population lived in nursing homes in 1996, the percentage increases dramatically with age, ranging from 1.1% for persons from 65 to 74 years old to 4.2% for persons aged 75 to 84 and 19.8% for persons over 85.[25,42]

Employment Status of the Aging US Population

About 3.7 million older Americans (12%) were in the labor force (working or actively seeking work) in 1998, including 2.2 million men (16%) and 1.6 million women (8%). They constituted 2.8% of the US labor force. About 3.2% were unemployed.[25]

Just over half (54%) of the workers over 65 years of age in 1998 were employed part-time: 48% of men and 62% of women.[25]

About 860,000 or 23% of older workers in 1998 were self-employed, compared to 7% for younger workers. Over two-thirds of them (71%) were men.[25]

Educational Status of the Aging US Population

The educational level of the older population is increasing. Between 1970 and 1998, the percentage who had completed high school rose from 28% to 67%. About 15% in 1998 had a bachelor's degree or more.[25] The percentage who had completed high school varied considerably by race and ethnic origin among older persons in 1998: 69% of whites, 43% of African Americans, and 30% of Hispanics.[25]

Health Status of the Aging US Population

Clinical measures clearly indicate the decline of health status with advancing age. The elderly are more likely to have chronic conditions that limit their activities, and they experience about twice as many days of restricted activity because of illness as the general population. However, to be aged in the United States today is not necessarily to be beset with numerous and complex disabilities. Life after age 65 years is not a period inexorably marked with massive physical deterioration.[43] Nevertheless, increasing life expectancy of those reaching age 65 years has had an important impact on the prevalence of disease and functional disability in the elderly population.

Life expectancy is a summary measure of the overall health of a population. It represents the average number of years of life remaining to a person at a given age if death rates were to remain constant. In the United States, improvements in health have resulted in increased life expectancy and contributed to the growth of the older population over the past century. In 1900, life expectancy at birth was about 49 years. By 1960, life expectancy had increased to 70 years, and in 1997, life expectancy at birth was 79 years for women and 74 years for men.[34] Life expectancies at age 65 and 85 have also increased. Under current mortality conditions, people who survive to age 65 can expect to live an average of nearly 18 more years, more than five years longer than persons aged 65 in 1900. The life expectancy of persons who survive to age 85 today is about seven years for women and six years for men.[25] Other variables come into play with health and well-being. Educational attainment is associated with higher life expectancy. The life expectancy of high school graduates at age 65 is approximately one year longer than the life expectancy at that age for persons who did not graduate from high school.[44,45,46] Overall, death rates in the US population have declined during the past century. For some diseases, however, death rates among older Americans have increased in recent years.[47,48] Between 1980 and 1997, age-adjusted death rates for heart disease and stroke declined by approximately one-third. Death rates for cancer, pneumonia, and influenza increased slightly over the same period. Age-adjusted death rates for diabetes increased by 32% since 1980, and death rates for chronic obstructive pulmonary diseases increased by 57%.[48-51]

In 1997, the leading cause of death among persons aged 65 or older was heart disease (1,832 deaths per 100,000 persons), followed by cancer (1,133 per 100,000), stroke (426 per 100,000), chronic obstructive pulmonary diseases (281 per 100,000), pneumonia and influenza (237 per 1000,000), and diabetes (141 per 100,000). Among persons aged 85 or older, heart disease was responsible for 40% of all deaths.[53-55]

Functioning in later years may be diminished if illness, chronic disease, or injury limits physical and/or mental abilities. Changes in disability rates have important implications for work and retirement policies, health and long-term care needs, and the social well-being of the older population. By monitoring and understanding these trends, policy makers are better able to make informed decisions.

The National Health Interview Survey conducted in 1981 by the National Center for Health Statistics provided national estimates of the level of functioning of the noninstitutionalized aged in the United States.[53] Table 1.2 provides a summary of the data collected in that survey. In 1981, about 20% of those community-dwelling elders aged 65 years of age or older reported some restrictions in their mobility. A similar trend is seen with respect to restrictions in elders' major daily activities. Forty-three percent reported some limitation in their amount or kind of functional activity.[57]

Figure 1.8 presents the percentage of Medicare beneficiaries aged 65 or older who were chronically disabled, by level and category of disability in repeat surveys by researchers.

Viewed as a homogeneous group, the majority of elders are free from disability. For most, the later years of life are characterized by substantial physical ability.[55]

DEMOGRAPHIC TRENDS AND PROJECTIONS IN THE MINORITY ELDERLY

The aging of the US population will affect every institution and every individual in our society. Projections of the proportion of the population 65 years of age and over

TABLE 1.2   Prevalence of Disability in Self-Reported Limitations in Functional Activities, Basic ADL and Instrumental ADL in Adults 65 and over: United States 1994

	Age		
Disability	*65–74(%)*	*75–84(%)*	*85+ (%)*
Self-reported functional limitations	27.8	42.6	60.8
Needs help in one or more Basic ADL	5.2	12.4	26.6
Needs help in one or more Instrumental ADL	15.6	28.2	53.0

Source: Compiled from National Center for Health Statistics (1996). Data File Documentation, National Health Interview Survey of Disability, Phase 1, 1994. Hyattsville, MD: National Center for Health Statistics. 1996.

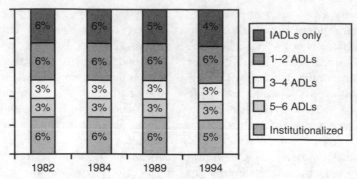

Figure 1.8   Percentage of Medicare beneficiaries aged 65 or older who are chronically disabled by level and category of disability. 1982 to 1994. (Source: National Long Term Care Survey 1982, 1984, 1989, 1994.)

anticipate dramatic increases over the next 50 years.[3] This phenomenon of population aging is of particular importance in minority groups in America.

In 1998, 15.7% of persons aged 65 and older were minorities: eight percent were African Americans, 2.1% were Asians or Pacific Islanders, and less than 1% were American Indians or Native Alaskans. Persons of Hispanic origin (who may be of any race) represented 5.1% of the older population.[56] Only 7.2% of minority race and Hispanic populations were aged 65 and older in 1998 compared with 14.8% of whites.

Minority populations are projected to represent 25% of the elderly population in the United States by 2030, up from almost 16% in 1998.[25] Between 1998 and 2030, the older white population is projected to increase by 79% compared with 226% of older minorities, including Hispanics (341%), African Americans (130%), American Indians, Eskimos, and Aleuts (150%), and Asians and Pacific Islanders (323%).[25]

Projected estimates of minority population growth indicate that the most significant and dramatic changes will occur between 2020 and 2050.[19,56] Currently, around 62% of the aged in all minority groups fall within the 65 to 74 years of age range. By 2050, the numbers in this age group will decrease to about 50% for Hispanics and other races, and to about 55% of the blacks.[56] Growth is projected to occur in the percent of the aged who are 85 and older. Currently, fewer than one in ten of the minority elderly are in the oldest-old age range, but it is anticipated that this ratio will increase to one in five by the year 2050.[19,57–66]

In light of the demographic trends, it appears that we can expect to see a large increase in the number of female-headed households among African Americans and Hispanics, and there seems likely to be an increase in minority elderly who live alone.[67–70] Both of these trends portend a substantial increase in the number of minority group elderly living in poverty.

Projected Trends in the World's Aging Population

Most of us probably are not aware of it, but the population of the world is undergoing an historic change. The older population is growing at a dramatic rate and the balance between the world's young and old is shifting. In many developed countries of Europe, the speed of population growth occurred gradually, taking fifty to one hundred years for the percent of the population aged 65 and over to double from 7% to 14%. However, in most developing countries of the world the same population increase will take place in less than thirty years. In approximately thirty years, there will be 850 million elderly worldwide.[71] Here are some pertinent facts:

- In most countries of the world there are declining fertility rates and people are living longer. This means that a country's population age structure will shift toward the older age population.
- Most of the growth in the numbers of elderly is taking place in developing countries.
- In developing countries the speed with which the elderly population is growing is very fast compared with the speed of the same changes in developed/industrialized countries. This contrast is particularly evident if you compare East Asia with Western Europe.
- Europe is the "oldest" world region, with the highest proportion of population aged 65 and older, and Africa is the youngest. Sweden is considered to be the oldest country with 18% of its population aged 65 and older.[72,73]

Life Expectancy.   There are several interesting trends in life expectancy. First, for most countries in the world, more babies are surviving infancy and childhood. Second, during the first half of the twentieth century, developed countries saw the average life expectancy of their population increase by over twenty years.

The Dependency/Support Ratio. How do we measure the impact of world aging? As mentioned above, dependency or support ratios are used. The dependency or support ratio is the ratio of the number of older people in the population to the population in the age categories most closely associated with employment (generally 20 to 64 years of age).[73,74] This ratio is intended to give an estimation of the size of the elderly population in comparison to the size of the population that can be expected to pay taxes to support benefits for the older group. This is a less than perfect measure since there are many people over the age of 64 still working and many younger people who are unemployed. It also does not take into consideration that many retired older people provide child care, which allows adult parents to enter or remain in the workforce. However, the ratio is a frequently cited statistic used by policy makers. The apparently favorable economic effect of slowing population growth in terms of total dependency/support ratio, actually increases the old-age dependency ratio.[75] Because older dependents lay claim to more public resources than do young dependents, the weight of the "old" component has great economic significance. For example, it is estimated that by the year 2025, in East Asia there will be about thirty-two older people for every one hundred working age people.[71] With change in the age structure of the population, consumption patterns of the people will change. The needs of older people are very different from the needs of middle-aged and younger people. Thus, businesses will have to reorient their policies. Entirely new products and marketing strategies will need to be developed.

Health and Disability. The number of disabled persons is likely to increase rapidly as populations grow older. Emerging morbidity patterns in developing countries may require a reevaluation of health services and service provision.

Given the nonmedical factors that can affect health status, the World Health Organization (WHO) takes a broad view of health, involving the health sector in the larger context of improving the quality of life. This is in accord with the organization's definition of health as complete physical, mental, and social well-being. In regard to the elderly segment of the world population, specific health goals that have been articulated include: promotion of maximum independence and productivity; and prevention of debilitating conditions in old age through healthier lifestyles, early diagnosis, environmental safety, and health education.

As might be anticipated, chronic conditions are more prevalent than acute disorders and infection among the world's elderly. However, on an international level there are substantial shortfalls in the provision of primary health care services to the aging, and in the provision of health aids,

particularly in underdeveloped countries and rural areas.[72] There is a high prevalence of physical disability, particularly with regard to sight, hearing, ambulation, and nutrition.

Among the world's elderly, arthritis, high blood pressure, foot problems, heart disease, lung disease, and stomach ulcers are the most common problems.[76] As an example of the prevalence of arthritis, for instance, cross-national surveys regarding morbidity indicate that 35.8% of all elderly persons in Myanmar reported suffering from arthritis, 11.9% in Korea, 49.1% in Indonesia, 31.3% in Sri Lanka, and 59.5% in Thailand. Quite substantial proportions of the elderly suffer from hypertension and heart disease, lung problems, foot ulcers, and stomach ulcers. These diseases, along with impaired vision and hearing, greatly affect their ability to carry out daily activities, self-care functions, and employment. Chronic illnesses also impose a huge burden on the national health expenditure in each country.[72,76,77]

While the overall picture still shows that in developing countries the elderly reside with their families and in developed countries the elderly reside on their own in the community, there are changes occurring that may alter these patterns. Urban migration in many developing countries is depleting the number of young people living in rural areas. This has led, or is leading, to large increases in the number of elderly who must shift for themselves. For example, in some areas of India, older people already have no children living with them to provide support.[78–81] Due to economic pressures in urban areas, their children are not able to send money back home to the village to support their parents. Until recently, the practice of apartheid frequently separated elderly blacks living in South African townships from their children.[82,83] Urban-dwelling blacks, who had lived and worked in townships for their entire adult lives, were not allowed to remain in those townships after retirement and were forced to return to their villages of origin. This separated them from their adult children who, for economic reasons, had to remain in the township.[84]

Institutionalization in nursing homes is low in most countries. In Japan, the proportion of the elderly aged 65 and older living in institutions is about 1.6%; in the United States, it is about 5%; in Germany, 4%; in Australia, 6%; and in Sweden, 9%.[81]

In some countries, fewer than one in ten older persons can read and write.[78] Secondary school completion rates of 2% or less are not uncommon among older populations, especially females. Literacy rates among the elderly, reflecting limited opportunities for education, were shown to be low in developing countries, primarily in the rural areas. This means that the elderly, particularly elderly women, tend to be disadvantaged in areas where education and adaptation to new roles may be an important factor, such as in reemployment, in knowledge of health and social issues, and in managing daily affairs without assistance.

References

1. Kinsella, K. Future longevity—Demographic concerns and consequences. *JAGS*. 2005; 53(9):299–304.

2. Vladeck, B. Economic and policy implications of improving longevity. *JAGS*. 2005; 53(9):304–307.

3. Angel JL, Hogan DP. The demography of minority aging populations. In: *Minority Elders: Longevity, Economics and Health: Building Public Policy Base*. Washington, DC: Gerontological Society of America; 1991.

4. Steel, K. The old-old-old. *JAGS*. 2005; 53(9): 312–316.

5. Gilford DM, ed. *The Aging Population in the Twenty-First Century*. Washington, DC: National Academy Press; 1988.

6. Rosenwaike I, Logue B. *The Extreme Aged in America: A Portrait of an Expanding Population*. Westport, CT: Greenwood Press; 1985.

7. United Nations. *The Aging of Populations and Its Economic and Social Implications*. New York: United Nations; 1956. (ST/SOA/SER.A/26).

8. Sundbarg G. *Grunddragen of befolkningslaren*. Stockholm. 1894.

9. Sundbarg G. Sur la repartition de la population par age et sur les taux de mortalite [On the separation of the population by age and the rates of mortality]. *Bul Internat Institute Statistics*. 1900; 12(99):89–94.

10. Dublin LI. *Health and Wealth: A Survey of the Economics of World Health: The Problem of Age*. New York: Harper; 1928: 149–168.

11. Pearl R. The aging of populations. *J Am Statistical Assoc Am*. 1940; 209:277–297.

12. Dublin LI, Lotka AJ. *Length of Life: A Study of the Life Table*. New York: Ronald Press; 1937.

13. Thompson WS, Whelpton PK. *Population Trends in the United States*. New York: McGraw-Hill; 1933.

14. Kinsella K. *Aging in the Third World*. Washington, DC: US Government Printing Office; 1988. US Bureau of the Census, International Population Reports, Series P-95, No. 79.

15. United Nations. *Economic and Social Implications of Population Aging*. New York: United Nations; 1988. (ST/ESA/SER.R/85).

16. Treas J, Logue B. Economic development and the older population. *Pop Dev Rev*. 1987; 12:645–673.

17. Winsborough HH. A demographic approach to the life cycle. In: Back KW, ed. *Life Course Integrative Theories and Exemplary Populations*. Boulder, CO: Westview; 1980. (AAAS Selected Symposium 41).

18. Soldo BJ. America's elderly in the 1980's. *Pop*. 1980; 35(1):1–48.

19. Spencer G. *Projections of the Population of the United States by Age, Sex, and Race: 1982 to 2050*. Washington, DC: US Bureau of the Census; 1989. Current Population Reports, Series P-25, No. 1007.

20. Rosenwaike I. A demographic portrait of the oldest-old. *Milbank Memorial Fund Quarterly Health and Society*. 1985; 63:187–205.

21. Preston SH, Himes C, Eggers M. Demographic conditions responsible for population aging. *Demography*. 1989; 26:691–704.

22. Grigsby JS. *The Demographic Components of Population Aging*. University of Michigan and Pomona College; 1988. Working paper.

23. US Bureau of the Census. *Population Estimates by Age, Sex, Race, and Hispanic Origin: 1980 to 1988*. Washington, DC: US Government Printing Office; 1990. Current Population Reports, Series P-25, No. 1045.

24. US Bureau of the Census. *Statistical Abstract of the United States. Profiles of Older Americans: 1999*. Washington DC: US Government Printing Office; 2000.

25. Administration on Aging. *Older Americans 2000: Key Indicators of Well-Being*. Federal Interagency. Forum on Aging-Related Statistics. Washington DC: Bureau of the Census; 2000.

26. Bourgeois-Pichat J. *Future Outlook for Mortality Decline in the World*. United Nations, Population Bulletin of the United Nations; 1978. No. 11; 12–41.

27. Crimmins EM. Implications of recent mortality trends for the size and composition of the population over 65. *Rev Public Data Use*. 1983; 11(l):37–48.

28. Rice DP. Long life to you. *American Demographics*. 1979; 1(9):9–15.

29. Taeuber C. Diversity: The dramatic reality. In: Bass SA, Kutza EA, Torres-Gil FM, eds. *Diversity in Aging*. Glenview, IL: Scott, Foresman; 1990.

30. US Bureau of the Census. *Current Population Reports: Poverty in the United States: 1998*. Washington DC: US Bureau of the Census; 1999. P60-207, September 1999 Report.

31. Kalache A, Keller I. The greying world: A challenge for the twenty-first century. *Sci Prog*. 2000; 83 (pt 1):33–54.

32. Soldo BJ, Agree EM. America's elderly. *Population Bull*. 1988; 43(3):1–51.

33. Myers G, Nathanson C. Aging and the family. *World Health Stat Quart*. 1982; 35:225–238.

34. Myers GC, Manton KG, Bacellar H. Sociodemographic aspects of future unpaid productive roles. *Productive Roles in an Older Society*. Washington, DC: National Academy Press. Committee on an Aging Society, Institute of Medicine and National Research Council; 1986; 110–147.

35. US Bureau of the Census. *Projections of the Number of Households and Families: 1979 to 1995*. Washington, DC: US Government Printing Office; 1989. Current Population Reports, Series P-25, No. 805.

36. Riley AG. *Aging and Society: Notes on the Development of New Understandings.* Ann Arbor: University of Michigan Press; 1983.

37. Gore T, Bottomley JM. Legislative and public policy issues related to elder homelessness. *Top Geriatr Rehabil.* 2001; 7(1):14–22.

38. Crane M, Warnes AM. Older people and homelessness: prevalence and causes. *Top Geriatr Rehabil.* 2001; 6(4)1–14.

39. Wright J, Rubin B, Devine J. *Beside the Golden Door: Policy, Politics and the Homeless.* New York: Aldine de Gruyter; 1998.

40. Cohen C. Aging and homelessness. *Gerontologist.* 1999; 39(1):5–14.

41. Burt M. Homelessness: Definitions and counts. In: Baumohl J, ed. *Homelessness in America.* Phoenix, AZ: Oryx Publications; 1996; 15–23.

42. US Bureau of the Census. *Population Projections of the United States by Age, Sex, Race and Hispanic Origin: 1995–2050.* Washington, DC: US Government Printing Office; 1999. Current Population Reports, Series P-25, No. 1130.

43. Jette AM, Branch LG. The Framingham disability study: II: Physical disability among the aging. *Am J Public Health.* 1981; 71:1211–1216.

44. Richards H, Berry R. U.S. life tables for 1990 by sex, race, and education. *J Forensic Economics.* 1998; 11:9–26.

45. Preston SH, Elo IT, Rosenwaike I, Hill M. African-American mortality at older ages: Results of a matching study. *Demography.* 1996; 33(2):193–209.

46. Manton KC, Stallard E, Wing S. Analyses of black and white differentials in the age trajectory of mortality in two closed cohort studies. *Stat Med.* 1991; 10:1043–1059.

47. National Center for Health Statistics. *Health, United States, 1999, with Health and Aging Chartbook.* Hyattsville, MD: National Center for Health Statistics, 1999; 36–37.

48. National Center for Health Statistics. *Health, United States, 1999, with Health and Aging Chartbook.* Hyattsville, MD: National Center for Health Statistics, 1999; 34–35.

49. Centers for Disease Control and Prevention. *Unrealized Prevention Opportunities: Reducing the Health and Economic Burden of Chronic Disease.* Atlanta, GA: Centers for Disease Control and Prevention, National Center for Chronic Disease Prevention and Health Promotion; 1997.

50. Wygaard HA, Albreksten G. Risk factors for admission to a nursing home. A study of elderly people receiving home nursing. *Scand J Primary Health Care.* 1992; 10:128–133.

51. Wells KB, Stewart A, Hays RD, et al. The functioning and well-being of depressed patients. Results from the Medical Outcomes Study. *JAMA.* 1989; 262:914–919.

52. Idler IL, Benyamini Y. Self-reported health and mortality: A review of twenty-seven community studies. *J Health & Social Behavior.* 1997; 38:21–37.

53. National Center for Health Statistics. *Current Estimates from the National Health Interview Survey: United States, 1981.* Washington, DC: US Government Printing Office; 1982. US Department of Health and Human Services Publication No. 10–141.

54. US Department of Health and Human Services. *Physical Activity and Health: A Report of the Surgeon General.* Atlanta, GA: Centers for Disease Control and Prevention, National Center for Chronic Disease Prevention and Health Promotion; 1996.

55. Butler RN, Davis R, Lewis CB, Nelson ME, Strauss E. Physical fitness: Benefits of exercise for the older patient. *Geriatrics.* 1998; 53(10):46–62.

56. US Census Bureau. *Projections of Population Trends.* Available from: http://www.census.gov/ population/projections/nation/summary/np-t3-a.txt.

57. Taeuber C, Smith D. Minority elderly: An overview of demographic characteristics and 1990 census plans. Presented to the National Council on Aging Symposium. Washington, DC; 1988.

58. Torres-Gil. Hispanics: A special challenge. In: Pifer A, Bronte L, eds. *Our Aging Society: Paradox and Promise.* New York: NW Norton; 1986: 219–242.

59. Cubillos HL, Prieto MM. *The Hispanic Elderly: A Demographic Profile.* Washington, DC: Policy Analysis Center, National Council of La Raza; 1987.

60. Agree E. *Portrait of Asian Elderly.* Washington, DC: American Association of Retired Persons, Minority Affairs Initiative. Georgetown University Population Research Center; 1985.

61. US Bureau of the Census. *Preliminary Estimates of the Population of the United States by Age, Sex, and Race: 1970 to 1981.* Washington, DC: US Government Printing Office; 1982. Current Population Reports, Series P-25, No. 917.

62. Agree E. *A Portrait of Older Minorities.* Washington, DC: American Association of Retired Persons, Minority Affairs Initiative. Georgetown University Population Research Center; 1985.

63. Siegel JS, Taeuber CM. Demographic perspectives on the long-live society. *Daedalus.* 1986; 115:77–117.

64. Saluter AF, Lugaila TA. *Marital Status and Living Arrangements: March 1996.* Washington, DC: US Government Printing Office; 1998. US Census Bureau, Current Population Reports, P60–207.

65. Kim PK. Demography of Asian-Pacific elderly: Selected problems and implications. In: McNeely RL, Colen JL, eds. *Aging in Minority Groups.* Beverly Hills, CA: Sage; 1983; 29–41.

66. Dalaker J. *Poverty in the United States: 1998*. Table 2. Washington, DC: US Government Printing Office; September 1999. US Census Bureau, Current Population Reports, P60–207.

67. Social Security Administration. *Income of the Population 55 or Older, 1998*. Tables VIII.4 and VIII.11. Washington DC: US Government Printing Office; 2000.

68. Smith JP. Wealth inequality among older Americans. *J Gerontol*. 1997; 52B(special issue):74–81.

69. Crystal S. Economic status of the elderly. In: Binstock RH, George LK, eds. *Handbook of Aging and the Social Sciences*. 4th ed. San Diego, CA: Academic Press, 1996.

70. Worobey JL, Angel RJ. Functional capacity and living arrangements of unmarried elderly persons. *J Gerontol*. 1990; 45(3):95–101.

71. Diczfalusy E. The third age, the Third World and the third millennium. *Contraception*. 1996; 53(1):1–7.

72. United Nations. *World Population Prospects: The 1998 Revision*. Vol. 1. Comprehensive Tables. New York: United Nations; 1999.

73. Wilmoth JR, Horiuchi S. Demography 1999. *Demograph*. 1999; 36:475–495.

74. Tuljapurkar SD, Li N, Boe C. Life expectancy in G-7 nations may exceed past predictions. *Nature*. June 15, 2000; 405:789–792.

75. Horiuchi S. Demography: Greater lifetime expectations. *Nature*. June 15, 2000; 405:744–745.

76. Butler RN. Global Aging: Challenges and opportunities of the next century. *Aging International*; Summer 1996.

77. Gilford DM. *The Aging Population in the Twenty-First Century: Statistics for Health Policy*. Washington DC: National Academy Press; 1998.

78. Restrepo HE, Rozental R. The social impact of aging populations: Some major issues. *Soc Sci Med*. 1994; 39(9):1323–1338.

79. Andrews GR. Aging in Asia and the Pacific: A multidimensional cross-national study in four countries. *Comparative Gerontology*. 1997; 1:24–32.

80. Hafez G. The "greying" of the nations. *World Health*. July–August 1994; 47(4).

81. Myers GC, Agree EM. The world ages, the family changes: A demographic perspective. *Aging International*. March 1994.

82. Allain TJ, Wilson AO, Gomo ZA, Mushangi E, Senanje B, Adamchak DJ, Matenga JA. Morbidity and disability in elderly Zimbabweans. *Age and Ageing*. 1997; 26:115–121.

83. Jette AM, Bottomley JM. The graying of America. *Am J Phys Ther*. 1987; 67(10):1527–1542.

Additional Recommended Reading

Berkman CS, Gurland GJ. The relationship among income, other socioeconomic indicators, and functional level in older persons. *J Aging Health*. 1998; 10:81–98.

Bureau of the Census. *Statistical Abstract of the United States. Profiles of Older Americans: 1998*. Washington DC: US Bureau of the Census; 1999.

Current Population Reports. In: *Developments of Aging: 1997*. Vol. 25. Washington DC: US Senate Special Committee on Aging; 1998.

Dey AN. Characteristics of elderly nursing home residents: Data from the 1995 National Nursing Home Survey. *Advance Data From Vital and Health Statistics*, No. 289. Hyattsville, MD: Public Health Service, DHHS Publication No (PHS) 97–1250; 1997.

Elo IT, Preston SH. Racial and ethnic differences in mortality at older ages. In: Martin LG, Soldo BJ, eds. *Racial and Ethnic Differences in the Health of Older Americans*. Washington DC: National Academy Press; 1997.

Jette AM, Branch LG. Inpairment and disability in the aged. *Chronic Dis*. 1985; 38:59–66.

Kalache A, Keller I. The greying world: a challenge for the twenty-first century. *Sci Prog*. 2000; 83(pt 1):33–54.

Kingston RS, Smith JP. Socioeconomic status and racial and ethnic differences in functional status associated with chronic diseases. *Am J Publ Health*. 1997; 87: 805–810.

Krauss NA, Altman BM. Characteristics of nursing home residents—1996. *MEPS Research Findings*. No. 5. Rockville, MD: Agency for Health Care Policy and Research, 1998; Pub No 99-0006.

Miller B. Minority use of community long-term care services: A comparative analysis. *J Gerontol*. 1996; 51B: S70–S81.

Norgard TM, Rodgers WL. Patterns of in-home care among elderly black and white Americans. *J Gerontol*. 1997; 52B(special issue):93–101.

Peck CW. Differences by race in the decline of health over time. *J Gerontol*. 1997; 52B:S336–S344.

Smith JP. Wealth inequality among older Americans. *J Gerontol*. 1997; 52B(special issue):74–81.

Tennstedt S, Chang B. The relative contribution of ethnicity versus socioeconomic status in explaining differences in disability and receipt of informal care. *J Gerontol*. 1998; 53B:S61–S70.

2

Comparing and Contrasting the Theories of Aging

Pearls

- Hayflick and Moorehead conducted a landmark study that showed that in culture human fibroblasts have a limited life span.
- Neuroendocrine and hormonal theory regard functional decrements in neurons and their associated hormones as central to the aging process.
- According to the free radical theory, free radicals accumulate with age and cause destruction to important biological structures through an oxidative process.
- Caloric restriction theory prescribes that an individual gradually loses weight until a point of maximum metabolic efficiency is reached for maximum health and life span.

- The error theory specifies that any error in the process of making proteins will cascade into multiple effects.
- Somatic mutation theory hypothesizes that genetic damage will result from radiation and that radiometric agents accumulate and create functional failure and death of the organism.
- In the cross-linkage theory, cross-linkage of macromolecules is responsible for secondary and tertiary aging.

INTRODUCTION

The search for the arcana of that nemesis called old age has enticed many scientists to theorize and experiment with explanations for the mechanisms involved in the aging process. What determines how we age? Are there some biological prognosticators that determine how quickly and/or how well we age? How do external factors affect our predisposed genetic makeup? The study of gerontology is a relatively young discipline, and the excitement of exploring new territory has seduced many scientific minds to delve into potential explications of how the human species ages. Several theories of aging have been proposed and the most prominent of these will be reviewed and compared in this chapter. With the decoding of the human genomes, new theories are evolving related to the potential of correcting gene coding that potentiates disease in old age and also to the possibility of extending the length of life. This critical look at current theories will provide a basic framework for understanding

and evaluating the subsequent chapters on normal and pathological aging as well as clinical observations and strategies for managing the care of elderly individuals.

HISTORICAL PERSPECTIVE

The study of aging has a long history. Much of the research in the biology of aging has focused on prolongation studies rather than on the actual mechanisms of aging.[1,2]

Research on aging began around the turn of the twentieth century.[3] Metchnikoff introduced the concept that aging was caused by the continuous absorption of toxins from intestinal bacteria; he received the Nobel Prize in 1908 for his contributions to biology and the study of aging.[4] Systematic studies that described the aging phenomenon in terms of cell morphology, physiology, and biochemistry began to flourish around 1950.[5] There were improvements in experimental designs in gerontological research which led to more accurate definitions of valid and reliable hypotheses. Two primary groups of aging theories evolved from the studies in the 1950s. Comfort[5] describes the first group of theories about aging as "fundamentalist" or *development-genetic theories.* These theories are based on the premise of "wear and tear,"[6] and aging is attributed to pathological decrements that are tissue-specific (e.g., connective, nervous, vascular, endocrine tissue). The second group of theories conceives of aging as an epiphenomenon in which environmental insults such as gravity, toxins, and cosmic rays impact the aging process. These theories are termed "nongenetic," environmental, or *stochastic theories* of aging. Many additional theories not contained in these two theoretical groups (though they could arguably be forced into one of the categories) view aging as a continuum with development and morphogenesis,[7] while others relate aging to a cessation of somatic cell growth[8] and energy depletion.[9]

Current modified versions of these theories have incorporated research on the immune system, the neuroendocrine system, failures in deoxyribonucleic acid (DNA) repair, random mutation in somatic cells, errors in protein synthesis, and random damage from free radicals.[10] Specific theories related to sleep and the rate of aging, growth hormone, dehydroepiandrosterone (DHEA), telomeres, and cell culture models of aging involving specific proteins have evolved. The most recent theories identify genetic characteristics (genotypes) and their effects on survival and the "rate-of-change."[11–15]

In 1961, a landmark study by two then unknown cell biologists, Hayflick and Moorehead,[16] turned the study of senescence of cultured cells completely around. They concluded from their in vitro studies of fetal fibroblast cells (lung, skin, muscle, heart) that human fibroblasts have a limited life span in culture. Hayflick and Moorehead reported that there was a period of rapid and vigorous cellular proliferation consistently followed by a decline in proliferative activity and characteristic senescent changes (e.g., decreased replication and wasting). They proposed that aging was a cellular as well as an organismic phenomenon. The loss in functional capacity of the aging person reflected the summation of the loss of critical functional capabilities within individual cells. For instance, the loss of type II fibers in the muscle with aging results in atrophy and a decrease in the muscle force production, thereby decreasing functional capacity. The Hayflick and Moorehead experiment altered the direction and interpretation of aging research and cellular biology. In essence, they were among the first scientists to set the course of the philosophy of modern biology and gerontology. From this basis, the subsequent theories evolved.

ANIMAL MODELS OF AGING

Dietary restriction (DR) has also been found to increase life span in many types of animals.[17–21] It has been suggested that the response to chronic dietary restriction may be an adaptation to environments with variable food levels. The ability to slow aging when food levels are low purportedly postpones reproductive senescence and therefore allows reproduction when food levels are high.[19] Harrison and Archer[19] predicted that the response to DR should be strongest in species with short reproductive life spans, because these species would be more likely to encounter periods of low food that are longer than their normal reproductive life spans. In contrast, Phelan and Austad[20] noted that reproductive senescence may be uncommon in nature and suggested that the increase in life span in response to DR is not an adaptation to variable food levels, but is instead a "secondary consequence of its effect in delaying age at maturity and decreasing the subsequent rate of reproduction." They predicted that the response to DR should be strongest in those species with early maturity and high reproductive rates. Recent investigations into animal models of aging with DR found that most, but not all, species responded by increasing mean life span, maximum life span, reproductive life span, mortality rate doubling time, and initial mortality rate.[18]

FUNDAMENTAL CONSIDERATIONS

Aging is developmental. This concept is very simple: we do not suddenly age. Our aging time capsules do not ignite at the age of 65. We evolve into mature adults and grow older developmentally, not chronologically. Aging is unique among all developmental stages. A 70-year-old person in chronological age may have the physiologic makeup of a 50-year-old person. Yet a 50-year-old person with chronic diseases may parallel the physiologic decline of a 90-year-old person.

Old age is a gift of twentieth-century technology and scientific advancement. The gerontologist James Birren has penned the notion that the extended life expectancy that we now have is really a gift of modern medicine and technology.[22] Some biologists argue that the "survivorship kinetics" of biological aging may be an artifact of civilization and domestication.

The effects of normal aging versus pathologic aging must be differentiated if possible. A confounding problem in understanding aging is the fact that there is a vast spectrum of aging changes. The process of aging is probably multifactorial in its regulation; however, it is virtually impossible to tell which changes are primary to a senescence-regulated event and which are secondary. Often we assume that a functional decline is due to aging. However, disease may often cause functional decline, which is not a normal aging process. For example, if one has adult-onset diabetes, then the probability of cardiovascular disease increases as a result of the effect of the diabetes. It is not "normal" to get diabetes; it is a function of lifestyle and heredity. The relationship between aging, disease, and dying is confusing.

Aging characteristically brings a loss in homeostasis and with it increased vulnerability to diseases, some of which result in death. Death has been used as the end point measurement of aging; however, death can occur from many causes, some of which are related to the aging process only secondarily, and in some cases totally unrelated to the process, as is true of accidents.

There is no universally accepted theory of aging. Aging does not occur in all species or in all organisms of the same species in exactly the same way. While one tissue may be losing functional capacity rapidly, others may be comparatively quite "young" functionally. Amid all these confusing assumptions of aging, a set of consistent aging characteristics has been identified. First, there is increased mortality with age.[23] Second, consistent changes in the biochemical composition of the body with age have been well documented,[24] including a decrease in lean body mass and an increase in fat. There are also characteristic increases in lipofuscin in certain tissues and an increase of cross-linkage in matrix molecules such as collagen.[23] Third, cross-sectional and longitudinal studies have provided evidence of a broad spectrum of progressive deteriorative changes.[25] Fourth, there is a reduced ability to respond adaptively to environmental change—perhaps the hallmark of aging. This can be demonstrated at all levels from an individual molecule to the complete organism.[26] Thus, the changes of age are not so much the resting pulse rate nor the fasting serum glucose, but the ability to return these parameters to normal after a physiological stress. Last, there is an increased vulnerability to many diseases with age,[25] which occurs even at the cellular level. Aging is a process that is distinct from disease. The fundamental changes of aging provide the substratum in which age-associated diseases can flourish.

Aging theories can be divided into two major categories: genetic (fundamentalist) and nongenetic (environmental). Genetic theories focus on the mechanisms for aging located within the nucleus of the cell, while nongenetic theories focus on areas located elsewhere, such as in organs, tissues, systems in the body, or extrinsic environmental causes. In order to understand both of the theories of aging, a basic understanding of three somatic cell types is necessary.

Not all somatic cells age at the same rate, nor do they have similar aging characteristics. Somatic cells are divided into three categories: (1) continuously proliferating or mitotic cells, (2) reverting postmitotic cells, and (3) fixed postmitotic cells.[27] Continuously proliferating mitotic cells never cease to replicate themselves, and injury done to these cells is healed through regeneration. Such cells can be found as superficial skin cells, red blood cells, cells of the lining of the intestine, and bone marrow cells. Reverting postmitotic cells have a slower rate of division than the continuously proliferating cells; but when there is injury, the rate of division is speeded up and regeneration

is possible. An example of these are kidney and liver cells. The final type of somatic cells, fixed postmitotic cells, never replicates once the cells reach maturity.[15,27] Muscle cells and nerve cells are primary examples of fixed postmitotic cells. Humans have all the fixed postmitotic cells they will ever get once they have reached biological maturity (for females at the time of menses; for males at the time they stop growing).

THEORIES OF AGING

Developmental-Genetic Theories

The developmental-genetic theorists consider the process of aging to be part of a continuum with development genetically controlled and programmed. The primary evidence of this is the species-specific maximum life span. Variation in life span is far greater among species than within species.[28] Because maximum life span is a species characteristic, it would seem evident that this is genetically determined. Further supporting evidence for the genetic basis of aging and maximal life span comes from the recognition of genetic disease of precocious aging, such as in genetic progeroid syndromes.[29] The classic progeria—Werner syndrome, Hutchinson-Guilford syndrome, and Down syndrome—are among these diseases. The precise mechanism of human aging is not replicated at an accelerated rate in these individuals; however, many of the commonly recognized aging changes occur more rapidly. These diseases are important probes in the study of aging.

Hayflick Limit Theory.   Hayflick and Moorehead[16] were able to show that a deterioration in cells (e.g., mitotic and mitochondrial activity) was not dependent on environmental influences, but rather, that cell aging was intrinsic to the cells. They found that there was a limited number of cell population doublings or replications ranging from forty to sixty, the average doubling being fifty per life cycle of the cell. The developmental senescence process of cultured cells includes three phases. Phase I is the beginning stage of cell life, phase II involves a rapid cell proliferation, and the final cessation of cell division occurs in phase III.[30] Hayflick and others have repeatedly shown that phase III is nearly always between forty and sixty population doublings for embryo cells.[31] Hayflick noted alterations and degeneration occurred within the cells before their growth limit,[32-36] evident in the cell organelles, membranes, and genetic material. Hayflick demonstrated that functional changes within cells are responsible for aging and that the cumulative effect of improper functioning of cells and eventual loss of cells in organs and tissues is probably responsible for the aging phenomenon.

Evolutionary Theory of Aging.   The evolutionary theory of aging is an expansion of the concept of natural selection as Darwin proposed decades ago.[37] This theory predicts that the frequency for deleterious mutations of genes will reach equilibrium from one generation to the next. In other words, there will be an increase in age of onset of mutation of a gene because of postponed selection. This makes each successive generation more resistant to mutations, and when mutations do occur, they occur at a later age.[38–40]

One theory under the evolutionary model, the network theory of aging, extends the argument that a global reduction in the capacity to cope with a variety of stressors and a concomitant progressive increase in proinflammatory status are major characteristics of the aging process.[41] This phenomenon, which Franceschi and associates[41] refer to as "inflamm-aging," is hypothetically provoked by a continuous antigenic load and stress. On the basis of evolutionary studies, these researchers argue that the immune and the stress responses are equivalent and that antigens are nothing other than particular types of stressors. This theory proposes that the persistence of inflammatory stimuli over time represents the biologic background (first hit) favoring the susceptibility to age-related diseases/disabilities. A second hit (absence of robust gene variants or the presence of frail gene variants) is likely necessary to develop overt organ-specific age-related diseases having an inflammatory pathogenesis, such as atherosclerosis, Alzheimer's disease, osteoporosis, and diabetes.[41,42] Following this perspective, these researchers found several paradoxes in healthy centenarians, such as an increase of plasma levels of inflammatory cytokines, acute phase proteins, and coagulation factors. Therefore, they conclude that the beneficial effects of inflammation devoted to the neutralization of dangerous and harmful agents early in life and adulthood become detrimental late in life.[41,42]

Stress Theory of Aging.   Along this same line of thought the stress theory of aging is also an evolutionary model. According to this theory, aging is considered in the context of the abiotic stresses to which free-living organisms are normally exposed.[43] Stress is defined in terms of adequate nutrition and degree of exposure to environmental strains and stressors. Assuming that the primary target of selection of stress is at the level of energy carriers, trade-offs under the rate-of-living theory of aging predict increased longevity from selection for stress resistance. Changes in longevity then become incidental to selection for resistance. Parsons[43] suggests that the primary trait inherited is resistance to stress. Consequently, at extreme ages those with inherited resistance to abiotic stress should dominate, and the reduction in homeostasis manifested by deteriorating ability to adapt to abiotic stress as aging proceeds should be slowest in those surviving the longest.[43] In other words, survival to old age is enhanced by high vitality and resilience associated with substantial physiological and morphological homeostasis. This is underlaid by genes for stress resistance, which confer high metabolic efficiency and hence adaptation to the energy costs of physiological and environmental stress.[44]

Neuroendocrine and Hormonal Theory.   The endocrine system regulates body composition, fat deposition, skeletal mass, muscle strength, metabolism, body weight, and physical well-being. Multiple endocrine changes evolve with aging in all species and, not surprisingly, some of the physiologic manifestations of aging are related to the effects of declining hormone levels. One of the earliest investigations into the possible role of the endocrine system in the aging process was conducted by Charles Edward Brown-Séquard (1817–1894),[45] a French-educated physician and professor of physiology and neuropathology at Harvard in the late nineteenth century.

The group of theories purporting the neuroendocrine basis of aging regards functional decrements in neurons and their associated hormones as central to the aging process. Given the major interactive role of the neuroendocrine system in physiology, this is an attractive approach. D. Donner Denckla, an endocrinologist turned gerontologist, believes that the center of aging is located in the brain.[45–50] He bases his theory on past studies of hypothyroidism, a disease that mimics mature aging (e.g., a depressed immune system, wrinkling of the skin, gray hair, and a slowed metabolic rate). Hypothyroidism can be fatal if untreated with thyroxine, inasmuch as all the manifestations of aging are evidenced.[53]

An important version of Denckla's theory proposes that the hypothalamic-pituitary-adrenal (HPA) axis is the master timekeeper for the organism and the primary regulator of the aging process. Functional changes in this system are accompanied by or regulated by decrements throughout the organism. The cascade effect of functional decrements in the hypothalamus, for example, and their potential sequelae have been documented in humans.[55] The neuroendocrine system regulates early development, growth, puberty, the control of the reproductive system, metabolism, and in part, the activities of all the major organ systems. Support of the neuroendocrine and hormonal theories of aging is evidenced by the decline in reproductive capacity due to a decrease in the release of gonadotropin releasing hormone by the hypothalamus, which appears to be the result of diminished activity of hypothalamic catecholamines.[55] Similarly, it has been shown that the release of pulsatile growth hormone declines with age.[56] These changes would have profound effects on estrogen and progesterone release and subsequently on functional capacity. Wise[56] has suggested that there is a loss of neurons in discrete areas of the brain and a loss of neurotransmitter responsiveness by the remaining neurons.

The Theory of Intrinsic Mutagenesis.   Another development-genetic theory is referred to as the theory of intrinsic mutagenesis.[57] This idea was first proposed by

Burnett[58] and is an attempt to reconcile stochastic theories of aging with the genetic regulation of maximum life span. Burnett suggests that each species is endowed with a specific genetic constitution that "regulates the fidelity of the genetic material and its replication." The degree of fidelity regulates the rate of appearance of mutations or errors, thereby affecting the life span. Alternatively, we can envision a case in which new "fidelity regulators" appear at different stages in an animal's life. Each successive evolutionary set of regulators could have a decreased capacity allowing an increase in mutational events. Another aspect of intrinsic mutagenesis is concerned with the increase in DNA excision repair associated with maximal life span.[59] There is evidence that the accuracy of DNA polymerase may decrease with age,[60–66] but the research in support of both of these hypotheses is rather controversial.

Immunological Theory.   The immunological theory of aging is another theory categorized as a developmental-genetic theory. This theory was proposed by Walford[67] and has two major observations: (1) that the functional capacity of the immune system declines with age as a result of reduced T-cell function[68] and a reduced resistance to infectious diseases, and (2) that the fidelity of the immune system declines with age as evidenced by the striking age-associated increase in autoimmune diseases. Walford[69] has related these immune system changes to the genes of the major histocompatibility complex genes in rats and mice. Congenic animals that differ only at the major histocompatibility locus appear to have different maximal life spans, suggesting that life span is regulated, at least in part, by this locus. Interestingly, this locus also regulates superoxide dismutase and mixed-function oxidase levels, a finding that relates the immunological theory of aging to the free radical theory of aging, which will be discussed subsequently.

Free Radical Theory.   There are more than 300 theories to explain the aging phenomenon. Many of them originate from the study of changes that accumulate with time. Among all the theories, the free radical theory of aging, postulated by Harman,[70] is the most popular and widely tested.[71] It is based on the chemical nature and ubiquitous presence of free radicals. This review aims to recapitulate various studies on the role of free radicals in DNA damage, both nuclear as well as mitochondrial, the oxidative stress they impose on cells, the role of antioxidants, the presence of autoantibodies, and their overall impact on the aging process.

The free radical theory is another example of development-genetic theory. This theory is attributed to Harman,[72–75] who proposed that aging changes are due to damage caused by radicals. Basically, free radicals are highly charged ions whose outer orbits contain an unpaired electron. Chemically, they are highly reactive species that are generated commonly in single-electron transfer reactions of metabolism. Free radicals have been shown to damage cell membranes, lysosomes, mitochondria, and nuclear membranes through a chemical reaction called lipid peroxidation. Both membrane damage and cross-linking of biomolecules result from free radical chain reactions.[76] The net result of free radical reactions, as summarized by Leibovitz and Siegel,[77,78] is a decline in cellular integrity caused by reduced enzyme activities, error-prone nucleic acid metabolism, damaged membrane functions, and the accumulation of aging pigments (lipofuscin) in lysosomes.

Free radicals are rapidly destroyed by protective enzyme systems, such as superoxide dismutase. According to this theory, however, some free radicals escape destruction and cause damage that accumulates in important biological structures. This accumulation of damage eventually interferes with function and ultimately causes death. The accumulation of age pigments is an example and does not refer to the dark brown spots on one's hands. Age pigments (lipofuscin) are seen at microscopic levels in self-selected tissues of the body, such as nerve and muscle tissue. Lipofuscin is the oxidation product of free radical action on polyunsaturated fatty acids. The rate of accumulation of age pigments is a good index of chronologic age and perhaps one of the few aging phenomena universally demonstrated in mammals. Age pigments as an entity are examples of degenerative change. When accumulated in tissue, they cut off oxygen and nutrient supplies to surrounding areas, causing further degeneration and eventual death of tissue.

The Caloric Restriction Theory.   Walford[79] is a staunch proponent of caloric restriction, also known as energy restriction (ER) or DR, as previously described. Dr. Walford himself serves as living evidence of the in vivo experiment and that a lifestyle committed to the high-nutrient/low-calorie diet, moderate vitamin and mineral supplementation, and a regular exercise regimen is beneficial. Caloric restriction and its effect on life span extension is perhaps one of the most promising probes of the mechanisms of aging. Caloric restriction may exert its effectiveness through the neuroendocrine system. Everitt[80] has shown a striking similarity between dietary restriction and hypophysectomy demonstrated in Denckla's neuroendocrine studies previously cited.[51,52]

This high-nutrient/low-calorie diet is a result of years of animal in vivo experimentation, exploring longevity and maximum life span potential. Dr. Walford's experiments have been well received and respected, and other noted theorists, such as Leonard Hayflick, have acknowledged Walford's work.[81,81a–84]

Walford's caloric restriction program prescribes that an individual gradually lose weight over several years until a point of maximum metabolic efficiency is reached for optimum health and life span.[81]

Paffenberger[85,86] has shown that greater caloric expenditure is positively correlated with increasing life span and health in humans. A caveat here, as with other statements, is that exercise could have beneficial effects in preventing disease while at the same time accelerating aging through increased free radical generation. On the other hand, disease prevention through exercise could completely obscure the effects of free radicals.

Stochastic Theories of Aging

The second category of theories is described as stochastic theories. These theories purport that aging at the molecular level is caused by an accumulation of insults from the environment. The result of these insults is that the organism eventually reaches a level incompatible with life.[87]

Error Theory.   The error theory, also known as the error catastrophe theory, was first presented by Orgel in 1963.[88] It states that, although random errors in protein synthesis may occur, the error-containing protein molecule will be turned over, and the next copy will be error free. If the error-containing protein is one that is involved in the synthesis of the genetic material or in the protein synthesizing machinery, however, then this molecule could cause further errors. If this is the case, the number of error-containing proteins expands to result in an "error crisis" that would be incompatible with proper function and life. The theory specifies that "any accident or error in either the machinery or the process of making proteins would cascade into multiple effects."[89–94]

Redundant DNA Theory.   Another dimension of the error theory is the premise that the ability to repair damage to the genetic material is somehow associated with aging or the rate of aging.[95] Medvedev[95] suggests that biologic age changes are a result of errors accumulating in functioning genes. As these errors accumulate, reserve genetic sequences with identical information take over until the system's redundancy is exhausted. This theory is known as the redundant message theory. Medvedev[95] writes that different species' life spans may be a function of the degree of repeated genetic sequences. If error occurred in a nonrepeated gene sequence, the chance of preserving a final intact gene product during evolution or a long life span would be diminished. Hart and Setlow[59] obtained evidence that the ability to repair DNA cells after ultraviolet damage in cell cultures derived from various species of different maximum life spans and was directly correlated to maximum life span potential.

The mitochondrial theory of aging, based on the redundant DNA theory, states that the slow accumulation of impaired mitochondria is the driving force of the aging process.[96] The discovery of age-related mitochondrial DNA deletions have shown that damaged mitochondria have a decreased degradation rate and tend to accumulate as a result. The underlying mechanism of the accumulation of defective mitochondria remains unclear; however,

this hypothesis solves inconsistencies of the current model of redundancy.[96]

Somatic Mutation Theory.   One of the most prominent theories in the stochastic theories category is the somatic mutation theory of aging.[97,98] This theory emerged following World War II as a result of increased research in the area of radiation biology. The theory hypothesizes that mutations or genetic damage results from radiation and that radiomimetic agents accumulate and eventually create functional failure and the death of the organism. The somatic mutation theory is based on the scientific observation that exposure to ionizing radiation shortens the life span. Szilard[98] showed that exposure to radiation was recessive. It requires two or more "hits" from radiation to inactivate a given locus, and the exposure must occur in a sufficient number of cells for the damage to be manifested. Comparison of chromosomal aberrations in dividing liver cells in mice supports this view.[99–100]

Interestingly, the caloric restriction theory supports the theory of somatic mutation. A key prediction of the somatic mutation theory of aging is that there is an invariant relationship between life span and the number of random mutations. A number of studies have shown that somatic mutations of a variety of types accumulate with age, and that dietary restriction prolongs life span by slowing the accumulation of mutant genes.[103]

Transcription Theory.   Other scientists have developed theories focused specifically on stages of genetic processing. One of these processes, transcription, is the first stage in the transfer of information from DNA to protein synthesis. It entails the formation of messenger RNA so that it contains, in the linear sequence of its nucleotides, the genetic information located in the DNA gene from which messenger RNA is transcribed. Hayflick's[54] theory maintains that with increasing age, deleterious changes occur in the metabolism of differentiated postmitotic cells. He also suggests that the alterations are the results of primary events occurring within the nuclear chromatin. A control mechanism responsible for the appearance and the sequence of the primary aging events exists in the nuclear chromatin complex.

Cross-Linkage Theory.   A theory related to the redundant DNA theory is based on cross-linking in macromolecules. In 1942, Johan Bjorksten first related the concept of cross-linkage to developmental aging.[104,105] Prior to the 1940s, cross-linking was used as a method to stabilize macromolecules for individual purposes, such as vulcanizing rubber. Although cross-linking is not restricted to proteins, most experimental research has been on collagen and elastin because these molecules are accessible, do not readily turn over, and show increased cross-linking with age. Bjorksten[104] looked at large reactive protein molecules within the body, such as collagen, elastin, and DNA molecules, and surmised that their cross-linkage was responsible for secondary and tertiary causes of aging. [106]

New Theories on Aging

Sleep and Aging.   Sleep, or the lack thereof, has been implicated as a factor in exacerbating the aging process. The importance of sleep is often overlooked. Sleep curtailment constitutes an increasingly common condition in industrialized societies and is thought to affect mood and performance, as well as physiological functions. [107,108] It is during the deepest levels of sleep (Stages III and IV) that the human species repairs tissues and synthesizes the neuroendocrines that comprise a homeostatic hormonal system.

There is evidence that prolonged sleep loss affects the homeostasis of the important hypothalamic-pituitary-adrenal (HPA) axis and increases the secretion of the so-called stress hormone, cortisol. Leproult and associates[107] evaluated the effects of acute partial or total sleep deprivation on the nighttime and daytime profiles of cortisol levels. Alterations in cortisol levels were demonstrated during the evening following the night of sleep deprivation. After normal sleep, plasma cortisol levels were found to be within normal limits. After partial and total sleep deprivation, plasma cortisol levels were found to be higher, and the onset of the quiescent period of cortisol secretion was delayed. Even partial acute sleep loss was found to delay the recovery of the HPA axis from early morning circadian stimulation and is likely to involve an alteration in negative glucocorticoid feedback regulation. [107] In other words, sleep loss could affect the resiliency of the stress response and accelerate the development of immunologic, metabolic, and cognitive consequences of glucocorticoid excess, thereby accelerating the breakdown of tissues.

The production of growth hormone (GH) is one of the most important neuroendocrine processes involved in the regulation and repair of tissues at the cellular level. The major daily peak in plasma growth hormone level normally occurs during the early part of nocturnal sleep. [108] Mullington and colleagues[108] investigated possible factors associated with nocturnal peaks of GH in the absence of sleep, including subjectively defined sleepiness; electroencephalographically defined drowsiness during short lapses into sleep (napping); measures of cortisol levels; and body temperature. In studying subjects aged 16 to 84 years old, the researchers found age to be a significant negative predictor of nocturnal GH peak levels in sleep-deprived subjects compared to subjects experiencing normal sleep. These results suggest that the well-known suppressive effect of sleep deprivation on GH secretion is an age-dependent phenomenon that evolves during early adulthood and increases with age.

Sleep fragmentation, prolonged sleep onset latency, and reduced rapid eye movement activity are evident in older adults. Some GH-releasing hormones and peptides can trigger sleep in rats, rabbits, and humans. [109] The drugs gamma-hydroxybutyrate and ritanserine can induce both slow-wave sleep and GH secretion, thereby relating sleep and GH release. [110] Conversely, the disordered sleep patterns associated with sleep-apnea syndrome suppress GH secretion. The normal relationship between deep sleep and GH secretion may be eroded in aging. Sleep deprivation in young men elicits some of the same neuroendocrine and metabolic features of aging, such as elevated evening cortisol levels, higher sympathetic tone, and decreased glucose tolerance. [110] These alterations are hypothesized to exacerbate the aging process.

Growth Hormone.   The hormonal imbalance–growth factor exposure theory (HI-GFE theory) has been hypothesized as a possible explanation for an exacerbation in the aging process. [111] According to this theory, there is too much growth hormone and not enough insulin. If true, the HI-GFE theory can account for two major aging phenomena: (1) a decline in mammalian reserve capacity (the ability to return to physiologic homeostasis following stress) with a consequent increase in diseases of maintenance, and (2) an increase in most age-associated proliferation of diseases, due to an imbalance of both growth hormone and insulin. According to this theory, the decline in the reserve capacity is due to a gradual decline in mitochondrial maximal energy production, which in turn accounts for the gradual redirection of energy production toward survival functions such as ion pumping. This results in the relative detriment of RNA and protein synthesis as seen in lesser synthetic rates and slower turnover with consequent gradual cellular impairment. [111] The hypothetical explanation is that this is triggered by developmental programming and also nutritionally driven. Growth hormone exposure in youth and middle age purportedly promotes events that lead to proliferative diseases that arise coincident to rapidly declining reserve capacity and the cumulative mutational status associated with age. Parr[111] suggests that one possible explanation for this is a lack of available insulin. He proposes that the declining mitochondrial energy production can be reversed, or at least greatly diminished, if there is an improvement in the insulin–growth hormone balance. The result of a lower overall growth factor exposure could potentially lead to a longer, healthier life span than that seen in calorie restricted models. [111]

In a study of centenarians, it was found that mean levels of insulin-like growth factor-1 (IGF-1) were relatively low, indicating that there is an age-associated decline in this substance even in the extremely old. [112–119]

Telomeres.   Telomeres have been implicated in the regulation of cellular senescence. Telomeres consist of tandem repeats of a short nucleotide sequence and are located on the ends of chromosomes. Their length limits the total number of attainable cell generations in a tissue or organ (the so-called "end-replication" problem—the inability of DNA polymerase to completely replicate the end of linear DNA).[120]

In 1971, Olovnikov published a theory in which he first formulated the DNA end-replication problem and explained how it could be solved.[3] The solution to this problem also provided an explanation for the Hayflick Limit, which underpins the discovery in vitro and vivo cell senescence. Olovnikov proposed that the length of the telomeric DNA, located at the ends of chromosomes, consists of repeated sequences, which play a buffer role and should diminish in dividing normal somatic cells at each cell doubling.[121] The loss of sequences containing important information could occur after buffer loss (shortening of telomeres) and could cause the onset of cellular senescence. According to this theory it was suggested that for germline cells and for the cells of vegetatively propagated organisms and immortal cell populations like most cancer cell lines, an enzyme might be activated that would prevent the diminution of DNA termini at each cell division, thus protecting the formation containing part of the genome. In recent years, Olovnikov's hypothesis has been authenticated by laboratory evidence. The DNA sequences that shorten in dividing normal cells are telomeres and the enzyme that maintains telomere length constant in immortal cell populations is telomerase.[121,121a] Shortening of the telomere occurs when there is insufficient telomerase. The length of the telomere is predictive of life span for that cell and ultimately predictive of the life span of the organism.

Progress of Cell Culture Aging Models.

At the cellular level, several new processes have been proposed as being involved in the physiology of aging and the development of some age-related diseases. "Apoptosis," a word coined in 1972, signifies the process of nontraumatic and noninflammatory cell death—and the opposite of cell mitosis—that balances cell proliferation and thus maintains homeostasis. This theme was adumbrated as early as the late 1800s in studies of ovarian follicular atresia. Specific gene products either promote or oppose regulated cell death via mitochondria effects.[122] Dysregulation of apoptosis has been implicated in the development of diseases that are more prevalent in older individuals, such as cancer and the neurodegenerative disorders of Alzheimer's and Parkinson's diseases.

Interest in the role of mitochondria in aging has intensified in recent years. This focus on mitochondria originated in part from the free radical theory of aging, which argues that oxidative damage plays a key role in degenerative senescence.[123] Among the numerous mechanisms known to generate oxidants, leakage of the superoxide anion and hydrogen peroxide from the mitochondria electron transport chain are of particular interest, due to the correlation between species-specific metabolic rate ("rate

of living") and life span. Phenomenological studies of mitochondrial function long ago noted a decline in mitochondrial function with age,[74,95] and ongoing research continues to add to this body of knowledge.[70,96,123] The extranuclear somatic mutation theory of aging proposes that the accumulation of mutations in the mitochondrial genome may be responsible in part for the mitochondrial phenomenology of aging. Recent studies of mitochondrial DNA deletions have shown that they increase with age in humans and other mammals.[70,96,124]

The Genome Project and Implications on Aging.

Aging is characterized as a breakdown process and the relevant events occur after reproduction, when the force of natural selection declines. Studies of life histories of species reveal that there is an association between resource allocation and longevity and that the aging process is retarded when animals are protected from the deleterious consequences of excess metabolic activity. Although the extent to which aging is caused by environmental or genetic factors is unresolved, our understanding of the field has been enriched by the rapid development of the tools of molecular biology.[125] In his pioneering work, Alex Comfort[5] has postulated a hierarchical clock system as a descriptive paradigm of the aging process, and investigations at the molecular level are bringing to light evidence of a genetic link to life span that seems consistent with Comfort's model. With the genome projects now coding the complex structure of genetic material, the appropriate context for these mechanistic observations is just starting to evolve. Although most studies agree that genetics influences longevity in humans, the magnitude of this effect is debated. A study of children of nonagenarians suggested a strong relation between genetic influences and longevity,[126] as did a study that compared the life span of adopted children with that of their adoptive and biological parents.[127]

Recent evidence supports a role for important genetic and environmental interactions on longevity in lower organsims.[126–132] Although less is known in humans, commonality in molecular and biological processes, evolutionary arguments, and epidemiological data would strongly suggest that similar mechanisms also apply. The completion of the Human Genome Project and the rapid innovations in technology will make possible the identification of human longevity–assurance genes.[132] Identification of specific traits relevant to the aging phenotype and genes that promote longevity will provide important mechanistic insights into the molecular basis of aging. Furthermore, these studies will provide insights into how these genes exert their phenotypic influences. The insights may lead to interventions that can be used to promote survival in people who were not fortunate enough to inherit a genome predisposing them to longevity.[133–138]

Werner Syndrome: Fast-Forwarding Aging.

Cataracts, osteoporosis, heart disease, and other such ills typically afflict the aged. A disease that mimics and exacerbates the aging process is called Werner syndrome. Though this is not normal aging per se, as it affects individuals early in the life cycle, it is a disease that has been studied in aging studies to determine causal effects of aging. For the unfortunate sufferers of Werner syndrome, the diseases of aging strike, not in the seventh or eighth decade of life, but as early as the third. Such people age abnormally fast and usually die before they reach the age of 50.

This disease is genetic and associated with a dysfunction in the eighth chromosome. It has been found in Werner syndrome that when the DNA sequence of the gene for Werner syndrome is compared with normal genes, it contains a unique class of enzymes called helicases, substances which unwind the double helix of DNA, which is unique to this disease.[1,132] Helicases, of which there are many different types, are crucial enzyme components of all living cells. They help repair DNA and enable messenger RNA molecules to ferry genetic instructions from the nucleus, where DNA resides, throughout the cell, where the instructions are biochemically translated into proteins.[4,7] Although most cellular functions that use DNA or RNA are going to involve a helicase, in order to replicate DNA, the two strands of DNA have to unwind before it can be copied or repaired.[132,139] When chromosomes segregate during cell division, untangling a bunch of chromosomes requires a helicase.[11,132] It is suspected that the enzyme identified in Werner syndrome is not essential to life, but is somehow conducive to a long and healthy one. It is hypothesized that the helicase is not required for DNA replication, but rather it is involved in DNA repair, or in preventing mutation during DNA synthesis. Damaged DNA from people with Werner appears to be capable of repairing itself; however, their DNA seems to accumulate mutations at a higher-than-normal rate. Understanding how the gene works could provide insight into normal aging. It may be that "normal" people carry variants of the gene that influence their life spans or predispose them to an earlier death. Studying Werner could help pinpoint the mechanism that underlies all diseases of aging, which appear in part to be due to the cell slowdown that is such a dramatic feature of this disease.[132,139]

Theories of Aging

Name	Author	Theory
Developmental-Genetic Theories Of Aging		
Hayflick Limit Theory	Hayflick and Moorehead	There is a limited amount of cell population doublings, the average being fifty per life cycle of the cell.
Evolutionary Theory of Aging	Darwin	An expansion of natural selection and states that each successive generation is more resistant to mutations and when mutations occur, they occur at a later age.
Stress Theory	Parsons	Survival into old age is enhanced by high vitality and resilience due to an underlying resistance to stress by the genes.
Neuroendocrine Theory	Denckla	Functional decrements in neurons and their associated hormones are central to the aging process.
Theory of Intrinsic Mutagenesis	Burnett	Each species has specific characteristics of its genes that regulate the rate of errors, thereby affecting the life span.
Immunological Theory	Walford	The functional capacity of the immune system declines with age as a result of reduced T-cell function.
Free Radical Theory	Harman	Aging changes are due to damage caused by free radicals.
Caloric Restriction Theory	Walford	A life committed to a high-nutrient and low-calorie diet is beneficial and longer.
Stochastic Theories of Aging		
Error Theory	Orgel	Any accident or error in either the machinery or the process of making proteins would cascade in multiple effects that would be incompatible with proper function and life.

(continued)

Theories of Aging (Continued)

Stochastic Theories of Aging

Redundant DNA Theory	Medvedev	Biological age changes are a result of errors accumulating in genes. An accumulation of these takes over the system until it is exhausted.
Somatic Mutation Theory	Szilard	Mutations or genetic damage result from radiation and these accumulate and create functional failure and death.
Transcription Theory	Hayflick	A control mechanism responsible for the appearance and the sequence of aging exists in the nuclear chromatin complex.
Cross-Linkage Theory	Bjorksten	The large reactive proteins such as collagen cross-link and are responsible for aging.

New Theories Of Aging

Sleeping and Aging	Leproult	Prolonged sleep loss effects homeostasis and the species' ability to repair tissue.
The Hormonal Imbalance–Growth Factor Exposure Theory	Parr	There is too much growth hormone and not enough insulin, which leads to a less healthy and shorter life.
Telemeres	Olovnikov	The length of the telemere is predictive of life span for that cell and ultimately of that organism.
Progress of Cell Culture Aging Models	Perez	Dysregulation of nontraumatic and noninflammatory cell death has been implicated in the development of diseases more prevalent in older persons.
Implications of the Genome Project	N/A	There is a strong relationship between genetic influences and longevity.
Werner Syndrome	Barzilai	Normal people carry variants of the gene that influence their life spans or predispose them to an early death.

References

1. Rose MR. Can human aging be postponed? *Sci Am.* 1999; 281(6):106–111.
2. Austad SN. Theories of aging: An overview. *Aging.* 1998; 10(2):146–147.
3. Freeman JT. *Aging, Its History and Literature.* New York: Human Science Press; 1979.
4. Harman D. Aging: Phenomena and theories. *Ann NY Acad Sc.* 1998; 845:1–7.
5. Comfort A. *The Biology of Senescence.* 3rd ed. New York: Elsevier; 1979.
6. Pearl R. *The Rate of Living.* New York: Vropfu; 1928.
7. Warthin AS. *Old Age, the Major Revolution: The Philosophy and Pathology of the Aging Process.* New York: Hoeber; 1929.
8. Weissman A. *Uber die dauer des lebens.* Germany: Jena; 1882.
9. Rubner M. *Das problem der lebensdaver und seine beziebungen zum wachstum und ernabrung.* Munich: Oldenbourg; 1908.
10. Rose MR. *Evolutionary Biology of Aging.* New York: Oxford University Press; 1991.
11. Cauley JA, Dorman JS, Ganguli M. Genetic and aging epidemiology. The merging of two disciplines. *Neurol Clin.* 1996; 14:467–475.
12. Carrel A, Burrows MT. On the physiochemical regulation of the growth of tissues. *J Experimental Med.* 1911; 13:562–569.
13. Carrel A, Ebeling T. On the permanent life of tissues outside the organism. *J Experimental Med.* 1912; 15:516–522.
14. Carrel A. Present condition of a strain of connective tissue twenty-eight months old. *J Experimental Med.* 1914; 20:1–13.

15. Hayflick L. Senescence and cultured cells. In: Shock N, ed. *Perspectives in Experimental Gerontology.* Springfield, IL: Charles C Thomas; 1966.

16. Hayflick L, Moorehead PS. The serial cultivation of human diploid all strains. *Exp Cell Res.* 1961; 25:585–593.

17. Stone D, Rozovsky I, Morgan T, Anderson C, Finch C. Increases synaptic sprouting in response to estrogen via an apolipoprotein E-dependent mechanism: Implications for Alzheimer's disease. *J Neurosci.* 1998; 18:3180–3185.

18. Kirk KL. Dietary restriction and aging: Comparative tests of evolutionary hypotheses. *J Gerontol.* 2001; 56A(3):B123–B129.

19. Harrison DE, Archer JR. Natural selection for extended longevity from food restriction. *Growth Dev Aging.* 1988; 52(2):65.

20. Phelan JP, Austad SN. Natural selection, dietary restriction, and extended longevity. *Growth Dev Aging.* 1989; 53(1):4–6.

21. Dozmorov I, Bartke A, Miller RA. Array-based expression analysis of mouse liver genes: Effect of age and longevity. *J Gerontol.* 2001; 56A(2):B72–B80.

22. Gadow S. Aging as death rehearsal: The oppressiveness of reason. *J Clin Ethics.* 1996; 7(1):35–40.

23. Strehler BL. *Time, Cells and Aging.* 2nd ed. New York: Academic Press; 1977.

24. Cristofalo VJ. Overview of biological mechanism of aging. *Annual Review of Gerontology and Geriatrics.* 1991; 6:1–22.

25. Shock NW. Longitudinal studies of aging in human. In: Finch CE, Schneider EL, eds. *Handbook of the Biology of Aging.* New York: Van Nostrand Reinhold; 1985: 721–739.

26. Adelman RC. Hormone interaction during aging. In: Schimke RT, ed. *Biological Mechanisms in Aging.* Washington, DC: US Department of Health and Human Services; 1980.

27. Fries I, Crapo L. *Vitality and Aging.* San Francisco: WH Freeman; 1981.

28. Kirkwood TB. Biological theories of aging: An overview. *Aging.* 1998; 10(2):144–146.

29. Martin GM, Turker M. Genetics of human disease, longevity and aging. In: Hazzard EG, ed. *Textbook of Genetic Medicine.* New York: McGraw-Hill; 1990.

30. Kallman JF, Jarvik LF. Twin data on genetic variations in resistance to tuberculosis. In: Gedda L, ed. *Genetica Della Tuberculosi e dei tumori.* Rome: Gregorio Mendel; 1957: 15–41.

31. Jarvik LF. Survival trends in a senescent twin population. *Am J Hum Gene.* 1960; 12:170–181.

32. Hayflick L. The cellular basis for biological aging. In: Finch C, Hayflick L, eds. *The Handbook of the Biology of Aging.* New York: Van Nostrand Reinhold; 1977.

33. Martin GM, Sprague CA, Epstein CJ. Replicative life span of cultivated human cells. *Lab Invest.* 1970; 23:26.

34. Schneider EL, Mitsui Y. The relationship between in vitro cellular aging and in vivo human age. *Proc Natl Acad Sci USA.* 1976; 73:3584–3597.

35. Rohme D. Evidence for a relationship between longevity of mammalian species and life span of normal fibroblasts in vitro and erythrocytes in vivo. *Proc Natl Acad Sci USA.* 1981; 78: 3584–3591.

36. Stanley JF, Pye D, MacGregor A. Comparison of doubling numbers attained by cultural anirnal cells with life span of species. *Nature.* 1975; 255:158.

37. Keller L, Genoud M. Evolutionary theories of aging. 1. The need to understand the process of natural selection. *Gerontology.* 1999; 45(6):336–338.

38. Gavrilova NS, Gavrilov LA, Evdokushkina GN, et.al. Evolution, mutations, and human longevity: European royal and noble families. *Hum Biol.* 1998; 70(4):799–804.

39. LeBourg E. Evolutionary theories of aging: Handle with care. *Gerontology.* 1998; 44(6):345–348.

40. LeBourg E, Beugnon G. Evolutionary theories of aging. 2. The need not to close the debate. *Gerontology.* 1999; 45(6):339–342.

41. Franceschi C, Bonafe M, Valensin S, Olivieri F, De Luca M, Ottaviani E, DeBenedictis G. Inflammaging. An evolutionary perspective on immunosenescence. *Ann NY Acad Sci.* 2000; 908:244–254.

42. Franceschi C, Ottaviani E. Stress, Inflammation and natural immunity in the aging process: A new theory. *Aging.* 1997; 9(4 suppl):30–31.

43. Parsons PA. Inherited stress resistance and longevity: A stress theory of aging. *Heredity.* 1995; 75(pt 2): 216–221.

44. Parsons PA. The limit to human longevity: An approach through a stress theory of aging. *Mech Ageing Dev.* 1996; 87(3):211–218.

45. Walford RL. The immunologic theory of aging: Current status. *Fed Proc.* 1974; 33:2020.

46. Pincus S, Mulligan T, Iranmanesh A, Gheorghiu S, Godschalk M, Veldhuis J. Older males secrete luteinizing hormone and testosterone more irregularly, and jointly more asynchronously, than younger males. *Proc Natl Acad Sci USA.* 1996; 93:14100–14105.

47. Veldhuis JD. Conference report: Endocrinology of aging. *Diabetes and Endocrinology.* 2000; 10:1–11.

48. Veldhuis JD, Iranmanesh A, Mulligan T. Current insights into hypothalamo-pituitary mechanisms of reproductive aging in men. In: Veldhuis JD. *Toward a Healthier Old Age: Biomedical Advances from Basic Research to Clinical Science.* Barcelona, Spain: Prous Science Publishers; 1999.

49. Veldhuis JD, Iranmanesh A. Pathophysiology of impoverished growth hormone (GH) secretion in aging. In: Veldhuis JD. *Toward a Healthier Old Age: Biomedical Advances from Basic Research to Clinical Science.* Barcelona, Spain: Prous Science Publishers; 1999.

50. Iranmanesh A, Veldhuis J. Functional alterations of the corticotropic axis with advancing aging. In: Veldhuis JD. *Toward a Healthier Old Age: Biomedical Advances from Basic Research to Clinical Science.* Barcelona, Spain: Prous Science Publishers; 1999.

51. Brody H, Jayashankar N. Anatomical changes in the nervous system. In: Finch CE, Hayflick L, eds. *Handbook of the Biology of Aging.* New York: Van Nostrand Reinhold; 1977.

52. Everitt AV. The hypothalamic pituitary control of aging and age-related pathology. *Experimental Gerontol.* 1973; 8:265–269.

53. Denckla WD. Role of the pituitary and thyroid glands in the decline of minimal O_2 consumption with age. *J Clin Investigation.* 1974; 53: 572–577.

54. Hayflick L. Theories of aging. In: Cape R, Coe R, Rodstein M, eds. *Fundamentals of Geriatric Medicine.* New York: Raven Press; 1983.

55. Finch CE, Landfield PW. Neuroendocrine and autonomic functions in aging mammals. In: Finch CE, Schneider EL, eds. *Handbook of the Biology of Aging.* New York: Van Nostrand Reinhold; 1985: 567–579.

56. Wise PA. Aging of the female reproductive system. *Rev Biol Res Aging.* 1983; 1:15–26.

57. Rosenfeld A. Are we programmed to die? *Saturday Rev.* 1976; 10(2):10.

58. Burnett M. *Intrinsic Mutagenesis: A Genetic Approach for Aging.* New York: John Wiley; 1974.

59. Hart RW, Setlow RB. Correlation between DNA excision repair and life span in a number of mammalian species. *Proc Natl Acad Sci USA.* 1974; 71: 2169–2183.

60. Krauss SW, Linn S. Studies of DNA polymerases alpha and beta from cultured human cells in various replicative states. *J Cellular Physiol.* 1986; 126:99–107.

61. Linn S. Decreased fidelity of DNA polymerase activity isolated from aging human fibroblasts. *Proc Natl Acad Sci USA.* 1976; 13:2818–2826.

62. Murray V, Holliday R. Increased error frequency of DNA polymerases from senescent human fibroblasts. *J Mol Biology.* 1981; 146:55–82.

63. Fairweather S. The in vitro life span of MRC-5 cells is shortened by 5-azacytidine induced derriethylation. *Experimental Cell Research.* 1987; 168:153–158.

64. Holliday R. Strong effects of 5-azacytidine on the in vitro life span of human diploid fibroblasts. *Experimental Cell Research.* 1986; 166:543–548.

65. Wilson VL, Jones PA. DNA methylation decreases in aging but not in immortal cells. *Science.* 1983; 220:1054–1071.

66. Wareham VA. Age related reactivation of an X-linked gene. *Nature.* 1987; 327:725–732.

67. Walford RL. Immunopathology of aging. In: Eisdorfer C, ed. *Annual Review of Gerontology and Geriatrics.* 2nd ed. New York: Springer; 1981:2.

68. Walford RL. *The Immunologic Theory of Aging.* Copenhagen: Munksgaard; 1969.

69. Walford RL. Multigene families, histocompatibility system, transformation, meiosis, stem cells and DNA repair. *Mech Ageing Dev.* 1979; 9:19–28.

70. Ashok BT, Ali R. The aging paradox: Free radical theory of aging. *Exp Gerontol.* 1999; 34(3):293–303.

71. Beckman KB, Ames BN. The free radical theory of aging matures. *Physiol Rev.* 1998; 78(2):547–581.

72. Banks D, Fossel M. Telomeres, cancer, and aging. Altering the human life span. *JAMA.* 1997; 278: 1345–1348.

73. Harmon D. Aging: a theory based on free radical and radiation chemistry. *J Gerontol.* 1956; 11: 298–311.

74. Harmon D. Prolongation of life: roles of free radical reactions in aging. *J Am Geriatr Soc.* 1969; 17:721.

75. Harmon D. The aging process. *Proc Natl Acad Sci USA.* 1981; 78:7124–7141.

76. Tappel AL. Lipid peroxidation damage to cell components. *Fed Proc.* 1973; 32:1870.

77. Leibovitz BE, Siegel B. Aspects of free radical reactions of biological systems: aging. *J Gerontol.* 1980; 35(1):45.

78. Sacher GA, Duffy PH. Genetic relation of life span to metabolic rate for inbred mouse strains and their hybrids. *Fed Proc.* 1979; 38:184–198.

79. Walford RL, Harris S, Weinciruch R. Dietary restriction and aging: Historical phases, mechanisms and current directions. *J Nutr.* 1987; 117:1650–1654.

80. Everitt AV. The effects of hypophysectomy and continuous food restriction, begun at ages 70 and 400 days, on collagen aging, proteinuria, incidence of pathology and longevity in the male rat. *Mech Ageing Dev.* 1980; 12:161–169.

81. Walford RL. *The 120-Year Diet.* New York: Pocket Books; 1986.

81a. Roth, G. Caloric restriction and conroic restriction mimetics: Current status and promise for the future. *JAGS;* 2005; 53(9): 280–284.

82. Weindruch R, Chia D, Barnett EV, Walford RL. Dietary restriction in mice beginning at complex levels. *Age.* 1982; 5:111–112.

83. Harmon D. Free radical theory of aging: Role of free radicals in the origination and evaluation of life, aging, and disease processes. In: Johnson JE, Walford RL, Harinon D, Miguel J, eds. *Free Radicals, Aging, and Degenerative Diseases.* New York: Alan Liss; 1986: 3–50.

84. Koizuini A, Weindruch R, Walford. RL. Influence of dietary restriction and age on live enzyme activities and lipid peroxidation in mice. *J Nutr.* 1987; 11(7):361–367.

85. Masoro EJ. Influence of caloric intake on aging and on the response to stressors. *J Toxicol Environ Health B Crit Rev.* 1998; 1(3):243–257.

86. Paffenberger RS. Physical activity, all-cause mortality, and longevity of college alumni. *N Engl J Med.* 1986; 314:605–609.

87. Pereira-Smith OM. Genetic theories of aging. *Aging.* 1997; 9(6):429–430.

88. Orgel LE. The maintenance of the accuracy of protein synthesis and its relevance to aging. *Proc Natl Acad Sci USA.* 1963; 49:517–531.

89. Sonnebom T. The origin, evolution, nature and causes of aging. In: Behnke J, Fince C, Moment G, eds. *The Biology of Aging.* New York: Plenum Press; 1979: 341.

90. Gallant J, Kurland C, Parker J, Holliday R, Rosenberger R. The error catastrophe theory of aging. *Exp Gerontol.* 1997; 32(3):333–346.

91. Ryan JM, Duda B, Cristofalo VJ. Error accumulation and aging in human diploid cells. *J Gerontol.* 1974; 29:616–627.

92. Holliday R, Tarrant GM. Altered enzymes in aging human fibroblasts. *Nature.* 1972; 238:26–34.

93. Holliday R. The current status of the protein error theory of aging. *Exp Gerontol.* 1996; 31(4):449–452.

94. Rothstein M. Age-related changes in enzyme levels and enzyme properties. In: Rothstein M, ed. *Review of Biological Research in Aging.* New York: Alan Liss; 1985; 1:421–444.

95. Medvedev Z. Possible role of repeated nucleotide sequences in DNA in the evolution of life spans of differential cells. *Nature.* 1972; 237: 453–454.

96. Kowald A. The mitochondrial theory of aging: Do damaged mitochondria accumulate by delayed degradations? *Exp Gerontol.* 1999; 34(5):605–612.

97. Failla G. The aging process and carcinogenesis. *Ann NY Acad Sci.* 1958; 71:1124–1130.

98. Szilard L. On the nature of the aging process. *Proc Natl Acad Sci USA.* 1959; 45:30–51.

99. Curtis HF, Miller K. Chromosome aberrations in lower cells of guinea pigs. *J Gerontol.* 1971; 26: 292–299.

100. Maynard-Smith J. Review lecturer on senescence: 1. The causes of aging. *Proceedings of the Royal Society of London.* 1962; (B):157:115–124.

101. Clark AM, Rubin NIA. The modification of X-irradiation of the life span of haptoid and diploid hagrogracon. *Radiation Research.* 1961; 14:244–251.

102. Fossel M. Cell senescence in human aging: A review of the theory. *In Vivo.* 2000; 14(1):29–34.

103. Morley A. Somatic mutation and aging. *Ann NY Acad Sci.* 1998; 854:20–22.

104. Bjorksten J. Cross-linkage and the aging process. In: Rockstein M, ed. *Theoretical Aspects of Aging.* New York: Academic Press; 1974: 43.

105. Bjorksten J. The cross-linkage theory of aging: Clinical implications. *Compr Ther.* 1976; 11:65.

106. Hall DA. *The Aging of Connective Tissue.* New York: Academic Press; 1976.

107. Leproult R, Copinschi G, Buxton O, Cauter E. Sleep loss results in an elevation of cortisol levels the next evening. *Sleep.* 1997; 20(10): 865–870.

108. Mullington J, Hermann D, Holsboer F, Pollmacher T. Age-dependent suppression of nocturnal growth hormone levels during sleep deprivation. *Neuroendocrinology.* 1996; 64(3):233–241.

109. Giustina A, Veldhuis J. Pathophysiology of neuroregulation of growth hormone secretion in experimental animals and the human. *Endocr Rev.* 1998; 19:717–797.

110. Van Cauter E, Plat L, Leproult R, Copinschi G. Alterations of circadian rhythmicity and sleep in aging: Endocrine consequences. *Horm Res.* 1998; 49: 147–152.

111. Parr T. Insulin exposure and unifying aging. *Gerontology.* 1999; 45(3):121–135.

112. Yasumichi A, Nobuyoshi H, Yamamura K, Shimizu K, Takayama M, Ebihara Y, Osono Y. Serum insulin-like growth factor-1 in centenarians: Implications of IGF-1 as a rapid turnover protein. *J Gerontol.* 2001; 56A(2):M79–M82.

113. Flynn MA, Weaver-Osterholtz D, Sharpe-Timms KL, Allen S, Krause G. Dehydroepiandrosterone replacement in aging humans. *J Clin Endocrinol Metab.* 1999; 84(5):1527–1533.

114. Morales AJ, Haubrich RH, Hwang JY, Asakura H, Yen SS. The effect of six months treatment with a 100 mg daily dose of dehydroepiandrosterone (DHEA) on circulating sex steroids, body composition and muscle strength in age-advanced men and women. *Clin Endocrinol.* 1998; 49(4):421–432.

115. Callies F. Influence of oral dehydroepiandrosterone (DHEA) on urinary steroid metabolites in males and females. *Steroids.* 2000; 65(2):98–102.

116. Barnhart KT, Freeman E, Grisso JA, Rader DJ, Sammel M, Kapoor S, Nestler JE. The effect of dehydroepiandrosterone supplementation to symptomatic perimenopausal women on serum endocrine profiles, lipid parameters, and health-related quality of life. *Clin Endocrinol.* 1998; 49(4):433–438.

117. Arlt W, Haas J, Callies F, Reincke M, Hubler D, Oettel M, Ernst M, Schulte HM, Allolio B. Biotransformation of oral dehydroepiandrosterone in elderly men: Significant increase in circulating estrogens. *J Clin Endocrinol Metab.* 1999; 84(6): 2170–2176.

118. Mazza E, Maccario M, Ramunni J, Gauna C, Bertagna A, Barberis AM, Patroncini S, Messina M, Ghigo E. Dehydroepiandrosterone sulfate levels in women. Relationships with age, body mass index and insulin levels. *J Endocrinol Invest.* 1999; 22(9): 681–687.

119. Tilvis RS, Kahonen M, Harkonen M. Dehydroepiandrosterone sulfate, diseases and mortality in a general aged population. *Aging.* 1999; 11(1):30–34.

120. Hayflick L. How and why we age. *Exp Gerontol.* 1998; 33(6):639–653.

121. Olovnikov AM. Telomeres, telomase, and aging: Origin of the theory. *Exp Gerontol.* 1996; 31(4): 443–448.

122a. Woodring. W. and Shay, J. Telomere biology in aging and cancer. *JAGS*. 2005; 53(9):292–295.

122. Perez G, Tilly J. Cumulus cells are required for the increased apoptotic potential in oocytes of aged mice. *Hum Reprod*. 1997; 12:2781–2783.

123. Beckman KB, Ames BN. Mitochondrial aging: Open questions. *Ann NY Acad Sci*. 1998; 854: 118–127.

124. Miquel J. An update on the oxygen stress-mitochondrial mutation theory of aging: Genetic and evolutionary implications. *Exp Gerontol*. 1998; 33(1–2): 113–126.

125. Carlson JC, Riley JC. A consideration of some notable aging theories. *Exp Gerontol*. 1998; 33(1–2): 127–134.

126. Abbott M, Abbey H, Bolling D, Murphy E. The familial component in longevity—A study of offspring of nonagenarians: III. Intrafamilial studies. *Am J Med Genetics*. 1978; 2(2):105–120.

127. Sorensen T, Nielsen G, Andersen P, Teasdale T. Genetic and environmental influences on premature death in adult adoptees. *N Engl J Med*. 1988; 318:727–732.

128. Ljungquist B, Berg S, Lanke J, McClearn GE, Pedersen NL. The effect of genetic factors for longevity: A comparison of identical and fraternal twins in the Swedish Twin Registry. *J Gerontol Med Sci*. 1988; 53A(4):M441–M446.

129. Herskind AM, McGue M, Iachine IA, et al. Untangling genetic influences on smoking, body mass index and longevity: A multivariate study of 2464 Danish twins followed for 28 years. *Hum Genet*. 1996; 98:467–475.

130. Perls TT, Burbrick E, Wager CG, Vijg J, Kruglyak L. Siblings of centenarians live longer. *Lancet*. 1998; 351(3):1560.

131. Robine JM, Allard M. The oldest human. *Science*. 1998; 279:1834.

132. Barzilai N, Shuldiner AR. Searching for human longevity genes: the future history of gerontology in the post-genomic era. *J Gerontol*. 2001; 56A(2): M83–M87.

133. Finch EF, Tanzi RE. Genetics of aging. *Science*. 1997; 279:1834.

134. Schachter F, Faure-Delanef L, Guenot F. Genetic associations with human longevity at the APOE and ACE loci. *Nat Genet*. 1994; 6:29–32.

135. Ivanova R, Henon N, Lepage V, Charron D, Vicaut E, Schachter F. HLA-DR alleles display sex-dependent effects on survival and discriminate between individuals and familial longevity. *Hum Mol Genet*. 1998; 7(1):187–194.

136. Mannucci PM, Mari D, Merati G. Gene polymorphisms predicting high plasma levels of coagulation and fibronolysis proteins. A study in centenarians. *Arterioscler Thromb Biol*. 1997; 17:755–759.

137. Van Orsouw N, Perls TT, Vijg J. Centenarians: Defining the "good" polymorphism of longevity enabling genes [abstract]. *Gerontologist*. 1999; 39(special issue)1:282. Session 182.

138. De Benedictis G, Rose G, Carrieri G. Mitochondrial DNA inherited variants are associated with successful aging and longevity in humans. *FASEB J*. 1999; 13:1532–1536.

139. Yu C, Oshim J, Wijsman E, et al. Mutations in the consensus helicase domains of the Werner syndrome gene. Werner's Syndrome Collaborative Group. *Am J Hum Genet*. 1997; 60:330–341.

3

Age-Related Changes in Physiology

Pearls

- Not all body cells age in the same way or at the same rate; however, in general, the total number of cells in the body decreases with age while remaining cells become less alike in structure and less organized in function.
- Cardiovascular cellular changes with age are numerous and range from lipofuscin accumulation at the poles of the nuclei of cardiac muscle to increased calcification in the media.
- In the pulmonary system, age changes can be organized according to mechanical properties, changes in flow, gas exchange, and impairment of lung defense.

- The decrease in aging muscle is associated with a selective loss of type II muscle fibers, a decrease in protein and nitrogen, and an increase in connective tissue and fat.
- Due to change in the thermal regulatory response, the aged have prolonged cooling time following increased activity, as well as a decrease of receptiveness to heat and cold.
- All five senses as well as proprioception/kinesthesia decline with age.
- The endocrine system plays a major role in the biologic variability of aging.

INTRODUCTION

The aging process occurs along the continuum of life. Beginning at conception and terminating in death, certain changes are recognized as transitional markers in the human aging process. Aging is viewed as characteristically decremental in nature and lacking in defined chronological points of transition, though linear with time.[1]

The notion of a "maximal achievable life span" is inherent in the concepts of aging.[2-4] Identifying and describing changes in function that are common to all individuals and not produced by pathology is a very difficult task. The use of the term "*eugeric*" distinguishes changes related to the natural aging process from changes related to pathology.[5] The hypothesis of eugeric death is that the decline of function continues linearly to the point where an internal environment compatible with cell life can no longer be maintained.

While the process of aging is complex and does not uniformly result in decreased functional capacity,[6] this survey of the body's systems will be based on the assumption that the losses associated with the aging process are due to declines in cellular functioning. In these cases, some functional units are lost, but the remaining units continue to

function normally. The kidney is an excellent example of this—function is diminished in proportion to the number of nephrons lost. Skeletal muscle is another example. While muscle mass decreases secondary to the loss of muscle fibers, the remaining muscle mass is capable of oxygenation and consuming metabolic substrates at a constant rate The most obvious aging changes are those in which function is totally lost: the capacity of the female to reproduce is an excellent example, while another would be the loss in ability to hear sounds above a certain frequency.

Homeostasis is a concept describing the "constancy of the internal environment."[7] This internal constancy enables humans to survive in many environments and to withstand many biological and physiological challenges, thereby expanding the habitable world of the human. Perhaps the single most salient and age-related difference is the diminishing ability of the body to respond to physical and emotional stress and return to the prestress level.[8,9] This decrease in homestatic capacity is seen in all the systems of the body but most marked in neuroendocrine interaction and in the systemic functional alteration in the responsiveness of the nervous and endocrine systems.[7]

The changes associated with aging through adulthood into old age are gradual. During adult life, in the absence of overt pathology, there is a slow decrement in function.

Homeostasis can be maintained, albeit at a lower level. Another observation is that the more complex the function, the more decline is seen. There are important differences between the young and old when considering interacting systems. Decrements are greater in the functions involving a number of connections between nerve and nerve, nerve and muscle, nerve and gland. For instance, the decrease in nerve conduction velocity is less than the decrease in maximum breathing capacity. In the former a single system is involved, while in the latter the coordination of a number of nerve and muscle activities is required.

Last, it is important to keep in mind that individuals age at different rates. Different tissues and systems within one person demonstrate different aging rates as well. Therefore, while it is useful to discuss the average declines of function, it is important to keep in mind that any one individual may show remarkable variability from his or her peers.

For information on cellular and anatomic changes, including cardiovascular changes see CD.

CARDIOVASCULAR CHANGES WITH AGE

Generally there is a decrease in cardiac output at rest, a decline in the cardiovascular system's response to stress, an increase in the systolic blood pressure, and a progressive increase in the peripheral vascular resistance to blood flow.

Heart rate, loading conditions, intrinsic muscle performance, and neurohumoral efficiency all affect cardiac output. The maximum heart rate achievable declines linearly with age at peak exercise levels.[10,11] Heart rate response is usually not affected at submaximal exercise levels. Heart rate response has been demonstrated to diminish in response to various physiological stimuli, such as coughing, postural changes, or during the Valsalva manuever.[12] The rate with which the heart rate peaks also becomes prolonged with increasing age.[10] Cardiac filling and vascular impedance are loading conditions that influence cardiac output. Diastolic filling rate has been shown to decrease with age,[13] and this is attributed to: prolonged isometric relaxation; thickening and sclerosis of the mitral valve, which impedes ventricular filling; and an age-associated decrease in left ventricular compliance.[13] Vascular impedance is affected by the central-aortic stiffness or compliance, peripheral vascular resistance, and the inertial properties of blood.[14] Systolic pressure in the aorta and pulse pressures are increased with age.[14,15] Late systolic pressure exceeds early systolic pressure in the elderly, and the index of elastance (characteristic impedance) and peripheral resistance are increased with age.[16] These changes are indicative of less aortic compliance and a reduced cross section of the peripheral vasculature, which causes an increase in pulse-wave velocity and an increase in wave reflection. Wei[10,15] hypothesizes that the consequent increase in vascular load could explain the age-associated reductions in stroke volume and cardiac output as well as the development of mild left ventricular hypertrophy and prolonged myocardial relaxation in the elderly.

Intrinsic muscle performance is estimated by the mean velocity of circumferential fiber shortening, and this does not change with age.[13] However, isometric relaxation and early diastolic relaxation are prolonged as age increases.[17] Left ventricular wall thickness may result from prolonged relaxation.[13]

Cardiac output is also affected by neurohumoral regulation. In the myocardium and in the peripheral vessels the end-organ responsiveness is decreased to beta-adrenergic stimulation.[14] The autonomic tone is increased based on plasma catecholamine levels.[18] Reflex activity of the cardiovascular system (e.g., Valsalva maneuver, orthostasis, and cough) are weaker in the aged cardiovascular system, due in part to a decreased baroreceptor sensitivity and associated with changes in the cardiopulmunary system.[10,12,19]

The ability of the body to maintain a homeostatic blood pressure is a function of: the autonomic nervous system; the arterial baroreceptor reflex; circulating neurohumoral factors; local vascular tone; and the extracellular fluid volume. There is an alteration in the homeostatic blood pressure regulatory role as a result of an altered autonomic nervous system with age.[14,19] According to Shimada, an elevation of blood pressure in the elderly can be attributed to an increase in plasma norepinephrine levels, which leads to an increase in the sympathetic responsiveness.[19] The functioning of the arterial baroreceptor reflex is lessened with age.[15,19] Atherosclerosis and the presence of hypertension also decrease the baroreceptor reflex.[19] Catecholamines and circulating neurohumoral factors assist in the maintainance of a homeostatic blood pressure.[20] These factors include renin, aldosterone, vasopressin, atrial natriuretic factor, and angiotensin II. The level of renin in the plasma has been found to remain unchanged or decrease in relation to age. It is hypothesized that this is due to a decrease in the concentration of active renin and not a result of the concentration of renin substrate in the plasma.[20] In proportion to the decreased renin activity in the plasma, there is a related decline in aldosterone and plasma-angiotensin II levels with increasing age.[20] Vasopressin remains unchanged or decreases with age. A decrease in vasopressin activity is most often related to blood loss or dehydration.[21] The level of plasma atrial natriuretic factor does not show a change with age. Vascular tone may show a local increase with age, though the constriction of the vessels is not changed in response to norepinephrine with age.[14]

The effect of these changes on the cardiovascular system is seen in changes in cardiac output, stroke volume, and blood pressure at rest and in response to stress. Resting heart rate does not show a consistent age-related change in humans.[15] Resting cardiac rate and cardiac output remain relatively unchanged, although peripheral resistance (blood pressure) is increased.[22] With age, myocardial weight tends to increase, and myocardial cells show an increase in lipofuscin deposition. Mitochondria decrease in size and myocardial cells are less responsive to catacholamine stimulation. A reduction in baroreceptor response and vascular elasticity combines to result in the tendency for older people to experience postural hypotension.[7,23] When sitting at rest, the cardiac output does not show a change with age; however, when supine there is often an age-related decrease in cardiac output.[15] There is also a similar position-associated change in stroke volume. This is explained by the changes with age in cardiac compliance and preload conditions.[14,15] Resting blood pressures, both diastolic and systolic, tend to show an increase with age.[15] It is not clear whether this increase in blood pressure is a reflection of eugeric aging or the result of heredity, environmental factors, or both.[15]

In response to stress, the cardiovascular system shows a decrease in heart rate acceleration and a decrease in ejection fraction with physical exertion.[15] Postural changes also affect cardiac output and blood pressure as previously discussed. Following a moderately sized meal, the elderly tend to show a decrease in systemic blood pressure.[15] With increasing levels of exercise, there is a concomitant rise in the systemic blood pressure. This rise is credited to the changes in preload conditions during cardiac filling.[15] In the absence of pathology, the cardiovascular responses to increased activity levels are consistently seen with increasing age; however, aerobic conditioning exercises may alter this. The effects of exercise on the cardiovascular system are positive and will be discussed in a subsequent chapter.

Cardiopulmonary Changes with age & Therapeutic Considerations

Body System	Changes with Age	Therapeutic Considerations
Cardiovascular	Changes in cardiac muscle fibers and electrolytes	Older persons are more prone to arrhythmias. Therefore, the physical therapist should check the pulse before and during the activity to determine any change in cardiac rhythm.
	Decline to the cardiovascular system's response to stress	In order to diminish stress on the cardiac muscle, warm-up and cool-down periods are necessary.
	Increase in systolic blood pressure	Check vitals before, during, and after activity. Significant changes should be documented. You may need to refer the patient back to the primary care physician before continuing with the exercise program.
	Increase in peripheral resistance	This change will be noticed in the increased effort of the left ventricle that will show in the BP by the end.
	Decreased maximum heart rate	Conventional heart rate formulas used for the young may need modification for older persons. Those formulas will demonstrate the target zone heart rate that will be allowed for the exercise routine.
	Decreased diastolic filling rate	Frequent rests may be needed with longer bouts of exercise. Check pulse and respiratory rate in order to adjust exercise intensity.
	Decreased ventricular compliance	Monitor heart rate and blood pressure when during exercise at higher levels.
Pulmonary	Decrease in chest wall compliance and decreased lung elastic recoil	Chest mobility is important to allow sufficient amount of air exchange; therefore they need sufficient oxygen during exercises. Therapists should monitor respiratory rate and pattern.
	Increased calcification of the ribs	Special consideration for mobilization techniques should be considered. Also be aware of osteoporosis and potential risk for fracture.

(*continued*)

Cardiopulmonary Changes with age & Therapeutic Considerations (Continued)

Body System	Changes with Age	Therapeutic Considerations
Pulmonary	Decreased intercostal muscle strength, decrease in diaphragmatic strength, decrease in abdominal muscle strength, and other ventilatory muscles' strength	Older population may present with diminished endurance, which will cause them to easily fatigue.
	Changes in spinal curvature	There will be diminished breathing capacity.
	Decreased maximum voluntary ventilation	Slowly progress exercise programs; gradually return to baseline when exercising.
	Vital capacity decreases	Persons will be unable to do the type of exercise they did at 20 years of age.
	Residual volume increases	There is more unused air in the lungs.
	Lung cilia less and less strong	Persons may be more prone to pulmonary dysfunction and infection; be aware of environmental changes.

PULMONARY CHANGES WITH AGE

In this chapter, aging changes defined by Butler as those changes that are "universal, intrinsic, progressive and irreversible" within the cardiopulmonary system will be discussed.[24] The pathologies of the lung will be further discussed in Chapter 5, Pathological Manifestations of Aging.

In the pulmonary system, age changes can be organized according to mechanical properties, changes in flow, changes in volume, alteration in gas exchange, and impairments of lung defense. Decreases in chest wall compliance and lung elastic recoil tendency are two mechanical properties that are altered with age. Increased calcification of the ribs, a decline in intercostal muscle strength, and changes in the spinal curvature all result in a lower compliance and in increased work of breathing.

At normal lung volume, airway resistance is not increased. However, normal aging results in a reduction of maximum voluntary ventilation, maximum expiratory flow, and forced expiratory volume in one second (alone and in relation to forced vital capacity). Though tidal volume remains fairly constant throughout life, vital capacity decreases while residual volume increases.

Ventilation, diffusion, and pulmonary circulation are the three major components of the respiratory system that lose efficiency with age. There is an increased thickening of the supporting membranes between the alveoli and the capillaries, a decline in total lung capacity, an increase in residual volume, a reduced vital capacity, and a decrease in the resiliency of the lungs. It is difficult to completely separate pulmonary changes resulting with age from those associated with the pathology of emphysema or chronic

bronchitis. Throughout a lifetime, exposure to occupational and environmental inhalants as well as cigarette smoke may result in chronic pulmonary changes and lung pathologies. These disease states closely parallel those of the aging process and also increase in incidence with advancing age.[25] "Normal" pulmonary aging includes a loss of elastic tissue leading to expiratory collapse of the larger airways, difficulty with expiration, and dilitation of the terminal air passages.[26]

There are changes in the diffusion efficiency of peripheral vascular system with age. Starting with the pulmonary system, impairment of gas exchange is illustrated by a reduced diffusing capacity of carbon monoxide, a lower resting arterial oxygen tension, and an increased alveolar-arterial oxygen gradient. Alveolar surface area and pulmonary capillary blood volume diminish with age. Small changes in red blood cell metabolism produce a decrease in 2,3 diphosphoglycerate (DPG). As a result, the oxygen dissociation curve shifts to the left, which makes oxygen less available at the tissue level.

The ability to provide oxygen to working tissues is altered as normal aging affects the cardiopulmonary system in a variety of ways. In the absence of pathology, the heart and lungs can generally meet the body's needs; however, reserve capacities are diminished. With any challenge, the body's demand for oxygen and perfusion may exceed available supply.

In an older person, normal changes result in an impairment of pulmonary defenses. Cilia are reduced in number, and those that remain become less strong. The mucous escalator and alveolar macrophages are less effective in removing inhaled particulate matter. In the absence of physiological challenges, the system maintains fairly adequate defenses. However, an older individual who is chronically exposed to air laden with particles will become at risk for pulmonary dysfunction.[7,27]

The recovery period following effort is prolonged in the elderly. Among other factors, this reflects a greater relative work rate, an increased proportion of anaerobic metabolism, a slower heat elimination, and a lower level of physical fitness. When exercising, elderly individuals need to lengthen the cool-down phase of exercise to allow for a more gradual return to the baseline vital signs. Abrupt cessation of exercise without considering an adequate recovery period could have negative effects for a person of any age, but it is particularly important in the elderly to provide adequate recovery time.

MUSCULOSKELETAL CHANGES WITH AGE

For information on Musculoskeletal Cellular Changes, see CD.

Changes in Cartilage

Other connective tissue also affected by aging includes bone, hyaline cartilage, elastic cartilage, and articular cartilage. Changes in bone will be presented separately.

Hyaline cartilage is found in the nose and the rings of the respiratory passages as well as in the joints. Elastic cartilage is found in parts of the larynx and the outer ear. Articular cartilage is found between the intervertebral discs, between the bones of the pelvic girdle, and at most articular joint surfaces.[28] With aging, cartilage tends to dehydrate, becomes stiffer, and thins in weight-bearing areas.

Cartilage is formed when the primitive mesenchymal cells are subjected to compressive forces in an environment of low oxygen concentration. The predominant secretions of the chondroblast are glycoprotein, chondroitin sulfate, and hyaluronic acid. Collagen is produced in lesser amounts than these. Cartilage is a unique connective tissue in that it has no direct blood supply. Blood flow in adjacent bones and synovial fluid provide nutrients to the chondroblasts. A strong osmotic force, created by glycoprotein secretions from the chondroblasts passing from the cells into the surrounding matrix, attracts water with dissolved gases, inorganic salts, and organic materials into the matrix providing materials necessary for normal metabolism. The concentration of glycoproteins in the matrix determines the amount of fluid drawn into the cartilage. Normal aging is accompanied by a reduction in the amount of chondroitin sulfate produced[29] and results in a decrease in osmotic attraction forces and impairment in the ability of the matrix to attract and retain fluids.

Nutrients enter the matrix of the cartilage only when compressive forces are absent.[29,30] In a loaded or compressed state, fluid and nutrient substances are squeezed out. To provide regular movement of substances in and out of the cartilage, it is necessary that alternating application and release of compressive forces occur. Metabolites remain in the matrix in the absence of compression. The presence of metabolites reduces the oxygen content, which results in a decrease in the secretion of glycoproteins and an increase in the amount of procollagen produced. With inactivity, hyaline cartilage is converted to fibrocartilage.[29,30] Therefore, weight-bearing exercises become particularly important in the elderly individual. The movement of nutritional substances in and out of the cartilage with activity could enhance the overall health of the cartilage and preserve the viability of the joints.[29]

In synovial joints the articular surfaces are covered by hyaline cartilage. Secretion of hyaluronic acid by the chondroblasts provides lubrication at the interface of the hyaline cartilage. Hyaluronic acid molecules form a viscous layer covering the hyaline cartilage. Compression facilitates production of hyaluronic acid ensuring continual lubrication of the joint during movement.[30] As previously noted, the secretion of hyaluronic acid decreases with age, thereby reducing the efficiency of the lubrication system of the joint.[29] Degenerative changes of the cartilage are not reversible and rehabilitation efforts need to be directed toward regular compression and release of compression in the aging joint. Normal weight-bearing exercises are recommended to maintain cartilagenous health.

The cartilage that normally covers body joints thins and deteriorates with aging. This especially occurs in the weight-bearing areas. Because cartilage has no blood supply or nerves, erosion within the joint is often advanced before symptoms of pain, crepitation, and limitation of movement are perceived. Decreased hydration, reduced elasticity, and increased fibrous growth around bony prominences contribute to increased stiffness and decreased functioning. Advanced stages of cartilage-joint deterioration are commonly known as osteoarthritis.[7,31,32]

For changes in body composition, see CD.

MUSCLE CHANGES WITH AGE

For information on cellular, anatomic and histological muscle changes with age, see CD.

Sarcopenia is the loss of muscle mass and strength that occurs with aging. It is a consequence of normal aging, and not necessarily related to disease, although muscle loss can be accelerated by chronic illness. Muscle wasting occurs in all humans, although it usually goes unnoticed. Sarcopenia results in muscle weakness, reduced activity level, increased prevalence of falls, morbidity, and loss of functional autonomy. It is the major cause of disability and frailty in the elderly.[33] There are many candidate mechanisms leading to sarcopenia, including age-related declines in alpha-motor neurons, growth hormone production, sex steroid levels, and physical activity. Age-related decreases in growth hormone, insulin-like growth factor I and II, estrogen, testosterone, and dehydroepiandrosterone and its sulfates play a major role in sarcopenia.[34,35] In addition, fat gain, increased catabolic cytokines, and inadequate intake of dietary energy and protein are also potentially important causes of sarcopenia. The relative contribution of each of these factors is not yet clear. Sarcopenia can be reversed with high-intensity progressive resistive exercise, which can also slow its development. A major challenge in preventing an epidemic of sarcopenia-induced frailty in the future is developing public health screening and interventions that deliver an anabolic stimulus to the muscle of elderly adults.

Skeletal Changes with Age

The skeletal system functions to support, protect, and shape the body. Additionally, bone has the metabolic functions of blood cell production, the storage of calcium, and a role in acid-base balance.

The most commonly known age-related change involving bone is calcium-related loss of mass and density. This loss ultimately causes the pathological condition of osteoporosis, in which bone density is lost from within by a process termed reabsorption. As we grow older, an imbalance occurs between osteoblast activity (bone buildup) and osteoclast activity (the breakdown of bone). Osteoclast activity proves to be the stronger. As one ages, a decline in circulating levels of activated vitamin D_3 occurs.[36] This causes less calcium to be absorbed from the gut and more calcium to be absorbed from the bones to meet body needs. In postmenopausal women, decreased estrogen levels influence parathyroid hormone and calcitonin to increase bone reabsorption, which in turn decreases bone mass. Certain factors such as immobility, decreased estrogens and progesterones, steroid therapy, and hyperthyroidism, to name a few, are known to accelerate bone erosion to pathological levels. Easily occuring fractures are the most common result.[7,23]

Osteoporosis is a critical disorder in the older adult, because it decreases the bone mineral content and, as a result, bone mass and strength decline with age. It is difficult to draw the line between what is normal and what is pathological in osteoporosis. Bone loss appears to be a normal aging process and has been characterized by a decreased bone mineral composition, an enlarged medullary cavity, a normal mineral composition, and biochemical normalities in plasma and urine. The rate of bone loss is about 1% per year for women starting at age 30 to 35 and for men at age 50 to 55. In elderly subjects, regions of devitalized tissue with osteocyte lacunae and haversian canals containing amorphous mineral deposits have been described.[7] These have been identified as micropetrotic regions and are noted to increase in frequency in the skeleton with age. Thus, it is clear that the mineral content of bone qualitatively changes with age.

Qualitatively, osteoporotic bone exhibits a reduction in bone mass with a resulting decrease in bone strength, and there is some evidence that alterations occur in the composition and structure of bone in the aged. Tensile strength of bone in man is related to the number and size of osteons. It has been found that bone from older humans has smaller osteons and fragments and more cement lines than younger bone, and this would account for some of the reduced bone strength of the older bone specimens. The remaining difference in strength results from the geometric structure of the bone in its distribution per unit area as a response to environmental stress placed on the bone. A more comprehensive discussion of osteoporosis is in the subsequent Chapter 5, Pathological Manifestations of Aging, and in Chapter 11, Orthopaedic Considerations.

Throughout life, red blood cells continue to be replaced after a life span of about 120 days. Some morphological changes do occur with aging. For instance, red cells are slightly smaller and more fragile; however, blood volume is well maintained until approximately 80 years of age. In the absence of pathology, few changes are seen in the white blood cells and in the platelet count. What is lost with aging is the functional reserve to quickly accelerate the production of red blood cells when needed.[7,37]

Musculoskeletal Changes with Age & Therapeutic Considerations

Body System	Changes with Age	Therapeutic Considerations with Age
Musculoskeletal		
Cartilage	Deteriorates	Persons will need more strength around the joints to decrease the stress.
	Decreased hydration	Shock-absorbing ability is less, so will need other ways to attenuate the force.

Musculoskeletal Changes with Age & Therapeutic Considerations (Continued)

Body System	Changes with Age	Therapeutic Considerations with Age
Musculoskeletal		
Cartilage	Reduced elasticity	Joint motion may take longer to stretch and need additional modalities and mobilizations for increasing motion.
	Increased fibrous growth around bony prominences	Joints may appear larger than when young.
Muscle	Atrophy in number of fibers especially type II fibers	Progressive resistive therapeutic exercise should be aimed at specifically identifying the type of weakness and appropriate exercise.
	Decline in alpha motor neurons	Quicker gains in strength may be seen in older persons versus young because of neurotrophic influences.
	Decreased maximal strength	Norms for increasing ages in all muscle groups will be less than for young.
	Decreased muscle mass	Girth measurements are not a reliable measure of improved strength.
Skeletal	Decreased calcium	Calcium supplements or medication must be taken in conjunction with exercise for significant results to occur.
	Decreased circulating levels of vitamin D	Persons must also get a minimum of ten minutes of sun exposure three times per week or take a vitamin D supplement to get the benefits of increased bone strength.
	Decreased bone strength	Weight-bearing muscle co-contractions, PRE exercises, etc. have been shown to improve bone strength. Also, persons with weaker bones are more prone to fracture, so care should be taken in exercise programming and persons should be screened for risk of falling.
	Decreased reserve to quickly accelerate the production of red blood cells when needed	Patients may become anemic more easily when stressed and may take longer to respond to medical management.

NEUROMUSCULAR CHANGES WITH AGE

Quantitatively, all muscle measures, including biological, anatomical, and physiological, decline after the age of 40.[38] Many of the changes associated with aging indicate a decrease in the number of active functional units (e.g., motor units or muscle fibers) and a loss in concentration of specific enzymes or fiber types.

CENTRAL NEUROLOGICAL CHANGES WITH AGE

After peaking in the early decades of life, brain mass or weight slowly decreases by as much as 6% to 7% by the time a person reaches 80 years old. Though the brain stem appears to be minimally affected by cell loss, widely varied but significant losses occur in the cerebral cortex lobes and cerebellar area. Central nervous system cells are postmitotic. The central neurons that remain continue to decline in numbers and efficiency of function.

Cell number and composition both decrease, and with aging, cells of the hippocampus undergo a degeneration caused by numbers of vacuoles surrounding dense central granules. Amyloid plaques develop, and lipofuscin is deposited within many remaining neuronal cells. After age 60, the number of neuronal microtubular structures may decrease and are often replaced by so-called neurofibrillary tangles. Though plaques and tangles occur with normal aging, they are most commonly associated with the occurrence of senile dementia of the Alzheimer's type (SDAT).

Impulse conduction and cerebral synaptic transmission are both delayed with aging, which affects the transmitter competence of the central nervous system. A particular explanation lies in the general decline of available neurotransmitters. Serotonin, catecholamines, and gamma-aminobutynic acid (GABA) are less prevalent in the older brain. A decrease in the neurotransmitter dopamine is found in normal elderly but is also associated with the pathology of Parkinson's disease.[39]

Conduction velocity of the central nervous system has been shown to decrease with advancing age. A loss of the myelin sheath and a loss of large myelinated fibers decreases axion abilities to transmit impulses, especially in the posterior spinal column tracts. These tracts provide for reflex positive-righting responses. Remembering that balance impairment partially results from cerebellar losses, and now coupled with central nervous system delays, one can begin to see why an older person has a greater tendency to fall and less ability to quickly correct a center of balance before injury occurs.[40]

INTERSYSTEM HOMEOSTASIS

Thermal Regulation

The role of the hypothalamus in homeostatic regulation is a major factor in age-related declines. With increasing age, the hypothalamus becomes less sensitive to the physiological feedback and consequently is less able to maintain the stability of the internal environment of the body. Processes ensue, such as increased body weight, increased serum cholesterol, and decreased glucose tolerance, followed subsequently by diseases.[41] The hypothalamic thermostat is the principal control center for regulating the body's response to ambient, locally applied, and internal temperature gradients. Many investigators have attributed the increased rate of heat stroke, hypothermia, and climate-related deaths among the aged population to faulty thermoregulation.[42]

Not only the hypothalamic thermostat and basal metabolic rate, but also the overall reactivity of the autonomic nervous system, declines with age, altering skin hydration and circulation in turn.[43] The vasomotor system is less responsive to warming and cooling, and the normal transient bursts of vasoconstrictor activity are reduced. It is unclear whether or not thermoreceptors in the skin are altered. Because cold receptors are dependent on a good oxygen supply, it may be reasoned that decreased circulatory supply may decrease perception of cold because of the vulnerability of cold receptors to hypoxia.

Age-related changes in the thermal regulatory response have clinical significance in the elderly individual's ability to maintain homeostasis with increasing exercise levels; the cooling time following exercise is often prolonged. In addition, a decrease in the receptiveness of temperature gradients impacts the application of heat and cold modalities in treatment interventions. Consideration of these changes needs to be employed when treating the elderly patient.

Hormonal Balance

Aging is marked by a deterioration not only in the function of individual cells and organs but also by a failure of mechanisms for the coordination of function between various parts of the body. A weakening of both neural and hormonal controls reduces the ability to adjust to external and internal stresses. Among other responsibilities, hormones contribute to (1) the regulation of circulating fluid volumes and cardiovascular performance, (2) the mobilization of fuels for exercise (maintenance of blood glucose, liberation of fat, and breakdown of protein), and (3) the repair of body structures with the synthesis of new protein (anabolism). All of the changes in these functions affect exercise tolerance and the healing process in the elderly. The aged are slower to reach homeostasis during exercise, and the return to a balanced homeostatic state following exercise is prolonged. In addition, the healing process is slower due to diminished synthesis of new protein.

Circulation

A blood flow rate of approximately 40mL/min/100 grams of brain tissue is regarded as minimally necessary to maintain adequate cerebral perfusion. As compared to the flow rate of 50–60mL/min/g experienced with youth, an older person may have as much as a 20% reduction in cerebral perfusion by the age of 70. Though cerebral perfusion is adequate if the body is not challenged, in the presence of pathology (e.g., arteriosclerosis, decreased cardiac output), the elderly experience increased risk of cerebral damage.[7]

PERIPHERAL NEUROLOGICAL CHANGES WITH AGE

Aging is often characterized by reduced sensibility, coordination, and cognitive abilities, as well as a reduced ability to react to changing circumstances. A general assumption is made that the loss of nerve tissue (i.e., reduced cell number) is a predominant feature of aging. In reality, although some loss of nerve cells does take place during the aging process, the extent to which this loss occurs is less than usually assumed. The reduced level of nervous system functioning in the elderly is better explained in terms of biochemical changes that take place in neurons during aging and senescence.

The ionic exchange across the nerve membrane to produce a nerve impulse is a relatively simple mechanism that is altered little during the aging process. In the elderly, there is no significant change in the conduction velocity along a specified portion of a nerve trunk compared to that found in younger adults. In the elderly, as in the younger person, if a reduction in conduction velocity is found, some narrowing of the fiber affecting the integrity of the nerve or some impairment of blood flow to the nerve sheath may be assumed.[44]

Sensory Changes with Age

In the body, information is gathered, interpreted, and transmitted through the integration of the neurosensory system, which includes the nervous system and each of the five senses (touch, smell, taste, vision, and hearing). Each of these systems is highly complex, and structural changes are known to occur with aging. The sum total of these changes results in a decline of neurosensory function.[45]

Touch

Peripheral receptors are responsible for the sense of touch. As with the other senses, touch also declines with age. Specific receptors for touch, pressure, pain, and temperature are found within the dermis and epidermis of the skin. Receptors can be freestanding or arranged in small corpuscular masses. Meissner's corpuscles (touch-texture receptors), Pacinian's corpuscles (pressure-vibration receptors), and Krause's corpuscles (temperature receptors), as well as peripheral nerve fibers, are noted to decline; therefore, sensitivity to touch, temperature, and vibration frequently decline with age. Though quantitative studies have produced inconclusive results, since free nerve endings remain relatively unchanged, the ability to sense pain should remain intact; however, the elderly person must take special care to avoid injury from concentrated pressures or temperature on the skin[28,31] (e.g., pressures from shoes that are too tight, bath water that is too hot, and so forth).

The skin is a very important element in touch. In general, skin wrinkles increase with advancing age, but the directional change of epidermal thickness remains controversial. The dermis becomes thinner, loses elasticity, and has a diminished vascularity.[45] Loss of tissue support for remaining capillaries results in fragility and easy bruising (*senile purpura*). Though tanning response diminishes, the appearance of flat pigmented lentigos (age spots) increases with exposure to the sun, and such exposure also increases the risk of neoplastic development from actinic keratosis. The previously reviewed decline in cellular division results in a slower rate and efficiency of tissue repair following any trauma.[46]

Changes in the dermal appendages (i.e., hair) also occur with age. The degree to which hair becomes gray is largely genetically determined, but in general, a reduction in hair follicles produces a reduction of hair. In contrast, after menopause, facial hair tends to increase in women. Nails grow more slowly and develop longitudinal ridges. The number and size of sweat glands is diminished, resulting in a reduction of sweat production.[46]

Health care providers need to be sensitive to the fact that some of the following changes may affect the self-esteem of an older person. If this is the case, sensitive psychological support must be provided in any interactions.

Vision

Though humans are strongly visual creatures, the eye is vulnerable to many age-related changes. Externally, the eyelids show an increase in wrinkling and in ptosis resulting from losses of elastic tissue and orbital fat, and a decrease in muscle tone. Very often the older person will develop an entropion (a turning inward of the eyelid) or an ectropian (an outward relaxation of the eyelid), which is particularly apparent with the lower lids. Aging results in diminished tear production, and ocular inflammation or infection may occur in some elderly people if supplementary artificial tears are not provided.

Arcus senilis, a deposit of lipids around the outer edge of the cornea, is a well-known, age-related phenomenon which does not interfere with vision. Arcus senilis has been associated with hyperlipidemia in younger people; however, no such association has been shown in the elderly.

In addition to becoming smaller with age, the ocular pupil reacts more slowly to light, and the ability to focus quickly from far to near declines. This loss of accommodation is termed presbyopia. The ability to focus is dependent on the ability of the ocular lens to change shape as needed. Presbyopia is partially caused by a decline in ciliary muscle efficiency; however, as a person ages, the ocular lens continues to grow while becoming more dense and inelastic. This change is associated with chronic dehydration of the tissues. Increased stiffness and less flexibility results in a decrease in the ability to change shapes and to focus on desired objects. Far vision is more easily achieved because the ciliary muscles relax and allow the lens to thin. Near vision requires the ciliary muscles to contract, increasing the thickness of the lens. This is why older people may require bifocals, which offer one prescription for far vision and another, stronger one for reading or close vision. Along with reduced accommodation, older people experience a decreased ability to adapt comfortably and quickly to changes of light and dark. Many older people say they had to give up driving at night because of this age-related change.

The older eye demonstrates a tendency toward increased intraocular pressure. As the lens continues to grow into the anterior chamber of the eye, the chamber becomes smaller, and the circulation of aqueous humor is reduced. Though the healthy older eye can tolerate this change, it is possible for a pathologic glaucoma to occur concurrently. The increased density of the lens may lead to a form of cataract which can result in the complete loss of useful vision. On a less serious note, the aqueous humor may also develop a yellowish pigmentation creating difficulty in distinguishing between greens and blues.

An older person may comment to you on the presence of "floaters" in his or her visual field. With aging, the vitreous body of the eye loses hydration and tends to demonstrate some clustering of collagen material. This clustering causes shadows or opacities to be projected on the retinal wall. Though the presence of these opacities is normally associated with dehydration, an increase in number and frequency of episodes can be indicative of retinal hemorrhage or detachment.

Age-related changes can ultimately produce a decline in visual acuity. Even when errors of aged refraction are corrected, a loss of visual receptors in the aging retina or macula will result in a decrease of acuity. Although there are some treatments, there is no cure. Fortunately, with modern technology, the majority of older people are able to maintain a high degree of visual function and independence.[47,48]

Hearing

Though a hearing loss may develop at any age, hearing losses do occur more frequently in the later years. A "sensorineural" hearing loss, called presbycusis, is most common in the elderly. With a sensorineural loss, sound is well conducted through the external and middle ear but age-related impairments of the inner ear or auditory nerve prevent the sound transmission to the brain. Age-related changes that may contribute to a sensorineural hearing loss include sclerotic changes in the tympanic membrane, cochlear otosclerosis, a loss of hair-like receptors in the organ of Corti, and a degeneration of the auditory nerve.

Presbycusis results in a decreased ability to hear and discriminate speech, particularly at higher and lower frequency levels. Because normal speech contains a broad range of frequencies, the older person may realize that he is being spoken to but may not understand all that is being said. The individual loses the ability to hear the "hard" sounds of language (e.g., the beginning and ending of most words). Difficulties increase when the speaker talks too quickly or when the hearing impaired individual is unable to observe the speaker's face.

Contrary to common belief, a sensorineural hearing loss does not always preclude the use of a hearing aid. Vision should be corrected so the skill of visual speech conception can be used as much as possible. When speaking with an elder with sensorineural loss, words should be spoken slowly in a medium pitched voice, and face-to-face communication should always be maintained.

Proprioception/Kinesthesia

Proprioception or kinesthetic sense is provided by sensory nerves which give information concerning movements and position of the body. These receptors are located primarily in the muscles, tendons, and the labyrinth system.[7] Though a greater degree of sensory-perceptual loss results from local system changes (e.g., impaired vision from increased lens density), cerebral cortex cell loss may result in less cellular availability for sensory interpretation.[49] This is of great clinical importance in that, as one ages, there may be a concomitant loss of position and movement sense. Coupled with losses in the other sensory systems, this could significantly affect an elderly individual's awareness of limb or body position, a safety concern during transfers and ambulation (see Chapter 12, Neurological Considerations).

Vestibular System

The vestibular system changes during the aging process. Degeneration occurs in the sensory receptors in both the otoliths and semicircular canals. The function of the vestibular system is to monitor head position and to detect head movements.[49] When an individual is deprived of visual and lower extremity somatosensory information, the vestibular system is left to provide sensation for control of balance. Healthy young adults are able to balance without meaningful visual or support surface information. Healthy elderly, on the other hand, lose their balance and might even fall when vestibular input is the only spatial orientation information available. All of the major sources of orienting information are compromised during the aging process. Dehydration and diseases further compound this problem. The vestibular system is discussed in more detail in Chapter 12, Neurological Considerations.

Taste and Smell

The senses of taste and smell become less acute with age.[50] As much as 80% of the taste buds may atrophy and perception of taste sensation (i.e., sweet, salty, bitter, and sour) becomes less sharp. A reduction of saliva flow occurs as a person ages, and this may aggravate an already dulled sense of taste. The olfactory bulb demonstrates age-related cell losses, which appear to be associated with decreased perceptions of various smells. It is proposed that the dulling of these sensations contributes to the appetite decline which is observed in and experienced by the majority of elderly people.[46]

Deficits in these chemical senses not only reduce the pleasure and comfort of food but also represent risk factors for nutritional and immune deficiencies, as well as adherence to specific dietary regimens. Chemosensory decrements can lead to food poisoning or overexposure to environmentally hazardous chemicals that are otherwise detectable by taste and smell.[50]

Neurosensory System Changes with Age & Therapeutic Considerations

Body System	Changes with Age	Therapeutic Considerations with Age
Intersystem Homeostasis	Hypothalamic thermostat declines	Older persons may need more time to accommodate to stabilizing body temperature whether due to changes in activity or the ambient temperature.
	Basal metabolic rate decreases	Body weight increases and weight gain is easier.
	Reactivity of the autonomic nervous system declines	Skin hydration and circulation may be slow to respond when necessary.
	Vasomotor system is less responsive to warming and cooling	Older person are more prone to hypo- or hyperthermia.
	Decreased hormonal balance	Exercise tolerance will be affected. Older persons will be slower to reach homeostasis during exercise, and the return to a homeostatic state following exercise is prolonged.
	Decreased blood flow to the brain	Blood is adequate for daily activities but may be insufficient when exercising. Monitor signs for decreased blood flow when exercising.
Peripheral Nervous System	Decreased nerve cells	Slower reaction time
	Decreased blood flow to the nerves	Increased activity improves blood flow to nerves.
Sensory		
Touch	Receptors and nerve fibers decline with age	Care should be taken when using hot or cold modalities as older persons may have decreased sensitivity.
	Skin changes such as dermal thinning, decreased elasticity, and vascularity	Older persons may bruise easily, repair skin injuries more slowly, and be at increased risk for adverse effects of sun exposure.
	The number and size of sweat glands are diminished	Older persons may not have an adequate sweat response so they should be checked for signs of hyperthermia when exercising.
Vision	Decrease in muscle tone	Less response to eye movements.
	Loss of elasticity and orbital fat around the eye	May affect self-esteem.
	Diminished tear production	Encourage the use of artificial tears if dryness is noted to avoid ocular inflammation or infection.
	Ocular pupil is smaller	The ability to focus far to near declines as does adapting quickly to light and dark
	Tendency toward intraocular pressure	More prone to glaucoma. Older persons should get their eye pressure checked once a year.
	Increased density of the lens	Difficulty distinguishing similar colors.
	Loss of visual receptors in the retina or macula	Decreased acuity; home programs should have larger print for ease of reading.
Hearing	Sclerotic changes in the tympanic membrane	Decreased ability to discriminate high frequency sounds—talk in lower tones.
	Cochlear oteosclerosis	Decreased ability to discriminate consonants—speak slowly and distinctly.

(continued)

Neurosensory System Changes with Age & Therapeutic Considerations (Continued)

Body System	Changes with Age	Therapeutic Considerations with Age
Hearing	Decreased receptors in the corti	Difficulty hearing softer sounds—speak more loudly.
	Degeneration of the auditory nerve	Difficulty localizing sound—face the person and use gestures when talking.
Proprioception/ Kinesthesia	Less cellular availability for sensory interpretation; less position and movement sense	Older persons will have lower scores on proprioceptive and kinesthethic tests. Special efforts should be made for safety in all mobility activities.
Vestibular	Degeneration in the sensory receptors in the otoliths and semicircular canals	Older persons may lose their balance more often due to dependence on decreased information. Programs to stimulate the vestibular system or compensate may be helpful.
Taste and Smell	80% of taste buds atrophy	A decline of appetite, which can lead to malnutrition.
	Decreased saliva	Difficulty digesting foods.
	Decreased cells in the olfactory bulb	Decreased interest in food; supplementing taste and smell with color and sound and socialization can enhance the eating experience.
	Chemosensory decrements	Food poisoning or hazardous chemicals can occur unless persons advised on proper food use.

GASTROINTESTINAL CHANGES WITH AGE

The gastrointestinal tract is subject to many changes throughout life. Though normal aging is not responsible for all gastrointestinal changes, it is sometimes difficult to differentiate the effects of aging from those that result from a lifetime of poor habits involving hygiene, food, and substance abuse. Epidemiological studies are beginning to implicate lifestyle more strongly in relation to some changes in the gut.

It is a fallacy to believe that teeth must be lost with aging. Improved dental hygiene and nutrition can prevent common pathologies of tooth loss such as dental caries and peridontal disease. With age, however, the tooth does lose masticating enameled surface area. Intermaxillary spaces decrease, and tooth pulp may atrophy and regress. If teeth are lost, the older person may experience a migration of the normally opposing teeth, with local oral trauma occurring as a result.[51]

The older esophagus demonstrates a reduction of motility and a hesitance of the lower esophageal sphincter to relax with swallowing. To define these changes, the term "*presbyesophagus*" was coined.[52] When eating, the older person may experience an often uncomfortable substernal sense of fullness as food entry into the stomach is delayed. In contrast, the lower esophageal resting pressure declines with age. This weakening allows gastric contents to more easily reflux into the lower areas of the esophagus causing heartburn to occur. Hiatal hernias frequently develop in the older person who has a reduced resting pressure of the lower esophageal sphincter.[53]

An age-related reduction in motility also affects the stomach, colon, and probably the small intestine. Gastric emptying time often is delayed.[54] Degeneration of gastric mucosa occurs in a small number of elderly and may cause a decrease of intrinsic factor, digestive enzymes, and hydochloric acid. Usually this "atrophic gastritis" is not the sole cause of B_{12} malabsorption and resulting pernicious anemia, but gastrointestinal digestion can be reduced. Medications activated by an acid gastric condition may be less effective in the more alkaline environment of an older stomach. Additionally, an older individual may interpret this gastric discomfort as acid indigestion and further diminish the available acid supply by taking over-the-counter antacids.

A reduced blood supply to the gut and a decrease in the number of absorbing cells can hinder nutrient absorption in the small intestine. Decreased motility in the colon and poor hydration cause the elderly to have a tendency to develop constipation. If the elderly person is particularly immobile or dehydrated, constipation can easily lead to the more serious conditions of fecal impaction and bowel obstruction. Diverticulosis is also common in the elderly. However, its occurrence is probably more related to a diet low in fiber and high in refined, low-residue foods than to aging.[7,53,55]

More on the gastrointestinal changes with aging will be covered in the Chapter 6, Exploring Nutritional Needs.

Internal Organ System Changes with Age & Therapeutic Considerations

Body System	Changes with Age	Therapeutic Considerations with Age
Gastrointestinal	Decreased motility of the esophagus	After eating a sense of substernal fullness is felt.
	Lower esophageal resting pressure and hesitance of the sphincter	More reflux and heartburn.
	Decreased motility in stomach and intestines	Increased incidence of constipation; encourage activity and hydration to combat this.
	Decreased blood supply to the gut	As above but can become more serious and cause fecal impaction.
Renal	Decreased mass and weight	Less effective.
	Protein binding of medications is decreased	Prolonged drug effects in older persons.
Hepatic	Liver mass and blood perfusion decline	Metabolism of many drugs is decreased.
	Decreased vascularity	Less productive.
	Decline in excretory and reabsorptive capacities	Prolonged drug effects.
	Decreased urine concentrating abilities	Urine will be less concentrated.
Urinary	Increase in residual urine	Difficulty completely emptying bladder and more urinary accidents.
	Increased reflux into ureters	More symptomatic and asymptomatic bacturiuria.

HEPATIC, RENAL, AND UROGENITAL CHANGES

It is generally accepted that liver mass and blood perfusion both decline with aging. Metabolism of many drugs is decreased and, following injury, regeneration of hepatic cells occurs more slowly. When compared to younger people, no significant differences are found in the serum indicators of liver status of older people. These indicators include measurement of bilirubin clearance, serum glutamic oxaloacetic transaminase (SGOT), serum glutamic pyruvic transaminae (SGPT), and alkaline phosphatase production. Though total serum protein remains relatively stable, reduced albumin to globulin (A/G) ratios result in a decline of colloidal osmotic pressure. Protein binding of medications may also be decreased. Alterations in protein binding and the prolongation of drug effects within the body are two of the more serious results of normal age changes in the liver.[7,56,57]

When discussing these systems, the gallbladder and pancreas should be mentioned, because they also demonstrate functional changes with aging. For example, the incidence of biliary stones increases in the elderly, which is probably related to a reduced efficiency of cholesterol stabilization in the body. Controversy exists over the reduction of pancreatic mass with age. A decline in mass may be hidden by an increase in pancreatic fat deposition. Pancreatic cells become less homogeneous, and studies have generally reported a decline in enzyme volume and concentration, though adequate amounts are available for normal digestive functions.[46,56] Another important endocrine age change is the decreased ability of the peripheral tissues to utilize available insulin produced by the pancreas.[58] The most important pancreatic age change, however, is the decreased ability of the beta cells to increase insulin production in response to a challenge of increased blood glucose.[56,57]

The aged kidney demonstrates both a loss of parenchymal mass and a reduction of total weight. By the time a person is 85 years old, the amount of remaining functioning nephrons may be decreased by as much as 30% to 40% of what was available in youth. Vascular changes, like a reduction in glomerular capillary loops and increased tortuosity of arcuate and interlobar arteries, have been reported. Renal perfusion declines as much as 50% by the later decades of life. The Bowman's capsule basement membrane thickens, glomerular filtration rate declines, and blood urea nitrogen (BUN) tends to show a rise. The renal tubules show a decline in excretory and reabsorptive capacities, and a loss of urine concentrating abilities occurs. Older kidneys can maintain acid-base homeostasis in an unchallenged environment; however, they are unable to handle increased loads of either acid or base. The structural changes observed in the normal aging kidney support the theory that one should expect a decline in renal function as one ages. Reports by renal physiologists, however, suggest that this is not always true.[59] The suggestion is made that vascular adaptations to structural changes may help to preserve glomerular filtration rate by producing a state of hyperperfusion and hyperfiltration in surviving nephrons.[59]

The urinary bladder demonstrates an increased number of uninhibited contractions frequently associated with cerebral arteriosclerotic changes and overconcentration of the urine. Increases in residual urine and reflux into the ureters provide an ideal environment for bacterial growth. Both asymptomatic and symptomatic bacteriuria are common in the elderly.[7,58,60]

For information on endocrine, sleep, memory, and intelligence changes with age, see CD.

For information on sleep, memory, and intelligence changes, see CD.

References

1. Eveleth PB, Tanner JM. *Worldwide Variation in Human Growth*. Cambridge, England: Cambridge University Press; 1976.
2. Cutler RG. Evolution of longevity in primates. *J Hum Evol*. 1976; 5:169–202.
3. Fries JF. Aging, natural death and the compression of morbidity. *N Engl J Med*. 1968; 303:113–123.
4. Kent S. The evolution of longevity. *Geriatrics*. 1980; 35:98–104.
5. Korenchevksy V. *Physiological and Pathological Aging*. New York: Hafner; 1961.
6. Andres R. Normal aging versus disease in the elderly. In: Andres EL, Bierman EL, Hazard WR, eds. *Principles in Geriatric Medicine*. New York: McGraw-Hill; 1985: 38–41.
7. Kenney RA. *Physiology of Aging*. Symposium of the Aging Process Clinics in Geriatric Medicine. February 1985; 1(1).
8. Shock NW. Physiological theories of aging. In: Rothstein JL, et al., eds. *Theoretical Aspects of Aging*. New York: Academic Press; 1974: 119–136.
9. Seyle HA. Stress and aging. *J Am Geriatr Soc*. 1970; 18(9):669–690.
10. Wei JY. Cardiovascular anatomic and physiologic changes with age. *Top Geriatr Rehabil*. 1986; 2(1): 10–16.
11. Rodeheffer RJ, Gerstenblith G, Becker LC, et al. Exercise cardiac output is maintained with advancing age in health human subjects: Cardiac dilatation and increased stroke volume compensates for diminished heart rate. *Circulation*. 1984; 69:203–213.
12. Shannon RP, Wei JY, Rosa RM, et al. The effect of age and sodium depletion on cardiovascular response to orthostasis. *Hypertension*. 1986; 4:229–242.
13. Gerstenblith G, Frederikson J, Yin FCP, et al. Echocardiographic assessment of a normal adult aging population. *Circulation*. 1977; 56:273–278.
14. Yin FCP. The aging vasculature and its effects on the heart. In: Weisfeldt ML, ed. *The Aging Heart*. New York: Raven Press; 1980: 2.
15. Wei JY. Heart disease in the elderly. *Cardiovasc Med*. 1984; 9:971–982.
16. Nichols WW, O'Rourke MF, Avolio AP, et al. Effects of age on ventricular-vascular coupling. *Am J Cardiol*. 1985; 55:1179–1184.
17. Miyatake K, Okamoto M, Kinoshita N, et al. Augmentation of atrial contribution to left ventricular inflow with aging as assessed by intracardiac Doppler flowmetry. *Am J Cardiol*. 1984; 53:586–589.
18. Ziegler MG, Lake CR, Kopin IJ. Plasma noradrenalin increase with age. *Nature*. 1976; 261:333–334.
19. Shimada K, Kitazumi T, Sadakne N, et al. Age related changes of baroreflex function, plasma norepinephrine, and blood pressure. *Hypertension*. 1985; 7:113–117.
20. Tsunoda K, Abe K, Goto T, et al. Effect of age on the renin-angiotensin-aldosterone system in normal subjects: Simultaneous measurement of active and inactive renin, renin substrate, and aldosterone in plasma. *J Clin Endocrinol Metab*. 1986; 62:384–389.
21. Shannon RP, Minaker KL, Rowe JW. Aging and water balance in humans. *Semin Nephrol*. 1984; 4: 346–353.
22. Weisfeldt ML, Gerstenblith G, Lakatta EG. Alterations in circulatory function. In: Andres R, ed. *Principles of Geriatric Medicine*. New York: McGraw-Hill; 1985.
23. Ham RS, Marcy ML. *Normal Aging: A Review of Systems/The Maintenance of Health in Primary Care Geriatrics*. Boston: John Wright, PSG, Inc.; 1983.
24. Butler RN. Current definitions of aging. In: *Epidemiology of Aging*. Bethesda, MD: National Institutes of Health Publication No. 80–969; 1980: 7–8.

25. Zadai CC. Cardiopulmonary issues in the geriatric population: Implications for rehabilitation. *Top Geriats Rehabil.* 1986:2(1):1–9.

26. Cummings G, Semple SG. *Disorders of the Respiratory System.* Oxford, England: Blackwell; 1973.

27. Wynne JW. Pulmonary disease in the elderly. In: Rossman I, ed. *Clinical Geriatrics.* 2nd ed. Philadelphia: Lippincott, 1979.

28. Hole JW. *Human Anatomy and Physiology.* Boston: Wm. C. Brown; 1988.

29. Walker J. Connective tissue plasticity: Issues in histological and light microscopy studies of exercise and aging in articular cartilage. *JOSPT.* 1991; 14(5):189–197.

30. Donatelli R, Owens-Burkart H. Effects of immobilization on the extensibility of periarticular connective tissue. *JOSPT.* 1981; 3(2):67–71.

31. Goldberg AL, Goodman HM. Effects of disuse and denervation on amino acid transport by skeletal muscle. *Am J Physiol.* 1975; 216:1116–1119.

32. Gardner DL. Aging of articular cartilage. In: Brocklehurst JC, ed. *Textbook of Geriatric Medicine and Gerontology.* New York: Longman Group Ltd.; 1978.

33. Roubenoff R. Sarcopenia: A major modifiable cause of frailty in the elderly. *J Nutr Health Aging.* 2000; 4(3):140–142.

34. Tseng BS, Marsh DR, Hamilton MT, Booth FW. Strength and aerobic training attenuate muscle wasting and improve resistance to the development of disability with aging. *J Gerontol.* 1995; 50: 113–119.

35. Booth FW, Weeden SH, Tseng BS. Effect of aging on human skeletal muscle and motor function. *Med Sci Sports Exerc.* 1994; 26(5):556–560.

36. Bidlack WR, Kirsh A, Meskin MS. Nutritional requirements of the elderly. *Food Technology.* 1988; 40:61–70.

37. Batata M, Spray GH, Bolton FG, Higgins G, Wollner L. Blood and bone marrow changes in elderly patients, with particular reference to folic acid, vitamin B12, iron and ascorbic acid. *Br Med J.* 1967; 2:667–669.

38. Jokl E. *Physiology of Exercise.* Springfield, IL: Charles C Thomas; 1984; 108–112.

39. Burchinsky SC. Neurotransmitter receptors in the central nervous system and aging: Pharmacological aspects (review). *Experimental Aging.* 1984; 19: 227–239.

40. Bohannon RW, Larkin PA, Cook AC, et al. Decrease in timed balance test scores with aging. *Phys Ther.* 1984; 64:1067–1070.

41. Besdine RW, Harris TB. Alterations in body temperature (hypothermia and hyperthermia). In: Andres R, Bierman EL, and Hazzard WR, eds. *Principles in Geriatric Medicine.* New York: McGraw-Hill; 1985: 209–217.

42. Asmussen E. Aging and exercise. In: Horvath SM, Yousef MK, eds. *Environmental Physiology, Aging,* *Heat and Altitude.* New York: Elsevier/North Holland; 1981.

43. Ajiduah AO, Paolone AM, Wailgum TD, Irion G, Kendrick ZV. The effect of age on tolerance of thermal stress during exercise. *Med Sci Spts Exerc.* 1983; 15:168. Abstract.

44. Grimby G. Physical activity and muscle training in the elderly. *Acta Med Scand.* 1986; 711(suppl): 233–237.

45. Corso JE. Sensory processes and age effects of normal adults. *J Gerontol.* 1971; 26:90–105.

46. Jacobs R. Physical changes in the aged. In: O'Hara-Devereaux M, Andrus LH, Scott CD, eds. *Eldercare.* New York: Grune & Stratton; 1981.

47. Kasper RL. Eye problems of the aged. In: Reichel PE, ed. *Clinical Aspects of Aging.* Baltimore: Williams and Wilkins; 1988.

48. Boyer GG. Vision problems. In: Camevali P, Patrick B, eds. *Nursing Management for the Elderly.* Philadelphia: Lippincott; 1989.

49. Woollacott MH, Shumway-Cook A, Nasner LM. Aging and posture control: Changes in sensory organization and muscular coordination. *Int J Aging Hum Dev.* 1986; 23:97–114.

50. Schiffman SS. Taste and smell losses in normal aging and disease. *JAMA.* 1997; 278(16):1357–1362.

51. Bennet J, Creamer H, Fontana-Smith DJ. Dentistry. In: O'Hara-Devereaux M, Andrus LH, Scott CD, eds. *Eldercare.* New York: Grune & Stratton; 1981.

52. Khan TA, Shragge BW, Crippen JS, et al. Esophageal mobility in the elderly. *Am J Digestive Dis.* 1977; 22:1049–1054.

53. Bartol MA, Heitkemper M. Gastrointestinal problems. In: Carnevali P, Patrick B, eds. *Nursing Management for the Elderly.* Philadelphia: Lippincott; 1989.

54. Horowitz M, Maddern GT, Chateron BE, et al. Changes in gastric emptying rates with age. *Clin Sci.* 1984; 67:213–218.

55. Morgan W, Thomas C, Schuster M. Gastrointestinal system. In: O'Hara-Devereaux M, Andrus LH, Scott CD, eds. *Eldercare.* New York: Grune & Stratton; 1981.

56. Goldman R. Decline in organ function with age. In: Rossman I, ed. *Clinical Geriatrics.* 2nd ed. Philadelphia: Lippincott, 1979.

57. Hyans DE. The liver and biliary system. In: Brocklehurst JC, ed. *Textbook of Geriatric Medicine and Gerontology.* New York: Longman Group Ltd.; 1978.

58. Fink RL. Mechanisms of insulin resistance in aging. *J Clin Invest.* 1983; 71:1523–1535.

59. Lindeman RD. Is the decline in renal function with normal aging inevitable? *Geriatr Nephrol Urol.* 1998; 8(1):7–9.

60. Sourander LB. The aging kidney. In: Brocklehurst JC, ed. *Textbook of Geriatric Medicine and Gerontology.* New York: Longman Group Ltd.; 1978.

4

Psychosocial Aspects of Aging

Pearls

- Full life development theories, such as Erickson's and Maslow's, discuss accomplishment stages throughout life for successful aging.

- Late life theories, such as those described by Peck, Neugarten, and Havighurst, focus on the state of late life and the older person's role in adapting to this stage of life.

- Intellectual performance in the aged can be enhanced by the therapist in many ways, including the mode of information presented, pacing, and feedback.

- Institutionalization causes changes in behavior and affects a person's performance. These effects can be countered with recognition of symptoms and behavioral and environmental interventions.

- Anxiety disorders, such as adjustment disorders, anxiety states, and phobic states, are often underreported and missed in the aged.

- Dementia affects millions of older persons and can be classified as acute disorders, chronic disorders, and presenile dementias. Assessment and treatment modification for working with these patients is based on behavioral and environmental modification by the therapist.

- Recognizing one's belief systems via the Facts on Aging Quiz can help the therapist work better with the aged.

INTRODUCTION

The aging process of human life is not one dimensional. Besides the obvious physical component, there exist the psychological, emotional, and spiritual components of aging. This chapter will address the psychosocial components. Even though physical health is extremely important, studies and life experience illustrate the effects of cognitive perception on life satisfaction and physical health.[1,2] One study on hip fracture outcomes for older persons showed that the most important variable in successful rehabilitation was the presence or absence of depression.[1,3] This study alone has tremendous implications for physical and occupational therapists, because it illustrates that unless the older person's emotional and mental abilities are addressed, the physical efforts may have minimal effect.

How does a physical or occupational therapist work in the psychosocial realm? Rehabilitation therapists are not psychologists and do not receive extensive training in the social and psychological sciences. Nevertheless, they can use specific information as an adjunct to daily treatment. For example, examining one's attitudes with respect to the various psychosocial theories of aging may provide information about a patient's satisfaction or motivation and enhance a therapist's ability to communicate with an older person. In addition, since the goal of therapy is to achieve optimal functioning, it is imperative that the therapist be able to recognize situations that require coping mechanisms and provide some assistance in these situations.

This chapter will explore the theories of aging and the cognitive changes in late life. Situations, both normal and pathological, that require coping mechanisms will be described in detail as well as society's view of aging and the lifestyle adaptations of older persons.

PSYCHOSOCIAL THEORIES OF AGING

In the last 30 years, many psychological theories of aging have been proposed. Prior to this time, however, few theories existed. The mainstream of thought centered around the theories of Freud and Piaget, which placed all the emphasis on the psychological development on the child while essentially ignoring the adult. The theories to be discussed in this section are either full life development theories or late life psychological development theories.

Full Life Development Theories

Erikson.   Eric Erikson was one of the first psychological theorists to develop a personality theory that extended into old age. Erikson viewed the process of human development as a series of stages that one goes through in order to fully develop one's ego.[4] Erikson describes eight stages in this process. These stages are listed in Table 4.1. Each of these stages represents a choice in the development of the expanding ego. The last two stages are of particular interest to the practitioner working with the older person.

A successful life choice of generativity, as Erikson calls it, consists of guiding, parenting, and monitoring the next generation. If an adult person does not experience generativity then stagnation will predominate. Stagnation is characterized by anger, hurt, and self-absorption. The final stage of Erikson's theory suggests that the older person must accept his or her life with the sense that "If I had to do it all over again, I'd do it pretty much the same."[5] At this stage the person experiences an active concern with life, even in the face of death, and learns to experience his or her own wisdom.

Jung.   Carl Jung was also a pioneer and designated adult stages on the basis of his own experience in clinical theory and practice.[6] His theory of development describes youth, from puberty to middle age, as a stage in which the person is concerned with sexual instincts, broadening horizons, and conquering feelings of inferiority. The adult period, between the ages of 35 and 40, involves the transport of the youthful self into the middle years. During this stage, Jung theorized that the person's convictions strengthen until they become somewhat more rigid at the age of 50.

TABLE 4.1   Erikson's Stages of Personality and Ego Development

Period in Life	Erikson's Stage
0–12 months	Trust vs. mistrust
2–4 years	Autonomy vs. shame
4–5 years	Initiative vs. guilt
6–11 years	Industry vs. inferiority
12–18 years	Identity vs. identity confusion
Young adulthood	Intimacy vs. isolation
Adulthood	Generativity vs. stagnation
Late life	Integrity vs. despair

Reprinted with permission from Erikson, E.H. Identity, Youth and Crisis. *New York: WW Norton; 1968.*

In later years, Jung suggests that activity levels decrease, that men become more expressive and nurturing, and that women become more "instrumental," providing care and continuation of the generations they have nurtured in their lives.[6,7] Jung also suggests that the later years are years in which the older person confronts his or her own death. Success in this involves the acceptance of death as a part of the cycle of life, not something to be feared.

Maslow.   Abraham Maslow's hierarchy of human needs is not a theory singular to aging, but it is an excellent framework for exploring growth, development, and motivation.[8] Maslow's hierarchy is a pyramid of needs, each of which builds on the other. In the lowest level, "biological and physiological integrity," the critical needs for an individual are food and clothing. At the second level, "safety and security," the primary need is protection against the elements and against other people. This cannot be achieved unless the person is first fed and clothed. At the third level, "belonging or love needs," the person begins to seek love from others, such as a parent or a significant other. When the person satisfies the need for love, he or she then progresses to the next level, "self-esteem," where the person in turn learns to cherish him- or herself, respects his or her own values and ideas, and feels good about who he or she is. Finally, at the level of "self-actualization," the person no longer worries about the lower needs, but is now able to give to others and has reached a higher level transcending the lower self-esteem needs. At the pinnacle of the pyramid of need, individuals can nurture and feed others, develop their own ideas, and actually live their own values and ideas in the community. According to Maslow, very few people in society are self-actualized. Some of our great leaders such as Martin Luther King, Winston Churchill, and Golda Meir were self-actualized people.

One must successfully fill each lower need before ascending to the next higher need. When one is at a given level, one's energies are consumed at that level.[9] One rarely stays at a higher level, but rather the person reverts to lower levels during periods when the lower needs are no longer being met. For example, a recently widowed woman may feel isolated or lonely and be unable to experience the higher levels of self-esteem or self-actualization until her grief has subsided.

This theory is particularly useful in the area of motivation. Since older persons are more likely to have physical decline, their needs will descend to the lower levels of the hierarchy. Therefore, motivation strategies should be aimed at the level of the person's needs. For example, if the person is unstable when walking, then strategies to encourage exercises in this area should appeal to his or her sense of safety if the person is at that level. If, however, the same person is more concerned about hunger during a treatment session, he or she will be unable to focus on the exercises.

Maslow believes, though, that it is the older person who truly has the knowledge and experience of life to be able to experience self-actualization, the highest level of the paradigm.[9]

Late Life Theories

Peck.   Robert C. Peck's theory describes tasks that must be accomplished to achieve integrity in old age. In this theory, the burden is placed on the older person to redefine the self, dismiss occupational identity, and go beyond self-centeredness. Peck's proposed tasks, in order to accomplish this, follow.

1. *Ego differentiation versus work role preoccupation.*In this instance, a retired person must look for new meaning and values beyond his or her previous work roles.
2. *Body transcendence versus body preoccupation.*Since old age may carry with it ill health, the older person must learn new ways to gain mental, physical, social, and spiritual pleasure that transcend physical discomfort.
3. *Ego transcendence versus ego preoccupation.*This last stage is a way of minimizing the prospect of death by giving to children and making charitable contributions to leave an enduring legacy.[10]

Buehler's Biophysical Model of Later Life.   Cheryl Buehler adopts a biophysical model of a living open system in which both maintenance and change of the organism are equally important.[7] She purports two kinds of maintenance: satisfying need and maintaining internal order. Two types of change are also proposed: adaptation and creativity. According to Buehler's theory, maturity is the age of fulfillment and in order to proceed successfully, these four basic elements (the two kinds of maintenance and the two types of change) must be met to ensure acceptance of old age. Successful passage through each of these stages requires integrating and balancing conflicting and competing trends from earlier stages. In middle age, self-assessment evolves and whatever order existed previously is questioned. Self-assessment succeeds when the self and others are accepted for what they are; when the individual attains a fresh appreciation of people and the world; and when he or she can be autonomous and serene. The final result is self-actualization. This introspection and reevaluation of maintenance and change determine how one faces old age: optimistically or pessimistically.

Neugarten.   Bernice Neugarten also describes the tasks that must be accomplished in order to be a successfully aging older person. The following are a few of her tasks that directly impact the rehabilitation milieu.

1. Accepting the increasing reality and imminence of death,
2. Coping with physical illness,
3. Coordinating the necessary dependence on support and accurately assessing the independent choices that can still be made to achieve maximum life satisfaction,
4. Giving and obtaining emotional gratification.[11]

Disengagement Theory.   The controversial disengagement theory credited to Cummings and Henry in the 1950s postulated that older people and society mutually withdraw. This withdrawal is characterized by a positive change in psychological well-being for the older person.[12] This theory, though not widely accepted at present, spawned much debate on the subject of late life adaptation. This theory is based on the sociologic perspective of functionalism; it is assumed that society has certain needs that must be met if stability and equilibrium are to be maintained. A structure is said to have a function if it contributes to the fulfillment of one or more of the social needs of the system.[13]

The disengagement theory depicts aging as a process of gradual physical, psychological, and social withdrawal. Disengagement is considered as functional during the aging process, purportedly preparing the person and society to face the inevitability of death. Changes in the personality of the individual are viewed as either the cause or the effect of decreased involvement with others. The authors of this theory claim that once this process starts it is irreversible, and that morale may remain high or improve as part of the process of disengagement.

Within this process, Cummings and Henry described three types of changes resulting in an older person's becoming less tied to the social system.[12] There are changes in the amount of interaction, the purposes of interaction, and the style of interaction with others. In outlining their theory, Cummings and Henry indicate that the process is both intrinsic and inevitable, and that the process is not only a correlate of successful aging but may also be a condition of it, since those who accept this inevitable reduction in social and personal interactions in old age are usually satisfied with their lives.[12]

Today, however, this theory has been largely discredited. Lipman and Smith,[14] while agreeing that a person's death may be dysfunctional for the social system if it is not prepared for, found that those who reduce their activities as they age tend to suffer a reduction in overall life satisfaction. This revised view is substantiated by recent studies of centenarians where successful aging includes, as the second most important factor, attitude, outlook, and social relationships.[15]

Functionalism versus Conflict Theory.   The challenge to functionalism and the disengagement theory came from several sources, one of which is called the conflict theory. It was believed that functionalism was too consensus oriented, with a built-in conservative bias, and that it treated both change and conflict in society negatively. Whereas the functionalists emphasized order, stability, and equilibrium, and therefore can devise an orientation that assumes that the person and the society mutually acquiesce to the withdrawal of the older adult, the conflict perspective is radically different. From the conflict perspective, consent and acquiescence take place through oppression, coercion, domination, and exploitation of one group by another. The conflict perspective stresses that there are always competing interests as groups struggle over claims to scarce resources, including status, power, and social class. While functionalists also assume that stratification is based on scarcity, the problem is often defined by functionalists as how to integrate the different sectors, groups, or classes. Conflict theorists, however, see the solution to this scarcity as occurring through the reduction of structural inequalities. These structural changes, they argue, will occur only in the presence of intense struggle.[16] This perspective is also shared by de Beauvoir,[17] who views aging as a class struggle. Estes, in her landmark analysis of the Older Americans Act, states that her research attempts to "make explicit how certain ways of thinking about the aged as a social problem . . . are rooted in the structure of social and power relations."[18(p2)]

Exchange Theory.   Another theoretical orientation that emerged as a reaction to functionalism is the exchange theory. Based on the belief that functionalism is too abstract and structural, and cannot explain actual human behavior, exchange theory is firmly rooted in rationalism. That is, human beings tend to choose courses of action on the basis of anticipated outcomes from among a known range of alternatives. Underlying this rational view of human behavior is the principle of hedonism, expressed in the contention that people tend to choose alternatives that will provide the most beneficial outcome. Everyone attempts to optimize gratification; that is, people continually try to satisfy needs and wants and to attain certain goals, and most of this occurs through interaction with other persons or groups. People attempt to maximize rewards, while reducing costs. Voluntary social behavior is motivated by the expectation of the return or reward this behavior will bring from others. One gives things in the hope of getting something in exchange.[19]

Another proposition essential to the exchange theory is the principle of reciprocity. In its simplest form it can be stated that a person should help (and not hurt) those who have helped her or him. The principle of reciprocity further assumes that a person chooses between alternative modes of behaving by comparing the anticipated rewards, the possible costs that may be incurred, and the magnitude of investment required to achieve those rewarding outcomes. Accordingly, rewards in human social interaction should be proportional to investment, and costs should not exceed rewards, or else the person will avoid that activity. Homans[20] has extended the principle of reci-

procity to include another concept, which he calls distributive justice. When rewards are not proportional to investments over the long term, Homan asserts, people tend to feel angry with social relations, instability is created, and the propensities for conflict increase.

People exchange not only tangible, material objects but also intangibles, such as the expression of love, admiration, respect, power, or influence. A good example of this theory might be that in the social exchange between the elderly and society, the elderly lose availability of resources. By losing power, the elderly are increasingly unable to enter into equal exchange relationships with significant others and all that remains for them is the capacity to comply.[21] Just as the conflict theorists focus on inequities and class struggle, the exchange theorists believe that to understand the situation of the aged, we must examine the role of society's stratification system in the aging process.[21]

Continuity and Activity Theories.   Two well-known theories that developed in response to the disengagement theory are the continuity and activity theories. The continuity theory proposes that activities in old age reflect a continuation of earlier life patterns,[22] while, in contrast, the activity theory states that successful adaption in late life is associated with maintaining as high a level of activity as possible. The older person should find substitutes when a meaningful activity, such as work, must be terminated. The person should develop an active rather than passive role toward his or her daily life as well as toward biological and social changes that are taking place.[23]

The continuity theory assumes that in the process of becoming adults, persons develop habits and preferences that become part of their personalities throughout their life experience and which are carried into old age. The continuity theory claims that neither activity nor inactivity assumes happiness. It posits that most older people want to remain engaged with their social environment and that the magnitude of this engagement varies with the person according to lifelong established patterns and self-concepts.[22] It further recognizes the interrelationships of biologic and environmental factors with psychological preferences. Positive aging becomes an adaptive process with interaction among all elements.

The activity theory, which is related to social role concepts, was advanced as an alternative interpretation to disengagement. It affirms that the continued maintenance of a high degree of involvement in social life is an important basis for deriving and sustaining satisfaction. It claims that those who maintain extensive social contacts, who engage in regular activities, similar to their engagement level in midlife, age most successfully. Declines in activity and role loss are thus associated with lower levels of satisfaction.[23]

In sum, continuity and activity theories assume the need for continued involvement throughout life; disengagement assumes mutuality in decline of involvement.

Exchange theory assumes neither. It posits that the degree of engagement is the outcome of a specific change relationship between the person and society in which the more powerful exchange partner dictates the terms of relationship.

Havighurst.   Robert J. Havighurst's theory on aging relates successful aging to social competence and flexibility in adaption to new roles. He believes in the importance of finding new and meaningful roles in old age, while maintaining comfort with the customs of the time.[24,25] Later, Neugarten and Havighurst noted that successful adaptation to age was related to personality and not age per se.[26] They noted the following four personality types.

1. *Integrated.* Shows a high degree of competence in daily activities and a complex inner life. This type is generally the best adapter.
2. *Passive dependent.* Seeks others to satisfy his or her emotional needs.
3. *Armored.* Attempts to control his or her environment and impulses and tends to be a high achiever.
4. *Unintegrated.* Shows poor emotional control and intellectual competency. This type tends to have the poorest adaptation in late life.[24]

Levinson.   While Erikson focuses on ego and personality development, Havighurst, Neugarten,[22] and Levinson[27] are concerned with the social tasks and roles that must be managed at each developmental stage of the person's life. Daniel Levinson[27] approaches the stages or "seasons" of adulthood as a developmental process involving occupation, love relationships, marriage and family, relation to self, use of solitude, and roles in various social contexts (e.g., relationships with individuals, groups, and institutions that have significance for their lives). According to Levinson, these components make up the underlying structure or pattern of a person's life. He refers to this pattern as the person's "life structure." Two basic types of developmental periods are hypothesized as determining life structure: structure building and structure change.

Levinson identifies a "novice" phase of adult development, which consists of three seasons: early adult transition (a structure-changing phase); entering the adult world (structure building); and transition (during which structure changing again takes place). The most important developmental tasks of early adulthood, according to Levinson, are: entering an occupation, developing mentor relationships, and forming a love or marriage relationship. During the transition phase, the primary task is reappraisal of the first part of adulthood and redirection and change as determined by this examination of earlier life choices. The transition may be relatively easy or difficult, but it is characteristic of this phase to either make new life choices or reaffirm old choices.

The next phase is the settling-down phase. Here the individuals establish their niche in society (e.g., occupation, family, community) and work toward advancement. This is followed by the midlife transition phase, which consists of reappraisal of the settling-down period, and dealing with and resolving polarities between the individual's sense of her- or himself and the world. Levinson offers some examples of polarities such as: young/old, destructive/creative, masculine/feminine, and attachment/separateness. The most important task is coming to terms with real or impending biologic decline, accompanied by the recognition of mortality, as well as the societal attitudes that denigrate or devalue the status of middle age in favor of youth.

The next phase is another structure-building period. Having faced the polarities of the midlife transition, the person now makes new choices or reaffirms old ones. As an individual moves to the end of this period, yet another structure-changing phase is entered as the person once again reevaluates on entry into "old age."

Positive aging is out of the hands of rehabilitation therapists. However, the more therapists understand stages that men and women are likely to undergo as they age, the more responsive they can be to persons in their care. Developing a meaningful context within which the transformations of aging can be understood will be aided by information offered by all who work with the elderly, especially those involved in their day-to-day rehabilitation.

COGNITIVE CHANGES IN LATE LIFE

Are cognitive declines an inevitable consequence of aging? Is there a continuum from normal aging to pathological states such as Alzheimer's dementia? According to the Seattle Longitudinal Study only 20% of adults exhibited reliable age-related decline from 60 to 67 years of age; 36% experienced decline between 67 and 74 years; and over 60% of elderly adults showed a decline between the ages of 74 and 81 years.[28] Community surveys indicate that over 50% of people over age 60 report memory problems,[29] and Crook and associates found the incidence is even higher in people referred *to a geriatric screening program*.[30] However, normative studies are difficult to accomplish without contaminating the data to a certain degree. Normative studies of the elderly, without longitudinal follow-up, typically have included individuals with preclinical dementia who have begun to decline cognitively but still perform within normal limits on neuropsychological testing.[31,32] This results in an underestimation of true level of normal cognitive performance. Estimates of variability are inflated due to the mix of individuals with and without preclinical dementia, and it is difficult to identify healthy elderly individuals who have unrecognized preclinical dementia.[32]

There is a significant variability in the pattern and rate of change in cognitive abilities. Verbal abilities reach peak performance in the sixth and seventh decades of life, and reliable age-related decline does not occur until the middle of the eighth decade.[28]

Table 4.2 summarizes the changes in cognition generally associated with normal aging.[33]

Memory

Memory has been extensively studied for many years, and yet no definitive conclusions have been obtained.[34,35] Some studies show a decrease in memory with age, while others show no change.[34,35] Studies agree that older persons do have poorer techniques for organizing new information into a usable form that will impact information retrieval.[36] In addition, older persons perform better on more familiar memory tasks.[37] Older adults perform at a lower level on most memory tasks and tend to use more external (physical) rather than internal (mental) memory strategies.[38]

For background on memory, see CD.

One's sense of competence and confidence related to a specific performance in a given domain has also been found to affect memory. Some studies have found a lack of correlation between self-reports and cognitive performance.[39] This is likely due to expectations about aging and memory loss rather than declining abilities. A self-perceived negative assessment of memory functioning was found to be associated with greater concern about developing disease.[39] If memory loss is not viewed as a problem by the elderly themselves, it does not interfere with their level of functioning and the achievement of everyday goals and cognitive performance scores remain within normal ranges. There is also evidence that learning occurs into advanced age.[39]

TABLE 4.2   Changes in Cognition with Normal Aging

Cognitive Abilities	Changes
Intelligence	Performance scale of the WAIS shows more decline than the verbal scale
Problem solving	Decline delayed until late sixth decade Older adults may be less proficient on laboratory tests
Memory	
Sensory memory	Little if any decline
Short term memory	No decline
Long term (secondary)	Some decline; deficits in encoding processes; deficits more pronounced in free recall than recognition
Long term (remote)	Little decline
Psychomotor skills	Decline may begin in the early 50s
Information processing	Decline may begin in the early 50s
Verbal skills	Declines do not occur until after age of 80 if at all
Abstract reasoning	Mental flexibility or set shifting in reasoning task have been shown to decline

Compiled from: Riley, K.P. Cognitive development. In Bonder, B.R., Wagner, M.B., eds. Functional Performance in Older Adults. Philadelphia: FA Davis; 1994.

RX

Treatment techniques for memory loss include the use of classes and educational strategies to assist memory. Classes in self-esteem, accurate record keeping, and the use of mnemonic devices can be helpful. Two additional hints in helping memory are to keep techniques as familiar as possible and to develop some type of reward system. (Refer to Chapter 18, Education and the Older Adult: Learning, Memory, and Intelligence, for learning strategies.)

Intelligence and Learning

The actual measurement of intelligence is not possible; what can be measured is the performance of the person's intelligence. Performance can easily be influenced by health, motivation, and sensory acuity. Even though the word "intelligence" is used, it is not singular. Intelligence can be subdivided into crystallized intelligence and fluid intelligence.[40]

Crystallized intelligence depends on sociocultural influence and involves the ability to perceive relations, engage in formal reasoning, and understand intellectual and cultural heritage.[41] The growth of crystallized intelligence, even after age 60, can be obtained through self-directed learning and education.[42]

Fluid intelligence depends primarily on the genetic endowment of the individual and the individual's ability to use short-term memory, create concepts, perceive complex relationships, and undertake abstract reasoning. This involves items that are mostly neuropsychologic in nature, which may decline after 60.[43]

The implications of this information for the therapist hoping to capitalize on intellectual performance and learning follow.

RX

1. Expect the intellectual ranges in older persons to be varied.
2. Poor performance may not mean poor learning.
3. Emphasize new knowledge that will be consistent with previous learning.[44]
4. Concentrate on one task at a time and be sure that the item is successfully learned before proceeding to the next.[43]
5. Reduce potential for distraction.
6. Space learning experiences sufficiently.
7. Allow for as much self-pacing as possible.
8. Assist older persons in organizing the information to be learned.
9. Present the information in the mode in which it will be used.[45]
10. Make the learning experience as concrete as possible.
11. Use supportive versus neutral instruction.
12. Use as many of the senses as possible to facilitate learning.
13. Provide as much feedback as possible.[46]

These suggestions have come from various studies[40-46] on changes in intelligence and performance, and are presented as techniques to improve performance.

Affect and reasoning appear to remain unchanged as one ages.[42,43] Again, dementia and drug complications are the major causes of decline in these areas.[42,43] (See section later in this chapter for specific changes associated with dementia. Also see Chapter 7, Pharmacology, for changes associated with drug interventions.)

SITUATIONS REQUIRING COPING MECHANISMS

Depression

The statistics on the prevalence of depression are varied. Nevertheless, the following quote aptly describes what many medical professionals may see in the health care setting, "Depression has been termed the common cold of the elderly."[47] Many older people cope with the depressive symptoms, and the statistics are quite significant. Depending on the source, cited depressive illness can be found in 5% to 65% of the older population.[48,49] Nevertheless, studies show that it is not aging per se that causes depression but the added variables of cognitive impairment, incontinence, chronic conditions, and disabilities, as well as significant personal and emotional losses.[50]

The DSM-IV[51] describes five categories of depression, all of which have relevance to geriatric patients. They are (1) major depression, (2) organic mood syndrome, (3) adjustment disorder with depression, (4) dysthymic disorder, and (5) dementia with depression.

A listing of symptoms of these disorders is found in Table 4.3. Major depression is characterized by having at least five of the symptoms listed for a period of at least two weeks. This type of disorder usually appears suddenly, and the symptoms are severe and are likely to end in a suicide attempt.[31] This disorder may occur in one single episode, or it may be recurrent with partial or full remissions between episodes. Mania, or euphoria, can occur between the episodes, but this is more characteristic of bipolar disease, which is much more severe.

For additional information on depression, see CD.

TABLE 4.3 Depressive Symptoms

Cognitive Symptoms:	Poor concentration
	Low self-esteem
	Indecisiveness
	Guilt
	Hopelessness
	Inability to concentrate
	Suicidal ideations
Somatic Symptoms:	Fatigue
	Altered sleep patterns
	Weight gain or loss
	Tearfulness
	Agitation
	Heart palpitations
	Overall weakness
Affective Symptoms:	Sadness
	Anxiety
	Irritability
	Fear
	Anger
	Depersonalization
	Feelings of isolation (loneliness)

RX

Anyone who talks to the patient in essence is providing psychotherapy. Therefore, the physical and occupational therapist should be aware of the treatment plans and goals for the individual patient. In addition, the therapist should be aware of some of the themes that emerge when working with the depressed older person. Older depressed patients must learn to adjust to new family roles, body image, and a measure of dependency, and they must learn to accept these changes without shame and continue to maintain intimacy with loved ones. In addition, patients must learn healthier coping mechanisms. For example, anticipating future discomfort, rather than denying future difficulties, is a healthier choice. Using humor, sublimation, and altruism helps the patient focus less on the illness and depression and more on other situations.

A Randomized Controlled Trial of Progressive Resistive Training in Depressed Elders; by Singh; *J Gerontol*; 05[52] High-intensity PRT is more effective than low-intensity for depressed patients.

PRT is an effective antidepressant in depressed elders, while also improving strength, morale, and quality of life.

Effects of Group Based Exercise Program on the Mood State of Frail Older Women after Discharge from Hospital; by Timonen; *Int J Geratric Psychiatry*; 02[53]

Group PRE ^ mood in frail women recovering from acute illness.

Effects of Exercise in Depressive Symptoms in Older Adults with poorly response depressive disease by Mather; A. *Brit J Psychiatry*, 02, Mg 180-411-415[56]

A program for 10 weeks, 2×/wk/45 min worked for depressed elders who responded poorly to meds.

Effects of Exercise Training on Older Patients with Major Depression; by Blumenthal; *Arch Intern Med*; 10-99[54]

An exercise training program may be considered an alternative to antidepressants for treatment of depression in older persons. Antidepressants may facilitate a more rapid response; however, at 16 weeks exercise was equally as effective in major depressive disorders.

The Effects of Resistance Training on Well-being and Memory in Elderly Volunteers; By Perig-Chiello; *A&A?* 9-98[55] age & ageing

An 8-week program of resistance training lessens anxiety and self-attentiveness and improves muscle strength.

Social Isolation

Social isolation can be divided into four types.[57,58] First is geographic isolation, which is a result of territorial restriction. The second, presentation isolation, results from an unacceptable appearance, while the third, behavioral isolation, results from unacceptable actions. Finally, attitudinal isolation arises from cultural or personal bound values. Any one of these types, or any combination of them, bars the older person from full acceptance by others. This will cause the person to feel alienated and out of step and will affect his or her self-esteem.

Geographic Isolation. Geographic isolation is usually a result of widowhood, urban crowding, rural lifestyle, or institutionalization. In all of these situations the older person may be alienated. For example, in the urban situation older people may be faced with a fast-paced, depersonalized lifestyle that gives them little opportunity to come in contact with close friends. (Institutionalization will be discussed in the next section.) The intervention techniques for geographic isolation include building on formal and informal support systems.

Table 4.4 lists formal and informal support systems.[58] In addition, older persons must examine the ramifications of any move they plan for an extended period of time in terms of the significance and size of the social support system they will be leaving behind versus the one they will be gaining.

Presentation Isolation. Unfortunately, in our society many judgments are made on superficial appearance, and as the body ages, its appearance no longer conforms to the

TABLE 4.4 Support Systems for Geographical Isolation

Formal Support Systems:	Involvement in social issues for seniors
	Senior centers
	Volunteer activities
	Friends of the library
	National Retired Teachers Association
	Retired Senior Volunteer Program
	Foster grandparenting programs
	Grandparenting (child care)
Informal Support Systems:	Neighbors/friends/family
	Social groups
	Home or nursing home therapists
	Medical visits (office or home)
	Pets
	Fictional kin (books-on-tape, soap operas)
	Beauty salons, restaurants, shops, etc.
	Housekeepers
	Retirement communities
	Churches

Madison Avenue stereotype. On top of this is the disfigurement that accompanies many physical disabilities associated with aging. The physical therapist can help older patients to deal with presentation isolation in several ways:

RX

1. By teaching them to avoid overexposure to individuals with similar image deficiencies, because the older persons may capitalize on their weaknesses rather than their strengths.
2. By helping them to establish new relationships with people who can accept them as they are now.
3. By giving lots of positive feedback on present strengths.
4. By asking questions to see what the older persons really think about themselves, and what experience they have had with similar conditions.
5. By teaching them to develop reasonable expectations.[57]

Behavioral Isolation. Behavioral isolation occurs when an older person displays behaviors that are unacceptable. The behaviors most likely to fall into this category are eccentricity, confusion, incontinence, and deviant behavior. The physical or occupational therapist can play a role by helping the person to identify the behavior and seek appropriate intervention for alleviating the problem.

Attitudinal Isolation. Attitudinal isolation is strongly entrenched in society's response to the older person. (Society's response will be discussed later in this chapter.) Ageism and the belief that it is acceptable and expected for older persons to be lonely are held by both the older person and the health professional. The intervention for this type of isolation is for both groups to evaluate their prejudices and misconceptions. In addition, the therapist must explore whether or not it is, in fact, desirable for the older person to be alone. To do this, the therapist should understand the difference between loneliness and being alone. Loneliness is a state of longing and emptiness, whereas being alone is being apart, solitary, and undisturbed. Figure 4.1 shows Maslow's factors of loneliness and isolation,[58] which may help the rehabilitation therapist in this assessment.

Institutionalization

Institutionalization appears to be a bizarre subheading under "situations requiring coping mechanisms." Nevertheless, organizational structure can have a profound impact on an individual's behavior. The classic text on the behavioral effects of institutionalization is *Asylums* by Goffman.[59] He identifies five aspects of a total institution (any institution where an individual spends 24 hours a day in residence):

1. A hierarchical authority exists with residents on the lowest rung. This type of authority results in situations where the staff is always right, and the residents are punished or reprimanded.
2. Total institutions take control of personal habits. For example, mealtimes are regulated, as well as urination and defecation. This makes it difficult for the resident to satisfy personal needs in an efficient way.
3. Residents of institutions are often made to feel humiliated, and an example of this is that many residents of institutions are not allowed to close their doors.
4. The setting often makes it impossible for the person to engage in face-saving behaviors. Any defensive behavior a resident may take after being rebuked may then become the focus of a new attack. For example, if a resident becomes angry because the doors must remain open, the staff may then begin to rebuke the resident for inappropriate anger.
5. The person's status within the institution is solely defined by his or her status within the institution and any outside roles are rarely counted. For example, a physical therapist who has worked hard for years to help people in an outside role will be treated the same as a criminal in an institution.

Interventions for helping the older person cope with institutionalization, short of changing the entire system, begin with the individual. The following list gives ways to help personalize the institutional setting for the clinician working with an older patient population.

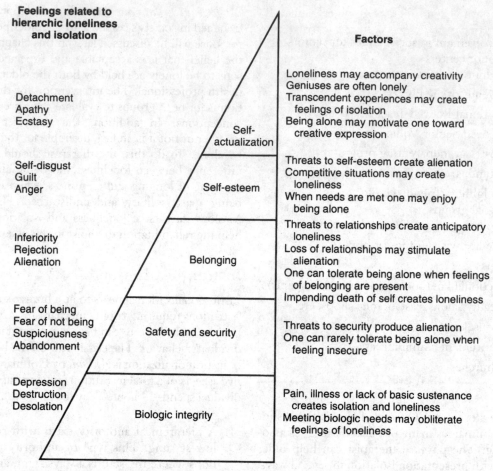

Feelings related to hierarchic loneliness and isolation

Detachment
Apathy
Ecstasy

Self-disgust
Guilt
Anger

Inferiority
Rejection
Alienation

Fear of being
Fear of not being
Suspiciousness
Abandonment

Depression
Destruction
Desolation

(pyramid levels, bottom to top:) Biologic integrity, Safety and security, Belonging, Self-esteem, Self-actualization

Factors

Loneliness may accompany creativity
Geniuses are often lonely
Transcendent experiences may create feelings of isolation
Being alone may motivate one toward creative expression

Threats to self-esteem create alienation
Competitive situations may create loneliness
When needs are met one may enjoy being alone

Threats to relationships create anticipatory loneliness
Loss of relationships may stimulate alienation
One can tolerate being alone when feelings of belonging are present
Impending death of self creates loneliness

Threats to security produce alienation
One can rarely tolerate being alone when feeling insecure

Pain, illness or lack of basic sustenance creates isolation and loneliness
Meeting biologic needs may obliterate feelings of loneliness

Figure 4.1   Factors of loneliness and isolation. *(Adapted from Ebersp., Hess, P. Towards healthy aging: Human needs and nursing response. St. Louis, Mosby Co.; 1981, with permission.)*

RX

1. Develop meaningful relationships.
2. Give accurate information.
3. Involve the family.
4. Recognize accomplishments with plaques, posters, and so forth.
5. Recognize and address people by their preferred name.
6. Recognize birthdays on the appropriate day.
7. Provide memorials for residents that have died.
8. Conduct life reviews.
9. Establish contacts with plants, pets, and children.
10. Every person must have some personal items with him or her.
11. Room sharing should be done only with a compatible resident.
12. Provide legal aid to protect the resident's rights.
13. Provide choices in all matters.

Anxiety Disorders

Anxiety disorders in the older person are frequently underreported and missed.[60] The incidence of anxiety disorders increases with age and is more frequent in women than in men.[61,62] Anxiety disorders present either with symptoms of fear, worry, or nervousness or as somatic problems without any physical cause. The DSM-IV of the American Psychiatric Association identifies three classes of disorders that share the characteristic of anxiety.[51] These are (1) adjustment disorders with anxious mood, (2) anxiety states, and (3) phobic states. Table 4.5 shows the most common anxiety disorders and their central features.

In the assessment of anxiety disorders, the clinician should be aware of the descriptions listed in Table 4.5, as well as some of the frequent symptoms associated with anxiety in the elderly. While the list is quite extensive, several symptoms are seen more frequently by occupational and physical therapists,[63] and these include tremor, headaches, chest pain, weakness and fatigue, neck and back pain, dry mouth, dizziness, paresthesia, and a nonproductive cough.[63] The presence of these symptoms does

TABLE 4.5 The Anxiety Disorders and Their Central Features

Disorder	Central Features
Adjustment disorder with anxious mood	Nervousness/anxiety in reaction to identifiable psychosocial stressor
Anxiety states	Persistent or recurrent anxiety not provoked by identifiable stimulus, generally nonsituational
Obsessive-compulsive disorder	Intrusive thoughts and/or repetitive behaviors performed under a sense of pressure
	Attempts to resist increased anxiety
Posttraumatic stress disorder	Acute and delayed reactions to a traumatic event
	Involves "reliving" the experience, emotional numbing, and development of somatic symptoms
Panic disorder	Sudden, unpredictable panic attacks involving intense apprehension and physical symptoms
Generalized anxiety disorder	Generalized, persistent anxiety for more than one month
	Includes three of the following: motor tension, autonomic hyperactivity, apprehension, and hypervigilance
Phobic disorders	Persistent, irrational fear or anxiety provoked by stimulus object, activity, or situation
	Avoidance of stimulus
	Fear recognized by patient as irrational or excessive
Agoraphobia	Feared stimulus: being alone or in a public place where escape would be difficult or help hard to find
	Occurs with or without panic attacks
Social phobia	Fear stimulus: social situations involving possible embarrassment or humiliation
Simple phobia	Fear stimulus: situations similar to a previous terrifying experience

Adapted and reprinted with permission from Geriatrics. *August 1985; 40(8):80.*

not mean that the older person has an anxiety disorder, because there may be physical causes as well as organic causes, such as caffeine, hypoglycemia, or thyroid disease. In addition, therapists should screen for the symptoms of depression already described, as depression may cause some of the symptoms of anxiety disorders.

Finally, physical and occupational therapists should seek additional information. For example, a patient may not tell you that she has a simple phobia; however, when you visit her at home, she may tell you that people are spying on her, listening to her through the walls, and tapping the phone. In further conversations, you discover that this patient had a terrifying experience as a child when she was left alone or when she was harassed and abused by Nazi soldiers. In this instance, the patient has developed a "simple phobic" reaction to always having people around—seen in terms of spying on her—to avoid her deep-seated fear of being alone.

RX

The treatment for anxiety disorders is condensed in Table 4.6. In treating anxiety disorders, the therapist can act in several ways. First, the physical or occupational therapist can alert the physician to the problem. Second, the therapist may be able to share additional information collected from the frequent rehabilitation therapy sessions. Third, the therapist can play an integral role in any of the behavioral therapies. Finally, the therapist can teach the patient stress management techniques, stress reduction interventions, and assertiveness ideas. These will be discussed in detail at the end of this chapter.

TABLE 4.6   Anxiety Disorders and their Management

Disorders	Management
Adjustment disorder with anxious mood	Supportive "brief psychotherapies"
	Stress management techniques
	Assertiveness training
	Interventions to eliminate or reduce stressors
Anxiety states	
Obsessive-compulsive disorder	Tricyclic antidepressants
	Avoid use of benzodiazepines
	Psychotherapy
Posttraumatic stress disorder	Crisis intervention techniques
	Supportive brief psychotherapies
Panic disorder	Short-acting benzodiazepines
	Frequent evaluations of medication effects; avoid abrupt withdrawal
	Shield eyes from fluorescent lights
	Stress management techniques
Generalized anxiety disorder	Short-acting benzodiazepines, with frequent evaluations; avoid abrupt withdrawal
	Supportive "brief psychotherapies"
	Stress management techniques
Phobic disorders	Avoid use of most benzodiazepines
Agoraphobia	Daily tricyclic antidepressants or MAO inhibitors
	With panic attacks, shield eyes from fluorescent lighting
Social phobia	Behavior therapies
Simple phobia	Behavior therapies

Adapted and reprinted with permission from Geriatrics. *August 1985; 40(8):80.*

Chronic Illness

As mentioned earlier in this chapter, the importance of coping with chronic illness is imperative for successful aging. In the older population, the percentage of persons with physical illness is staggering. According to Weg, 70% of people over the age of 65 have some type of chronic illness.[64] The three major illnesses for older persons are (1) heart conditions, (2) visual impairments, and (3) arthritis.[65] These types of chronic illnesses can be mild, thereby causing only minimal adaptations or lifestyle changes, or they can be devastating and cause major lifestyle modification. Serious illness or a devastating life event can cause profound changes in a person's appreciation of life,[66] and often this will result in a shift in goals, relationships, and values.

Physical and occupational therapists can recognize their roles in this area by enhancing the older patient's new realizations and thought processes. The following list offers some suggestions to enhance this process.

1. Realize that patients may have a heightened sense of beauty and of caring relationships.
2. Provide opportunities for the patient to talk about these new changes in values.
3. Encourage the patient in these new realizations, and let him or her know that these types of thoughts are part of the growth process.
4. Foster communication between the patient and his or her family, especially in light of the patient's new values.
5. Suggest participating in discussion groups for patients recovering from similar conditions.

Death, Dying, Grief, and Multiple Losses

These final situations that require coping mechanisms fit together well because the insights, manifestations, and mechanisms of coping for each are similar. The legal and ethical aspects of death and dying will be discussed in Chapter 17.

Many people think of aging as a time of loss. In reality, aging represents not only one loss; rather it is a time of multiple losses. Some of the most common losses include the loss of the patient's mobility, productivity, usefulness, body image, time left to live, health, income, and status. These and other losses occur throughout life; however, their frequency increases with old age, and their cumulative effect increases the emotional impact as a person ages. Another very important variable affecting loss is the person's general personality and ability to tolerate loss. Some people view loss as giving up what one had, while others focus happily on what they have.

The physical or occupational therapist constantly works with people who have lost something, whether it is health, mobility, body image, or independence. The therapist's role is extremely important. To evaluate the loss, the therapist must consider if the loss is simple, compound, or symbolic. Losing $10.00 might be simple—if the person is financially healthy. However, if that $10.00 was borrowed with high interest to pay a long-standing debt, then it becomes compound and more emotional. In another situation, the $10.00 may be the first money ever received in a business and, therefore, may be symbolic. When evaluating a loss, first check for its type by assessing its significance and by discussing it with the patient and family.

To assist the person, be sure to review the loss with the person and any supportive family and friends. Remember to constantly reorient the person to the reality of the situation. The therapist should not make false promises and set unrealistic goals (see Chapter 14 for treatment suggestions to assist patients with limb loss). Be realistic and set short-term, attainable goals. Watch for signs of chronic grief.

Symptoms of a single loss should subside in six weeks, however, it may take longer in old age to resolve grief.[66] The symptoms are weakness, tiredness, sighing, and digestive symptoms. The patient may exhibit feelings of anger, deprivation, and guilt, but chronic grief in the older person may be much more subtle. For example, they may not cry, but they may sigh frequently when talking or complain of constant tiredness. The most useful treatment suggestion for the physical or occupational therapist working with a grief-stricken patient is to listen and care. This can help bridge the isolation. A recommendation for psychological counseling is also imperative.

To some, the death of an older person is viewed as a blessing or the final chapter in a full and rich life. This, unfortunately, does not hold for all older people, because many older people feel they are not ready to die and that they have not fulfilled their lives. According to Kalish, though, the fear of death diminishes as one ages.[67] This may be due to the increased exposure to dying with the aging of family and friends.

Dying has a special significance for the older patient. The following list gives six areas that are different for the older versus the younger patient.

1. Older persons tend to reminisce as a way of integrating their life prior to dying.

2. Older people are less likely to have an advocate. This is especially true for older women, because they tend to outlive their husbands.

3. Older persons are less able to be communicative than younger patients when dying because of brain syndromes or confusion. This lack of communicative ability makes it more difficult for the health team to provide caring without a reciprocal response.

4. Older people may get less than optimum care because of the belief that they will die soon anyway.

5. The social value of an older person's life is thought to be less than that of younger person's.[67]

Much has been written about the process of dying. The most well-known author in this area is Kübler-Ross. She is most well known for her stages of dying, which are (1) denial, (2) anger, (3) bargaining, (4) depression, and (5) acceptance.[68] Even though her stages have not been proven to be consistent, they have received great acceptance. In interpreting her stages, it is important to note that not all people go through all the stages. For example, someone may not experience anger and go straight from denial to bargaining. In addition, there are no time limits on these various stages. Other studies have postulated stages of the dying or grief process. Bowlby[69] and Engel,[70] for example, have similar stages but end their stages with the process of reorganization.

The interventions for therapists working with the dying patient are to enhance the older person's ability to die with dignity and achieve final growth, which can be done by recognizing impediments to growth. (These impediments are described in the sections on isolation and institutionalization.)

RX

In addition, the physical or occupational therapist can help to fulfill the unmet needs of the dying person. The most common unmet needs are freedom from pain and loneliness, conservation of energy, and maintenance of self-esteem. Physical therapists are well versed in pain management, and a full discussion of loneliness can be found in the isolation section.

Physical and occupational therapists can also provide environmental and ergonometric assessment by evaluating an older patient's daily program and offer helpful suggestions to the patient and caregiver to reduce excessive energy expenditure. Finally, there are a few helpful hints for bolstering the self-esteem of an older person who is dying. Be sure that the person's physical comfort is assured (e.g., cleanliness, personal appearance, and lack of odor). Therapists should use as much sensory feedback as possible in the visual, auditory, and tactile realms. Also, therapists should focus on the immediate future and present opportunities; they should not confuse their values with those of the dying person's. Dying is very individual, and everyone perceives it differently.

The final topic under death, dying, grief, and loss focuses on the health care provider. It is imperative that the provider working with dying patients realizes the extreme amount of stress in this situation. Harper has developed stages that health care providers may experience when working with dying patients for a one- to two-year period.[71] They are

1. *Intellectualization* usually occurs in the beginning of employment. The health professional is quite accurate about his or her job; however, the provider avoids discussions about death.
2. *Emotional survival* is characterized by an understanding of the pain and suffering. Here the provider may be unable to face—and may question—his or her own mortality.
3. Depression is a stage where the provider accepts the reality of death or quits. Feelings of grief are classic here.
4. *Emotional arrival* is characterized by a deeper awareness of and sensitivity to the dying person.
5. *Deep compassion* is characterized by full maturity. Here the provider is extremely constructive and has clear emotions on his or her own and others' issues of death.[66]

DELIRIUM

The syndrome of delirium is a common, serious, and often life-threatening condition in the elderly patient. Often unrecognized, it is the second most common syndrome involving cognitive failure in the geriatric population.[72] It may be the most common adverse outcome of hospitalization and surgery in older patients.[73,74]

Though there are many synonyms used to describe this clinical state (e.g., acute brain syndrome, acute confusional state, metabolic encephalopathy, toxic or exogenous psychosis[75]), the DSM-IV[40] defines delirium as an abrupt change in mental status and behavior, with global, fluctuating impairment in cognitive processes and alterations in attention. There is disturbed psychomotor activity, disorientation, disordered thinking, and inability to correctly process information from the environment. As a result, memory is impaired and the patient is easily distracted and has difficulty concentrating and following commands. Behavioral changes may range from withdrawal to agitation, with or without psychotic symptoms. Illusions and paranoid ideation frequently occur due to misinterpretation of visual or auditory stimuli. Sleep-wake disturbances and sundowning (increased agitation in late afternoon and early evening) are common.[72,74]

For additional information on delirium, see CD.

RX

General principles of managing patients with delirium include the first element, which is to provide enough fluids and nutrition to keep the patient from becoming dehydrated. A calm and quiet environment that enhances cognitive function, maximizes comfort, and minimizes environmental stress should be provided. A low level of lighting without shadows that can induce perceptual disturbances is optimal. Exposure to natural lighting through a window may be beneficial. Reorienting the individual frequently with simple, clear explanations for activities taking place is important. Having familiar objects, clocks, and calendars present will help with orientation. Eyeglasses and hearing aids should be in place to correct sensory deficits. Presence of familiar individuals, such as family members and friends, is usually reassuring, and they can often help provide one-to-one observation when staffing is inadequate.

It is preferable to avoid restraining the agitated patient with delirium. Attempts to "escape" restraints often place the delirious patient at great risk for injury and falls.

Dementia

Millions of older Americans are victims of dementias. Because of this, dementia or cognitive impairment is the major cause of disability in older persons. The statistics are staggering: in the United States the estimated number of people suffering moderate to severe dementia ranges from 1.5 million to 2.3 million.[76,77] One study equates these figures to "One family in every three will see one of their parents succumb to this disease."[76] The prevalence of dementia also increases with age. The estimate for people over 65 is 5%, but for those over 75, it is estimated that 20% will have some degree of cognitive impairment.[76] In addition, in the nursing home setting it is estimated that the prevalence reaches 50%.[78] Besides the amazing emotional burdens, the economic burdens are immense. The care for persons with Alzheimer's disease alone in 1999 was 100 billion.[79]

The categorization of Alzheimer's disease as a cognitive impairment emphasizes the need for precision when describing and categorizing pathologies. The categorization and description of the cognitive impairments of older persons is probably the most important aspect of its assessment and treatment, and yet descriptions and classifications are not always in perfect agreement.[80,81]

1. *Acute disorders.* These are potentially reversible. Under this subheading are delirium, depression, multiple causes, and accidents.
2. *Chronic disorders.* These are the irreversible cognitive impairments, including Alzheimer's disease, vascular disease, and subcortical disorders.
3. *Presenile dementias.* These diseases tend to be rarer and to occur in younger populations. They are also not reversible.

Acute cognitive disorders have been romanticized in American society. While acute disorders are reversible, their prevalence is not as great as was once reported.[82] In an article entitled "The Reversible Dementias: Do They Reverse?" the results showed only a 3% full resolution and an 8% partial resolution of the dementias.[83]

Despite the less than impressive response rates to treatment, it is still important to understand this aspect of dementia, because it can be reversed. Acute disorders often have multiple causes. Among these causes are drugs, translocation, infection, neoplasm, trauma, malnutrition, toxic states, metabolic imbalances, and depression. According to Clarfield, the most common reversible causes were drugs (28.2%), depression (26.2%), and metabolic changes (15.5%).[83]

The symptoms of this type of cognitive impairment (except for the acute delirium caused by depression) are characterized by a rapidly developing confusion state. The person will often display clouded, fluctuating consciousness accompanied by agitation. In addition the patient will have alterations in the following processes:

1. *Perception.* The person may be hypersensitive to light or sound and suffer from visual, auditory, or tactile hallucinations.
2. *Memory.* This can be significantly impaired—more so in the short term than in the long term. New information may be difficult to learn, possibly because of the delirious patient's decreased attention span.
3. *Thinking.* Delirious patients tend to have illogical and disjointed thoughts. They may have difficulty with problem solving and word finding. Finally, these patients may also have persecution delusions, which they may forget when they recover.
4. *Orientation.* Delirious patients classically are disoriented to time. They may lose orientation to place as the disease progresses; however, they rarely lose orientation to person.
5. *Alertness.* Delirious patients may be either hypo- or hyperalert. They may display increased pulse or pressure or decreased alertness.

The manifestation of delirium due to depression differs in several major aspects. The depressed patient will have a slower onset of these symptoms, a longer history of so-

matic complaints, and a lower self-esteem. The depressed patient will tend to be on the hypo side of alertness. The greatest cognitive decline in the depressed patient will be the ability to process information, which will be blunted.

For more information on dementia, see CD.

Physical Activity and Risk of Cognitive Impairment and Dementia in Elderly Persons; by Laurin; *Arch Neurol*; 3-01[84]

- Regular physical activity was associated with lower risks of cognitive impairment.
- The higher the activity, the better.
- High = 3×/wk ^ walking.
- Mod = 3×/wk, = walking.
- Why? -^ blood flow, metabolic demands, aerobic capacity, cerebral nutrient supply.

Does participation in Leisure Activities Lead to Reduced Risk of Alzheimer Disease? A Perspective of Swedish Twins; by Crowe; *J. Gerontol*; 03[85]

Participation in leisure activities was associated with a lower risk of Alzheimer's disease.

Physical Activity; Including Walking and Cognitive Function in Older Women; by Weuve *JAMA*; 9-04[86]

Walking is associated with a reduced risk of dementia in men (Abbott) and women (Weuve).

The general characteristics of chronic brain syndrome can be summarized by the following mnemonic device, JAMCO.[5]

J—*Judgment.* The person may show inappropriate behavior as a result of improper information processing. For example, the patient walks out of his or her room undressed.

A—*Affect.* The person's affect is more labile, causing the patient to laugh or cry easily or uncontrollably. An example might be the patient who constantly giggles or weeps.

M—*Memory.* The person will lose his or her memory, first short-term and then long-term. An example might be the patient who evades current questions by relating anecdotes from the past; however, when forced to answer the current questions the patient is unable to do so.

C—*Cognition.* Cognition will be disjointed and illogical, as well as delusional and hallucinatory. The therapist may be talking to the patient about the patient's exercises and the patient may relate a story about the FBI watching the nursing home.

O—*Orientation.* The person may, in general, have a flat level of awareness. The therapist may find that if the patient is left alone to do exercises, he or she falls asleep or into a daydreaming state.[5]

Alzheimer's disease deserves additional description in terms of manifestations. Typically, three stages of AD are recognized. Occasionally a fourth stage is identified.[87] Hayter has described various stages of Alzheimer's disease.[88] The first stage lasts two to four years and is characterized by moodiness, hypochondriasis, time disorientation, lack of spontaneity, poor judgment, blaming others, and a sense of helplessness and worthlessness. Generally, the person has difficulty with social adaptation and may display catastrophic reactions to stressful events.

The second stage may last several years, and it is characterized by an increase in symptoms. At this point the person is usually in the health care system (e.g., hospital or nursing home) due to unsafe behaviors, such as constant movement, paranoia and hallucinations, and physical abusiveness. The person may display sleep pattern disturbances, as well as incontinence. The third or final stage has no time limit and is characterized by irritability, seizures, disorientation on all spheres, illogical communication, severe anorexia, rigid postures, and explosive sounds and behaviors.

RX

What is the physical or occupational therapist's role in working with the patient with cognitive impairment? A diagnosis of Alzheimer's is often a cause for denial of payment for physical and occupational therapy. Many intermediaries cite the inability of Alzheimer's patients to learn as a reason for denial; because rehabilitation is structured around learning, the benefits derived would be minimal. While this argument has its merits, Alzheimer's patients can learn. In addition, therapy is more than learning. A large part of rehabilitation is environmental and physical modification. For example, if a patient with Alzheimer's disease is sent to physical therapy because of muscle weakness in the legs and an increased incidence of falls, then the physical therapist would be judicious in administering a strengthening program on a daily basis to the weakened muscles. Also, an environmental assessment for potential falls might be indicated. Occupational therapy may often be involved in activities that assist the demented patient in reorienting to his or her surroundings. Therefore, it is appropriate to design and execute programs for the cognitively impaired elderly with treatable functional decline. In addition, the training and education of the family is crucial to any in-home rehabilitation program.

Some general guidelines for working with the cognitively impaired elderly follow.[89]

1. *Simplify.* That includes simplifying the instructions, programs, and environment.
2. *Explain.* This should be done thoroughly, frequently, constantly, and repetitively, if necessary.
3. *Reorient.* In normal conversation, if possible, remind the patient of the time, place, and activity. Have clocks, calendars, and orienting pictures in view.
4. *Slow down.* Take your time in all aspects. Have a slow, low voice.
5. *Avoid change.* Change should be avoided in the environment, with the personnel, and in all aspects of programming, if possible.
6. *Encourage familiarity.* The environment should have as many familiar objects as possible, exercises should mimic familiar activities, and familiar people should be encouraged to visit.
7. *Touch.* Encourage as much touching as possible. This conveys caring and support to a patient who is going through an uncontrollable change and may desperately need support.
8. *Encourage independence.* This may necessitate simplifying commands and labeling items for ease of recognition.
9. *Respect individual dignity.* Encourage the patient to discuss and demonstrate previous successes and accomplishments. Display pictures of the patient in memorable moments. Respect modesty and dignity.
10. *Educate and support the family.* Be prepared to confront denial in the family and patient. Provide information on additional support services for cognitively impaired patients. Frequently bring up the topic of additional support. (Families frequently refuse initial offerings of help.) Reinforce that the patient's behavior is not volitional. Offer helpful suggestions for ways to tell others about the disease when the family is ready.
11. *Listen to the patient.* Even if the patient is not making sense, try to listen. Every once in a while a lucid statement will be verbalized.
12. *Take care of yourself.* Working with cognitively impaired patients can be emotionally exhausting. If a patient is combative or abusive, tell the patient that this type of behavior upsets you and take time out from the patient.

Facts on Aging Quiz

Please take this short "Facts on Aging Quiz"

T   F   1. The majority of old people (past age 65) are senile (i.e., defective memory, disoriented, or demented).

T   F   2. All five senses tend to decline in old age.

T   F   3. Most old people have no interest in, or capacity for, sexual relations.

T   F   4. Lung capacity tends to decline in old age.

T   F   5. The majority of old people feel miserable most of the time.

T   F   6. Physical strength tends to decline in old age.

T   F   7. At least one-tenth of the aged are living in long-stay institutions (i.e. nursing homes, mental hospitals, homes for the aged, etc.)

T   F   8. Aged drivers have fewer accidents per person than drivers under age 65.

T   F   9. Most older workers cannot work as effectively as younger workers.

T   F   10. About 80% of the aged are healthy enough to carry out their normal activities.

T   F   11. Most old people are set in their ways and unable to change.

T   F   12. Old people usually take longer to learn something new.

T   F   13. It is almost impossible for most old people to learn new things.

T   F   14. The reaction time of most old people tends to be slower than reaction time of younger people.

T   F   15. In general, most old people are pretty much alike.

T   F   16. The majority of old people are seldom bored.

T   F   17. The majority of old people are socially isolated and lonely.

T   F   18. Older workers have fewer accidents than younger workers.

T   F   19. Over 15% of the US population are now age 65 or older.

T   F   20. Most medical practitioners tend to give low priority to the aged.

T   F   21. The majority of older people have incomes below the poverty level (as defined by the Federal Government).

T   F   22. The majority of old people are working or would like to have some kind of work to do (including housework and volunteer work).

T   F   23. Older people tend to become more religious as they age.

T   F   24. The majority of old people are seldom irritated or angry.

T   F   25. The health and socioeconomic status of older people (compared to younger people) in the year 2000 will probably be about the same as now.

Figure 4.2   Facts on Aging: A short quiz. *(Reprinted with permission Palmore, E. Facts on aging: A short quiz. Gerontologist. Aug 1977; 17:3150320. © The Gerontology Society of America.)*

BELIEF SYSTEMS REGARDING THE AGING PROCESS

"Ageism" is the term Butler coined to denote a prejudice against a person or group of persons due to their age.[90] A myth is a belief that a person holds with or without the appropriate facts to gain control of an ambiguous situation. Society holds many of these beliefs. The current belief that is biased toward youth sprung out of the post-Depression era. The focus for hope shifted from the older generation to the new, bright-futured baby boomers. The parents who had nothing growing up in the Depression could now give it all to their children with the hope that they would make a better world. The focus unfortunately shifted from the older population. This shift has combined with the birth of high technology and self-absorption and has led to low self-esteem and negative attitudes for older people.

The Facts on Aging Quiz, by Erdman Palmore (Figure 4.2) is an important tool for assessing bias against older persons.[91] To score this quiz, all the odd-numbered questions are false, and all the even-numbered questions are true. This quiz can be used to test a person's myths, biases, and knowledge.

The problem of ageism or negative attitudes toward older people is particularly pronounced in the health arena. Older patients may be seen as complaining, somatasizing, uninteresting, or helpless. In addition they may not receive the same services as younger persons. In the United States, for example, physicians are often overaggressive with diagnostic tests for older persons but less aggressive in providing rehabilitation services,[92] and physical therapists have been shown to be less aggressive in goal setting for older patients.[93]

The evaluation and treatment of the social misinterpretation of aging is not an easy task. Both the evaluation and the treatment must begin on a personal level. Self-evaluation of myths, belief systems, and the personal evaluation of individual patients must be done daily.

A simple treatment is to show others (by example) healthy and positive ways of working with older persons. The ultimate goal is not to display negative prejudices to other groups in hopes of valuing the older population, but to develop a society with a healthy mixture and respect for all groups. A society to strive for would be one of bright youths, secure middle-aged adults, and wise older persons.

For more information on lifestyle adaptation, stress, see CD.

References

1. Mossey J, Murtan E, Knott K, et al. Determinants of recovery 12 months after hip fracture: The importance of psychosocial factors. *Am J Public Health*. March 1989; 79:279–286.

2. Magaziner J. Predictions of functional recovery one year following hospital discharge for hip fracture: A prospective study. *J Gerontol*. 1990; 45:101–107.

3. Gilford, DM, ed. *The Aging Population in the Twenty-First Century*. Washington, DC: National Academy Press; 1998.

4. Erikson EH. *Identity, Youth and Crisis*. New York: WW Norton; 1968.

5. Lewis CB. Psychological aspects of aging. In: Lewis CA, ed. *Aging: Health Care's Challenge*. Philadelphia: FA Davis; 2002.

6. Jung CG: *The Stages of Life. The Structure and Dynamics of the Psyche*. New York: Pantheon; 1960.

7. Buehler C. Theoretical observations about life's basic tendencies. *Am J Psychother*. 1959; 13: 561–581.

8. Maslow A. *Motivation and Personality*. New York: Harper & Row; 1954.

9. Maslow A. *Toward a Psychology of Being*. Princeton: Van Nostrand Co.; 1962.

10. Peele B. Psychological developments in the second half of life. In: Neugarten B, ed. *Middle Age and Aging*. Chicago: University of Chicago Press; 1975.

11. Neugarten B. *Middle Age and Aging*. Chicago: University of Chicago Press; 1975.

12. Cummings E, Henry W. *Growing Old: The Process of Disengagement*. New York: Basic Books; 1961.

13. Lipman A. Latent function analysis in gerontological research. *Gerontologist*. 1969; 5:256–259.

14. Lipman A, Smith KJ. Functionality of disengagement in old age. *J Gerontol*. 1968; 23:517–521.

15. Perls TT, Burbrick E, Wager CG, Vijg J, Kruglyak L. Siblings of centenarians live longer. *Lancet*. 1998; 351(3):1560.

16. Brodsky DM. The conflict perspective and understanding aging among minorities. In: Manual RC, ed. *Minority Aging*. Westport, CT.: Greenwood Press; 1982.

17. De Beauvoir S. *The Coming of Age*. New York: Putnam Books; 1972.

18. Estes CL. *The Aging Enterprise*. San Francisco: Jossey-Bass; 1979.

19. Lipman A. Minority aging from the exchange and structural-functionalist perspectives. In: Manual RC,

ed. *Minority Aging*. Westport, CT: Greenwood Press; 1982.

20. Homans G. *Social Behavior in Elementary Forms*. New York: Harcourt Brace & World; 1961.

21. Dowd JJ. Aging as exchange: A test of the distributive justice proposition. *Pacific Sociol Rev*. 1978; 21: 351–375.

22. Havighurst R, Neugarten B, Tobin S. Disengagement and patterns of aging. In: Neugarten B, ed. *Middle Age and Aging*. Chicago: University of Chicago Press; 1975.

23. Butler R, Lewis M. *Aging and Mental Health*. St. Louis: Mosby-Year Book; 1982: 33–35.

24. Havighurst RJ. Flexibility and the social role of the retired. *Am J Sociol*. 1954; 59:399.

25. Neuhaus R, Neuhaus R. *Successful Aging*. New York: John Wiley; 1982: 9–12.

26. Havighurst RJ. *Developmental Tasks and Education*. New York: David McKay; 1972.

27. Levinson D. *Seasons of a Man's Life*. New York: Knopf; 1978.

28. Schaie KW. *Intellectual Development in Adulthood: The Seattle Longitudinal Study*. New York: Cambridge University Press; 1996.

29. Bolla KI, Lindgren KN, Bonaccorsy C, Bleecker ML. Memory complaints in older adults: Fact or fiction? *Arch Neurology*. 1991; 48:61–64.

30. Crook TH, Feher EP, Larrabee GJ. Assessment of memory complaint in age-associated memory impairment: The MAC–Q. *International Psychogeriatrics*. 1992; 4:165–176.

31. Linn RT, Wolf PA, Bachman DL, Knoefel JE, Cobb JL, Belanger AJ, Kaplan EF, D'Agostino RB. The "preclinical phase" of probable Alzheimer's disease. *Arch Neurol*. 1995; 52:485–490.

32. Sliwinski M, Lipton RB, Buschke H, Stewart W. The effects of preclinical dementia on estimates of normal cognitive functioning in aging. *J Gerontol*. 1996; 518:217–225.

33. Riley KP. Cognitive development. In: Bonder BR, Wagner MB, eds. *Functional Performance in Older Adults*. Philadelphia: FA Davis; 1994.

34. Cockburn J, Smith P. The relative influence of intelligence and age on everyday memory. *J Gerontol*. 1991; 46(l):31–35.

35. Hultoch D, Masson M, Small B. Adult age differences in direct and indirect test of memory. *J Gerontol*. 1991; 46(l):22–30.

36. Craik F, Masani P. Age differences in the temporal integration of language. *Brit J Psychology*. 1967; 58:291–299.

37. Botwinck J. *Aging and Behavior*. 2nd ed. New York: Springer; 1978.

38. Larrabee GJ, Crook TH. Estimated prevalence of age-associated memory impairment derived from standardized tests of memory function. *International Psychogeriatric*. 1994; 6:95–104.

39. Johansson B, Allen-Burge R, Zarit SH. Self-reports on memory functioning in a longitudinal study of the oldest old: Relation to current, prospective, and retrospective performance. *J Gerontol*. 1997; 52: 139–146.

40. Labouvie–Vief G. Intelligence and cognition. In: Birren JE, Schaie KW, eds. *Handbook of the Psychology of Aging*. New York: Van Nostrand Reinhold; 1985.

41. Cattell RB. Theory of fluid and crystallized intelligence: A clinical experiment. *J Educ Psychol*. 1963; 54:1.

42. Knox AB. *Adult Development and Learning*. San Francisco: Jossey-Bass; 1977.

43. Botwinick J. *Aging and Behavior: A Comprehensive Integration of Research Findings*. New York: Springer; 1978.

44. Hayslip B, Kennelly KJ. Cognitive and noncognitive factors affecting learning among older adults. In: Lumsden BD, ed. *The Older Adult as a Learner*. Washington, DC: Hemisphere Publishing; 1985.

45. Eisdorfer C, Nowlin F, Wilke F. Improvement of learning in the aged by modification of autonomic nervous system activity. *Science*. 1970; 170:1327.

46. Schultz NR, Hoyer WJ. Feedback effects on spacial egocentrism in old age. *J Gerontol*. 1976; 31:72.

47. Bettes S. Depression: The "common cold" of the elderly. *Generations*. Spring 1979; 3:15.

48. Epstein L. Symposium of age differentiation in depressive illness: Depression in the elderly. *J Gerontol*. 1976; 31:278.

49. Gurland B. The comparative frequency of depression in various adult age groups. *J Gerontol*. 1976; 31:283–292.

50. Ferucci LI, Guralnik J, Marchionni N, et al. Aging and prevalence of depression. *Gerontologist*. October 1990; 30:314A.

51. American Psychiatric Association. *Diagnostic and Statistical Manual of Mental Disorders*. 4th ed. Washington DC: American Psychiatric Association; 1994: 124.

52. Singh NA, Clements KM, Fiatarone MA. "A Randomized Controlled Trial of Progressive Resistive Training in Depressed Elders." *Journal of Gerontology: Medical Sciences*. (1997); 52(1):M27–M35.

53. Timonen L, et al. "Effects of a Group-based Exercise Program on the Mood State of Frail Older Women After Discharge From Hospital." *Int J Geriatric Psychiatry*, 2002 Dec; 17(12):1106–11.

54. Blumenthal JA, Babyak MA, Moore KA, Craighead WE, Herman S, Khatri P, Waugh R, Napolitano MA, Forman LM, Applebaum M, Doraiswany PM, Krishnan KR. "Effects of Exercise Training on Older Patients With Major Depression." *Arch Intern Med*, 159:2349–2356; 1999.

55. Perrig-Chiello P, et al. "The Effects of Resistance Training on Well-Being and Memory in Elderly Volunteers." *Age and Ageing* 27:469–475; 1998.

56. Mather A. "Effects of exercise on depressive symptoms in older adults with poorly responsive depressive disorder" Br J. Psychiatry, 2002 May; 180: 411–415

57. Goffman E. *Stigma: Notes on the Management of Spoiled Identity.* Upper Saddle River, NJ: Prentice Hall; 1963.

58. Ebersole P, Hess P. *Towards Healthy Aging: Human Needs and Nursing Response.* St. Louis: Mosby; 2003: 387.

59. Goffman E. *Asylums: Essays on the Social Situations of Mental Patients and Other Inmates.* Garden City, NY: Doubleday; 1961.

60. Shader R, Goodman M. Panic disorders: Current perspectives. *J Clin Psychopharmacol.* 1982; 2:2–105.

61. Carey G, Gottesman I, Robins E. Prevalence and rates for the neurosis: Pitfalls in the evaluation of familiarity. *Psychol Med.* 1980; 10:437–443.

62. Kleen D, Robkin J, eds. *Anxiety: New Research and Changing Concepts.* New York: Raven Press; 1981.

63. Tumball J, Tumball S. Management of specific anxiety disorders in the elderly. *Geriatrics.* 1985; 40:875–881.

64. Weg R. *The Aged: Who, Where, How Well.* Los Angeles: Ethel Percy Andrus Gerontology Center; 1979.

65. Frankel V. *Man's Search for Meaning.* Boston: Beacon Press; 1959.

66. Ebersole P, Hess P. *Towards Healthy Aging: Human Needs and Nursing Response.* St. Louis: Mosby; 2003: Philadelphia, 389.

67. Kalish R. *Death, Grief and Caring Relationships.* Monterey, CA: Brooks/Cole; 1981.

68. Kübler-Ross E. *On Death and Dying.* New York: Macmillan; 1969.

69. Bowlby J. Process of mourning. *Int J Psychoanal.* 1961; 42:317.

70. Engel G. Grief and grieving. *Am J Nursing.* 1964; 64:93.

71. Harper B. *Death: The Coping Mechanisms of the Health Professional.* Greenville, NC: Southeastern University Press; 1977.

72. Shua-Haim JR, Sabo MR, Ross JS. Delirium in the elderly. *Clin Geriatr.* 1999; 7(3):47–64.

73. Dobmeyer K. Delirium in elderly medical patients. *Clin Geriatr.* 1996; 4:43–68.

74. Berkow R. Cognitive failure: Delirium and dementia. In: Abrams WB, Beers MH, Berkow R, eds. *The Merck Manual of Geriatrics.* 2nd ed. Whitehouse Station, NJ: Merck & Co., Inc.; 1995: 1139–1146.

75. Pompei P, Casall CK. Delirium in hospitalized elderly patients. *Hosp Proc.* 1993; July 15:49–56.

76. Glenner G. Alzheimer's disease (senile dementia) a research update and critique with recommendations. *J Am Geriatc Soc.* 1982; 30:59–62.

77. Rocca W, Amaducci LA, Shoenberg BS, et al. Epidemiology of clinically diagnosed Alzheimer's disease. *Ann Neurol.* 1981; 19:415.

78. Gurland B, Cross P. Epidemiology of psychopathology in old age: Some implications for clinical services. *Psychiatric Clinics in N Am.* 1982; 5:11–26.

79. National Institute of Health 2001–2002 Alzheimer's Disease Progress Report Publisher Number 03-5333, July 2003, p. 2.

80. Rossman J. *Clinical Geriatrics.* 2nd ed. Philadelphia: Lippincott; 1979.

81. Eisdorfer C, Cohen D. The cognitively impaired elderly: Differential diagnosis. In: Storandt M, Seigler I, Elias M, eds. *The Clinical Psychology of Aging.* New York: Plenum Press; 1985.

82. Delaney P. Dementia: The search for reversible causes. *South Med Journal.* 1982; 75:707–709.

83. Clarfield A. The reversible dementias: Do they reverse? *Ann Intern Med.* September 1988; 476–486.

84. Laurin D, Verreault R, Lindsay J, MacPherson K, Rockwood K. "Physical activity and risk of cognitive impairment and dementia in elderly persons." *Arch Neurol,* 2001 Mar, 58:498–504.

85. Crowe M, Andel R, Pedersen NL, Johansson B, Gatz M. "Does Participation in Leisure Activities Lead to Reduced Risk of Alzheimer's Disease? A Propectibe Study of Swedish Twins." *Journal of Gerontology: Physical Sciences* 2003, Vol 58B, No. 5 P249–255.

86. Weuve J, Kang JH, Manson JE, Breteler MMB, Ware JH, Grodstein F. "Physical Activity, Including Walking and Cognitive Function in Older Women." *JAMA* 2004; 292:1454–1461.

87. Forsyth E, Ritzline PD. An overview of the etiology, diagnosis, and treatment of Alzheimer disease. *Phys Ther.* 1998; 78(12):1325–1331.

88. Hayter J. Patients who have Alzheimer's disease. *Am J Nurs.* 1974; 74:1460.

89. Mace NL, Rabins PV. *The 36-Hour Day.* 3rd ed. Baltimore: John Hopkins University Press; 1999.

90. Butler R. Agen-ism: Another form of bigotry. *Gerontologist.* 1969; 9:243.

91. Palmore E. Facts on aging—A New York, New York Springer Publish co., 2006 (in press): 17:4.

92. Kemp B. The psychosocial context of geriatric rehabilitation. In: Kemp B, Brummel–Smith K, Ramsdell JW, eds. *Geriatric Rehabilitation.* Boston: Little, Brown; 1990.

93. Kvitek S, Dr Shaver BJ, Blood H, et al. Age bias: physical therapists and older patients. *J Gerontol.* 1986; 41:702.

5

Pathological Manifestations of Aging

Pearls

- The death rate for certain diseases increases more steeply than the overall death rate, which arouses the suspicion that aging predisposes one to the development of the condition or a fatal outcome.

- There are no clinically significant effects on heart function that can solely be ascribed to aging. Therefore, the numerous pathologies seen in the cardiovascular system (e.g., ischemic heart disease, cardiomyopathy, conductive system disease, valvular disease, hypertension, myocardial degeneration, and peripheral vascular disease) account more for the decrements in the function of the system.

- The two most common types of diseases affecting the respiratory system are pneumonias, which compromise gas exchange and serve as a source for sepsis, and chronic obstructive lung disease and emphysema, which affect the amount of airflow in the lungs.

- The most commonly seen conditions affecting bone in older adults include osteoporosis, osteopenia, osteomalacia, Paget's disease, and joint changes (e.g., degenerative arthritis or os-

teoarthritis, rheumatoid arthritis, gout, temporal arteritis or polymyalgia, and spondyloarthropathies).

- Diseases of the neuromuscular system (e.g., CNS and peripheral nervous system dysfunction, confusion, dementia and delirium, Alzheimer's disease, cerebrovascular disease, Parkinson's disease, Huntington's disease, amyotrophic lateral sclerosis, normal pressure hydrocephalus, cervical spondylosis, spinal cord injury, and peripheral nervous system problems), like those of the cardiovascular system, are much more responsible for the decrements seen in aging than the effects of aging.

- Vestibular problems in the elderly are numerous and include benign paroxysmal positional vertigo, acute vestibular neuritis or labyrinthitis, Ménière's disease, and bilateral vestibular disorders.

- Two life-threatening conditions, hypothermia and hyperthermia, need to be recognized and treated in the elderly. The regulation of body temperature will greatly impact an individual's homeostatic well-being during activity and exercise and must be considered when prescribing exercise.

Introduction

Aging is considered a normal physiological process because of its universality. As much as the aging process may influence the predisposition to disease, aging in and of itself is not considered to be pathological. This distinction seems conceptually clear; however, the fine line between aging and disease is often blurred when applied to specific cases, and some degree of decreasing biological, physiological, anatomical, and functional capabilities occurs as one ages. (See Chapter 3.) Some degree of atrophy is evident in all tissues of the body. A variety of degenerative processes are called "normal aging" until they proceed far enough to cause clinically significant disability.

Recent epidemiological genetic study findings indicate pathologic significance of age-related changes such as vascular stiffening and loss of muscle mass,[1] which are genetically driven and were, until recently, considered normal aging. Genes with effects on unrecognized pathologies could be detected through genome scans to identify loci affecting broader outcomes.

Genetic factors may influence not only physiologic functions but also their rates of change with age, which can influence whether and when disease occurs. Rates of change with age in many physiologic functions directly affect risk of age-related morbidity (e.g., changes in bone density, vital capacity, cognitive function, lens opacity, and blood pressure). Another important group includes rates of decline in homeostatic functions, such as glucose tolerance, blood pressure stability, and balance. Rates of change in cellular biochemical properties implicated in age-related pathologies could also be studied, as data are needed on the predictive validity of such changes for mortality, age-related diseases, or functional status.

The incidence of many diseases is influenced markedly as age advances (Fig. 5.1).[2] The death rates for atherosclerosis, myocardial degeneration, hypertension, and cancer all increase more steeply than the overall death rate, which arouses the suspicion that aging predisposes an individual either to the development of the condition or to a fatal outcome. With some conditions, such as respiratory infections, the incidence is not increased in the elderly, but the likelihood of fatality from the insult is greater than in younger persons.[3] In a child or young adult, death is most commonly caused by some form of accident (Fig. 5.2); however, in the elderly, the main problems are coronary heart disease, cerebrovascular accidents, respiratory diseases, diabetes, peripheral vascular diseases, and neoplasms.[4]

The purpose of this chapter is to review those pathologies that are manifested in the aged population, but it will not cover a detailed consideration of every possible geriatric pathology; rather, it will examine some of the more common conditions that afflict the elderly and affect functional activities of daily living.

AGING AS DISEASE

There is always the tacit implication that aging, like growth and development, is a normal physiological process lying outside the domain of disease. Though aging may not be considered a disease process, the time-dependent loss of structure and function in all organ systems leads to pathological end states. There is a general

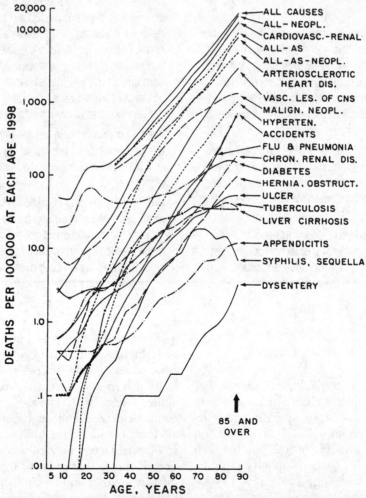

Figure 5.1   Age-specific death rates from selected causes. (Created graph from statistics garnered from: US Bureau of the Census. Statistical Abstract of the United States. Profiles of Older Americans: 1999. Washington DC: US Bureau of the Census. 2000.)

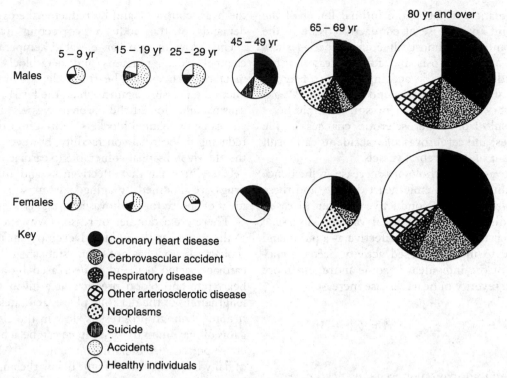

Figure 5.2   Principal causes of death for each sex at different ages. (Created from statistics garnered from: Administration on Aging. Older Americans 2000: Key Indicators of Well-Being. Federal Interagency. Forum on Aging-Related Statistics. Washington DC: US Bureau of the Census. 2000.)

decline in structure, function, and number of many kinds of cells with age. Cellular aging is accompanied by denaturation of extracellular proteins. The collagen and elastin of the skin become irreversibly crystalline and broken. The hyaline cartilage on articular surfaces of joints becomes fibrillar and fragmented, and the beautifully ordered structure of the lens of the eye becomes brittle and chaotic as lens protein is gradually denatured.

The aging process proceeds slowly and ubiquitously over the life course resulting in a loss of structure and function within every organ or tissue. Countless microtraumas occur and accumulate in small increments as imperceptible injuries. Over a lifetime, the skin elastin is exposed to microinsults from ultraviolet rays from the sun, repetitive mechanical stresses cause degeneration of articular cartilage, and reactions with metabolites diminish the opacity of the lens of the eye. The most important aging changes occur at the molecular level, as reviewed in Chapter 2, Comparing and Contrasting the Theories of Aging. Small injuries occurring within the cell result in the loss of genetic memory and progressive cross-linking of collagen, the chief structural protein in the body.

Wiley Forbus, a pathologist, defined disease as the reaction to injury.[5] If aging is a gradual accumulation of incompletely repaired injuries due to microtrauma through the life course, it may not be normal, despite its universality. Perhaps "aging" is a pathological process resulting from tissue reactions to imperceptible, avoidable injuries.

Physical and occupational therapists could play a major role in preventing the disabilities that result from these insidious microtraumas. Preventive strengthening and conditioning exercises, positioning, joint and tissue mobilization, and the numerous modalities that could be employed all impact functional capabilities, especially in an aged population. From the authors' clinical perspective, preventing disabilities that can result from pathological processes greatly improves the level of function and the quality of life. There are certainly changes that occur in aging that don't need to be inevitable.

CARDIOVASCULAR MANIFESTATIONS OF AGING

There are no clinically significant effects on heart function which can be ascribed to aging alone. Cardiovascular dysfunction attributed to the aging process closely mimics the decline in cardiac function seen with inactivity.[6–8] "Arteriosclerosis" is a generally used term to describe any form of vascular degeneration associated with a thickening and loss of resilience in the arterial wall.[9] Atherosclerosis is a more specific type of degeneration that is associated with an accumulation of fat in the intimal lining of the blood vessels and an increase of connective tissue in the underlying subintima.[9] Almost all animal species show some degree of atherosclerosis, and, for this reason, it has been considered an inevitable accompaniment of aging. The pathological consequences depend on the site. Weakness in the aorta can cause an aneurysm; ischemic heart disease can result from atherosclerotic changes in the coronary arteries; and cerebrovascular accidents can result from involvement of the cerebral vessels.[10]

Other cardiovascular pathologies increase in incidence with age in addition to ischemic heart disease, and these include cardiomyopathies, conductive system diseases, valvular heart disease, and peripheral vascular disease.[11] The result is that the heart is less effective as a pump and has less reserve to meet increased activity needs. Functional abilities of the individual become more and more restricted as the severity of heart disease increases.

Ischemic Heart Disease in the Elderly

For background information on ischemic heart disease, see CD.

In the elderly, anginal pain is not a consistent symptomatic indicator of ischemia of the cardiac tissue. The elderly more commonly report dyspnea (shortness of breath). Clinically, shortness of breath is a much more reliable indicator of ischemia than is anginal pain in the elderly individual.[12] There is a general correlation between ST segment depression on the EKG and the onset of anginal symptoms,[9] though in the elderly, marked ST segment depression occurs with dyspnea without the development of the characteristic anginal pain.[12]

Early intervention in ischemic heart disease takes several forms. The most important is to reduce the risk factors that predispose individuals to the development of coronary artery disease, such as cigarette smoking, high blood pressure, and serum cholesterol. Secondary prevention of heart attacks, once CAD is established, requires the reduction of risk factors as well as the use of aspirin to prevent platelet aggregation, which may initiate obstruction of a coronary artery, and beta-blockers, which appear to limit the extent of muscle injury. Management of symptomatic coronary artery disease is similar in all age groups, and consists of medical and surgical interventions. Since the pathophysiology of coronary artery disease is the mismatch between the metabolic demands of the heart muscle and the ability of the coronary arteries to supply blood, interventions are directed at decreasing the metabolic needs of the heart muscle or increasing the ability of the coronary arteries to carry blood. The metabolic demands of heart muscle can be reduced by lowering the pressure against which the heart has to push, by reducing the rate at which the heart contracts, and by reducing the overall metabolic demands of the body by correcting hyperthyroidism, anemia, low oxygen, or elevated temperature. Calcium channel blocking agents and beta-blockers reduce the metabolic demands on heart muscle, and nitroglycerine reduces the pressure against which the heart has to pump by causing dilitation of the coronary vessels. Beta-blockers[13] and calcium channel blockers[14] often improve function by reducing myocardial contractility; however, this may leave the elderly individual vulnerable to cardiac failure. It is still debated how far the effectiveness and toxicity of these drugs are modified by aging.[15] Exercise is still the treatment of choice for cardiovascular diseases.

There are a number of reasons why exercise is helpful to the patient with angina.[9] Development of an enhanced "collateral" flow has not been established.[16] However, the cardiac oxygen demand is decreased by a drop in both heart rate and blood pressure at a given workload. The lengthening of the diastolic phase facilitates coronary perfusion.[9] Though progress is slow in the elderly, dramatic gains of maximum oxygen intake can be achieved if the exercise periods are of sufficient lengths.[9,17] Many activities of daily living can be brought below the anginal threshold by exercise training. Strengthening of the skeletal muscles may help to reduce blood pressure and, therefore, to reduce the likelihood of developing anginal symptoms during functional activities of daily living.

Cardiomyopathy/Congestive Heart Failure

Cardiomyopathies are conditions in which the heart muscle hypertrophies and cardiac function is impaired, often resulting in congestive heart failure.[10] The muscle of the heart weakens because of poor nutrition, toxins, infections, or genetic factors.[5] The weakening results in dilation of the heart and can lead to congestive heart failure because the heart cannot contract strongly enough to empty a sufficient amount of blood into the peripheral vasculature to meet the body's needs. Hypertrophy of cardiac muscle tissue can be the end results of hypertension, outflow obstruction, or genetic factors.[10] The cardiovascular changes imposed by cardiomyopathies impair function through several pathological mechanisms. The hypertrophied heart is stiff and does not easily fill with blood. As a result, the heart contracts vigorously but there is little forward circulation to show for the effort and the body's energy and oxygen needs are not met. In hypertrophic cardiomyopathy, the muscle abnormally contracts, actually creating an obstruction to the outflow of blood from the heart. The more strongly the heart contracts, the greater is the obstruction.

Exercise has historically been contraindicated in the patient with cardiomyopathy; however, that perspective is rapidly changing as the benefits of exercise in this condition are documented and acknowledged.[18–20] Medical treatment is directed at correcting or ameliorating the pathophysiology of the underlying cause of the heart failure. Rehabilitative efforts need to be directed toward maintaining and improving the maximal functional capabilities of the elderly individual and preventing the debilitating effects of immobility.

> For more background on congestive heart failure (CHF), see CD.

Here are two evidence-based strategies:

Hemodynamic Responses During Aerobic and Resistance Exercise; by Karlsdotter; *J Cardiopulm Rehabil*; 6-02[21]

- Left ventricular function remains stable during moderate intensity resistance exercise even in patients with CHF.
- This form of exercise can be used safely in a rehabilitation program.

Exercise Training in Patients with Heart Failure; by Keteyian; *Ann Intern Med*; 96[22]

- Compensated heart failure due to left ventricular dysfunction benefits significantly from regular moderate aerobic exercise.
- The program—3×/wk, 12 weeks.
- How it works:
  - in cardiac output
  - reduction in vascular resistance
  - amelioration of muscle metabolism on the cellular level

Conduction System Diseases

Conduction system diseases are those which affect the rate and rhythm of the heart's contractions.[10] The propagation of the electrical wave which results in the coordinated contraction of the heart muscle is initiated in the two pacemaker sites in the heart and carried initially along specialized pathways that spread the wave throughout the heart, also known as the conduction system. These pacemakers and pathways can be damaged by many different agents, including those that result in cardiomyopathies and myocardial infarction.[23] The most common consequences of pacemaker dysfunction are extremely rapid (tachycardic) contractions, poorly coordinated (dysrhythmic) contractions, or extremely slow (bradycardic) contractions that are less effective in moving blood and result in diminished cardiac output.[9] Low cardiac output can result in confusion, fatigue, poor exercise tolerance, and congestive heart failure. Rapid reductions in cardiac output can cause syncope.

Tachycardias and poorly coordinated rhythms, such as atrial fibrillation, are usually treated with medication to control the rate and convert the rhythm back to normal. Occasionally, electrical cardioversion is required.[10] Bradycardia is usually managed by surgical implantation of an artificial pacemaker, which can be set to trigger a heartbeat at a predetermined rate. Age, per se, is not a contraindication to pacemaker therapy, and the surgery is minor and well tolerated.

Valvular Disease of the Heart

The heart valves, which function to keep the blood flowing in one direction, tend to withstand many microtraumas throughout the life course. Defects of the heart valves are of two types. Stenosis or narrowing of the valve restricts blood flow,[10] and insufficiency or regurgitation results in the backward flow of blood. Both conditions increase the workload on the heart and greatly reduce its efficiency.[9] Two valves are most frequently involved: the mitral valve between the left atrium and ventricle, and the aortic valve, which moves the blood into the systemic circulation.

Rheumatic valve disease, caused by earlier episodes of rheumatic fever, is the most common cause of mitral stenosis and insufficiency in the aged.[23] Congestive heart failure, arrhythmias, and embolization of blood clots from the heart to the brain and other organs are the most common complications of mitral valve disease. These patients require attentive medical management, which includes the use of anticoagulants to prevent emboli, diuretics to control congestive heart failure, and digitalis or other medications to control the heart rate.[10] Nutritional support is often required to assure compliance with a low sodium diet. Because of the potentially serious side effects from too much anticoagulant (bleeding, hemorrhagic stroke) and digoxin (arrhythmias), the narrow range of effective dosages, and the deleterious effect of inadequate dosage, exercise must be gradually implemented and progressed slowly. Protective intervention should focus on skin protection and maintenance of maximal functional capabilities, with close monitoring of the individual's vital signs and subjective responses of perceived tolerance to increasing activity levels.

> For additional information on valvular disease of the heart, see CD.

Hypertension

Hypertension is another common condition affecting the cardiovascular system. It is clear that the aged with systolic blood pressures above 160 mm Hg and diastolic pressures above 95 mm Hg are at increased risk for stroke, congestive heart failure (hypertensive cardiomyopathy), and renal failure. Isolated systolic hypertension carries a similar risk,[10] because much of the cardiovascular morbidity and mortality in the elderly is related to hypertension.[2] This is true for both isolated systolic hypertension and systolic-diastolic blood pressure elevations.[24] In addition to accelerated atherogenesis (myocardial infarction and congestive heart failure), hypertension adversely affects cardiac performance, renal function, and cerebral blood flow. It also increases aortic aneurysm rupture and dissection, and increases the incidence of cerebrovascular bleeding.[25]

Treatment to lower blood pressure significantly reduces the risks of developing these complications. Medical and dietary management are important in controlling hypertension. In the elderly, most recommendations are for drug treatment for blood pressure readings in excess of 160/95.[25] There is little proof that antihypertensive drug therapy alters the course of asymptomatic elderly individuals without evidence of end-organ damage from isolated systolic hypertension.

Nevertheless, isolated systolic hypertension doubles the risk of cardiovascular complications, so that the risk, expense, and inconvenience of drug therapy must be compared with the benefits of lower systolic blood pressure. Compliance with medication and the early identification and avoidance of drug-induced side effects, such as dizziness, hypokalemia, depression, syncope, and confusion, are major challenges to the health care team. Complications of antihypertensive therapy are more frequent in the elderly individual, both because the diminution of renal function increases the incidence of drug toxicity and because the aged patient with less sensitive baroreceptor responses is more susceptible to the orthostatic complications of volume depletion. Assuming the upright posture gradually may help avert dizziness and syncope. Exercise has been shown to have positive effects in reducing high blood pressure.

Here are three evidence-based treatment studies.

The Effects of Aerobic Exercise and T'ai Chi on Blood Pressure in Older People: Randomized Trial; by Young; *J Am Geriatr Soc*; 99[26]

- Blood pressure improved in both groups, more so in the aerobic group.
- Aerobic capacity improved in only the aerobic exercise group.

Effect of Aerobic Exercise Training in Community Based Subjects Aged 80 and Older; by Vaitkevicius; *J Am Geriatr Soc*; 02[27]

Subjects aged 80 and older can improve aerobic capacity and reduce systolic blood pressure in an aerobic exercise program.

Progressive Resistance Exercise and Resting Blood Pressure; by Kelley; *Hypertension*; 2000[28]

Progressive resistive exercise is efficacious for reducing resting systolic and dyastolic blood pressure.

Myocardial Degeneration

The general decline of cardiac performance with age and with inactivity affects the ability of elderly individuals to function at their maximum. The recognized changes in cardiac function include a decrease in right ventricular work rate and a variable change of left ventricular work rate depending on the relative magnitudes of the reduction in maximum cardiac output and the increase of systemic blood pressure.[9,29] While a young person readily accepts a sustained increase of cardiac work rate, in old age an equivalent relative stress may give rise to cardiac failure, particularly if there are other circulatory problems such as a high systemic blood pressure, a minor disorder of the heart valves, or an excessive intake of fluids. Complaints of shortness of breath in the elderly frequently reflect problems with getting enough oxygen to the working muscle through a failing circulatory system.

For more information on myocardial degeneration, see CD.

Peripheral Vascular Disease

Peripheral vascular disease is frequently the result of untreated hypertension, cigarette smoking, diabetes mellitus, and elevated serum cholesterol.[23] Atherosclerosis and other forms of peripheral vascular disease can lead to partial or complete obstruction of the main arterial supply to the limbs. The consequences are intermittent claudication with walking and skin lesions which may lead to amputation.[9] When early intervention to reduce risk factors is unsuccessful, management is through the modification of diet to reduce weight and cholesterol, medications to enhance blood flow and reduce blood pressure, and behavior modifications to reduce cigarette consumption. Exercise is particularly helpful in treating peripheral vascular disease from a preventative perspective.[9,30–33]

For more information on peripheral vascular disease, see CD.

Here are the evidence-based studies for PAD.

The Effect of Exercises on Walking Distance of Patients with Intermittent Claudication: A Study of Randomized Clinical Trials; by Brandsma; *Phys Ther*; 3-98[34]

- Analysis of literature.
- All studies showed that walking exercises improved walking distance.
- Patients should be encouraged to exercise to point of maximum claudication pain.

Intermittent Claudication: Implementation of an Exercise Program; by Hunt; *Physiotherapy*; 99[35]

- Non-weight-bearing warm-up and cool down and stretching exercise for lower extremity.
- Main session (past pain).
  - alternating heel raises
  - simultaneous heel raises
  - step-ups on low bench
  - toe walking
- Patients were encouraged to walk (past pain).

Exercise Training for Patients with Peripheral Artery Disease; by Gardner; *Phys and Sports Med*; 8-01[36]

Recommended Exercise Program for Patients Who Have Peripheral Artery Disease

Exercise Component	Detail
Frequencey	3 sessions per week
Intensity	Progression from 50% of peak exercise
	Capacity to 80% by program's end
Duration	Progression from 15 min of exercise
	Per session to more than 30 min by program's end
Mode	Walking, non-weight-bearing tasks (bicycling)
	May be used for warm-up and cool down
Type of Exercise	Intermittent walking to near maximal, claudication pain
Program Length	At least 6 months

Treatment Efficacy of Intermittent Claudication by Surgical Intervention, Supervised Physical Exercise Training Compared to No Treatment in Unselected Randomised Patients; by Gelin; *Eur J Endo Vasc Surg*; 8-01[37]

Invasive treatment increased walking capacity, leg blood flow, and pressure. Supervised physical exercise training offered no therapeutic advantage compared to untreated controls.

Increasing Exercise Tolerance of Persons Limited by Claudication Pain Using Polestriding; by Langbein; *J Vasc Surg*; 5-02[38]

RCT of 24-weeks polestriding significantly improves measures of exercise tolerance limited by intermittent claudication pain. (Polestriding simulates cross-country skiing.)

Exercise Rehabilitation Improves Functional Outcomes and Peripheral Circulation in Patients with Intermittent Claudication; by Gardner; *J Am Geriatr Soc*; 01[39]

Exercise is beneficial well into a 12-month maintenance program (3x/wk for 30 min).

The Effects of Exercise Training on Walking Function and Perception of Health Status in Elderly Patients with PAD; by Tsai; *J Intern Med*; 02[40]

- Significant improvements in claudication (walking time, pain, and function)
- Rx:
  - 12 weeks
  - 5 min warm-up and cool down
  - begin 10 min and increase the grade of treadmill
  - encouraged to walk to 30 min and a grade of 2–3 pain (moderate)

Efficacy of a Short-Course Intensive Rehabilitation Program in Patients with Moderate-to-Severe Intermittent Claudication; by Ambrosetti; *Ital Heart J*; 02[41]

Treatment and outcomes are the same as above but 4 weeks long.

PULMONARY MANIFESTATIONS OF AGING

For a review of pulmonary manifestations of aging see CD.

Pneumonia

Pneumonia is the most common infectious cause of death in the elderly[42] and the most common infection requiring hospitalization. It is often the means of death for patients with other serious conditions, such as diabetes, cancer, stroke, congestive heart failure, dementia, and renal failure. The increased incidence of pneumonia with aging is due in part to the weakening of the local pulmonary defenses; however, the high mortality of pneumonia is largely due to its more subtle presentation in the elderly. Typical symptoms such as a productive cough, fever, and pleuritic chest pain are frequently absent, but subtler symptoms, such as confusion, alteration of sleep-wake cycles, increased congestive heart failure, anorexia, and failure to thrive, are more common. A typically lower core temperature in an older, inactive adult, results in a failure to recognize that the individual has a fever. Misdiagnosis and late diagnosis are common and contribute to the high mortality of pneumonia in the elderly.[42]

Successful treatment of pneumonia requires early recognition and institution of proper antibiotic therapy. The identification of causative bacteria in the examination of a sputum sample is the single most important diagnostic test for determining initial antibiotic therapy. Unfortunately, such samples are often difficult to obtain in a dehydrated and confused elderly patient, and, as a result, therapy is often empirical and not as specifically directed or effective as possible. Hydration, nutritional support, chest physical therapy, and treatment of complicating illnesses are often required in addition to antibiotics.

Cardiovascular Pathologes & Therapeutics Conducts

Pathology	Definition	Difference in the Aged	Therapeutic Considerations with Age
Ischemic Heart Disease (CAD)	Insufficient blood flow to the cardiac muscle	Fatigue and dyspnea are more common complaints than angina	Observe changes in respiratory rate and patients complaint of fatigue. May use Borg scale as a form of monitoring exertion. Progressive aerobic exercises and strengthening exercises may be used. Avoid isometric activities leading to Valsalva maneuver.
Congestive Heart Failure	Inability of the heart muscle to contract strongly enough to meet the vascular demands of the body	Very common with age	Exercise is prescribed per client tolerance and disease stage (mild to moderate CHF). Supervised aerobic and resistance training program are important to improve functional capacity. Avoid isometric activities leading to Valsalva maneuver. Monitor fatigue, dyspnea, and systolic blood pressure.
Conduction System Problems	Changes in heart rate and rhythm	Very common with age	Monitor pulse rate and especially rhythm. Blood pressure monitoring during activity is also very important. Continue monitoring patient after activity. Cool-down phase is important to avoid a sudden decrease in venous return. Exercise to patient's tolerance. Always observe for signs of confusion, fatigue, and syncope.

Cardiovascular Pathologes & Therapeutics Conducts (Continued)

Pathology	Definition	Difference in the Aged	Therapeutic Considerations with Age
Valvular Disease	Defects in the heart valves which can restrict or cause backward flow of the blood in the heart. Valve disease usually increases workload of the heart	Very common with age	Exercise within rate of perceived exertion (RPE) of 11 to 14. During exercise observe for dyspnea, fatigue, weakness, pallor, and/or confusion. Stop exercise with pronounced coughing of patients with mitral valve disease. Medication may blunt heart rate and make it difficult to monitor. Slowly progress aerobic exercise. Alternate days of activity to ensure maximal recuperation.
Hypertension	Increased blood pressure: Stage I (mild) 140–159/90–99 Stage II (moderate) 160–179/100–109 Stage III (severe) >180/> 110	Tends to increase with aging and associate cardiac and peripheral diseases	Beware of adverse effects of antihypertensives. Medications can contribute to orthostatic hypotension, arrythmias, and agina during exercise. Use progressive aerobics with longer periods of warm-up and cool down. Monitor blood pressure before, during, and after activity. Be aware of abnormal symptoms such as dizziness, syncope, headaches, weakness, and fatigue.
Myocardial Degeneration	General decline of cardiac performance with age	Slow HR recovery and possible absence of anticipated ^ in SBP with exercise	Need for frequent rest with exercise. Encourage exercise but go slowly.
Peripheral Vascular Disease	Partial or complete obstruction of blood flow to the limbs. May be arterial or venous disease	More common with age, inactivity, and disease. Very common in patients with CAD	Encourage progressive exercise to tolerance. Patients with intermittent claudication should exercise until symptoms are present, followed by rest and return to activity as soon as symptoms decrease. Monitor heart rate and blood pressure during exercise routine.
Pneumonia	Lung infection	Most common infectious cause of death in the elderly. Sudden change in mood may be indicative of infection	Hydration and chest PT. Elder patients may be more susceptible to broken ribs.

Obstructive and Resistive Lung Disease

Conditions that cause obstruction to airflow within the lungs are called obstructive airway diseases, while conditions that result in resistance to airflow are called resistive airway diseases. They share the common characteristic of increased resistance to airflow within the airways.[43]

For background on obstructive and resistive lung disease, see CD.

The treatment goal of individuals with COPD is to prevent smoking and maintain optimum functioning for as long as possible. This usually involves chest physical therapy, medication, oxygen therapy, and environmental changes designed to conserve energy and reduce exertion. The depression that accompanies chronic illness of all types can be particularly significant in COPD patients, many of whom feel that they have brought it on themselves by smoking. Because of its complexity, COPD is an excellent example of a health problem that requires an interdisciplinary approach.

Here are a few evidence-based studies showing the efficacy of rehabilitation for COPD.

Improvement in Exercise Tolerance and Spirometric Values in Stable Chronic Obstructive Pulmonary Disease Patients After an Individualized Outpatient Rehabilitation Program; by Alfaro; *J Sports Med Phys Fitness*; 9–96[44]

Individualized outpatient rehabilitation programs are able to improve exercise tolerance in stable COPD patients affected by dyspnea during exercise, through reconditioning of both skeletal and respiratory muscles and improved gas exchange during exercise, thus reducing the ratio of dead space to tidal volume.

Physiological Benefits of Exercise Training in the Rehabilitation of Patients with Severe COPD; by Casaburi; *Am J Resp Crit Care Med*; 97[45]

- Rigorous exercise training for patientsts with COPD yields more efficient exercise breathing pattern and improved exercise tolerance.
- Program = 3d/wk, for 8 weeks, 80% work rate, 45 minutes.

The Cost/Benefits of Outpatient-Based Pulmonary Rehabilitation; by Rosenbaum, *Arch Phys Med Rehabil*; 3–97[46]

- Program consisted of education, training, group therapy, and individualized home exercise.
- Patients cycled 2x/day, 7d/wk, active range of motion, used inspiratory muscle trainer, 2x/day.
  - weekly patient education on energy conservation, relaxation, smoking etc.
- Results: Patients improved on cardiopulmonary parameters and activities of daily living.
- Cost of 10 sessions $650.

Musculoskeltal Manifestations of Aging

For background on musculoskeletal manifestations of aging, see CD.

Fibromyalgia/Myofibralgia

Fibromyalgia, also called myofibralgia, is a common form of nonarticular rheumatism with diffuse musculoskeletal aching and multiple tender points at characteristic sites.[47]

For more information on fibromyalgia/myofibralgia, see CD.

Short-term exercise and educational programs can produce immediate and sustained benefits for patients with fibromyalgia.[48] Here are some evidence-based studies for fibromyalgia.

Prescribing Exercise for Fibromyalgia Patients; by Clark; *Arthritis Care Res*; 12-94[49]

- Avoid eccentric exercise.
- Avoid high-intensity exercise.
- Prescribe stretching after exercise.
- Exercise at 60% to 70% of max HR.
- Use active range of motion as a warm-up.

Effects of Pool-Based and Land-Based Aerobic Exercise; by Jentoff; *Arthritis Care Res*; 02-01[50]

- Pool and land exercise beneficial[50]
- –1×/wk for 20 weeks
- Improve strength, fatigue
- Improve cardiovascular parameters
- Decrease pain

The Effects of Progressive Strength Training and Aerobic Exercise; by Rooks; *Arthritis Rheum*; 2-03[51]

- 60 min/session, 3x/wk, for 20 weeks
- 4 weeks of active range of motion in the pool
- 16 weeks of land cardiovascular exercise, progressive resistive exercise, and flexibility that progressed as the person tolerated

---

Biofeedback/Relaxation Training and Exercise Interventions for Fibromyalgia: A Prospective Trial; by Buckelew; *Arthritis Care Res*; 6-98[52]

- 120 patientsts assigned to 1 of 4 groups.
  - biofeedback/relaxation
  - exercise training
  - combination
  - education/attention
- All three groups improved in self-efficacy.
- The exercise and combination group improved in physical activity and kept benefit longest.

Effects of a 1.5 Day Multidisciplinary Outpatient Treatment Program for Fibromyalgia; by Pfeiffer; *Am J Phys Med Rehabil*; 3-03[53]

- Rx = education, self-management, OT and PT
- Rx group = improved in function

A Comparative Evaluation of a Fibromyalgia Rehabilitation Program; by Bailey; *Arthritis Care Res*; 10-99[54]

- Fibro-Fit was effective in improving physical impairments and function.
- Fibro-Fit:
  - 12 weeks, 3x/wk
  - PT, OT, SW
  - orientation, self-management, goal setting, stretching strengthening, aerobics
  - counseling—sleep, stress, fatigue, nutrition, coping

SKELETAL MANIFESTATIONS OF AGING

For more information on the skeletal manifestations of aging, see CD.

Osteoporosis

Osteoporosis is a heterogeneous condition characterized by an absolute decrease in the amount of normal bone (i.e., loss of bone). Osteoporosis is defined as a metabolic bone disease "characterized by low bone mass and microarchitectural deterioration of bony tissue leading to enhanced bone fragility and a consequent increase in fracture risk."[55] Osteoporosis results when the production of new bone mass is exceeded by the reabsorption of old bone; in other words, osteoporosis is the failure of bone formation to keep pace with bone resorption. This is termed coupling. The result is that bone becomes structurally weakened.

For more information on osteoporosis, see CD.

Bone mineral density (BMD) as measured by dual x-ray absorptiometry (DXA) is expressed as absolute BMD (g/cm^2) and may be designated by either the number of standard deviations (SD) from the mean of age-matched controls (known as Z score) or the number of SD from the young normal mean (T score).[56] The World Health Organization (WHO) developed guidelines for the clinical diagnosis of osteoporosis, which are based on the T score, with a T score of less than –1.0 being defined as osteopenic and a T score of less than –2.5 being referred to as osteoporosis. An outline of these diagnostic criteria for osteoporosis is shown in Table 5.1.[57]

The WHO guidelines for T scores are as follows: (1) a T score above −1.0 is defined as "normal"; (2) a T score between −1.0 to −2.5 is defined as "osteopenic"; (3) a T score below −2.5 is defined as "osteoporotic"; and (4) a T score below −2.5, plus one or more fragility fractures, is defined as "severely osteoporotic." This classification is particularly important for the physical or occupational therapist prescribing exercise and determining levels of risk for fractures and frailty. The authors of the book have added preventive "actions" to those prescribed by WHO in Table 5–1, in addition to expanding the criteria to provide suggested prescriptions for rehabilitative interventions.

Osteopenia

The term "osteopenia" describes an evenly systemic decrease in bone density below an expected level. Therefore, bone loss is not unilateral or limited to one area of the skeleton. Osteopenia is the prelude to osteoporosis. Table 5.1 indicates the BMD range that differentiates osteopenia from osteoporosis.

For more information on osteomalacia and osteonecrosis, see CD.

Paget's Disease

Paget's disease (PD, also called osteitis deformans) is a disorder of bone remodeling characterized by increased bone resorption and increased formation. It usually presents

TABLE 5.1   Modified WHO Criteria for Osteoporosis (Added Enhanced "Action" and "Rehabilitation Prescription")[57]

Category	Fracture Risk	Action	Rehabilitation Prescription
Normal BMD < 1 SD below young adult reference range	Below average	Be watchful for "clinical triggers" Preventive interventions: diet and exercise	Trunk extension exercises Resistive exercises Weight-bearing exercises Deep breathing exercises Aerobic exercise
Osteopenia BMD 1–2.5 SD below young adult reference range	Above average	Consider hormone replacement therapy Be watchful for "clinical triggers" Nutritional supplements Drug therapy as warranted Repeat investigations 2–3 years	Trunk extension exercises Resistive exercises Weight-bearing exercises Deep breathing exercises Aerobic exercise Functional activities Environmental modifications Fall prevention program
Osteoporosis BMD > 2.5 SD below young adult reference mean	High	Exclude secondary causes Therapeutic intervention indicated: Diet, exercise, supplementation, drug therapy as warranted Hormone replacement therapy	Trunk extension exercises Resistive exercises Weight-bearing exercises Deep breathing exercises Functional activities Environmental modifications Fall prevention program
Severe Osteoporosis BMD > 2.5 SD below young adult reference mean, plus one or more fragility fractures	Extremely high	Exclude secondary causes Therapeutic intervention indicated: Diet, exercise, supplementation, drug therapy as warranted Established osteoporosis	Trunk extension exercises Weight-bearing exercises Deep breathing exercises Functional activities Environmental modification Fall prevention program Protective clothing as warranted

Source: World Health Organization (see ref 57)

after the fourth decade of life and its prevalence increases with age to affect 1% to 2% of individuals over age 60 in the United States, with a slight male predominance.[58] It is usually a focal disease involving one bone (monostotic), but it can involve several bones (polystotic). In rare cases, PD can become generalized, especially in familial disease. Osteogenic sarcoma is a dreaded complication of PD in the elderly.[58]

Increased and abnormal osteoclastic bone resorption is the initiating event in PD. There is accumulating evidence that a slow virus plays a role in its pathogenesis. Increased interleukin-6 (IL-6) production may be a contributing factor to the development of PD. Genetic mechanisms are also likely to be important in familial cases, with possible linkage to chromosome 6 or 18.[58,59]

The rate of bone resorption in PD can be as much as tenfold to twentyfold the normal rate. This is reflected in increased biochemical indices of bone resorption, including urinary excretion of collagen catabolites, like hydroxyproline and collagen cross-linked peptides, and osteoclast products, notably serum acid phosphatase. Osteoblastic new bone formation responds appropriately to the increased resorption, and this is reflected in increased osteoblast products such as alkaline phosphatase and osteocalcin. The increased cellular activity produced highly vascular and cellular bone, and collagen is deposited by overworked osteoblasts in an abnormal and disorganized pattern of "woven bone."[59]

Because the tight coupling of formation and resorption is maintained in PD despite the increased skeletal turnover, systemic mineral homeostasis is usually unperturbed and serum calcium is usually normal. However, when patients with PD are immobilized, as can occur on fracture or surgery, they may become hypercalciuric or even hypercalcemic. This occurs because muscle stimulation of bone formation is decreased and bone resorption proceeds relatively unopposed. Hypercalcemia may also signal the presence of hyperparathyroidism, which is commonly reported with an increased level of calcium in the serum plasma of a patient with PD.[59]

Joint Changes with Aging

For more information on joint changes with aging, see CD.

Degenerative Arthritis/Osteoarthritis

There are several different types of arthritis, but all lead to a common final pathway known as degenerative joint disease (DJD) or osteoarthritis.[60] Recurrent joint trauma leads to intra-articular damage, resulting in the release of proteolytic enzymes, which often causes bleeding. A cycle is set up with increased cartilage damage, bleeding, and the release of potentially distructive enzymes. Over time, cartilage is eroded, new bone growth is stimulated, and the joint gradually loses its ability to respond to trauma, making it even more susceptible to additional trauma and damage.[61] Pain develops because of irritation of the periostium, joint capsule, and fibrotic changes of the periarticular muscles. Unlike rheumatoid arthritis, the synovial membrane in osteoarthritis is not the primary site of involvement. However, over time it can become fibrotic as a result of the primary degenerative process.[60]

The joints most often affected by DJD are the hands, knees, hips, lumbar, and cervical spine. It is manifested clinically by stiffness and pain that increase with use. Impaired mobility makes it difficult to accomplish routine activities of daily living (ADLs).[62]

The onset of symptoms in osteoarthritis can occur insidiously or suddenly. Generally, joint destruction occurs gradually and progresses slowly. Pain is described as a deep ache, can occur at rest, and often awakens the individual at night with nocturnal discomfort. Stiffness of the involved joint(s) after periods of inactivity occurs and usually is resolved in a relatively short period of movement. Loss of flexibility is associated with soft tissue contractures, intra-articular loose bodies, ostephytes, and loss of joint surface congruity.[63]

The development of effective anti-inflammatory medications and improvement of surgical interventions in joint disease has changed the current management of end-stage DJD. Joint replacement can be very effective in restoring function and limiting pain, and joint fusion and anti-inflammatory medications are often effective in pain control.

Rehabilitative treatment is focused on protection of the involved joint from excessive mechanical stresses with the use of an assistive ambulatory device; foot orthotics that provide shock absorption and proper joint positioning; and patient education on nutrition, hydration, and reduction of wear and tear on the joint. Maximizing joint function through flexibility and strengthening exercises is important.

Rheumatoid Arthritis

Rheumatoid arthritis (RA) can occur at any age and is characterized by the abrupt onset of symmetrical joint swelling, erythema, and pain. Inflammation of the synovial membrane results in the release of proteolytic enzymes which perpetuate inflammation and joint damage.[61] A biochemical marker for RA is a positive rheumatoid factor, which is an antibody that reacts with immunoglobulin antibodies found in the plasma. Rheumatoid factor is also often found in the synovial fluid and synovial membranes of individuals with the disease. It is hypothesized that the interaction between rheumatoid factor and the immunoglobulin triggers events that initiate an inflammatory reaction. The leukocytes, monocytes, lymphocytes, and phagocytes attracted in the immune system response lead to the release of lysosomal enzymes, which cause articular cartilage destruction and synovial hyperplasia. These changes also result in the development of destructive vascular granulation tissue called pannus. This tissue proliferates, gradually diminishing the joint space.[62] The pannus contains inflammatory cells which destroy the cartilage, bone, and periarticular tissues leading to joint instability, deformity, or ankylosis.

Symptoms are usually insidious and progress slowly as the disease progresses. Complaints of joint pain, muscle fatigue and weakness, weight loss, and general loss of stamina are common. Inflammation and musculoskeletal symptoms are localized to the specific joint, though multiple joints are usually involved. Morning stiffness is more pronounced and of longer duration than in osteoarthritis. Intense pain can occur following periods of rest. The involved joints tend to be the small joints of the hands and feet, the wrists, shoulders, elbows, hips, knees, and ankles. Essentially every joint is involved in this autoimmune, systemic condition. Eventually deformities occur affecting mobility and basic ADLs. Rheumatoid arthritis is a systemic disease; therefore, other signs and symptoms are often present, including: fever, fatigue, malaise, poor appetite, weight loss, nutritional deficiencies, weakness, anemia, enlarged spleen, and lymphadenopathy (disease of the lymph nodes).[60]

Response to therapy is usually quite good. Treatment needs to focus on reducing pain, maintaining mobility, and minimizing joint restrictions, edema, and joint damage. Given the ease with which the aged develop muscle atropy with disuse, aggressive physical therapy is essential to maintain strength and joint mobility during phases of remission; and occupational therapy is required to focus on joint protection and basic ADLs. During exacerbation, physical and occupational therapy should be directed toward pain management through decreasing swelling in the joint (ice, electrical stimulation), maintaining joint mobility and decreasing discomfort (oscillation joint mobility techniques, active motion), and encouraging participation in functional ADL. Foot orthotics are recommended to reduce shock and reposition the foot to lessen the stresses on the involved lower extremity joints.[64]

For more information on gout temporal arteritis/polymyalgia rheumatica, and spondyloarthropathies, see CD.

NEUROMUSCULAR MANIFESTATIONS OF AGING

For move information on the neuromuscular manifestations of aging in the central nervous system, see CD.

Confusion/Delirium

Cognitive disorders of all types account for nearly two-thirds of nursing home admissions and a significant majority of those elderly persons who are incapacitated by illness.[65] Severe cognitive dysfunction may not impair an individual's longevity, especially with meticulous attention to treatable complicating illnesses. As a result, the aged with cognitive dysfunction make up the largest group of functionally disabled individuals.

Those conditions resulting in alterations in cognitive function can be divided into several groups on the basis of reversibility and chronicity. Acute cognitive dysfunction of rapid onset without underlying damage to brain tissue carries the best prognosis for recovery. This usually results from toxic or metabolic derangements, which affect the normal functioning of the brain, or from psychiatric illness, such as depression, which also has a metabolic basis. The term "delirium" is used to describe these acute confusional states. Susceptibility to toxic/metabolic delirium (toxic encephalopathy) is not limited to the elderly; however, the more limited metabolic reserve of the aging brain makes the elderly person more sensitive than younger persons to minor stresses.

Confusion, restlessness, agitation, poor attention span, reversal of sleep-wake cycles, hallucinations, and paranoia can all be manifestations of delirium. Subtle changes resulting from correctable toxic/metabolic abnormalities can persist for extended periods before they are recognized as resulting from potentially reversible causes. Appropriate interventions are frequently delayed. It is particularly important for these reversible conditions to be identified by the health care team because failure to intervene in a timely manner can result in permanent cognitive dysfunction. Equally important is the risk that inappropriate treatment will result in further functional impairment or a greatly increased risk of injury. Pathological brain dysfunction resulting from toxic/metabolic causes usually has a good prognosis for recovery when the underlying abnormality is corrected. Table 5.2 lists the more common causes of toxic confusion/delirium in the elderly.

Interventions are directed at identifying and correcting the underlying metabolic abnormality. Although

TABLE 5.2   Common Causes of Toxic/Metabolic Confusion/Delirium in the Elderly.[65]

Drugs	Metabolic Abnormalities
Alcohol	Hypoglycemia
Psychotropics (tranquilizers, antipsychotics, antidepressants)	Hyponatremia
Over-the-counter sleep, cold, and allergy medications	Hypocalcemia
Analgesics	Hypothermia
Antihypertensives	Hypothyroidism
Beta-blockers (propranolol)	Hypoxia
Antiparkinsonian medications	Vitamin B_{12} deficiency
Anticonvulsants (phenobarbital, phenytoin, carbamazepine)	Hepatic failure (elevated ammonia)
Digoxin	Renal failure (elevated BUN, creatine)
H_2 blockers (cimetadine)	Elevated cortisol
Amphetamines	Cortisol deficiency
	Pulmonary failure (elevated carbon dioxide)

Source: Wedgewood (see ref 65)

the prognosis for return to baseline CNS function is usually good with correction of the abnormality, the patient's overall prognosis is often determined by the underlying disease that causes the metabolic abnormality rather than the degree of brain dysfunction. During a confusional state, however, the individual is more prone to accidental injury, complications such as aspiration pneumonia, and further cognitive dysfunction due to inappropriate use of sedatives that may aggravate rather than relieve the agitation. The occurrence of any of these complications may worsen the overall prognosis for recovery. Acute toxic/metabolic delirium may coexist with chronic progressive forms of brain dysfunction, such as Alzheimer's disease.

Dementias

Dementias are characterized by slow onset of increasing intellectual impairment, including disorientation, memory loss, diminished ability to reason and make sound judgments, loss of social skills, and the development of regressed or antisocial behavior.[66] Frequently, depression is superimposed on dementia as a reaction to the perceived loss of intellectual skills, which leads to further cognitive impairment.[67]

Alzheimer's disease and multi-infarct dementia are the two most common forms of irreversible dementia. Each has a fairly characteristic pattern of onset and findings. Alzheimer's disease is usually slowly progressive and begins insidiously. It is not associated with focal neurological deficits or abrupt changes in severity. Patients typically begin with short-term memory deficits that progress to severely regressed behavior, an inability to learn or remember new tasks, and the loss of ability to perform ADLs.[68] Multi-infarct dementia is usually of more rapid onset, occurs in younger individuals, and progresses in a stepwise fashion with abrupt worsening and subsequent plateaus of function. Frequently, there are focal neurological deficits such as paresis and parethesias.[69] Often, the individual is hypertensive, diabetic, or both. He or she may also show evidence of generalized atherosclerosis.[70]

It is important to distinguish between Alzheimer's and multi-infarct dementias. The prevention of recurrent cerebral infarction may arrest the progression of multi-infarct dementia, which has as its pathophysiological basis irreversible brain damage resulting from repetitive ischemic injury caused by emboli or bleeding. Normalization of blood pressure is the most effective intervention known. Other types of reversible dementia, such as those resulting from hypothyroidism, vitamin B_{12} deficiency, and normal pressure hydrocephalus, can become "fixed" and unresponsive to treatment unless identified and treated at an early stage. Early identification of these correctable dementias is essential. Unfortunately, though no such therapeutic imperative currently exists for Alzheimer's disease, recent research on Alzheimer's has produced promising results, and the potential for delaying

and perhaps preventing the onset of this dreaded dementia looms on the horizon.

Regardless of the etiology of dementia, once reversible causes have been ruled out, the main tasks of the clinical team are to minister to the patient's emotional needs, assist in the act of grieving for lost function, alter the environment so that the patient's remaining skills can be used, augment the patient's capacity to successfully undertake ADLs, educate the family, provide emotional and physical support for the family and caretakers, and provide the patient and family with a realistic prognosis. Any superimposed illness can cause a rapid and prolonged decline in mental status, which may totally resolve as the underlying illness is treated.

Alzheimer's Disease: A Special Consideration

Striking with cruel randomness across an increasingly elderly population, Alzheimer's disease (AD) afflicts some 4 million Americans, most of them over the age of 65.[71] They may range from a former president to a neighbor next door, but the ailment is always the same: it clutters the brain with tiny bits of protein, slowly robbing victims of their mental power until they are no longer able to do even the simplest chores or recognize their closest friends and kin. So far, medical science has been stymied, unable to treat the disease or slow its fatal progression. However, recent research is encouraging. Strategies to prevent or delay the onset of symptoms, as well as to prevent the decline into the advanced stage of AD, are being explored. While these strategies do not yet exist in a proven and clinically applicable form, the science is progressing rapidly.[72] There may yet be a light at the end of that long, dark tunnel called Alzheimer's.

Alzheimer's disease is the form of dementia that is most common in the elderly population. Currently it has been diagnosed in approximately 4 million Americans, and if the present trend continues, it is projected that the number will increase to 14 million by the year 2050. Women are more likely to suffer from AD, with a women to men ratio of 2.8:1.0 for those aged 75 and older. Alzheimer's is the fourth leading cause of death following heart disease, cancer, and stroke.[73–75] One in every ten persons over the age of 65 has Alzheimer's, and approximately half those over the age of 85 are diagnosed with AD.[73,74]

Alzheimer's disease is a progressive, degenerative disease that affects the hippocampus, neocortex, and transcorticol pathways of the spinal cord, resulting in impaired memory and thinking, behavioral changes, and progressive return of primitive motor patterns that were encephalized during late fetal and early childhood development. The classic appearance of neurofibrillary plaques and tangles progressively impedes synaptic connections and results in neuronal death.[76] The neuritic plaques are comprised of amyloid precursor protein (APP), which is encoded for by a gene on chromosome 21. Smaller fragments of APP called amyloid beta peptides (Aβ) have also been identified.[77] The gene carries the code for APP and appears to be one link in the chain of events that leads to deposits of beta amyloid. The neurofibrillary tangles are composed of paired helical filaments that consist of tau proteins and develop in the cytoplasm of pyramidal cells.[77] Neuritic plaques and neurofibrillary tangles are located in the areas of the cerebral cortex linked to intellectual function and sensory integration (just posterior to Wernicke's area) and the hippocampus and neocortex, the two most primitive areas of the brain.[71,78,79]

Some scientists believe that as many as half of all cases of Alzheimer's may have a genetic component. In addition to the abnormality on chromosome 21, chromosome 14 defects have also been identified in individuals with early onset AD. Further support of this theory is the recent discovery of a gene on chromosome 19 that appears to be defective in many people with the more common, late-onset form AD. It has also been found that one form of the apolipoprotein E4 (APOE4) gene is inherited at an increased rate among patients with late-onset Alzheimer's.[77,80] This apolipoprotein is involved in cholesterol metabolism. Chromosome 1 has also been identified to carry a "presenile" gene associated with early-onset AD.[80]

The protease theory of Alzheimer's is also being explored. An enzyme called protease has been identified and isolated in individuals with AD and may play a key role in creating the biochemical chaos in the brain that causes Alzheimer's. This enzyme has become the target of many drug designers. Just as protease inhibitor medications are currently used to block the activity of the autoimmune deficiency (AIDS) virus by targeting proteins (e.g., beta-secretase), it is hypothesized that protease inhibitors may also be effective in blocking amyloid plaque formation.[79] Protease has long been postulated to act as a chemical scissors that helps snip away excess protein from brain cells, thereby inhibiting the buildup of protein debris that accumulates into amyloid plaques.

Nongenetic, environmental factors, such as an infectious agent (e.g., virus), nutritional components, or toxic environmental substances (e.g., metals or industrial chemicals), are also being evaluated for their potential roles in the development of this disease. An example of potential nutritional factors in AD is provided by the Nun Study. Previous studies suggested that low concentrations of folate in the blood are related to poor cognitive function, dementia, and Alzheimer's disease–related neurodegeneration of the brain. Nutrients, lipoproteins, and nutritional markers were measured in participants of the Nun Study who later died between the ages of 78 and 101 years old (mean: 91 years). At autopsy, several neuropathic indicators of AD were determined including atrophy of the neocortex (frontal, temporal, and parietal) and the number of neocortical lesions (senile plaques and neurofibrillary tangles). There was a strong correlation between serum folate and severity of atrophy of the neocortex. Low serum folate was associated with atrophy of the cerebral cortex.[81] Other nutrients, such as the low circulating levels of antioxidants, have been identified as potentially contributing to the development and progression of the disease.

Scientists have now learned that Alzheimer's disease begins at least 20 years before symptoms appear, and prevention and early intervention could potentially improve the quality of life of people predisposed to this disease. Some of the major scientific discoveries related to Alzheimer's disease over the past few years include

- Genes associated with Alzheimer's have been identified on four chromosomes;
- Diagnostic techniques have improved to a 90% accuracy rate (without autopsy);
- The Food and Drug Administration has approved several drugs for the treatment of Alzheimer's, an effective first step toward effective therapies;
- Mounting evidence that readily available treatments, such as estrogen, vitamin E, folate, ibuprofen, and exercise, may help slow or prevent Alzheimer's;
- Associations between higher levels of education and reduced risk of Alzheimer's have been observed;[77] and
- Scientists have learned that Alzheimer's is not caused by a single factor but probably by a number of genetic and environmental factors.

Sister Mary, the gold standard for the Nun Study, was a remarkable woman who had high cognitive test scores before her death at 101 years of age. What is more remarkable is that she maintained this high status despite having abundant neurofibrillary tangles and senile plaques. Findings from Sister Mary and all 678 participants in the Nun Study may provide unique clues about the etiology of aging and Alzheimer's disease, exemplify what is possible in old age, and show how clinical expression of some diseases may be averted.[82]

Cerebrovascular Diseases

In contrast to the dementing illnesses which result in "global" brain dysfunction, cerebrovascular disease more commonly results in focal brain dysfunction.[70] There are several different types of cerebrovascular disease, each with a different pathophysiological mechanism, prognosis, and treatment. The mechanisms include the rupture of small blood vessels from hypertension; abrupt blockage of vessels by emboli from the heart or atheramatous plaques in the large arteries leading to the brain; and spontaneous formation of blood clots within the blood vessels due to local increases in coaguability. The pathophysiology of cerebrovascular disease is the interruption of blood flow to brain tissue with resultant cell damage or death from ischemia.[9] Decreases in the heart's ability to pump blood can lead to ischemia, as can blockage of the blood vessels to or within the brain from atheromatous plaque, emboli, or inflammation of the lining of the blood vessels. Uncontrolled hypertension, diabetes mellitis, smoking, and elevated cholesterol contribute to cerebrovascular disease directly by affecting the entire circulatory system. (See Chapter 11 for EBM strategies.)

Preventive interventions must be specifically directed at the underlying pathophysiology. Hypertension can be controlled by medication, diet, and exercise. The prevention of emboli usually requires the use of anticoagulants such as aspirin, diperiadamole, and warfarin. The risk of bleeding, both into the brain and into other organs, increases with the use of these agents and often limits their use in certain patients. If emboli result from cardiac arrhythmias, prevention results from a return to normal sinus rhythm through the use of electrical cardioversion or antiarrhythmics such as quinidine, procainamide, and digoxin.[23] Because of the heightened risk of intracerebral bleeding, anticoagulants are avoided in the presence of hypertension and in cerebral vascular accidents resulting from bleeding into brain tissue.

Recurrent, small cerebral vascular accidents can result in multi-infarct dementia. More commonly, however, limited areas of the brain are damaged and result in more focal disabilities, including loss of motor or sensory function over the right or left side of the body and alterations in vision, speech, and the ability to interpret sensory inputs. The extent of the deficit following a stroke depends on the location and function of the injured part of the brain, the degree of damage, and the availability of unaffected regions of the brain which can assume the lost function. Residual effects can be so subtle as to be functionally negligible or so extensive that only the most basic brain functions, such as the control of respiration and blood pressure, are preserved.

Parkinson's Disease

Parkinson's disease (PD) is the most prevalent type of parkinsonism, a clinical syndrome caused by lesions in the basal ganglia, predominantly in the substantia nigra, that produce deficits in motor behavior.[83] Parkinsonism is a clinical rather than an etiologic entity, since it is associated with several pathological processes that damage the extrapyramidal system. Its many causes are divided into four categories:[83]

- Primary, or idiopathic (PD)
- Secondary parkinsonism (associated with infectious agents, drugs, toxins, vascular disease, trauma, brain neoplasm)
- Parkinson-like syndromes
- Heredodegenerative diseases.

Parkinson's disease is a progressive, degenerative disease of unknown cause resulting in the loss of melanin-containing brain cells in the substantia nigra and locus caeruleus and a decrease of dopamine in the caudate nucleus and putamen. The term "Parkinson's disease" is reserved for those cases of unknown etiology.[84] Parkinson's disease makes up approximately 80% of cases of parkinsonism.[83] The syndrome results in a reduction in muscle power, rigidity, and slowness of movement (akinesia), crucial to the characteristic tetrad known as **TRAP:**

Resting **T**remor
Cogwheel **R**igidity
Bradykinesia/**A**kinesia
Postural reflex impairment

For more information on Parkinson's disease, Huntington's disease, amyotrophic lateral sclerosis, normal pressure hydrocephalus, and spinal cord injury, see CD.

Peripheral Nervous Systems

With aging, the number and size of peripheral nerve fibers diminish with a concomitant decrease in conduction velocity.[85] There is often a clinically insignificant decrease in touch and vibration sense. The peripheral nerves, however, are easily affected by nutritional deficiencies, toxins, and endocrine disorders.[23] The resulting neuropathies can cause marked loss of position sense, resulting in instability, falls, chronic pain, and dysesthesia (painful and persistent sensation induced by even a gentle touch of the skin).

The common nutritional deficiencies which lead to neuropathy are folic acid (caused by poor diet or folic acid antagonists, such as diphenylhdantoin, sulfonamides), vitamin B_{12} (caused by pernicious anemia due to malabsorption of B_{12}), and alcohol-related deficiencies of thiamine, pyridoxine, and other B vitamins.[43,86] Toxic neuropathies can result from heavy metal exposure (such as lead and arsenic), from medications (such as nitrofurantoin, disulfiram, diphenylhydantoin), or from uremia. Replacement of the deficiency and removal of the toxin are the cornerstones of therapy. Prognosis is good for resolution.[87]

Diabetic neuropathy can take several forms. There is a distal sensory polyneuropathy which affects the hands and feet with diminished sensation and burning pain; a proximal motor neuropathy resulting in proximal muscle wasting and weakness; and a diffuse autonomic neuropathy resulting in orthostatic hypotension, neurogenic bladder, obstipation (intractable constipation), and bowel immotility.[88] In addition to these diffuse forms of neuropathy, single nerves can be affected. The resulting mononeuropathies can cause loss of ocular muscle function and painful nerve root and branch dysfunction wherever an involved nerve travels.[89] Treatment is symptomatic and may involve analgesics, specific physical therapy, and possible splinting. Relief from painful dysesthesias may be obtained in some cases with the use of diphenylhydantoin, amitriptyline, or carbamazepine. Tight control of the blood sugar appears neither to prevent nor to lessen diabetic neuropathy.[90] Rarely, another endocrine disease, hypothyroidism, can present with neuropathy. It responds to thyroid hormone replacement. Other causes of neuropathy in the aged include paraneoplastic syndromes (lung, ovary, multiple myeloma) and amyloid.[91]

NEUROSENSORY MANIFESTATIONS OF AGING

Vestibular Problems

Vestibular complaints have been reported in over 50% of elderly people.[92] The central mechanisms that are involved in the control of balance do not appear to change excessively with age, but are more likely to be affected by degenerative neurologic diseases such as Alzheimer's or Parkinson's disease. However, there are age-related changes in the peripheral vestibular system. Hair cell receptors decrease in number and there is a loss of the vestibular receptor ganglion cells. The myelinated nerve cells of the vestibular system decrease by as much as 40%. There is a reported increase in the incidence of benign paroxysmal positioning vertigo (BPPV) with complaints of dizziness with head movements. This may be due to an increase in the deposits in the posterior semicircular canal. Partial loss of vestibular function in the elderly can lead to complaints of dizziness, with less ability of the nervous system to accommodate to positional changes.[92]

Coupled with the vestibular losses, there is concomitant loss in vision and somatosensation, which severely affects sensory input necessary for the maintenance of balance. In addition, there are longer response latencies and delayed reaction times. Vision changes include loss of acuity, decreased peripheral fields, and loss of depth perception. The loss of input from this combination is slow, with compensation developing through the years. Therefore, compensatory strategy in response to postural instability is not the same as in the person with acute vestibular insufficiency. There is an overall loss of functional reserve so that the threshold for clinical loss is lowered. This is demonstrated by the increased number of falls in older people with a history of falls compared to age-matched groups with no history of falls when they are tested with increased challenges to balance.[93] There is an apparent decrease in the ability to integrate the conflicting sensory information to determine appropriate postural responses. Since there are changes as well in motor output, the loss of balance, in addition to lack of sensory organization, may be due to a poor response to vestibulospinal stimulation.[93]

Various pathological conditions will affect the peripheral vestibular system to produce vertigo or disequilibrium. Benign paroxysmal positional vertigo is the most common cause of vertigo with changes in head position in an older adult population. Generally, BPPV is associated with the deposition of otoconial material in the cupula of the posterior semicircular canal. The otoliths adhere to the cupula in some cases and retard its return to a resting position after head rotation, or obstruct the flow of endolymph, producing symptoms from the affected posterior semicircular canal by impeding or ceasing stimulation to the vestibular nerve. It can be unilateral or bilateral. Prolonged inactivity can also lead to symptoms of BPPV. Habituation exercises (placing the person in positions that provoke vertigo) and balance exercises have been found to be very effective in the treatment of this disorder. These exercises are discussed in Chapter 12, Neurological Considerations.

Acute vestibular neuritis, also known as *labyrinthitis*, is the second most common cause of vertigo in the elderly.[94] It is associated with a viral infection causing inflammatory changes of branches of the vestibular nerve. In the elderly, onset is usually preceded by upper respiratory or gastrointestinal tract infections. The chief complaint is the acute onset of prolonged severe rotational vertigo that is exacerbated by movement of the head. Symptoms include spontaneous horizontal-rotatory nystagmus beating toward the good ear, postural imbalance, and nausea.[94] Antiviral medications are used in this condition, and habituation exercises help to quickly resolve this condition once the infection clears.

Ménière's disease is a disorder of the inner-ear function that can cause hearing problems and vestibular symptoms in the elderly.[94] The patient complains of a sensation of fullness of the ear, a reduced ability to hear, and tinnitus. These symptoms are accompanied by rotational vertigo, postural imbalance, nystagmus, and nausea and vomiting that can last for extended periods of time. A phenomenon identified in Ménière's disease is endolymphatic hydrops, a condition in which malabsorption of endolymph results in an increase in endolymphatic fluid pressure in the endolyphatic duct and sac. Medical intervention includes a salt-restricted diet and the use of diuretics to maintain the fluid balance in the ear. Vestibular suppressant medication is sometimes used during the acute phases and the patient is advised to avoid caffeine, alcohol, and tobacco. In severe cases surgical intervention is to insert a shunt to drain excess fluid from the ear; however, the effectiveness of this procedure is questionable.[94] Ménière's disease presents a challenge to rehabilitation efforts. Until the fluid imbalance is controlled, patients with this disease do not respond well to typical vestibular rehabilitation programs. Emphasis should be on safety and balance exercises.[95] Challenging the balance to recruit the other systems, such as the cervico-ocular reflex and proprioceptive and visual mechanisms for controlling posture during stance and ambulation, may be effective.

Bilateral vestibular disorders may occur secondary to other diseases in the elderly or could be drug induced.

Routine for:
Created by:

STANDING DYNAMIC-3
Weight Shift: Diagonal

Slowly shift weight forward over right leg. Return to starting position. Shift backward over right leg.

Hold each position _____ seconds.
Repeat _____ times per session.
Do _____ sessions per day.
___Repeat on compliant surface _____.

STANDING DYNAMIC-5
Weight Shift: Lateral (Righting/Equilibrium)

With feet shoulder width apart, slowly shift weight over right leg, bending head and trunk slightly to left. Let left arm hang out from side. Return to starting position. Shift weight over left leg, bending head and trunk slightly to right. Let right arm hand out from side.

Repeat _____ times per session.
Do _____ sessions per day.

STANDING DYNAMIC -11
Turning in Place: Compensatory Strategy

Standing in place, first move eyes to target at eye level. Keeping eyes fixed on target, turn head and then body toward target. Repeat sequence with a target on each wall to complete a full turn.

Repeat _____ times per session.
Do _____ sessions per day.

STANDING DYNAMIC-9
Turning in Place: Compliant Surface (Pillow)

Standing on pillow, lead with head and turn slowly making quarter turns toward right.

Repeat _____ times per session.
Do _____ sessions per day.
___ Repeat _____ turns with eyes closed.

OTOLITH STIMULATION -1
Sit to Stand: Varied Speeds (With Head Tilts)

With head __upright__, stand up slowly with eyes __open__.
Repeat ____ times per session. Do ____ sessions per day.

HABITUATION-4
Diagonals

In __sitting__ __slowly__ bring head down with nose in direction of __right__ knee. Maintain position until symptoms subside, plus _____ seconds. __Slowly__ come up diagonally, extending back of head toward __right__ shoulder. Maintain position until symptoms subside, plus _____ seconds.

Repeat _____ times per session.
Do _____ sessions per day.

Copyright © 1999 VHI

85

Routine for:
Created by:

EYE EXERCISES-3
Visuo-Vestibular: Head / Eyes Moving in Same Direction

Holding a single target, keep eyes fixed on target. Slowly move target, head and eyes in same direction _up-down_ for _____ seconds each direction.

Perform in _____ position. Repeat _____ times per session. Do _____ sessions per day.
___ Repeat using full field stimulus _____.

EYE EXERCISES-5
Oculomotor: Smooth Pursuits

Holding a single target, keep eyes fixed on target. Slowly move it <u>side to side</u> while head stays still. Move _____ seconds each direction.

Perform in _____ position.
Repeat _____ times per session.
Do _____ sessions per day.

EYE EXERCISES-4
Visuo-Vestibular: Head / Eyes Moving in Opposite Direction

Holding a single target, keep eyes fixed on target. Slowly move target _up-down_ while moving head in opposite direction of target for _____ seconds each direction.
Perform in _____ position. Repeat _____ times per session. Do _____ sessions per day.
___ Repeat using full field stimulus _____.

EYE EXERCISES-7
Compensatory Strategies: Corrective Saccades

1. Holding two stationary targets placed _____ inches apart, move eyes to target, keep head still.
2. Then move head in direction of target while eyes remain on target.
3/4. Repeat in opposite direction.
Perform in _____ position.
Repeat sequence _____ times per session.
Do _____ sessions per day.

GAIT-2
Side to Side Head Motion

Walking on solid surface with head and eyes straight ahead, turn head and eyes toward _right_ for _____ steps. Return with head and eyes straight ahead. Repeat, turning head and eyes to other side.

Repeat sequence _____ times.
Do _____ sessions per day.

___ Repeat while at mall or grocery store.

GAIT-3
Up / Down Head Motion

Walking on solid surface with head and eyes positioned straight ahead, move head and eyes toward ceiling for _____ steps. Return with head and eyes straight ahead. Repeat, moving head and eyes toward floor. Maintain a straight path and postural control throughout activity.

Repeat sequence _____ times.
Do _____ sessions per day.

___ Repeat while at mall or grocery store.

Conditions that may lead to vestibular problems include meningitis, labyrinthine infections, oteosclerosis, Paget's disease, polyneuropathy, bilateral tumors (acoustic neuromas in neurofibromatosis), endolymphatic hydrops, bilateral vestibular neuritis, cerebral hemosiderosis, ototoxic drugs, inner-ear autoimmune disease, or congenital malformations of the inner ear.[94] Autoimmune conditions such as rheumatoid arthritis, psoriasis, ulcerative colitis, and Cogan's syndrome (iritis accompanied by vertigo and sensorineural hearing loss) can lead to a progressive, bilateral sensorineural hearing loss often accompanied by bilateral loss in vestibular function. Additionally, alcohol may cause an acute vertigo as the dehydration created by alcoholic substances can change the specific gravity of the endolymph. Other agents that may cause vertigo include organic compounds of heavy metals and aminoglycosides.[94,95,96] Controlled physical exercises can improve the condition in patients with bilateral vestibulopathy by recruiting nonvestibular sensory capacities such as the cervico-ocular reflex and proprioceptive and visual control of stance and gait.

Pathogens in the Aged & Therapeutics

Pathology	Definition	Difference in the Aged	Therapeutic Considerations with Age
Obstructive and Resistive Lung Disease	Alteration of airflow in the lungs. Changes in lung volumes and capacities	More common with age and risk factors	Progressive aerobic activities, accessory muscles stretch, use of inspiratory muscle training, and breathing retraining. Be careful with signs of dizziness, pallor, cyanosis, and changes in respiratory and heart rate that may be signs of deoxygenation.
Fibromyalgia	Systemic disorder with diffuse muscular aching and multiple trigger points	Not very common in older persons. Sometimes associated with rheumatoid arthritis and chronic fatigue syndrome	Encourage progressive aerobic exercise. However, do not allow fatigue levels because they promote an inverse effect.
Osteoporosis	Decrease in bone mass leading to bone fragility and fracture. Main sites of fracture are hip, spine, and wrist	Significantly increased incidence with age	Rehab is very effective. It helps in maintaining bone mass. Encourage weight bearing. Progressively resistance training is very effective in preventing bone loss. Core and scapular stabilization exercises help prevent vertebral fractures. Balance and flexibility activities are also necessary to help prevent falls and therefore decrease risk for fracture. Exercises should vary in intensity from low-load to high-load activities to help obtain the maximal osteogenic effect. Avoid flexion activities.
Paget's Disease	Disorder of bone remodeling with increased bone reabsorption and formation	Prevalence with age	Bone deformities, fractures, arthritis, and pain are complication of the disease. Muscle weakness and pain as well as fatigue are usually present. Heart may be overloaded due to the increased peripheral resistance. Patients with chronic headaches and diffuse ache pain may be experiencing the first symptoms of Paget's disease. Also, be aware of the side effects of anti-inflammatory medication.
Osteoarthritis	Degenerative joint disease	80% of people in their 70s have it	Rehab is very effective. Must minimize mechanical stress. Water aerobics, rowing, and elliptical machines may be preferable types of exercise. Strengthening exercises are very important. Patient education on prevention and decrease of mechanical stress are fundamental for quality of life (mobilization, PRE, aquatics, ROM).

(cont.)

Pathogens in the Aged & Therapeutics (Continued)

Pathology	Definition	Difference in the Aged	Therapeutic Considerations with Age
Rheumatoid Arthritis	Chronic systemic inflammatory disorder	Can get in early adulthood or have late onset	Rehab is effective as noted with osteoarthritis. Patients may present with chronic fatigue and malaise. Focus of exercise training is to maintain proper range of motion, strength, and flexibility, preventing contractures and deformities. Progressive aerobic training is very important to decrease the systemic effect of fatigue. During acute phases therapy should balance rest with sufficient activity to maintain conditioning. Can participate even during exacerbation phase.
Confusion/ Delerium	Confusion, restlessness, agitation, hallucination	Aged more sensitive to toxic and metabolic causes. May be related to polypharmacy	Check for toxic or metabolic causes. Rehab protocol should be well structured with the same therapist at the same place and at the same time.
Dementia/ Alzheimer's	Progressive degenerative disease with slow onset of motor and cognitive impairment	^ incidence with age. 50% over age 85 have it	Rehabilitation encouraging functional activities and therapeutic exercise is effective. Group activities also promote social interaction and are effective to decrease depression.
Cerebral Vascular Accident (CVA)	Vascular event that leads to brain tissue death	More common with age. Number-one neurological diagnosis for rehab	Sensory, motor, and cognitive impairments may be present. Aerobic activities are important to maintain cardiovascular endurance. Physical therapy should focus on preventing deformities as well as regaining functional independence. Numerous rehab techniques are shown to be effective. Constraint induced therapy, ES, Ther ex, Bobath, PNF, partial body-weight supported treadmill training, and muscle power training are some of the various examples of therapeutic techniques.
Parkinson's Disease	Chronic progressive degeneration of the basal ganglia	It is more common with aging	Rigidity, tremor, and brady kinesia are common signs and symptoms. Postural impairments progress with the disease and may be prevented by scapular and core stability program as well as flexibility activities. Cardiovascular endurance is very important. Therefore, progressive aerobic activities should be included in the rehab program. Monitor heart rate and rhythm throughout activities. Balance and proprioception activities should be included in the protocol. Rehab is very effective, more so if started earlier.
Peripheral Neuropathies	Can broadly include neuropathies and myopathies	Aging causes a decrease in conduction velocity, which can ^ process	Be aware of signs and symptoms such as numbness, tingling, and muscle weakness. Fatigue may be present due to correlation of other diseases. Due to the correlation with other metabolic diseases, progressive aerobic activity to increase cardiovascular endurance has to be well monitored. Rehab program should include balance and proprioceptive activities, functional activities, strengthening, and flexibility.

Pathogens in the Aged & Therapeutics (Continued)

Pathology	Definition	Difference in the Aged	Therapeutic Considerations with Age
Vestibular Dysfunction	Group of disorders of the vestibular system causing problems in appropriate postural response, balance, head position, and eye movement	Affects 50% of the elderly	Vestibular exercises, including habituation, is effective. Be aware of signs of dizziness, nausea, and vomit. Advise patient to perform home exercise habituation activities under supervision.

Skin Pathologies

The skin is the largest organ of the body and functions to protect the interior of the body from the effects of pathogens, toxins, environmental extremes, trauma, and ultraviolet irradiation. With age, and often as the result of the accumulated effects of repeated injury, the skin changes. It grows and heals more slowly, becomes more sensitive to most toxins, and is less able to resist injury.[97] It becomes less effective as a barrier to infections. The specialized appendages, such as sweat and sebum glands, pressure and touch sensors, and hair follicles, atrophy. This results in dryness, a decrease in ability to alter body temperature through sweating, and loss of hair. The small blood vessels in the skin diminish with age, which contributes to less effectiveness as a barrier to infection, diminished reserve for repair, and altered ability to assist in thermoregulation.[98]

There are several skin diseases that are common in the aged and which have significant effects on function. These include malignant tumors, herpes zoster, and decubitus ulcers. A great deal of data have accumulated to demonstrate an association between cutaneous aging and the development of skin cancers, infections, and ulcers.[97] Many of the factors that appear to predispose individuals to the development of pathological manifestations in the aged are similarly operative in the development of skin problems.[99] These include cumulative exposure to carcinogens, diminished DNA repair capacity, and decreased immunosurveillance. In addition, the reduced epidermal density in the skin that is seen with senescence is likely to play a role in the development of skin lesions, infections, and ulcerations.

For more information on tumors, herpes zoster, and decubitus ulcers, see CD.

Disturbances of Touch and Vision

For more background information on disturbances of touch and vision, see CD.

Macular Degeneration

Age-related macular degeneration (AMD) causes loss or blurriness of central vision creating a blind spot. Peripheral vision remains intact. Age-related macular degeneration results in an inability to see fine details, such as colors or a person's facial features.[100] Age-related macular degeneration is a progressive, degenerative disorder of the retina, and it is the leading cause of new cases of blindness in people aged 65 and older. In this country, nearly 11% of the population between 65 and 74 have AMD to some degree, as do 28% of those older than 75.[101]

Immediately beneath the sensory retina lies a single layer of cells called the retinal pigment epithelium. These cells provide nourishment to the portion of the retina where they are in contact. In AMD, the maintenance of this contact is threatened. A small hemorrhage may break through and accumulate between the retinal pigment epithelium and the sensory retina. This leads to disruption of the photoreceptor cells' nutrition and to their death, with attendant loss of central vision.[102] This type of age-related maculopathy is referred to as the *wet type* because of the leaking vessels and edema or blood that detaches the retina. The *dry type* consists of disintegration of the retinal pigment epithelium because of nutritional loss. The light-sensitive cells of the macula break down over time and a yellow deposit called drusen accumulates under the retina.[103]

A *cataract* is an opacity of the lens that reduces visual acuity (to 20/30 or less).[104] An early sign is the complaint of "glare" from bright lights at night or even during the day, the result of rays of light being scattered by the opacities. Over time, the lens opacities progress and eventually interfere with vision so that reading becomes difficult even with glasses. The hallmark of all cataracts is painless, progressive loss of vision. Though the cause has not been elucidated, there appears to be a strong nutritional link related to low levels of antioxidants.[105] Cataract surgery, the removal of the lens from the eye, is the treatment of choice.[106]

Glaucoma is a disorder characterized by increased intraocular pressure that can lead to irreversible damage to the optic nerve, with the accompanying impairment of blindness. It is a pathological process in the eye that anatomically or functionally blocks the outflow channels. The most common type of glaucoma in the elderly is the open-angle glaucoma accounting for 90% of all cases.[107] Onset is insidious and usually asymptomatic causing slow loss of visual field, affecting both eyes, and occurring more commonly in blacks.[108] Secondary glaucoma is associated with diabetes (diabetic retinopathy), uveitis, and with occular tumors that affect the optic nerve.[108]

The leading causes of visual impairment are age related, but appropriate care can preserve useful vision for most older adults.[109] Vision loss due to macular degeneration cannot be delayed in all patients; however, it can sometimes be postponed through laser therapy. Low-vision rehabilitation can maximize the usefulness of remaining sight. Cataract surgery is highly successful. Early detection and treatment of glaucoma can prevent vision loss. Laser treatment is remarkably effective in treating diabetic retinopathy.[109] Otherwise, the low vision state is best addressed with vision-enhancing devices, adaptive equipment, and patient education available through occupational therapy. Referral to a low-vision rehabilitation program is needed for a comprehensive evaluation and intervention. Individual adaptation and supportive services often result in a significant improvement in function and quality of life for those elders with low vision.

Hearing Pathologies with Age

For more information on age changes to hearing, see CD.

The hearing losses that occur with presbyacusis affect the higher, pure tone frequencies.[110] Basically, the individual loses the hard sounds of language. This leads to a decrease in ability to understand speech where parts of words or whole words are lost because of higher tones as well as the interference of background noise. The use of hearing aids and surgical implants has provided relief for some, but the process of presbyacusis is such that these steps can only blunt the effects of the problem. Because most cases of presbyacusis are of mixed etiology, as has already been noted, intervention will not completely correct the loss. Thus, the clinical focus should be on improving and maintaining as much of the hearing capability as possible, and helping the older person and the family adapts to the limitations necessitated by substituting other forms of communication and environmental stimuli to compensate for the loss that remains.[111]

The clinician needs to be mindful of the effects of hearing loss on all aspects of the older patient's life. Failure to consider the effects of hearing loss when evaluating such problems as depression, confusion, possible attention span deficits, and a variety of other clinical problems may lead to less than adequate clinical intervention.

Tinnitus is the diagnosis given to a variety of "ear noise" disorders. A small percentage of the elderly suffer from this condition to varying degrees,[110] and it is an annoying problem. Patients often report constant or intermittent noises, such as buzzing, ringing, or hissing, that result in a distortion of accurate reception of environmental sounds and voices. If patients complain of tinnitus, considerations for a quiet treatment environment should be made to decrease the bombardment of external noise sources superimposed on the internal sources.

Otalgia is ear pain that results from an otologic process or may be referred along neural pathways, including the trigeminal, glossopharyngeal, vagus, and cervical nerves. Inflammation of the pinna, external auditory canal, tympanic membrane, or middle ear can result in otalgia. With eustachian tube obstruction, negative pressure in the middle ear may produce painful retraction of the tympanic membrane. In the elderly, it is common for pain in the temporomandibular joint (TMJ) to be referred to the ear.

Massive accumulation of cerumen (wax) is frequently seen in the elderly. The individual is usually dehydrated, complains of hearing loss and a feeling of fullness in the ear, and often reports dizziness.

An effusion in the middle ear, usually related to obstruction of the eustachian tube, is called serous otitis media. In the elderly, this condition generally occurs unilaterally and the patient perceives a sensation of aural fullness and hearing loss.

Dizziness, encompassing the sensations of vertigo, dysequilibrium, and unsteadiness, is a common complaint in elders with ear disorders. Evaluation of balance problems should include an assessment of hearing pathologies.

For more information on proprioceptive and vestibular dysfunction, see CD.

For more information on sensory changes in smell and taste, see CD.

GASTROINTESTINAL PATHOLOGIES IN AGING

For background information on gastrointestinal pathologies in aging, see CD.

Dysphagia

Dysphagia is difficulty in swallowing. It commonly results from neuromuscular disorders, such as cerebral vascular accident, Parkinson's disease, diabetes, or other neuropathies. Malnutrition results from decreased intake; aspiration of oral contents is a common accompaniment that frequently leads to pneumonia. Siebens and colleagues[112] have identified a fairly high incidence of swallowing problems involving the mouth, pharynx, and upper esophageal sphincter in the elderly population.

For background information on dysphagia, see CD.

True esophageal dysphagia, where the transport of the ingested material down the esophagus is impaired, is common in the elderly.[113] Carcinoma of the esophagus, which occurs with increasing frequency in the elderly, usually presents with dysphagia. The most common symptom is the sensation of food "hanging up" in the esophagus. It has a poor prognosis for cure and usually requires extensive palliative treatment. Hiatus hernia, another cause of dysphagia, is also increasingly common in the aged. Few, however, are symptomatic, and medical management with antacids and H_2 blockers is effective.[114] It is important to understand that achalasia can initially present in the elderly, and that other motility disorders, such as diffuse esophageal spasm and scleroderma, do occur in these individuals.[113] Another cause of esophageal dysphagia that is unique to the elderly population is dysphagia aortica, in which the transport of material down the esophagus is impaired by a markedly tortuous and enlarged aorta, heart, or both.[115]

The role of the physical and occupational therapist in treating dysphagia is to coordinate the team efforts of speech pathology, dietary, and nursing to provide a comprehensive positioning and feeding program. The physical therapist is involved in evaluating and treating head and trunk control; neck range of motion; neck weakness; sitting balance; abnormal postural reflex activity interfering with head control, sitting balance, or both; gross facial muscle test; ability to handle secretions; voluntary deep breathing ability, breath control, and voluntary cough; and gross motor upper extremity ability. The occupational therapist is involved in some of the same interventions, and additionally provides adaptive equipment as warranted. Specific emphasis needs to be placed on wheelchair and bed positioning, and respiratory status.

For information on ulcer disease, anemia, gastrointestinal cancer, and bilary tract disease, see CD.

BOWEL AND BLADDER PROBLEMS

Urinary Incontinence

Urinary incontinence can affect both men and women. It afflicts more than half of nursing home residents and is often the reason for admission.[116] The causes of incontinence can be divided into two broad categories: established and transient.[117] Established incontinence is usually the result of neurological damage or intrinsic bladder or urethral pathology. By contrast, incontinence caused by transient causes, such as a medication or diet, is generally reversible if the underlying problem can be addressed adequately.

Incontinence is not a normal sequela of aging and characteristics of what is commonly called "overactive bladder" include decreases in bladder capacity, urethral compliance,

maximal urethral closure pressure, and urinary flow rate.[117] In both sexes, postvoid residual volume and the prevalence of involuntary detrusor contractions probably increase, while urethral resistance increases in men.[118]

The various types of urinary incontinence identified are stress, urge, mixed, overflow, and functional incontinence. Stress incontinence refers to the loss of bladder control due to the physical stress of increased pressure in the abdomen from such activities as coughing, sneezing, laughing, jogging, or straining on a lift or during a bowel movement. Urge incontinence is defined as the sudden urge to urinate without the ability to hold the urine long enough to reach a bathroom. Mixed incontinence is a combination of stress and urge incontinence. Overflow incontinence is the accidental loss of urine from a chronically full bladder. This may occur as the result of a cystocele (a vaginal hernia or bulge due to weakened vaginal muscles), an enlarged prostate, or a tumor, all of which block the flow of urine through the urethra. Other causes of overflow incontinence might include damage to the bladder nerves from diabetes, loss of adequate estrogen or progesterone,[119] or a herniated lumbar disc. Functional incontinence is the inability to get to the bathroom because of physical limitations, or the inability to manage clothing once the individual has made it to the bathroom. In the older adult, a combination of these conditions may exist.

The causes of transient incontinence may be denoted by the mnemonic DIAPPERS:[120]

- **D**elirium
- **I**nfection (especially urinary tract infection)
- **A**trophic vaginitis
- **P**harmaceuticals
- **P**sychological factors (e.g., depression, poor motivation)
- **E**xcess fluid output (e.g., diuretics, diabetes)
- **R**estricted mobility (e.g., Parkinson's disease, arthritis)
- **S**tool (constipation or impaction)

Any condition that impairs cognition, mobility, or the ability to hold urine can contribute to functional incontinence. Although such causes potentially may be reversible, in reality, many patients' functional status may not improve, and therefore incontinence becomes established. Many of the causes of established incontinence involve urinary tract dysfunction. These include overactivity of the bladder with involuntary contraction; failure of the bladder to contract at the appropriate time or as strongly as it should; low resistance to urinary flow when it should be high (stress incontinence); and high resistance to urinary flow when it should be low (urinary obstruction).[121] Detrusor instability is characterized by a sudden and urgent need to empty the bladder. The volume emptied is variable but may be large. Often in the elderly, the detrusor muscle contracts, but the bladder does not empty completely, leaving residual urine and an increased risk for urinary tract infection.[117]

There are numerous interventions for urinary incontinence that rehabilitation therapists can offer the older person with this condition.[122,123] Behavioral treatments are considered appropriate for patients with stress, urge, and mixed incontinence. Physical therapy may include biofeedback, therapeutic exercise, neuromuscular reeducation, therapeutic activity, and gait training. Instruction in pelvic floor exercises, commonly known as Kegels, is helpful in regaining strength of the pelvic floor musculature.[122] Occupational therapy may be involved in training for functional activities that facilitate toileting as well as the modification of clothing (i.e., replacing buttons or zippers with Velcro) to enhance the ease of disrobing and eliminate incontinence resulting from functional limitations.

Evidence-based treatment strategies are as follows.

Behavioral versus Drug Treatment for Urge Urinary Incontinence in Older Women; by Burgio; *JAMA*; 12–98[124]

- Randomized and controlled trial = safe and effective
- Behavioral training
  - Visit 1—anorectal feedback
  - Visit 2—urge strategies (when urged, pause, relax, contract pelvic muscles; then proceed to toilet.)
  - Visit 3—muscle biofeedback, if not 50% better with above
  - Visit 4—fine-tune
  - Home program—15 Kegels, 3x/day, for 10 seconds, lying, sitting, standing . . . interrupting or slowing urine flow

---

Single Blind RCT of Pelvic Floor Exercises, ES, Vaginal Cones, and No Treatment in Management of Genuine Stress Incontinence in Women; by Bo; *British Medical Journal*; 3-02[125]

- 4 groups
  - Pelvic floor exercise.
    - 8–12 contractions, 3x/day
    - 1x/wk with PT in a group (supine, sitting, etc.)
  - Electrical stimulation.
    - intermittent stimulation 30 minutes a day
  - Vaginal cones 20 minutes a day.
  - Control—untreated.
  - All groups had a once-a-week meeting with the PT.
- Improvements in leakage and strength were greater in the exercise-only group; no side effects (discomfort and bleeding).

Vaginal ES of the Pelvic Floor; by Spruijt; *Acta Obstet Gynecol Scand*; 03[126]

Study on electrical stimulation in elderly showed no difference if exercise or exercise and electrical stimulation. Electrical stimulation has high physical and emotional cost.

Fecal Incontinence

The inability to control bowel movements is termed fecal incontinence. This condition may have psychological causes such as depression, anxiety, confusion, or disorientation. Physiologic contributors to fecal incontinence that are most commonly seen in the elderly include neurological impairments that involve sensory and motor function (such as cerebral vascular accident, Parkinson's, spinal cord injury, or later stages of Alzheimer's disease), anal dysfunction resulting from giving birth, hemorrhoids, rectal prolapse, anal dilatation, altered levels of consciousness, and severe diarrhea. Diabetes and autonomic neuropathy may produce internal sphincter dysfunction as well. Fecal impaction is a common cause of diarrhea in the geriatric population. The stool proximal to the obstructing fecal mass becomes liquefied and oozes around the obstruction. Since elders with long-standing constipation cannot sense the movement of stool in the rectal vault and the fecal impaction tonically inhibits the internal anal sphincter, this may lead to fecal incontinence. The preservation of continence is complex, and its failure is usually multifactoral.[127]

Treatment includes hydration and in the presence of a fecal impaction an enema may be warranted. From a medical perspective, nonspecific diarrhea is treated with bulking agents and antidiarrheal drugs. Physical therapy may implement sphincter exercises to restrengthen the weakened muscle. Biofeedback treatment is very successful in the treatment of fecal incontinence. The visual or auditory feedback provides sufficient sensory input (for a patient with good cognition) to often resolve the problem in one treatment session. Biofeedback has been found to be helpful in more than 70% of individuals with incontinence due to sensory or motor impairment.

For information on other GI problems, see CD.

The Medical Pathology of the Aged & Therapeutic Considerations

Pathology	Definition	Changes with Age	Therapeutic Considerations with Age
Macular Degeneration	Degenerative changes in the macula causing blurring or loss of central vision	11%—ages 65–75, 28%—age 85. Leading cause of blindness among individuals over 55	Low-vision rehabilitation. Patient education on environmental changes such as proper lighting and removing clutter to prevent falls.
Cataracts	Opacity of the lens reduces visual acuity	Difficulty seeing objects clearly. Commonly affects distal distance	Surgery is very effective. Patient education on environmental changes such as proper lighting and removing clutter to prevent falls.
Glaucoma	^intraocular pressure that leads to damage of the optic nerve and blindness	Patients over 60 must get checked annually for this	Prevention and continued treatment imperative. Patient education on environmental changes such as proper lighting and removing clutter to prevent falls.
Presbyacusis	Loss of hearing that occurs with normal aging. Inability to hear high-frequency sounds	60% of people over age 65	Speak slowly and loudly and use visual cues to supplement the verbal.
Tinnitus	A constant crackling, buzzing, ringing, or whistling in one or both ears	10% of people over age 65	Decrease external noise, encourage the use of hearing aides. May be related to balance issues.
Dysphagia	Difficulty swallowing	Higher incidence in elderly	Evaluate head, neck, and trunk control. Work on proper positioning when eating. Patients who also have cognitive problems may need supervision while eating. Be aware of signs and symptoms of bronchoaspiration.
Incontinence	Difficulty or inability to control urine or bowel	Affects more than half of nursing home residents	Kegels, urge strategies, and electrical stimulation shown to be effective. Patient education on emptying bowel before exercise routine. Avoid Valsalva manauver.

KIDNEY PROBLEMS

Renal Disease

The kidneys are the major modulators of the amount of water, sodium, and potassium found in the extracellular fluid of the body. They also are a major route of drug excretion and are important in maintaining an appropriate blood pressure.[128] Alterations in renal function can have profound effects on all of these essential functions.

With age, the amount of blood that can be filtered by the kidneys declines steadily.[115] This is in part due to a decline in the amount of blood that arrives at the kidney because of heart disease or narrowing of the blood vessels. It is also caused in large part by the decrease in the number and size of the glomeruli, which are the areas of the kidney that filter plasma. The ability of the kidney to reabsorb water and solutes from the filtered plasma also declines.[129] Although these reabsorptive capacities remain, they are at a significantly lower level in the aged and help to account for the decreased capability of the aged person to excrete an excessive amount of water or to prevent the loss of water in the face of dehydration.

There are eight commonly encountered problems in the aged to which altered renal function contributes: too much or too little water; too much or too little sodium; too much potassium; drug intoxication; and acute and chronic renal failure.[130] All of these disruptions of body homeostasis can result in altered mental status and can be life threatening.

Acute and Chronic Renal Failure

Acute cessation of renal function can occur at any age, but the diminished blood supply of the aging kidney renders it more susceptible to injury.[130] Hypotension is the usual precipitating cause and can result from dehydration, overmedication, surgery, or sepsis. Acute injury from certain antibiotics or from contrast dye used in radiology can also result in acute renal shutdown.

Acute renal failure is associated with the rapid buildup of toxic waste products and drugs, fluid overload, and elevation of serum potassium. Any of these complications can be fatal if not managed correctly. In addition, the immune system is impaired, and patients with acute renal failure frequently die with infections.[131,132]

Chronic renal failure is marked by the slow deterioration of renal function and is usually detected when the presence of another illness stresses the renal system and elevated blood urea nitrogen (BUN), hyponatremia, or increased fluid retention leads to an evaluation of renal function.[133] The functional side effects of chronic renal failure result primarily from anemia and congestive heart failure. Patients with renal disease severe enough to cause significant chronic mental status changes have a poor prognosis and often require dialysis or transplantation—a touchy subject in light of possible rationing of health care imposed by health care reforms.

The clinical implications of problems in the kidney in relation to exercise and activity tolerance center around the electrolyte balance and the potential inability of the kidney to facilitate homeostasis. Increasing energy expenditure through exercise is positively correlated with an improvement in mortality and morbidity through a number of mechanisms.[134] Despite these benefits some are relevant, especially for the elderly with renal failure, to recommend fitness programs because of the fear that exercising too intensely will provoke cardiac arrhythmias, myocardial infarction, or increased blood pressure.[135] Regular eccentric training can increase protein turnover (37% higher muscle catabolism) in older people and can require a higher protein intake.[136]

Combined with a calorie-appropriate diet, regular exercise maintains a reasonable body weight, delays loss of lean muscle mass, and promotes good physical performance. Activity level is a predictor of survival for people aged 60 years and beyond.[137,138]

Here are three evidence-based strategies.

Exercise Training in Patients with End-Stage Renal Disease on Hemodialysis: Comparison of Three Rehabilitation Programs; by Konstantinidou; *J Rehab Med*; 02[139]

- 4 groups finished a 6-month program.
  - group. A = outpatient rehabilitation; 3x/wk/ PRE and aerobic on nondialysis days
  - group B = 60 min aerobic and PRE and flexibility; 3x/wk
  - group C = followed a home exercise program (cycle and exercise)
  - group D = control
- Only groups A and B improved on cardiovascular exercise tests.

Exercise for the Dialyzed; by Oh-Park; *Am J Phys Med Rehabil*; 11-02[140]

- An exercise program during dialysis can be performed safely and improve strength, fitness, and function.
- During first 2 hours of dialysis, 2–3x/wk, HR and BP nurse/PT monitored every 5 minutes.
- Strength (while in chair) 50% of the one repetition maximum; lower extremity—3 sets of 10.
- Aerobic—cycle in chair, Borg scale used to monitor; 5 min cycle/1 min rest; 6 to 30minutes.

Low-Volume Exercise Rehabilitation Improves Functional Capacity and Self-Reported Functional Status of Dialysis Patients; by Mercer; *Am J Phys Med Rehabil*; 2-02[141]

- 2x/wk for 12 weeks
- Treated on dialysis days before treatment
- PT, RN, and MD supervision
- Program:
  - warm-up and cool down
  - 3–5 minute bouts of aerobics
  - PRE to all muscles

For information on additional types of altered Renal function, see CD.

ENDOCRINE DISEASES

For background information on endocrine diseases, see CD.

Glucose Metabolism and Diabetes Mellitus

The number of insulin receptors found on cell membranes decreases with age.[142] Reflecting this change, the incidence of glucose intolerance increases with age and reaches nearly 25% by age 80.[143] In the aged, it is important to identify glucose intolerance, not only to prevent the complications of untreated diabetes (neuropathy, retinopathy, nephropathy, and accelerated atherosclerosis) but also, even more so, to identify those individuals at risk for nonketotic hyperosmolar coma or severe hyperglycemia, which can be precipitated by infection, dehydration, or other physiologic stress.

Symptoms of diabetes include increased urination, thirst, hunger, fatigue, and lethargy; weight loss; and numbness or tingling in the feet and hands. Though no clear understanding of the cause of diabetes has been found and there is no cure, the disease can be controlled by achieving and maintaining normal blood glucose levels.[89] This requires a carefully balanced utilization of four critical components: diet, exercise, education for self-monitoring, and drug therapy.

Here are some evidence-based strategies:

Physical Activity and Reduced Occurrence of Non-Insulin-Dependent Diabetes Mellitus; by Helmrich; N Engl J Med; 7-91[144]

Conclusion: Increased physical activity is effective in preventing NIDDM, and the protective benefit is especially pronounced in persons at the highest risk of the disease.

Low Cardio-respiratory Fitness and Physical Inactivity as Predictors of Mortality in Men with Type II Diabetes; by Wei; Ann Intern Med; 2000[145]

- Physically inactive men increase mortality by two-fold.
- Progressive resistive training and aerobic exercise improve longevity.

Resistance Training in the Treatment of Non-Insulin-Dependent Diabetes Mellitus; by Eriksson; Int J Sports Med; 97[146]

- Significant improvement in:
  - glycemic control
  - muscle endurance increased 32%
  - muscles hypertrophied 21%
- The program:
  - 3 months
  - 2x/wk
  - 50% 1RM , 15–20 Repetitions

Effects of Long-Term Resistive Training on Mobility and Strength in Older Adults with Diabetes; by Brandon; J Gerontol Med Sci; 03[147]

- Increased mobility and strength after 2 years.
- Program—3x/wk
  - 3 sets of 8–12 Repetitions
  - 50% to 70% 1RM
  - 50 minutes of PRE
  - 10-minute warm-up/cool down and flexibility

For background information on thyroid disease, see CD.

CANCER

As the U.S. population becomes increasingly elderly, cancer rates have gone up and are expected to continue that increase. Currently 50% of all malignancies occur in the 12% of the population aged 65 and older.[148] While mortality from cardiovascular disease has been declining in this age group over the past two decades, cancer-related mortality has remained constant.[149] Age is the single most significant risk factor for cancer. Cancer incidence and mortality rates increase exponentially with age until the age of 84 years. At this point, it has been found that the occurrence of cancer plateaus (survival of the fittest?).

Simply defined, cancer refers to a large group of diseases characterized by uncontrolled cell growth and spread of abnormal cells. Cancer is called by many other terms, including malignant neoplasm, malignancy, carcinoma, and tumor. In its various forms it is a genetic disease, characterized by changes in the normal genetic mechanisms that regulate cell growth and division.[150] *Differentiation* is the process by which normal cells undergo physical and structural changes as they develop into different tissues with specialized physiologic function. In malignant cells, differentiation is altered and may be entirely lost so that the cell no longer resembles its parent cell. When this occurs it is called an undifferentiated or *anaplastic* malignancy. *Dysplasia* is a category of tumor in which there is a disorganization of cells from their normal shape, size, or organization. *Metaplasia* is the first stage of dysplasia, which is reversible and benign. This stage is the stage targeted for early detection screenings. *Hyperplasia* refers to an increase in the number of cells in tissue resulting in an increase in tissue mass. A *tumor*, or a *neoplasm*, is a new growth and may be benign or malignant.

Two nonmutually exclusive hypotheses may account for higher cancer rates among the older population. First, carcinogenesis is a time-consuming process. Therefore, cancer is more likely to become detectable in older individuals.[149] Second, a number of molecular changes occur with aging. These changes are similar to those of carcinogenesis and prime the aging cells to the effects of late-stage carcinogens.[150,151] Aging cells, when copying their genetic material, may begin to err, giving rise to mutations, but the aging immune system may not recognize these mutations as foreign, thus allowing them to proliferate and form a malignancy. Research has reported findings that indicate that mutations linked with lymphoma and leukemia accumulate with age.[151] For example, individuals 60 years of age and older have a 40-fold risk of developing non-Hodgkin's lymphoma compared to younger populations. Older individuals are more likely to develop cancer after exposure to environmental carcinogens than are younger individuals. Both experimental and epidemiological data support this hypothesis.[151,152] The clinical consequences are important. Increased likelihood of developing cancer makes older persons ideal candidates for preventative interventions. The older individual may be a candidate for all forms of primary cancer prevention, from elimination of environmental carcinogens to increased activity, modification of diet, and in some cases chemoprevention.

Cancers that exhibit the most consistent increases in rate with age are leukemia and cancers of the digestive system, breast, prostrate, and urinary tract.[148] The incidence of myelodysplastic syndrome (MDS), a group of hematopoietic stem cell disorders leading to leukemia, appears to be increasing in the aging population.[150,151] Several neoplasms may behave differently in the older patient. Simply put, older people may develop "different" cancers. In addition, patient age may influence tumor growth and affect the individual's responsiveness to treatment.[153]

Two primary approaches to the treatment of elderly cancer patients include curative and palliative interventions.[149] Curative cancer treatment includes surgery, radiation, chemotherapy, biotherapy, and hormone therapy. Surgery, aimed at tumor removal, is frequently used in combination with other treatment modalities listed above. Adjuvant therapy following surgery is used to decrease the potential proliferation of any residual cancer cells. Surgical interventions in the elderly carry the negative consequences of confusion and weakness related to the use of anesthesia and prolonged bed rest and immobility following the procedure. Radiation therapy is used to eradicate cancer cells. The success of this intervention is dependent on the localization of the tumor and the fact that malignant cells respond differently to radiation depending on blood supply, oxygen satuation, previous irradiation, and immune system status. Side effects may include nausea and vomiting leading to more attention to nutrition, and overall weakness results in functional declines. Chemotherapy is generally used when there is widespread metastatic disease, such as in leukemia, with the aim of destroying cancer cells through the use of potent chemical agents. The side effects are similar to those of radiation. In addition, chemotherapy usually dramatically alters the status of red blood cell and platelet counts, leaving the individual in a particularly compromised immune state.[149] Patients often are required to reside in protective environments (significantly limiting functional activities) in order to protect them from exposure to potential infectious agents. Biotherapy, also called immunotherapy, relies on biologic response modifiers (BRM) to change or modify the relationship between the tumor and the host by strengthening the host's immune system response.[150,151] The most widely used agents include interferons (which have a direct antitumor effect) and interleukin-2 (one of the cytokine proteins released by the macrophage to trigger the immune response). Other forms of biotherapy include bone marrow transplantation (used for cancers that are unresponsive to high levels of chemo or radiation therapy), monoclonal antibody therapy (β lymphocytes that bind to and destroy cancer cells), the injection of colony-stimulating factors (used as hematopoietic growth factors which guide the division and differentiation of normal cells in individuals with particularly low blood counts), and hormonal therapy (used in cancers that are affected by specific hormones). Hormonal therapy is being utilized more and more to good effect in an older population. For example, the luteinizing-release hormone leuprolide is used in the treatment of prostrate cancer. It has been found that this hormone inhibits testosterone release and tumor growth. Likewise, the use of tamoxifen, an antiestrogen hormonal agent, is used in breast cancer to block estrogen receptors in tumor cells that require estrogen to survive.[150,151]

Palliative care, providing symptomatic relief, may include radiation or chemotherapy, physical therapy (e.g., physical agents, exercise, positioning, relaxation techniques, biofeedback, manual therapy), medications, acupuncture, chiropractic care, alternative medicine (e.g., homeopathic and naturopathic treatment), nutritional therapy, and hospice care. It is primarily end-of-life care with the emphasis on minimizing pain and helping to make patients as comfortable as possible as they approach their impending death.

Numerous symptoms and functional losses in the older cancer patient require attention by physical and occupational therapy. The management of pain and a minimization of functional loss are imperative in treating the elderly cancer patient. Treatment approaches for the management of pain by the rehabilitation professional may include noninvasive physical agents, such as cryotherapy, thermotherapy, electrical stimulation, immobilization, exercise, massage, biofeedback, and relaxation techniques. Often functional mobility exercises are helpful in relieving pain and improving a cancer patient's outlook. As the individual becomes older the level of frailty increases dramatically. In frail elderly patients, functional reserves are exhausted and tolerance of physical stress is poor.[154] Although chronological age alone cannot be used to make a clinical assessment of patient age, in the majority of people over the age of 75 with a cancer diagnosis, frailty needs to be addressed.[154] It has been determined that, even in the frailest elderly patient newly diagnosed with cancer, the life expectancy is greater than two years.[154] While frail patients seem candidates only for palliative measurements, exercise and pain management have been found not only to improve functional capabilities and decrease pain but also to serve to improve the quality of life. These patients require continuous and effective treatment of their symptoms no matter what the prognosis. Here are some evidence-based studies for cancer rehabilitation.

Physical Activity, Physical Function, and the Risk of Breast Cancer in a Prospective Study Among Elderly Women; by Cerhan; *J Gerontol*; 98[155]

Postmenopausal physical activity level is inversely associated with breast cancer.

Function in Elderly Cancer Survivors Depends on Comorbidities; by Garman; *J Gerontol Med Sci*; 03 Vol 58A, No 12, pg 1119-1124[156]

In the older cancer survivor, regardless of duration following diagnosis, the presence of comorbidity rather than history of cancer correlates with function.

Functional Recovery in Cancer Rehabilitation; by Cole; *Arch Phys Med Rehabil*; 5-00[157]

Is rehabilitation effective for patients with cancer?
- You bet!
- Results: Inpatient rehabilitation improves both motor and cognitive function in patients with disability.

Exercise as an Intervention for Cancer-Related Fatigue; by Watson; *Phys Ther*; 8-04[158]

- Reviews studies on topic.
- Gives recommendations for exercise programs for patients with CRF.
- Gives link information to guidelines (www.nccn.org).

For information on immune system diseases, see CD.

HYPOTHERMIA

Hypothermia is an often fatal environmental emergency. Deaths due to hypothermia are usually accidental and are the result of exposure to extreme environmental temperatures.[159] Exposure to cold, together with the elderly person's decreased ability to cope with the effects of changes in ambient temperature because of decreased metabolism and body fat, less efficient peripheral vasocontriction, often poor nutrition, and concomitant medical disorders, presents a problem of significant dimensions.[160] Other factors contributing to the development of hypothermia are drugs, alcohol, metabolic disorders, stroke, and sepsis.

The ability to perceive cold diminishes with age. The ability to detect environmental temperature differences varies between 2.5° C and 10°C (4.8°F and 18°F) in the elderly as compared with a discrimination threshold of 0.8°C (1.4°F) in the young.[160] Due to lower activity levels and poor circulation, the elderly individual's basal metabolic rate is often significantly decreased, and this is reflected in a lower core temperature. Body water acts as a thermal buffer and heat reservoir, but in the elderly, total body water is decreased, reducing this protective mechanism. Shivering occurs in only 10% of the elderly and, coupled with decreased resting metabolic rate, results in an inability to maintain normal core temperature.[160] These problems, together with concomitant problems (e.g., heart failure, diabetes mellitus, hypothyroidism, movement disorders, and drugs), result in a mortality rate of approximately 50% in the elderly with hypothermia.[159]

Determining that an elderly individual is suffering from hypothermia requires a certain degree of suspicion in conjunction with physical and laboratory examination. Because standard clinical thermometers do not record temperatures below 34.4°C (94°F), a special thermometer may be required to establish core temperature. Skin color is usually pale and cold to the touch, and the individual may be experiencing sleepiness, confusion, and disorientation. Often hypothermia is accompanied by cardiovascular changes, such as hypotension, bradycardia, artrial flutter, and ventricular tachycardia. Pulmonary manifestations are slow, shallow breathing and a decreased cough reflex. Hypothermic individuals frequently present with atelectasis and pneumonia.[159] Changes in laboratory and diagnostic tests include electrolytes (decreased CO_2), creatinine and glucose (increased), CBC (increased Hb, Hct, and WBC), platelets (decreased), PT and PTT (decreased), and arterial blood gases (increased PO_2 and PCO_2 and decreased pH). Neurological symptoms include thick, slow speech, ataxic gait, and depressed reflexes.[160]

Therapy for accidental hypothermia can be divided into primary intervention by rewarming and secondary treatment of the direct effects and complications of hypothermia. From a rehabilitation perspective, activity above the resting level helps to enhance circulation and promote warming of the tissues.

It is not uncommon to see an elderly person wearing a sweater on a hot summer day. With advancing age, the efficiency of mechanisms that regulate heat production and loss declines, placing many older people at high risk for cold discomfort and hypothermia, even in warm environments. Whereas healthy elders compensate by turning up the thermostat and adding extra clothing, the frail elders with impaired environmental awareness, physical abilities, and communication may be dependent on caregivers to provide the extra warmth they require. Education of the caregiver is crucial.

HYPERTHERMIA

Abnormally high body temperature due to pathologic changes, inadequate or inappropriate responses of heat-regulating mechanism, and high environmental temperature represent an important health risk for older people.[161–163] Both chronic diseases exacerbated by heat and heatstroke itself can lead to death in an elderly population. Under usual environmental conditions, convection and radiation, as well as evaporation from skin and lungs, provide adequate heat loss. The hypothalamus regulates heat loss via neuroendocrine and autonomic mechanisms.[161,162] Heat causes blood vessels of the skin to dilate, and increased sweating due to cholinergic discharge occurs. Vasodilation, in turn, increases heart rate and cardiac output (CO).[161] When environmental temperature exceeds body surface temperature, heat loss by convection and radiation stops and heat absorption begins. Evaporation of sweat becomes a means of heat loss, but increased humidity prevents cooling by this mechanism.

Aging appears to reduce the effectiveness of sweating in cooling the body. The sweat glands become fibrotic, and surrounding connective tissue becomes less vascular. In addition, the remaining anatomically normal glands may not function normally. Older individuals require a higher core temperature to initiate sweating and produce lower maximal sweat output.[161,162] Because physiologic responses to heat include vasodilation and associated increases in cardiac work and output, the high prevalence of heart disease in older persons increases their risk of heat stress. Heart failure worsens this problem when ambient heat and humidity are increased. Thus, changes seen both with normal aging and as the consequence of diseases more common in the elderly combine to impair optimal heat regulation.[161,162]

Risk factors for hyperthermia include ambient temperature and humidity, low socioeconomic status (can't afford air-conditioning for home), impaired ability to perform self-care, alcoholism (dehydration), cognitive decline, and concomitant disorders (e.g., cardiovascular or cerebral vascular disease, diabetes, COPD). Some drugs predispose the elderly to heat stroke. Anticholinergic agents, phenothiazines, tricyclic antidepressants, antihistamines, to name a few, impair both hypothalamic function centrally and sweat output peripherally. By altering awareness of heat, these drugs, as well as narcotics, sedative-hypnotics, and alcohol, diminish the ability to respond to heat stress. Amphetamines can increase body temperature by direct action on the hypothalamus. Diuretics (by causing fluid loss) and β-adrenergic blockers (by impairing cardiovascular responsiveness) can increase the risk of heat stroke.[162] Therefore, it is important that the therapist pay close attention to the drugs that the exercising elderly individual is on. Hyperthermia is often a complication of activity and exercise, especially in a hot environment. Sensible environmental manipulation includes having the patient wear light clothing and monitoring the ambient temperature. Adequate fluid intake and avoidance of overexercise are important. Prevention is preferable to treatment, since morbidity and mortality are high due to hyperthermia.

More Medical Pathologies of the Aged of the Aged & Therapeutic

Pathology	Definition		Therapeutic Considerations with Age
Acute and Chronic Renal Failure	Improper kidneys function with associated buildup of toxic waste and fluid kidneys	Decreased blood supply with age and unbalanced diet render elders more susceptible to injury of the	Exercise with monitoring of individuals with chronic renal failure who often show signs of fatigue, muscle weakness, and reduced cardiovascular endurance. Exercise is prescribed per client tolerance. Monitor HR and BP due to associated conditions.

More Medical Pathologies of the Aged & Therapeutic Considerations

Pathology	Definition		Therapeutic Considerations with Age
Diabetes	Inability to produce or properly use insulin causing hyperglycemia	Glucose intolerance ^ with age	Associated diseases such as retinopathy, neuropathy, and musculoskeletal problems need to be considered when creating exercise program. Cardiovascular complications, fatigue, and muscle wasting are common complications. Longer periods of exercise may lead to hypoglycemia. Monitor sugar levels before, during, and after 15 minutes of activity. Be aware of confusion, lethargy, sudoresis, headache, hyperventilation, fruity odor to breath, polyuria, thirst, excessive weakness, increased heart rate, changes in heart rhythm, palpitation, alterations in vision, hunger, shakiness, and numbness of lips and tongue. Exercise should be scheduled to avoid peak insulin time and periods of fasting. Do not administer insulin on muscle groups that will be exercised. Proper footwear is needed.
Cancer	A large group of diseases characterized by abnormal and uncontrolled cell growth that may spread to other body parts	Neoplasms behave differently in older persons	Rehabilitation is effective for patients with cancer (relaxation training, pain management, biofeedback). Be careful with bone metastasis and risk of fracture. Check blood results of patients under chemotherapy or radiotherapy to better prescribe exercise routine. Fatigue and cardiovascular deconditioning may be present. Patient education in energy conservation techniques may be important.
Hypo-/ Hyperthermia	Elevated or lowered core body temperature	Elders more susceptible due to decreased activity and poor nutrition and circulation	Cooling or heating as needed (appropriate clothing layers, lots of fluid). Careful management of physical agents and electrotherapy modalities. Exercise activities should be performed on a comfortable well aired environment. Humidity increases the effect of heat because it limits your ability to sweat. Warm-up and cool-down phases are very important. Cramps and fatigue may be signs of heat exhaustion.

References

1. Holloszy JO, ed. Workshop on sarcopenia: Muscle atrophy in old age. *J Gerontol A Biol Sci Med Sci.* 1995; 50A(special issue):1–161.

2. US Bureau of the Census. *Statistical Abstract of the United States. Profiles of Older Americans: 1999.* Washington DC: US Bureau of the Census; 2000.

3. Kohm RR. Human aging and disease. *J Chron Dis.* 1963; 16:5–21.

4. Administration on Aging. *Older Americans 2000: Key Indicators of Well-Being.* Federal Interagency. Forum on Aging-Related Statistics. Washington DC: US Bureau of the Census; 2000.

5. Johnson HA. Is aging physiological or pathological? In: Johnson HA, ed. *Relations Between Normal Aging and Disease.* Aging Series Vol. 28. New York: Raven Press; 1985: 239–247.

6. Dieftick JE, Whedon GD, Shorr E. Effects of immobilization upon various metabolic and physiologic functions of normal men. *Am J Med.* 1948; 4:3–9.

7. Lamb LE, Stevens PM, Johnson RL. Hypokinesia secondary to chair rest from 4 to 10 days. *Aerospace Med.* 1965; 36:755.

8. Miller PB, Johnson RL, Lamb LE. Effects of four weeks of absolute bed rest on circulatory functions in man. *Aerospace Med.* 1964; 35:1194.

9. Shepard RJ. *Physical Activity and Aging.* 2nd ed. Gaithersburg, MD: Aspen Publishers; 1987.

10. Ragen PB, Mitchell J. The effects of aging on the cardiovascular response to dynamic and static exercise. In: Weisfelt ML, ed. *The Aging Heart*. New York: Raven Press; 1980: 269–296.

11. Ham RJ, Marcy ML, Holtzman JM. The aging process: Biological and social aspects. In: Wright J, ed. *Primary Care Geriatrics*. Boston: PSG, Inc.; 1983.

12. Ewing DJ, Campbell IN, Clarke BF. Heart-rate response to standing as a test for automatic neuropathy. *Brit Med J*. 1978; 1(6128):1700.

13. Thadani U, Davidson C, Singleton W, Taylor SH. Comparison of the immediate effects of five beta-adrenoceptor blocking drugs with different ancillary properties in angina pectoris. *N Engl J Med*. 1989; 300:750–755.

14. Cairns JA. Current management of unstable angina. *Can Med Assoc J*. 1988; 119:477–480.

15. Gerstenblith G, Weisfeldt ML, Lakatta EG. Disorders of the heart. In: Andres R, Bierman EL, Hazzard WR, eds. *Principles of Geriatric Medicine*. New York: McGraw-Hill; 1985: 515–526.

16. Kattus A, Grollman J. Patterns of coronary collateral circulation in angina pectoris: Relation to exercise training. In: Russek HI, Zohman BL, eds. *Changing Concepts of Cardiovascular Disease*. Baltimore: Williams and Wilkins; 1972: 352–376.

17. Larson EB, Bruce RA. Health benefits of exercise in an aging society. *Arch Intern Med*. 1987; 147:353.

18. Webb-Peploe KM, Chua TP, Harrington D, Henein MY, Gibson DG, Coats AJ. Different response of patients with idiopathic and ischaemic dilated cardiomyopathy to exercise training. *Int J Cardiol*. 2000; 74(2–3):215–224.

19. Thomson HL, Morris-Thurgood J, Atherton J, McKenna WJ, Frenneaux MP. Reflex responses of venous capacitance vessels in patients with hypertrophic cardiomyopathy. *Clin Sci*. 1998; 94(4): 339–346.

20. Harrington D, Clark AL, Chua TP, Anker SD, Poole-Wilson PA, Coats AJ. Effects of reduced muscle bulk on the ventilatory response to exercise in chronic congestive heart failure secondary to idiopathic dilated and ischemic cardiomyopathy. *Am J Cardiol*. 1997; 80(1):90–93.

21. Karlsdotter AE, Foster C, Porcari JP, Palmer-McLean K, White-Kube R, Backes RC. Hemodynamic responses during aerobic and resistance exercise. *J Cardiopulm Rehabil*. 2002; 22:170–177.

22. Keteyian SJ, et al. Exercise training in patients with heart failure. *Ann Intern Med*. June 15, 1996; 124 (12):1051–1057.

23. Schneider EL, Reed JD. Modulations of aging processes. In: Finch CE, Schneider EL, eds. *Handbook of the Biology of Aging*. New York: Academic Press; 1985.

24. NIH. *National High Blood Pressure Education Program Coordinating Committee, 1989: Statement on Hypertension in the Elderly*. Bethesda, MD: National Institutes of Health; 1989.

25. Abrams WB. Pathophysiology of hypertension in older patients. *Am J Med*. 1988; 85(suppl 3b):7–13.

26. Young D, Appel L, Lee S, Miller E. The effects of aerobic exercise and T'ai Chi on blood pressure in older people: Results of a randomized trial. *J Am Geriatr Soc*. 1999; 47:277–284.

27. Vaitkevicius PV, et al. Effects of aerobic exercise training in community based subjects 80 and older: A pilot study. *J Am Geriatr Soc*. 2002; 50:2009–2013.

28. Kelley GA, Kelley KS. Progressive resistance exercise and resting blood pressure: A meta-analysis of randomized controlled trials. *Hypertension*. 2000; 35:838–843.

29. Toscani A. Physiology of muscular work in the aged. In: Huet JA, ed. *Work and Aging*. Second international course in social gerontology. International Centre of Social Gerontology, Paris; 1971.

30. Garner AW, Poehlman ET. Exercise rehabilitation programs for the treatment of claudication pain. *JAMA*. 1995; 274:975–980.

31. Patterson RB, Pinto B, Marcus B, Colucci A, Braun T, Roberts M. Value of a supervised exercise program for the therapy of arterial claudication. *J Vasc Surg*. 1997; 25(2):312–319.

32. Regensteiner JG, Steiner JB, Hiatt WR. Exercise training improves functional status in patients with peripheral arterial disease. *J Vasc Surg*. 1996; 23(1): 104–115.

33. Ubels FL, Links TP, Sluiter WJ, Reitsma WD, Smit AJ. Walking for training for intermittent claudication diabetes. *Diabetes Care*. 1999; 22(2):198–201.

34. Brandsma JW, Robeer BG, van den heuvel S, et al. The effect of exercises on walking distance of patients with intermittent claudication: A study of randomized clinical trials. *Phys Ther*. 1998; 78:278–288.

35. Hunt D, Leighton M, Reed G. Intermittent claudication: Implementation of an exercise programe. *Physiotherapy*. March 1999; 85(3).

36. Gardner AW. Exercise training for patients with peripheral artery disease. *Phys and Sports Med*. August 2001; 29(8):25–35.

37. Gelin J, Jivegard L, Taft C, Karisson J, Sullivan M, Dahllof AG, Sandstrom R, Arfividsson B, Lundholm K. Treatment efficacy of intermittent claudication by surgical intervention, supervised physical training compared to no treatment in unselected randomised patients I: One year results of functional and physiological improvements. *Eur J Endo Vasc Surg*. 2001; 22:107–113.

38. Langbein WE, Collins EG, Orebaugh C, Maloney C, Williams KJ, Littooy FN, Edwards LC. Increasing exercise tolerance of persons limited by claudication pain using polestriding. *J Vasc Surg*. 2002; 35(5):887–893.

39. Gardner AW, Katzel LI, Sorkin JD, Bradham DD, Hochberg MC, Flinn WR, Goldberg AP. Exercise rehabilitation improves functional outcomes and peripheral circulation in patients with intermittent claudication: A randomized controlled trial. *J Am Geriatr Soc.* 2001; 49:755–762.

40. Tsai JC, Chan P, Wang CH, Jeng C, Hsieh MH, Kao PF, Chen YJ, Liu JC. The effects of exercise training on walking function and perception of health status in elderly patients with peripheral arterial occlusive disease. *J Int Med.* 2003; 252:448–455.

41. Ambrosetti M, Salerno M, Tramarin R, Pedretti RFE. Efficacy of a short-course intensive rehabilitation program in patients with moderate-to-severe intermittent claudication. *Ital Heart J.* 2002; 3(8): 467–472.

42. Gladman JRF, Barer D, Venkatesan P, et al. The outcome of pneumonia in the elderly: A hospital survey. *Clin Rehab.* 1991; 5:201–204.

43. Kenney RA. *Physiology of Aging: A Synopsis.* Chicago: Year Book Medical Publishers; 1982.

44. Alfaro V, et al. Improvement in exercise tolerance and spirometric values in stable chronic obstructive pulmonary disease patients after an individualized outpatient rehabilitation programm. *J Sports Med Phys Fitness.* 1996; 36:195–203.

45. Casaburi R, et al. Physiologic benefits of exercise training in rehabilitation of patients with severe chronic obstructive pulmonary disease. *Am J Resp Crit Care Med.* 1997; 155:1541–1551.

46. Rosenbaum R, Bach JR, Penek J. The cost/benefits of outpatient-based pulmonary rehabilitation. *Arch Phys Med Rehabil.* 1997; 78:240–244.

47. Gowin KM. Diffuse pain syndromes in the elderly. *Rheum Dis Clin North Am.* 2000; 26(3):673–682.

48. Gowans SE, de Hueck A, Voss S, Richardson M. A randomized, controlled trial of exercise and education for individuals with fibromyalgia. *Arthritis Care Res.* 1999; 12(2):120–128.

49. Clark SR. Prescribing exercise for fibromyalgia patients. *Arthritis Care Res.* December 1994; 7(4).

50. Jentoft ES, Kvalvik AG, Mengshoel AM. Effects of pool-based and land-based aerobic exercise on women with fibromyalgia/chronic widespread muscle pain. *Arthritis Rheum.* February 2001; 45(1): 42–47.

51. Rooks DS, Silverman CB, Kantrowitz FG. The effects of progressive strength training and aerobic exercise on muscle strength and cardiovascular fitness in women with fibromyalgia: A pilot study. *Arthritis Rheum.* February 2003; 47(1):22–28.

52. Buckelew SP, et al. Biofeedback/relaxation training and exercise interventions for fibromyalgia: A prospective trial. *Arthritis Care Res.* 1998; 11(3): 196–209.

53. Pfeiffer, A, Thompson JM, Nelson A, Tucker S, Luedtke C, Finnie S, Sletten C, Postier J. Effects of

54. Bailey A, Starr L, Alderson M, Moreland J. A comparative evaluation of a fibromyalgia rehabilitation program. *Arthritis Care Res.* 1999; 12(5):336–340.

55. Consensus Development Conference. Diagnosis, prophylaxis and treatment of osteoporosis. *Am J Med.* 1993; 94:646–650.

56. Lees B, Banks LM, Stevenson JC. Bone mass measurements. In: Stevenson JC, Lindsay R, eds. *Osteoporosis.* Philadelphia: Chapman & Hall Medical; Lippincott Williams and Wilkins; 1998: 137–160.

57. World Health Organization Study Group on Assessment of Fracture Risk and Its Application to Screening and Postmenopausal Osteoporosis. Report of a WHO Study Group. Technical Report Series (No. 84); 1994.

58. Mundy G. Bone remodeling. In: Favus MJ, ed. *Primer on the Metabolic Bone Diseases and Disorders of Mineral Metabolism.* American Society for Bone and Mineral Research. 4th ed. Philadelphia: Lippincott Williams and Wilkins; 1999: 30–38.

59. Deftos W. *Clinical Essentials of Calcium and Skeletal Disorders.* Caddo, OK: Professional Communications; 1998.

60. Klein FA, Rajan RK. Normal aging: Effects on connective tissue metabolism and structure. *J Gerontol.* 1985; 40(5):579–585.

61. Walker J. Connective tissue plasticity: Issues in histological and light microscopy studies of exercise and aging in articular cartilage. *JOSPT.* 1991; 14(5):189–197.

62. Donatelli R, Owens-Burkart H. Effects of immobilization on the extensibility of periarticular connective tissue. *JOSPT.* 1981; 3(2):67–71.

63. Schiller AL. Bones and joints. In: Rubin E, Farber JL, eds. *Pathology.* 2nd ed. Philadelphia: Lippincott; 1994: 1273–1347.

64. Herman HH, Bottomley JM. Anatomical and biomechanical considerations of the elder foot. *Top Geriatr Rehabil.* 1992; 7(3):1–13.

65. Wedgewood, J. The place of rehabilitation in geriatric medicine: An overview. *Int Rehabil Med.* 1985; 7:107.

66. Molsa PK, Paljarvi L, Rinne JO, et al. Validity of clinical diagnosis in dementia: A prospective clinicopathologic study. *J Neurol Neurosurg Psychiatry.* 1985; 48:1085–1090.

67. Alexopoulos GS, Abrams RC, Young RC, Shamoian CA. Cornell scale for depression in dementia. *Biol Psychiatry.* 1988; 23:271–284.

68. Hughes CP, Berg L, Danziger WL, et al. A new clinical scale for the staging of dementia. *Brit J Psychiatry.* 1982; 140:566–572.

69. Cummings JL, Miller B, Hill MA, Neshkes R. Neuropsychiatric aspects of multi-infarct dementia and dementia of the Alzheimer type. *Arch Neurol.* 1987; 44:389–393.

70. Hachinski VC, Illiff LD, Zilhka E, et al. Cerebral blood flow in dementia. *Arch Neurol.* 1975; 32: 632–637.

71. Gilman S. Alzheimer's disease. *Perspect Bio Med.* 1997; 40:230–245.

72. Post SG. Future scenarios for the prevention and delay of Alzheimer disease onset in high-risk groups. An ethical perspective. *Am J Prev Med.* 1999; 16(2): 105–110.

73. National Center for Health Statistics. *Health, United States, 1999, with Health and Aging Chartbook.* Hyattsville, MD: National Center for Health Statistics; 1999: 36–37.

74. National Center for Health Statistics. *Health, United States, 1999, with Health and Aging Chartbook.* Hyattsville, MD: National Center for Health Statistics; 1999: 34–35.

75. Centers for Disease Control and Prevention. *Unrealized Prevention Opportunities: Reducing the Health and Economic Burden of Chronic Disease.* Atlanta, GA: Centers for Disease Control and Prevention, National Center for Chronic Disease Prevention and Health Promotion; 1997.

76. Forsyth E, Rizline PD. An overview of the etiology, diagnosis, and treatment of Alzheimer disease. *Phys Ther.* 1998; 78:1325–1331.

77. Snowdon DA, Greiner LH, Markesbery WR. Linguistic ability in early life and the neuropathology of Alzheimer's disease and cerebrovascular disease: Finding from the Nun Study. *Ann NY Acad Sci.* 2000; 903:34–38.

78. Small GW, Rabins PV, Barry PP. Diagnosis and treatment of Alzheimer disease and related disorders. *JAMA.* 1997; 278:1363–1371.

79. Wolf DS, Gearing M, Snowdon DA, Mori H, Markesbery WR, Mirra SS. Progression of regional neuropathology in Alzheimer disease and normal elderly: Findings from the Nun Study. *Alzheimer Dis Assoc Disord.* 1999; 13(4): 226–231.

80. Riley KP, Snowdon DA, Saunders AM, Roses AD, Mortimer JA, Nanayakkara N. Cognitive function and apolipoprotein E in very old adults: Findings from the Nun Study. *J Gerontol B Psychol Sci Soc Sci.* 2000; 55(2):S69–S75.

81. Snowdon DA, Tully CL, Smith CD, Riley KP, Markesbery WR. Serum folate and the severity of atrophy of the neocortex in Alzheimer disease: Finding from the Nun Study. *Am J Clin Nutr.* 2000; 71(4):993–998.

82. Snowdon DA. Aging and Alzheimer's disease: Lessons from the Nun Study. *Gerontologist.* 1997; 37(2):150–156.

83. Waters CH. *Management of Parkinson's Disease.* 2nd ed. Caddo, OK: Professional Communications; 1999.

84. Schoenberg BS. Epidemiology of movement disorders. In: Marsden CD, Fahn S, eds. *Movement Disorders.* London: Butterworth; 1987: 17–32.

85. Baloh RW. Neurology of aging: Vestibular system. In: Albert ML, ed. *Clinical Neurology of Aging.* New York: Oxford University Press; 1984.

86. Batata M, Spray GH, Bolton FG, et al. Blood and bone marrow changes in elderly patients, with particular reference to folic acid, vitamin B_{12}, iron and ascorbic acid. *Brit Med J.* 1967; 2:667–669.

87. Burchinsky, SG. Neurotransmitter receptors in the central nervous system and aging: Pharmacological aspects (review). *Experimental Aging.* 1984; 19: 227–239.

88. Gambert SR. *Diabetes Mellitus in the Elderly: A Practical Guide.* New York: Raven Press; 1990.

89. Bergman M. *Principles of Diabetes Management.* New York: Medical Examination Publishing; 1987.

90. Riddle MC. Diabetic neuropathies in the elderly: Management update. *Geriatrics.* 1990; 45(9):32–36.

91. Gutmann E, Hanzlikova V. Basic mechanisms of aging in the neuromuscular system. *Mech Ageing Dev.* 1972; 1:327–349.

92. Chandler JM, Duncan PW. Balance and falls in the elderly: Issues in evaluation and treatment. In: Guccione AA, ed. *Geriatric Physical Therapy.* St. Louis, MO: Mosby-Year Book; 1993: 237–252.

93. Shumway-Cook A, Woollacott MH. *Motor Control: Theory and Function.* Baltimore: Williams and Wilkins; 1995.

94. Fetter M. Vestibular system disorders. In: Herdman SJ, ed. *Vestibular Rehabilitation.* Philadelphia: FA Davis; 1994: 80–89.

95. Allison L. Balance disorders. In: Umphred DA, ed. *Neurological Rehabilitation.* 3rd ed. St Louis: Mosby-Year Book; 1995: 802–837.

96. Epley JM. Aberrant coupling of otolithic receptors: Manifestations and assessment. In: Arenberg IK, ed. *Dizziness and Balance Disorders.* New York: Kugler Publications; 1993: 183–202.

97. Gilchrest BA. *Skin and Aging Processes.* Boca Raton, Fla: CRC Press; 1984: 67–81.

98. Silverberg N, Silverberg L. Aging and the skin. *Postgrad Med.* 1989; 86:131–136.

99. Pollack SV. Skin cancer in the elderly. In: Cohen FU, ed. Cancer II: Specific neoplasms. *Clin Geriatr Med.* 1987; 3(4):715–728.

100. Swagerty DL Jr. The impact of age-related visual impairment on functional independence in the elderly. *Kans Med.* 1995; 96(1):24–26.

101. Hawkins BS, Bird A, Klein R, West SK. Epidemiology of age-related macular degeneration. *Mol Vis.* 1999; 5:26.

102. Fong DS. Age-related macular degeneration: Update for primary care. *Am Fam Physician*. 2000; 61 (10):3035–3042.

103. Silvestri G. Age-related macular degeneration: Genetics and implication for detection and treatment. *Mol Med Today*. 1997; 3(2):84–91.

104. McCarty CA, Nanjan MB, Taylor HR. Attributable risk estimates for cataract to prioritize medical and public health action. *Invest Ophthalmol Vis Sci*. 2000; 41(12):3720–3725.

105. Taylor A. Nutritional influences on risk for cataract. *Int Ophthalmol Clin*. 2000; 40(4):17–49.

106. Storr-Paulsen A, Bernth-Petersen P. Combined cataract and glaucoma surgery. *Curr Opin Ophthalmol*. 2001; 12(1):41–46.

107. Elolia R, Stokes J. Monograph series on aging-related diseases: XI. Glaucoma. *Chronic Dis Can*. 1998; 19(4):157–169.

108. Willis A, Anderson SJ. Effects of glaucoma and aging on photopic and scotopic motion perception. *Invest Ophthalmol Vis Sci*. 2000; 41(1):325–335.

109. Kalina RE. Seeing into the future. Vision and aging.*West J Med*. 1997; 167(4):253–257.

110. Zegeer LJ. The effects of sensory changes in older persons. *J Neuroscience Nurs*. 1986; 18:325–332.

111. Christenson MA. Designing for the older person by addressing the environmental attributes. *Phys Occup Ther Geriatrics*. 1990; 8:31–48.

112. Siebens H, Trupe E, Siebens A, et al. Correlates and consequences of eating dependency in institutionalized elderly. *J Am Geriatr Soc*. 1986; 34(3):192–198.

113. Castell DO. Dysphagia in the elderly. *J Amer Geriatr Soc*. 1986; 34(3):248–249.

114. Bidlack WR, Kirsch A, Meskin MS. Nutritional requirements of the elderly. *Food Technology*. 1988; 40:61–70.

115. Bartol MA, Heitkemper M. Gastrointestinal problems. In: Carnevali P, and Patrick, B, eds. *Nursing Management for the Elderly*. Philadelphia: Lippincott; 1989.

116. Brandeis GH, Baumann MM, Hossain M, Morris JN, Resnick NM. The prevalence of potentially remediable urinary incontinence in frail older people: A study using the Minimum Data Set. *J Am Geriatr Soc*. 1997; 45(2):179–184.

117. Dillon L, Fonda D. Medical evaluation of causes of lower urinary tract symptoms and urinary incontinence in older people. *Top Geriatr Rehabil*. 2000; 15 (4):1–15.

118. Fonda D. Nocturia: A disease or normal ageing? *Brit J Urol Int*. 1999; 84(1):13–15.

119. Vliet EL. Hormone connections in urinary incontinence in women. *Top Geriatr Rehabil*. 2000; 15(4): 16–30.

120. Resnick NM. Urinary incontinence in the elderly. *Medical Grand Rounds*. 1984; 3:281–290.

121. Resnick NM. Urinary incontinence. *Lancet*. 1995; 345:94–99.

122. Meadows E. Physical therapy for older adults with urinary incontinence. *Top Geriatr Rehabil*. 2000; 16 (1):22–32.

123. Fantl JA, Newman DK, Colling J. *Urinary Incontinence in Adults: Acute and Chronic Management. Clinical Practice Guideline No. 2, 1996 Update*. Rockville, MD: US Department of Health and Human Services, Agency for Health Care Policy and Research; 1996. AHCPR Pub No. 96-0682.

124. Burgio, Kathryn L. et al. Behavioral versus drug treatment for urge urinary incontinence in older women. *JAMA*. December 1998; 280(23): 1995–2000.

125. Bo K, Talseth T, Holme I. Single blind, randomised controlled trial of pelvic floor exercises, electrical stimulation, vaginal cones, and no treatment in management of genuine stress incontinence in women. *Brit Med J*. 1999; 318:487–493.

126. Spruijt J, Vierhout M, Verstraeten R, Janssens J, Burger C. Vaginal electrical stimulation of the pelvic floor: A randomized feasibility study in urinary incontinent elderly women. *Acta Obstet Gynecol Scand*. 2003; 82(11):1043–1048(6).

127. Snape WJ. Disorders of gastrointestinal motility. In: Wyngaarden JB, Smith LH, Bennett JC, eds. *Cecil Textbook of Medicine*. 19th ed. Philadelphia: WB Saunders; 1992: 671–680.

128. Andres R. Normal aging versus disease in the elderly. In: Andres EL, Bierman EL, Hazzard WR, eds. *Principles in Geriatric Medicine*. New York: McGraw-Hill; 1985: 38–41.

129. Goldman R. Decline in organ function with age. In: Rossman I, ed.*Clinical Geriatrics*. 2nd ed. Philadelphia: Lippincott; 1979.

130. Goyal VK. Changes with age in the human kidney. *Exp Gerontol*. 1982; 17:321–331.

131. Lindeman RD, Goldman R. Anatomic and physiologic age changes in the kidney. *Exp Gerontol*. 1986; 21:379–406.

132. Lindeman RD, Tobin JD, Shock NW. Longitudinal studies on the rate of decline in renal function with age. *J Am Geriatr Soc*. 1985; 33:278–285.

133. Fine LG. Preventing the progression of human renal disease: Have rational therapeutic principles emerged? *Kidney Int*. 1988; 33:116–128.

134. Nieman DC. *The Sports Medicine Fitness Course*. Palo Alto, CA: Bull Publishing; 1986.

135. Drinkwater BL: *The Role of Nutrition and Exercise in Health. Continuing Dental Education*. Seattle: University of Washington; 1985.

136. Suominen H, Heikkinen E, Liesen H. Effect of 8 weeks endurance training on skeletal muscle metabolism in 56–70 year old men. *Eur J Appl Physiol*. 1987; 37:173–180.

137. Kaplin GA, Seemah TE, Cohen RD. Mortality among the elderly in the Alameda County study: Behavioral and demographic risk factors. *Am J Public Health*. 1987; 77(3):307–312.

138. Stones MJ, Dorman B, Kozma A. The prediction of mortality in elderly institution resident. *J Gerontol Psychol Sci*. 1989; 44(3):72–79.

139. Konstantinidou E, Koukouvou G, Kouidi E, Deligiannis A Tourkantonis. Exercise training in patients with end-stage renal disease on hemodialysis: Comparison of three rehabilitation programs. *J Rehabil Med*. 2002; 34:40–45.

140. Oh-Park M, Fast A, Gopal S, Lynn R, Frei G, Drenth R, Zohman L. Exercise for the dialyzed aerobic and strength training during hemodialysis. *Am J Phys Med Rehabil*. 2002; 814–821.

141. Mercer TH, Crawford C, Gleeson NP, Naish PF. Low-volume exercise rehabilitation improves functional capacity and self-reported functional status of dialysis patients. *Am J Phys Med Rehabil*. 2002; 81:162–167.

142. Lipson LG. Diabetes in the elderly: Diagnosis, pathogenesis and therapy. *Am J Med*. 1986; 80(suppl 5A):10–21.

143. Morley JE, Mooradian AD, Rosenthal MJ, et al. Diabetes mellitus in elderly patients: Is it different? *Am J Med*. 1987; 83:533–544.

144. Helmrich SP, Ragland GR, Leung RW, Paffenbarger RS. Physical activity and reduced occurrence of non-insulin-dependent diabetes mellitus. *N Engl J Med*. July 1991; 325(3):147–152.

145. Wei, J. Low cardio-respiratory fitness and physical inactivity as predictors of mortality in men with Type 2 diabetes. *Ann Intern Med*. 2000.

146. Eriksson J, et al. Resistance training in the treatment of non-insulin-dependent diabetes mellitus. *Int J Sports Med*. 1997; 18:242–246.

147. Brandon JL, Gaasch DA, Boyette LW, Lloyd AM. Effects of long term resistive training on mobility and strength in older adults with diabetes. *J Ger Med Sci*. 2003; 58A(8):740–745.

148. Yancik R, Ries LA. Cancer in the older person: Magnitude of the problem. In: Balducci L, Lyman GH, Ershler WB. *Comprehensive Geriatric Oncology*. Amsterdam,: The Netherlands: Harwood Academic Publishers; 1998: 95–104.

149. Duthie EH. Physiology of aging: Relevance to symptoms, perceptions, and treatment tolerance. In: Balducci L, Lyman GH, Ershler WB. *Comprehensive Geriatric Oncology*. Amsterdam, The Netherlands: Harwood Academic Publishers; 1998: 247–262.

150. Campisi J. Aging and cancer: The double edged sword of proliferative senescence. *J Am Geriatr Soc*. 1997; 45(4):482–490.

151. Anisimov V. Age as a risk factor for multistage carcinogenesis. In: Balducci L, Lyman GH, Ershler WB. *Comprehensive Geriatric Oncology*. Amsterdam, The Netherlands: Harwood Academic Publishers; 1998: 157–178.

152. Barbone F, Bonvenzi M, Cavallieri F. Air pollution and lung cancer in Trieste, Italy. *Am J Epidemiol*. 1995; 141:1161–1169.

153. Balducci L. Prevention and Treatment of Cancer in the Elderly. *Oncol Issues*. 2000; 15:26–28.

154. Balducci L, Beghe C. The application of the principles of geriatrics to the management of the older person with cancer. *Crit Rev Oncol Hematol*. 2000; 35(3):147–154.

155. Cerhan JR, et al. Physical activity, physical function, and the risk of breast cancer in a prospective study among elderly women. *J Gerontol*. 1998; 53A(4): M251–M256.

156. Garman KS, Peiper CF, Seo P, Cohen P, Cohen HJ. Function in elderly cancer survivors depends on co-morbidities. *J Geront Med Sci*. Vol 58A No. 12 pp. 1119–1124.

157. Cole RP, Scialla SJ, Bednarz L. Functional recovery in cancer rehabilitation. *Arch Phys Med Rehabil*. 2003; 81:623–627.

158. Watson T, Mock V. Exercise as an intervention for cancer-related fatigue. *Phys Ther*. 2004; 84(8): 736–743.

159. Ward ME, Cowley AR. Hypothermia: A natural cause of death. *Am J Forensic Med Path*. 1999; 20 (4):383–386.

160. Worfolk JB. Keep frail elders warm! *Geriatr Nurs*. 1997; 18(1):7–11.

161. Stauss HM, Morgan DA, Anderson KE, Massett MP, Kregel KC. Modulation of baroreflex sensitivity and spectral power of blood pressure by heat stress and aging. *Am J Physiol*. 1997; 272(2 pt 2):H776– H784.

162. Vassallo M, Gera KN, Allen S. Factors associated with high risk of marginal hyperthermia in elderly patients living in an institution. *Postgrad Med J*. 1995; 71(834):213–216.

163. Fehrenbach E, Niess AM. Role of heat shock proteins in the exercise response. *Exerc Immunol Rev*. 1999; 5:57–77.

6

Exploring Nutritional Needs

Pearls

- The age-related changes in the gastrointestinal system, such as decreased saliva, poor dentition, decrements of taste and olfaction, gastromucosal atrophy, and reduced intestinal mobility, will have the most impact on nutritional status because this system is directly involved in digestion.

- Obesity is common in the aged and can be due to decreased activity, medication, and poorly balanced diet. This problem is associated with numerous medical disabilities, such as osteoarthritis, diabetes, hypertension, and heart disease, and can greatly hinder an older person's independence.

- The clinical evaluation of nutritional status can be done by the use of anthropometric measures, functional assessment tools, physical signs of nutrition deficiencies, or a combination of these.

- The elderly require a higher quality, more nutrient dense (i.e., more nutrients per calorie) diet.

- The recommended daily allowance of nutrients changes with advancing age.

- Drugs may affect nutritional status in the simplest sense by their effect on appetite, but more commonly, absorption, metabolism, and excretion of dietary constituents are altered.

- Despite the fact that the way to get an abundant supply of nutrients is through healthy eating (a variety of foods on a daily basis), many elderly individuals do not consume a balanced diet and require supplementation.

- Programs such as the Federal Food Assistance program, federal food stamps, and congregate and home-delivered meals can assist the older person in attaining adequate nutrition.

INTRODUCTION

As the population ages, it is increasingly important to understand the factors that affect the nutritional status and thus the health status of older adults. Many factors contribute to inadequate nutrition, including health status, financial capacities, mobility, exercise, and physiologic needs.[1,2]

Nutritional manifestations often overlap normal aging and disease and facilitate their progression. In fact, nutritional deficits frequently mimic and exacerbate the aging process. With the elderly, under- and overnutritional problems and concerns are of great importance in accurately determining overall fitness and functional levels of activity. The Department of Health and Human Services (DHHS) has continued earlier efforts begun by the Surgeon General with *Healthy People 2010*. The benefits of better nutrition (in addition to increased levels of physical activity) have been realized with resulting increases in longevity and a compression of morbidity.[3–5]

This chapter will address the changes related to aging that affect the nutritional well-being of the elderly by looking at common deficiencies and risk factors. Guidelines for good nutrition in the elderly and the impact of poor nutrition on the physical, emotional, and cognitive well-being of the elderly will also be addressed. In addition, components of nutritional programs for the elderly will be presented to provide the necessary guidelines for nutritional measures and the insights essential to assessing the nutritional status of the elderly to promote health, prevent or reduce risks of certain diseases, support other medical interventions, and improve the quality of life in old age.

There is no clear demarcation to indicate where on the spectrum of "healthy old age" nutrition begins and ends. There is clearly a state produced by normal aging, but there is great difficulty in identifying this conceptually "healthy" state in the absence of overt or occult disease. As each cohort ages there is a progressive variability in biological efficiency. This variability is a result of a combination of the disparate influences of activity, disease, environment, time, genetic profile, and nutrition on an individual's aging process.

AGE-RELATED CHANGES IN THE GASTROINTESTINAL SYSTEM

Changes in the digestive system will have the most impact on nutritional status as the gastrointestinal tract is most directly involved in ingestion, absorption, transport, and excretion of food products.[1,6]

> For more information on the age-related physiological changes that affect nutrition, see CD.

Changes in the Liver

There is a decrease in the liver enzyme activity with aging. This directly affects the metabolism of carbohydrates and the breakdown of drugs and alcohol in the system. Alterations in synthetic, excretory, or metabolic processes can affect the response to disease and the disposition of drugs. This is more thoroughly covered in the subsequent chapter on pharmacology (Chapter 7, Geriatric Pharmacology).

Liver weight decreases and this parallels the anthropometric changes of decreased body weight and muscle mass. In advanced age, the liver becomes disproportionately small and there is a reduction in the numbers of hepatocytes. Other changes in liver morphology are nonspecific and may be due to extrahepatic processes. There is an increase in portal and periportal fibrosis, and liver cells tend to be larger. It is suggested that the enlargement of the liver cells may be due to compensatory hypertrophy.[1] An increased amount of lipofuscin pigment is present in the Kupffer's cells, and changes in the Golgi apparatus and rough and smooth endoplasmic reticulum may parallel hepatic functional changes seen in older individuals.[7]

Decreases in liver blood flow occur with age resulting in the potential for changes in drug metabolism. Levels of albumin, a product of hepatic synthesis, are frequently reduced in the elderly and result in a decreased rate of total body protein synthesis.[1]

Other Age-Related Changes

Other age-related changes or chronic diseases influencing food habits are those affecting the musculoskeletal, neuromuscular, cardiovascular, and pulmonary systems. Problems creating pain, weakness, paralysis, breathing difficulties, or fatigue create loss of function and resulting immobility. Shopping, opening food containers, and cooking can often become insurmountable obstacles.

Changes in body composition and weight and a decline in physical exercise and activity levels also influence nutritional needs. With aging, as with inactivity, there is an increase in adipose tissue, a decrease in lean body mass, a decrease in basal metabolism (only a problem from the prospective of obesity), a decrease in caloric requirements, and a decrease in total body water.[8]

Predictors of potential malnutrition include recent weight loss, depression, bereavement, loneliness, multiple medications and long-term medication use, and functional losses.

CHRONIC DISEASE AND NUTRITION IN THE ELDERLY

Aging processes and lifelong eating patterns are often associated with diseases and disorders that influence the life span, such as atherosclerosis, hypertension, osteoporosis, diabetes, cancer, Alzheimer's disease, renal disease, dental disease, obesity, and immunity.[9] The prevalence of many chronic degenerative diseases increases with advancing age. These disease states may have synergistic negative effects on individuals whose physiological function is already compromised by the aging process. Many chronic conditions have dietary implications that alter the need for nutrients, the physical and metabolic form in which nutrients are delivered, and the activities of daily living related to food and eating. Modifications in the type or amount of energy, or in the energy-providing nutrients, vitamins, and minerals, may all be called for in order to provide nutritional support or to control the progression of chronic degenerative diseases. Unfortunately, manifestations of malnutrition, such as cracks in the mouth or a bright red tongue, are overt signs of a problem that is far advanced. For example, physical signs of dehydration are usually not apparent until it's in the advanced stages. With decreased nutrient intake, there is gradual tissue depletion with evolving biochemical abnormalities before an overt deficiency surfaces. Table 6.1 summarizes the most frequently encountered conditions and the related nutritional problems.

> For additional information on chronic disease in the elderly, see CD.

Obesity and Nutrition in the Elderly

Obesity is common in persons aged 65 years or older. A diet that is higher in calories than required for the body's energy needs leads to energy storage and fat deposition. Excess calories from fat, carbohydrate, and protein foods lead to obesity. Some drugs promote appetite (hyperphagic

TABLE 6.1   Chronic Conditions and Related Nutritional Problems

Chronic Condition	Related Nutritional Problems
Alzheimer's disease, other dementias	Cachexia and emaciation due to poor eating habits and self-care
Celiac sprue	Malabsorption, diarrhea, weight loss, malabsorption with secondary vitamin deficiencies
Cerebral vascular accident	Suppressed cough reflex, increased risk of choking, dysphagia
Chronic mesenteric ischemia	Abdominal pain after eating, weight loss, malabsorption
Constipation	Prolonged transit time especially with immobility, decreased colonic motility
Gastroenteritis	Malabsorption, protein and vitamin B complex deficiencies, poor absorption of calcium and all other nutrients, loss of appetite
Colitis	Decreased elasticity of rectal wall, abdominal discomfort, fecal impaction
Coronary artery disease	Dyspnea, drugs lead to suppressed appetite and constipation
Diabetes mellitus	Glucose intolerance, poor energy utilization
Diverticular disease	Gastrointestinal pain, bowel discomfort, possible bleeding, infection, lack of appetite, weight loss
Emphysema	Dyspnea leading to lack of appetite and difficulty eating
Gallbladder disease	Gallstones, cholecystitis, pancreatitis, food restriction, some foods repugnant, undernutrition
Gastritis/duodenitis	Malabsorption of proteins, vitamin B_{12} and iron, some food restrictions, other foods repugnant, undernutrition
Hiatal hernia	Gastroesophageal reflux, heartburn, dysphagia
Liver diseases	Foods repugnant, restricted protein, drug level changes
Obesity	Energy intakes usually low, need for essential nutrient intake
Osteoarthritis	Difficulty in food shopping and preparation
Osteoporosis	Dyspnea with vertebral collapse, distortion of thorax and abdominal compression, lack of appetite, difficulty eating, decreased intake
Peptic ulcer	Obstruction, bleeding, and perforation, dysphagia, dyspepsia, retrosternal discomfort, antacid overuse and undernutrition
Pernicious anemia	B_{12} deficiency, spinal cord degeneration
Renal disease	Limited ability to handle protein, sodium, potassium, and water

Modified and used with permission: Dwyer, J.T. Nutritional concerns and problems of the aged. In: Satin, D.E., ed. The Clinical Care of the Aged Person: An Interdisciplinary Perspective. *New York: Oxford University Press; 1993.*

drugs) leading to obesity because of increased food intake. Alcohol intake, in addition to a diet that provides sufficient food-energy to meet caloric needs, can also lead to obesity. Reduction in body weight in obese persons is commonly retarded or impeded by a disinclination for exercise. Exercise may also be restricted as a result of secondary effects of obesity, such as osteoarthritis and cardiovascular dysfunction leading to physical disabilities.

Obesity is associated with numerous medical disabilities. Causal relationships have been identified between obesity and the development of late-onset diabetes, essential hypertension, and hypertensive heart disease. Obesity increases the risk of cardiovascular disease. Data from the Framingham Heart Study demonstrate a continuous rela-

tionship between obesity and coronary morbidity and mortality (greater in men than in women). Obesity is associated with increased blood pressure and serum lipoprotein levels.[10] The effects of weight change on blood lipid profiles are considerable. The Framingham Study has shown that weight reduction results in modest increases in high-density lipoprotein (HDL) cholesterol.[11] It appears that both blood lipids and blood pressure are sensitive to the degree of obesity.

Obesity is the most common nutritional problem of public health concern in the United States.[12] While gross obesity is uncommon in the very old (because persons who are morbidly obese are more likely to die at an earlier age), obesity is still a serious disability in the elderly.

Obesity is also associated with the development of abdominal hernias. Gallbladder disease and gout are more common in obese individuals, and most importantly, obesity is associated with increased symptoms of degenerative osteoarthritis. Other complications include varicose veins with stasis dermatitis and stasis ulcers and bacterial and yeast infections between fat folds.[10,11]

In general, obesity is a hindrance to independent living in the elderly. Despite the limitations of modern actuarial reports and experimental finding, the data do show that obesity shortens life span and that limitation in food or caloric intake can result in a longer life.[13]

Nutrition and Immunity in the Elderly

Immune function declines with age, leading to increased infection and cancer rates in aged individuals.[14,15] In fact, recent progress in the study of immune system aging has introduced the idea that rather than a general decline in the functions of the immune system with age, immune aging is mainly characterized by a progressive appearance of immune dysregulation throughout life.[15,16] Nutritional factors play a major role in the immune responses of aged individuals and are of great consequence even in the very healthy elderly.

Systemic studies have confirmed that nutrient deficiencies impair immune system response and lead to frequent severe infections resulting in increased mortality, especially in the elderly.[16–19] Protein-energy malnutrition results in reduced number and function of T cells, phagocytic cells, and secretory immunoglobin A antibody response. In addition, levels of many complement components are reduced.[16,18] Similar findings have been reported for moderate deficiencies of individual nutrients such as trace minerals and vitamins, particularly zinc, iron, selenium, vitamins A, B_6, C, and E.[16,17] For example, zinc deficiency is associated with profound impairment of cell-mediated immunity such as lymphocyte stimulation response and decreased chemotaxis of phagocytes. In addition, the level of thymulin, which is a zinc-dependent hormone, is markedly decreased.[16,20] The use of nutrient supplements, singly or in combination, stimulates immune response and may result in fewer infections in the elderly, as well as reducing the problems associated with malnourished, critically ill elderly patients.

Malnutrition is often one of the consequences of chronic and neoplastic diseases.[17–19] Additionally, secondary immunological changes occur as the result of environmental factors other than diet, including drug intake, physical activity, and stress, or are alternatively due to underlying diseases. For instance, the effects of high lipid intake as well as the impact of diseases, such as Alzheimer's disease and atherosclerosis, underline the complexity of immunological alterations to be expected in old age.[20] Because aging and malnutrition exert cumulative influences on immune responses, many elderly people have poor cell-mediated immune responses and are therefore at greater risk for infection and complications associated with an immunosuppressed response.[21]

Both excessive thinness[22] and severe obesity are associated with impaired immune responses, and obesity increases the risk of infection.[23] All forms of sugar (including honey) interfere with the ability of white blood cells to destroy bacteria. Diets high in sucrose impair immune system response.[24,25] Alcohol intake, including single episodes of moderate consumption, has an immunosuppressive effect.[26,27]

Excessive intake of total dietary fat impairs immune response, but some types of fat (monounsaturated fats, as found in olive oil) have no detrimental effects and may even be beneficial.[28,29] Research on the effect of the omega-3 fats abundant in fish, fish oils, and flaxseed oil, has shown that they improve immune system function and reduce infections in critically ill patients.[30] The positive effects of omega-3 fats have been demonstated to be further improved with the addition of antioxidants, especially vitamin E.[31]

As previously discussed, zinc supplements have been reported to increase immune function and this effect is particularly potent in the elderly, most of whom have zinc deficiencies.[32,33] Vitamin A plays an important role in immune system function and helps mucous membranes, including those in the lungs, resist invasion by microorganisms.[34] Beta-carotene and other carotenoids have increased immune cell numbers and activity in human research, an effect that appears to be separate from their role as precursors to vitamin A.[35] In the elderly, supplementation may increase natural killer cell activity.[36] Vitamin C stimulates the immune system by elevating interferon[37] levels and enhancing the activity of immune cells.[38] Vitamin E enhances all measures of immune cell activity in the elderly.[39] A combination of antioxidant vitamins A, C, and E has been found to significantly improve immune cell number and activity compared to placebo in a group of hospitalized elderly people.[40] Most double-blind studies find that elderly people have better immune function and reduced infection rates when taking a multivitamin.[41,42]

CLINICAL EVALUATION OF NUTRITIONAL STATUS

There are several physical findings related to nutritional status, and many of the normal changes of aging mimic clinical findings described as pathognomic of malnutritive states in the elderly.[2] Clinically overt malnutrition is rarely caused by a primary deficit in nutritional intake; rather, it is more likely associated with gastrointestinal tract dysfunctions or with one of the chronic debilitating illnesses common to the elderly. In contrast, subclinical malnutrition,[43] by definition, undetectable by physical findings on clinical evaluation, is probably frequent in certain at-risk elderly populations. These subgroups might include those who are institutionalized, those with mental disturbances or gross central nervous system disease, or those at or below the poverty level. In subclinical malnutritive states, an elderly individual may manifest depleted nutritional reserves as a failure to thrive. Diminished nutritional reserves may contribute to postoperative confusion, delayed recovery times of homeostatic function, slow wound healing, and increased susceptibility to infection.[44]

Anthropometric variables provide estimates of body composition that can be utilized as indicators of nutritional status. The most relevant of anthropometric measures are weight and skin-fold thickness.[45] Weight is a measure of all the constituents of the body. Weight, however, does not reflect any of the alterations or changes in the relative proportions of body constituents which accompany aging, specifically the increase in fat and decline in lean muscle mass. Variables, such as food or fluid intake, constipation, or problems producing edema, are not accounted for by weight measures.[46,47] *Weight/height* measures have been standardized to define "ideal" weights. Another measure utilizing weight is a *weight/stature* measure. This measure provides a moderate correlation with percent of body fat and a high degree of correlation with total body fat in the elderly.[48] A third weight measure is *relative weight.* Height decreases approximately 3 cm during an average life span as a result of loss of bony mass secondary to osteoporosis, loss of joint space resulting from intervertebral disk shrinkage and wearing of articular cartilage, and postural changes, such as kyphosis due to anterior vertebral wedge fractures. Because of the potential inaccuracies in the estimation of height, other related measures are employed. For example, recumbent length or arm span measures are used for comparison to actual height measures. Arm span is a reasonable equivalent to height during all stages of the life span. The measure of "wing span" reflects the height prior to loss of stature with age. Relative weight is then determined utilizing adjusted height tables which have been standardized to account for possible height reduction adjusted for age.[49,50]

Other anthropometric measures include triceps/subscapular skin-fold thickness and upper arm circumference. The accuracy of skin-fold thickness measures in the elderly is questionable due to age-related changes in the skin and altered skin compressability. Upper arm circumference is a good measure of total body fat in edematous patients in cases where weight might be misleading. There are, however, progressive muscular changes associated with aging, specifically an increase in fibrous tissue, loss of muscle fibers, and an increase in intramuscular fat, that may confound the accuracy of this measure. Measuring skin-fold thickness at the inferior angle of the scapula is more precise than triceps caliper measures as a result of these confounding factors. It is important to recognize that all of these anthropometric measures do not actually measure nutritional status; rather, they provide an indicator of nutritional status. When compared with standardized norms, these measures provide a percentile nutritional rank for the individual patient.[51,52]

Laboratory evaluations that may contribute to nutritional evaluation or appropriate nutritional intervention include assessment of visceral protein status (serum transferrin or albumin), renal and liver function, pancreatic endocrine function (glucose), serum electrolytes and minerals (calcium, magnesium, and phosphorus), and hematologic evaluation (total lymphocyte count and red cell indices). Although not routinely used, delayed cutaneous hypersensitivity testing (skin test antigens) may be helpful to gauge systemic immune function. Determination of nitrogen balance by 24-hour urinary urea nitrogen (UUN) is helpful in nutritional intervention regimens, particularly in the use of enteral or parenteral nutrition. The aim of nutritional intervention is to minimize the degree of negative nitrogen balance (i.e., excessive loss of body protein not compensated by adequate nutritional intake). If nitrogen intake is less than output, the patient is considered to be in negative nitrogen balance, with a net loss of body protein. This contributes to progressive muscle wasting, fatigue, and immune compromise. Therefore obtaining this information is imperative in comprehensive nutritional assessment of elderly individuals.[51,52]

Functional assessment tools are also valuable in assessing the elderly individual's nutritional status. Increasingly, attention has been paid to the importance of maintaining essential activities of daily living among the aged. Simple questionnaires have been developed that appear to be closely associated with nutritional risk.[46,51–53] These provide another type of assessment tool important in assessing the overall nutrition-related functional status. Functional assessment tools such as those evaluating basic activities of daily living and instrumental activities of daily living provide important insights into the well-being of the aged.[46,51,54]

The clinical or physical examination may reveal findings associated with nutritional deficiencies.[51,52] The history and physical examination are the most important components of assessment of nutritional status. This should include weight history (current, usual, and ideal); assessent of oral intake changes (type and duration); symptoms impacting nutrition (including anorexia, nausea and vomiting, diarrhea, constipation, stomatitis/mucositis, dry mouth, taste/olfactory abnormalitites, and pain); medications that may affect intake or metabolic requirements; other medical conditions that may affect nutritional intake or nutrition intervention options; and performance status evaluation. Physical examination entails a general assessment of physical condition, including evidence of weight loss, loss of subcutaneous fat, muscle wasting, presence of sacral or tibial edema, or ascites.

Table 6.2 provides possible clinical manifestations of nutritional deficiencies that can occur in the aged. It is

TABLE 6.2   Physical Manifestations of Malnutrition

Nutrient Deficiency	Physical Manifestation
Protein	Edema; hypoalbuminemia; enlarged liver; diarrhea
Protein/Energy	Muscle wasting; sparse, thin, dry, brittle hair; dry, inelastic skin; muscle weakness
Vitamin A	Poor visual accommodation to dark; Bitot's spots (eyes); dryness of the eyes; hair loss; impaired taste; gooseflesh
Vitamin D	Bowed legs, beading of ribs, and other skeletal deformities (rickets)
Vitamin K	Bleeding (poor coagulation of blood)
Thiamin B_1	Cardiac enlargement; mental confusion; irritability; calf muscle tenderness and foot drop; hypoflexia; hyperesthesia; paresthesia
Riboflavin B_2	Fissures around mouth; reddened, scaly, greasy skin around the nose and mouth; magenta-colored tongue
Niacin B_3	Bright red, swollen, painful tongue; pellagrous dermatitis; depression, insomnia, headaches, dizziness; dementia; diarrhea
Pyridoxine B_6	Neuropathies; glossitis; nasolabial seborrhea
Folic Acid	Red, painful, shiny, smooth tongue; skin hyperpigmentation
Vitamin B_{12}	Mild dementia; sensory losses in hands and feet; red, smooth, shiny, painful tongue; mild jaundice; optic neuritis; anorexia; diarrhea
Vitamin C	Joint tenderness and swelling; hemorrhages under the skin; spongy gums that bleed easily; poor wound healing; petechiae
Essential Fatty Acids	Sparse hair growth; dry, flaky skin; depression and psychosis, dementia
Calcium	Poor reflexes; poor cardiovascular accommodation to activity; slow mental processing; depression; dementia
Magnesium	Lethargy and weakness; anorexia and vomiting; tremor; convulsions
Iodine	Goiter
Iron	Pallor; pale, atrophic tongue; spoon-shaped nails; pale conjunctivae
Zinc	Sluggish muscle contraction; poor wound healing; diminished taste and appetite; dermatitis, hair loss, diarrhea

important to keep in mind that before ascribing any physical findings elicited on physical examination to nutritional problems, the clinician should consider whether the findings are consistent with normal aging or with an underlying disease state.

Obtaining a quantitative as well as a qualitative dietary history can be helpful in dietary assessment, especially as a means of demonstrating to the elderly person or his or her family or caregiver that changes can be made to increase calorie, protein, and micronutrient intake. Useful data also include specific likes, dislikes, and intolerance of specific foods by the person. The latter may help to determine the need for specific supplemental nutrients or enzymes (lactase, other disaccharidases, or pancreatic enzymes).

Malnutrition is an important predictor of morbidity and mortality. In the elderly, various subjective nutritional assessments have been developed that provide high interrater agreement, correlate with other measures of nutritional status, and predict subsequent morbidity. Familiarizing the

rehabilitation professional with the information garnered from such tools is helpful in synchronizing nutritional with functional goals. Standardized staging criteria for degree of nutritional deficit or risk have been developed and validated in two commonly utilized tools.[52,55–57]

The Subjective Global Assessment (SGA) is a reproducible and valid tool for determining nutritional status in the institutional[55] and community-dwelling elderly.[51] This evaluation tool has been validated in a number of patient populations including surgical, human immunodeficiency virus (HIV), acquired immunodeficiency syndrome (AIDS), renal dialysis, and cancer populations.[57] With appropriate training, the method is sensitive, specific, and has little interobserver variability. Figure 6.1 provides an example of information obtained by the SGA.[56] It is comprised of a patient survey and clinician evaluation that correlates with physical measures of skin-fold caliper, weight and height measures, and nutritional status and has been determined to be highly predictive for morbidity and mortality.[51] The SGA has been found to be particularly

Patient Name (Last Name, First Name): _____   **Date:** _____

History

1. <u>Weight change:</u> Overall loss in past 6 months: amount = _____ kg _____ %

   Change in past 2 weeks: ☐ increase   ☐ no change   ☐ decrease

2. <u>Dietary intake change</u> (relative to normal)   ☐ no change

   ☐ change duration = _____ weeks

   type: ☐ suboptimal solid diet   ☐ full liquid diet

   ☐ hypocaloric liquids   ☐ starvation

3. <u>Gastrointestinal symptoms</u> (that persisted for > 2 weeks)

   ☐ none   ☐ nausea   ☐ vomiting   ☐ diarrhea   ☐ anorexia

4. <u>Functional capacity</u>   ☐ no dysfunction (i.e., full capacity)

   ☐ dysfunction   duration = _____ weeks

   type: ☐ working suboptimally   ☐ ambulatory   ☐ bedridden

Physical (for each trait specify: 0 = normal, 1+ = mild, 2+ = moderate, 3+ = severe)

_____ loss of subcutaneous fat (triceps, chest)

_____ muscle wasting (quadriceps, deltoids)

_____ ankle edema

_____ sacral edema

_____ ascites (accumulation of fluid in the peritoneal cavity of abdomen)

Subjective Global Assessment rating (select one)

YA = well nourished

YB = moderately (or suspected of being) malnourished

YC = severely malnourished

Figure 6.1   Subjective Global Assessment (SGA). (Source: Sacks, G.S., Dearman, K., Replogle, W.H., Cora, V.L., Meeks, M., Canada, T. Use of Subjective Global Assessment to identify nutrition-associated complications and death in geriatric long-term care facility residents. *J Amer Coll Nutrition.* 2001; *19(5):570–577.)*

sensitive in identifying elderly individuals who are undernourished or at risk for developing undernutrition.[56] Similarly, the Mini Nutritional Assessment (MNA) is designed and validated to provide a single, rapid assessment of nutritional status in elderly patients in outpatient clinics, hospitals, and nursing homes.[52] The MNA has been found to be an efficient method for detecting malnutrition in the elderly and also accurately predicts the one-year mortality.[58] It has been translated into several languages and validated in many clinics around the world. The MNA is composed of simple measurements and brief questions that can be completed in about ten minutes. Figure 6.2 provides a sample of the information collected by the MNA in its various formats.[58,59] Like the SGA, the MNA scale has also been found to be predictive of mortality as well as predictive of hospital cost.[52] Most important, it is possible to identify people at risk for malnutrition be-

fore severe changes in weight or albumin levels occur. These individuals are more likely to have a decrease in caloric intake that can be easily corrected by nutritional intervention.[52]

NUTRITIONAL REQUIREMENTS OF THE ELDERLY

Many studies have been done on nutrition in institutionalized elders, but there are inherent difficulties in assessing the nutritional status of community elderly. As a group, there is very little information available relating to the nutritional quality of diets consumed by the elderly compared to any other age group. Major nationwide surveys, such as the USDA Food Consumption Surveys, the Department of Health and Human Services Ten State Nutrition Survey,

---

Last name: **First name**   **Sex:**   **Date:**

Age: **Weight, kg:**   **Height, cm:**   **I.D. Number:**

Complete the screen by filling in the boxes with the appropriate numbers. Add the numbers for the screen. If score is 11 or less, continue with the assessment to gain a Malnutrition Indicator Score.

Screening

Has food intake declined over the past 3 months due to loss of appetite, digestive problems, chewing or swallowing difficulties?
☐   0 = severe loss of appetite
     1 = moderate loss of appetite
     2 = no loss of appetite

Weight loss during the last 3 months?
☐   0 = weight loss greater than 3 kg (6.6 pounds)
     1 = does not know
     2 = weight loss between 1 and 3 kg (2.2 and 6.6 pounds)
     3 = no weight loss

Mobility
☐   0 = bed or chair bound
     1 = able to get out of bed/chair but does not go out
     2 = goes out

Has suffered psychological stress or acute disease
☐   0 = yes 2 = no

Neuropsychological problems
☐   0 = severe dementia or depression
     1 = mild dementia
     2 = no psychological problems

Body Mass Index (BMI) (weight in kg)/(height in m)^2
☐   0 = BMI less than 19
     1 = BMI 19 to less than 21
     2 = BMI 21 to less than 23
     3 = BMI 23 or greater

Screening score (subtotal max. 14 point)

12 points or greater = Normal—not at risk—no need to complete assessment

11 points or below = Possible malnutrition—continue assessment

Assessment

Lives independently (not in a nursing home or hospital)
☐   0 = no   1 = yes

Takes more than 3 prescription drugs per day
☐   0 = no   1 = yes

Pressure sore or skin ulcers
☐   0 = no   1 = yes

Figure 6.2   Mini Nutritional Assessment (MNA). (Sources: Riogo, S.P., Sanchez-Vilar, O., Gonzalez de Villar, N. Geriatric nutrition: Studies about MNA. Nutr Hosp. 1999; 14(5)suppl 2:32S–42S. Guigoz, Y., Vallas, B., Garry, P.J. Mini Nutritional Assessment: A practical assessment tool for grading the nutritional state of elderly patients. *Facts and Research in Gerontology.* 1994; suppl 2:15–59.)

and the National Health and Nutrition Examination Survey (NHANES), have been used to assess the nutritional status of the elderly. Findings vary depending on the age, sex, and economic status characteristics of the group surveyed and the methods used for study (e.g., clinical signs, biochemical measurements, or dietary intake surveys). These studies are hampered by the lack of anthropometric, biochemical, and clinical norms that are specific to the elderly.

In spite of this, some generalizations can be made. Diets of the elderly living independently in the community have

How many full meals does the patient eat daily?

☐   0 = 1 meal
    1 = 2 meals
    2 = 3 meals

Select consumption markers for protein intake

☐ • ☐ –At least one serving of dairy products (milk, cheese, yogurt) per day?   ☐ yes   ☐ no
        –Two or more servings of legumes or eggs per week?   ☐ yes   ☐ no
        –Meat, fish, or poultry every day?   ☐ yes   ☐ no
        0.0 = if 0 or 1 yes
        0.5 = if 2 yes
        1.0 = if 3 yes

Consumes two or more servings of fruits or vegetables per day

☐   0 = no 1 = yes

How much fluid (water, juice, coffee, tea, milk . . .) is consumed per day?

☐ • ☐ 0.0 = less than 3 cups
        0.5 = 3 to 5 cups
        1.0 = more than 5 cups

Mode of feeding

☐   0 = unable to eat without assistance
    1 = self-fed with some difficulty
    2 = self-fed without any difficulty

Self view of nutritional status

☐   0 = views self as being malnourished
    1 = is uncertain of nutritional state
    2 = views self as having no nutritional problem

In comparison with other people of the same age, how does the patient consider his/her health status?

☐ • ☐ 0.0 = not as good
        0.5 = does not know
        1.0 = as good
        1.0 = better

Mid-arm circumference (MAC) in cm

☐ • ☐ 0.0 = MAC less than 21
        0.5 = MAC 21 to 22
        1.0 = MAC 22 or greater

Calf circumference (CC) in cm

    0 = CC less than 31
    1 = CC 31 or greater

Assessment (max. 16 points)   ☐ ☐•☐

Screening score   ☐ ☐

Total Assessment (max. 30 points)   ☐ ☐•☐

Malnutrition Indicator Score

17 to 23.5 points   at risk of malnutrition   ☐
Less than 17 points   Malnourished   ☐

Figure 6.2   (Continued)

been found to be more nutritionally adequate than those who are institutionalized or in nursing homes.[60,61] Dietary intake data reveal that a substantial portion of diets for the elderly are low in vitamins C and A, thiamine, calcium, iron, folate, and zinc compared to the recommended dietary allowances (RDA). The prevalence of nutritional problems among the aged arising from low dietary intakes appears to be quite high. In national population and community-based surveys, intakes were low among those 65 years of age, especially among the poor, for protein, calcium, thiamine, vitamin D, folic acid, vitamin B_6 and zinc.[62] Many diets were found to have very low caloric intakes. Twenty-one percent of the white population and 36% of the black population had daily intakes of less than 1000 calories. Conversely, 25% of the lower-income black and white women aged 45 to 75 years of age were found to be obese. Protein was reported to be near or above the RDA with the exception of some low-income groups. In fact, the elderly appear to maintain approximately the same ratio of protein, fat, and carbohydrate in their diets compared to younger cohorts, namely: 13% to 30% protein; 50% to 55% carbohydrate; and 30% to 35% fat. When biochemical methods were used, vitamins C, A, and B_6, thiamine, riboflavin, iron, zinc, and calcium were most likely to be below RDA standards.[2] Despite the reporting of the inadequate dietary intake of these nutrients, there was a relative lack of clinical symptoms indicating nutrient deficiencies. Clinical signs other than iron deficiency were infrequently found. This leads one to question the appropriateness of RDA standards for good nutrition in an elderly population.

The aged are highly vulnerable to malnutrition because there is little direct experimental evidence available from which to establish nutritional standards or necessary dietary intake, especially for those aged 85 years and over. Information on the nutritional needs of the elderly have been derived by extrapolation from investigations using young adults.[12] Table 6.3 provides the most recent RDAs for individuals aged 40 years and older.

Because elderly adults have distinct metabolic characteristics that alter various nutrient requirements, simple extrapolations of nutrient requirements for younger adults are not warranted. Gastrointestinal function is well preserved with aging regarding the digestion and absorption

TABLE 6.3   Recommended Daily Allowances (Revised 2000)

Males	40–50 years	51–70 years	70+ years	Females	40–50 years	51–70 years	70+ years
Weight (kg)[a]	70	70	70	Weight (kg)	58	58	60
Height (cm)[a]	173	171	170	Height (cm)	160	157	154
Energy (kg)	2600	2400	2200	Energy (kg)	1850	1700	1650
Protein (gr)	65	65	65	Protein (gr)	55	55	55
Fat-Soluble Vitamins				**Fat-Soluble Vitamins**			
Vitamin A (I.U.)	5000	5000	5000	Vitamin A (I.U.)	5000	5000	5000
Vitamin D (I.U.)	400	400	400	Vitamin D (I.U.)	400	400	400
Vitamin E (I.U.)	30	30	30	Vitamin E (I.U.)	25	25	25
Vitamin C (mg)	60	60	60	Vitamin C (mg)	60	100	100
Folate acid (mg)	0.4	0.4	0.4	Folate acid (mg)	0.4	0.4	0.4
Niacin (mg equiv)	18	17	17	Niacin (mg equiv)	13	12	12
Riboflavin (mg)	1.7	1.7	1.7	Riboflavin (mg)	1.5	1.5	1.5
Thiamine (mg)	1.3	1.2	1.2	Thiamine (mg)	1.0	1.0	1.0
Water-Soluble Vitamins				**Water-Soluble Vitamins**			
Vitamin B_6 (mg)	2.0	2.0	2.0	Vitamin B_6 (mg)	2.0	2.0	2.0
Vitamin B_{12} (µg)	5	5	5	Vitamin B_{12} (µg)	5	6	6
Calcium (mg)	800	800	800	Calcium (mg)	1500	1500	1500
Phosphorus (gm)	0.8	0.8	0.8	Phosphorus (gm)	1.5	1.5	1.5
Iodine (µg)	125	110	100	Iodine (µg)	100	90	80
Iron (mg)	10	10	10	Iron (mg)	18	10	10
Magnesium (mg)	350	350	350	Magnesium (mg)	300	300	300
Zinc (µg)	15	15	15	Zinc (µg)	15	15	15
Selenium (µg)	60	60	60	Selenium (µg)	55	55	55

Weights and heights represent actual median weights and heights for age groups derived from national data collected by the National Center for Health Statistics. From Committee on Dietary Allowances of the Food and Nutrition Board of the National Academy of Science/Nutrition Research Council, 2000.

of macromutrients, but the aging gastrointestinal tract becomes less efficient in absorbing vitamin B_{12}, vitamin D, and calcium.[63,64] The new dietary reference intakes considered recent studies in aging adults and concluded that the RDAs should be between 1200 mg and 1500 mg and 15 microg for calcium and vitamin D, respectively, for persons over the age of 70 years.[63-65] The new RDAs for riboflavin, niacin, thiamine, folate, vitamin B_6, and vitamin B_{12} are not different for persons in the oldest age category (> 70 years) than for those aged 40 to 70 years.[63-65] Because this line of study is a quickly advancing field, it will be important to closely follow new research on nutrient requirements and aging over the next several years.

The increasing relative and absolute number of elderly in most countries and the high prevalence of disease in the higher age groups make the lack of nutritional standards an important concern. Both the aging process per se and the effects of disease on nutritional status add difficulties to determining RDAs based on chronological age. Not only disease but also factors such as impaired vision, presbycusis, oral health, smoking, and alcohol use or misuse may complicate nutrition in the elderly. Cohort differences may have a marked impact on nutrition regarding several factors. In many countries meal habits and intake of energy and nutrients in at least young elderly are on average acceptable.[61] However, variation is marked. Standardizing nutient requirements from the perspective of prevention and dietary habits becomes an ominous task.

Lowenstein[66] reviewed the problem of lack of nutrient standards for the aged. It was found that the quality of the diet required by the aged is higher. Caloric needs decrease because of reduced metabolic rates and lower levels of physical activity, while needs for protein, vitamins, and minerals stay more or less constant. Thus, nutrient density (i.e., nutrients per calorie) necessary to fulfill recommended dietary allowances is higher for the aged when compared to younger adults.[66] The fact that separate guidelines have not been established for advancing age (except for extrapolations for the 55 and over age group) reflects the lack of solid knowledge of the needs of the elderly. This, coupled with the facts, that (1) the elderly are much less uniform compared to other age groups with respect to biological, anatomical, and physiological aging; (2) the elderly have an increased susceptibility to disease and chronic illness; and (3) there are a variety of other social and psychological influences that affect diet, makes it unlikely that a specific standard can be devised that accounts for all these factors.[61]

The aged are vulnerable and at high risk of developing nutritional problems because of various social, psychological, and physical factors,[12] including living alone (especially if there has been a recent bereavement or significant negative life event), lack of an effective family or community support network, and low income. Psychological factors such as depression, mental deterioration, and impaired self-concept, increase the risk of nutritional deficiencies. Physical factors, such as functional dependence,

sensory impairment, and limited mobility (especially when they are associated with severe chronic degenerative diseases), also have a negative influence. Indices of nutritional risk using these factors are proving useful in identifying the aged with more nutritional deficits than their hospitalized or institutionalized peers.[51]

The elderly generally have a progressive decline in exercise levels and a proportional decrease in energy expenditure, which, when linked to the decrease in their BMR, suggests the need to progressively reduce caloric intake.[67]

Recommendations for dietary intake according to the food pyramid have been altered for those individuals aged 70 and older. Figure 6.3 is the modified food pyramid for the mature (70 and over) adult.

COMMON NUTRITIONAL DEFICIENCIES IN THE AGED

The need for the forty-two essential nutrients remains qualitatively similar over the life span. However, quantitative changes for some nutrient requirements are of importance to the elderly individual. When diet-related disorders are present, additional alterations in nutrients may also be necessary. When mean population intakes of a nutrient are below a standard, such as the RDA, nutritionists regard it as a "problem nutrient." Surveys of the aged reveal that mean intakes of calories and calcium are low and often problematic, and that, while mean intakes of protein are adequate, at least a third of those surveyed have intakes below the standard, especially in certain subgroups of the population.[62,68] Other vitamins and minerals present special problems for certain groups of the aged and will be discussed. Although vitamin and mineral deficiencies are presumed to be more common in the elderly, there is little experimental data on which to estimate exact daily requirements of these so-called micronutrients in the diet. Increased need, with age, for vitamins and minerals may result from less efficient absorption, altered metabolism and excretion, and increasing use of certain medications. It is important to remember that any nutrient may be insufficient or in excess and can constitute a problem for the elderly.

For specific information on nutritional deficiencies in the aged, see CD.

DRUGS' EFFECTS ON NUTRITION

The frequent use of pharmacologic agents increases the vulnerability of the elderly to malnutrition. Drug-diet interactions occur at all ages, but are more common in the elderly because of prescription and over-the-counter drug use on a regular basis. In addition, age-related changes in

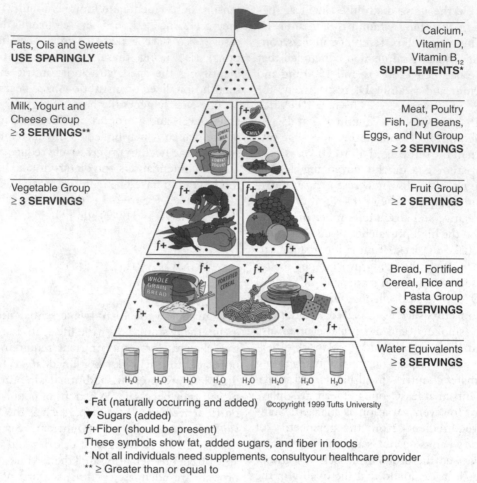

Fats, Oils and Sweets
USE SPARINGLY

Calcium,
Vitamin D,
Vitamin B_{12}
SUPPLEMENTS*

Milk, Yogurt and
Cheese Group
≥ 3 SERVINGS**

Meat, Poultry
Fish, Dry Beans,
Eggs, and Nut Group
≥ 2 SERVINGS

Vegetable Group
≥ 3 SERVINGS

Fruit Group
≥ 2 SERVINGS

Bread, Fortified
Cereal, Rice and
Pasta Group
≥ 6 SERVINGS

Water Equivalents
≥ 8 SERVINGS

• Fat (naturally occurring and added)   ©copyright 1999 Tufts University
▼ Sugars (added)
f+Fiber (should be present)
These symbols show fat, added sugars, and fiber in foods
* Not all individuals need supplements, consult your healthcare provider
** ≥ Greater than or equal to

Figure 6.3   Modified Food Pyramid for Mature (70+) Adults.

gastrointestinal function, liver and renal function, and body composition alter drug and nutrient metabolism. Coexisting disease, undernutrition, and malnutrition may further complicate these interactions.[69,70]

Drugs may affect nutritional status in the simplest sense by their effects on appetite, but more commonly, absorption, metabolism, and excretion of dietary constituents are altered. Dietary factors such as water consumption, amount of food consumed, timing of meals in relation to drug intake, and the constituents consumed may affect absorption and oxidative drug metabolism.[69]

Drugs cause malabsorption of nutrients by exerting an effect on the ability of the gastrointestinal mucosa to absorb. These effects can be limited and specific for a particular nutrient, or they may affect an entire class of nutrients, such as fat-soluble vitamins or trace minerals. For instance, drugs may decrease nutrient bioavailability by repelling the nutrient, therefore inhibiting the intestinal phase of fat digestion and absorption.[71] Drugs may also interfere with nutrient absorption through secondary mechanisms. For example, drugs can impair absorption of nutrients by adverse effects on gastric or intestinal, pan-

creatic, or hepatic bile secretion. H_2 blockers (such as cimetidine) inhibit gastric acid production, thereby reducing the liberation of vitamin B_{12} from its protein-bound state, making it less available for association with intrinsic factors.[71] This could result in vitamin B_{12} deficiency and resulting pernicious anemia.

Several over-the-counter drugs may induce adverse nutritional effects. Antacids are associated with impaired absorption of riboflavin, copper, and iron, and may induce hypophosphatemia[72] with the development of proximal limb muscle weakness, malaise, paresthesias, anorexia, and secondary syndromes of hypomagnesemia/tetany[73] and osteomalacia.[74] Excessive use of sodium bicarbonate can result in sodium overload and render the pH of the gut sufficiently alkaline to decrease the absorption of folic acid.[75] Commonly used drugs that increase calcium need include aluminum-containing antacids, which decrease phosphorus absorption, lowering plasma phosphorus and ultimately increasing calcium excretion.[76] Thiazide diuretics, on the other hand, decrease calcium needs by decreasing urinary calcium losses and may have a positive effect on bone mass.[77]

Laxatives, if taken at mealtime or in the postprandial absorptive period, prevent absorption of carotenes and fat-soluble vitamins via solubilization. Overuse of stool softeners may result in malabsorption of glucose, calcium, potassium, vitamin D, and protein. Laxative use has been linked to an increased incidence of osteomalacia.[78] In the elderly patient, the risks of hypokalemia and potassium deficiency, with the attendant hazards of cardiac arrhythmias, digitalis toxicity, and hyperglycemia, are associated with concurrent use of laxatives and diuretics.[71]

Anti-inflammatory drugs, commonly used by elderly individuals, produce small hemorrhages of the gastrointestinal mucosa, leading to iron-deficiency anemia and decreased absorption of vitamin C. Chronic aspirin use is associated with folic acid deficiency and macrocytic anemia.[71]

Drugs may act to inhibit the essential intermediary metabolism of a nutrient or to promote its catabolism. For example, drug interference of vitamin D metabolism with a secondary impairment of calcium absorption can result in osteomalacia. Drugs that increase hepatic enzymes for drug metabolism (e.g., sedatives, hypnotics, and anticonvulsants) may increase the demand for specific nutrients, such as folic acid, B_6, and B_{12}.

Drugs may also increase the excretion of some nutrients by displacement from plasma protein-binding sites, chelation, or reduction of renal reabsorption. For example, aspirin competes for folic acid-binding sites on serum proteins and enhances the vitamin's excretion.[79] Long-term use of aspirin results in chelation of essential minerals such as copper and zinc. Although diuretic therapy effectively decreases the resorption of sodium, it also reduces renal absorption and enhances renal excretion of calcium, chromium, magnesium, potassium, and zinc.[71]

Table 6.4 provides a summary of drug-induced effects on nutrient absorption, metabolism, and excretion.[71]

Drugs have an effect on nutrition and, conversely, diet has been shown to affect the metabolism and response to many drugs. Food may influence both the absorption and the presystemic metabolism of drugs. These effects may be caused by food intake or by different nutrients or additives, food/fluid volume, or polycyclic hydrocarbons present in grilled foods.

Food and its constituents can influence drug absorption as a result of physical or chemical interactions between the food product and the drug or because of physiologic changes in the gastrointestinal tract. The net effect of this interaction may be that drug absorption is reduced, slowed, or increased by food intake.[80] Food can act to alter the rate of gastric emptying and drug dissolution. It can act as a mechanical barrier, preventing drug access to the mucosal surface. For example, acetaminophen absorption is more rapid after fasting than after consumption of a high-carbohydrate meal containing pectin.[71] Foods interfere with the mucosal transfer of drugs, such as levodopa, a drug whose chemical structure is similar to that of amino acids. Competition for transport between the drug and amino acids from protein in the diet diminishes drug uptake and appears responsible for the "on-off" phenomenon of levodopa in Parkinson's patients.[81]

Nutritional influences on drug distribution may be limited in the elderly who are poorly nourished because of a reduction in plasma albumin. Even in well-nourished, healthy elders, albumin concentrations have been found to be lower compared to younger adults.[71] As a result, the extensively protein-bound drugs, such as warfarin and diazepam, are not as readily distributed due to a reduced binding capacity in old age.

Metabolism of drugs may also be affected by nutrient intake, particulary the composition of the diet. Research indicates that the total caloric input and the percentage of calories obtained from different sources (e.g., carbohydrates, proteins, fats) will influence pharmacokinetics of various drugs.[82,83] For example, the rate of drug breakdown and elimination is affected by the type of diet consumed. Comparing high-carbohydrate, high-fat, or high-protein diets, the rate of drug elimination is slowest with the high-carbohydrate diet and fastest with the high-protein diet.[71] Reduced drug clearance is demonstrated in elders whose diets are low in protein.[71]

Specific dietary constituents such as cruciferous vegetables and charcoal-broiled beef can also alter drug metabolism.[84] Certain foods should not be ingested when specific drugs are on board. As one among many examples, fermented cheese and wine inhibit the monoamine oxidase enzymes (MAO inhibitors). High amounts of tyramine contained in these foods stimulate the release of catecholamines (norepinephrine, epinephrine), which confounds the action of MAO inhibitors whose purpose is to suppress these elements. As a result, consumption of tyramine-containing foods in the presence of MAO inhibitors can cause a dramatic and life-threatening increase in blood pressure.[83]

Under normal circumstances, most vitamin-rich foods are good for us. However, as discussed above, certain medications can have an increased or decreased absorption when taken with food, thereby affecting their efficiency. For example, tetracycline antibiotics are not effective when taken within an hour of milk or dairy products. Hismanal (astermizole), Plendil (felodipine), or Procardia/Adalat (nifedipine) should not be taken with acid-containing juices, such as grapefruit juice, which may increase blood levels of these drugs and result in harmful side effects.[71,84] Individuals taking blood pressure medications, particularly ACE inhibitors or potassium-sparing diuretics, should avoid potassium salt substitutes because of the danger of potassium overload. One of the most serious interactions occurs when Coumadin (warfarin) is taken with foods high in vitamin K. Coumadin interferes with the body's ability to make blood clots. Vitamin K helps the body form blood-clot factors; thus it decreases the effectiveness of Coumadin.

TABLE 6.4   Mechanism of Drug Effects on Specific Nutrient Absorption, Metabolism, and Excretion

Drug Group	Nutrient Influenced	Mechanism of Nutritional Alteration	Kinetic Alteration
Antibiotics (general)	Vitamin B_1, B_2, B_6, B_{12}, K, biotin	Δ Bacterial flora	Absorption
Cephalosporins	Vitamin K	$\Downarrow$ Reductase/carboxylation	Metabolism
Tetracyclines	CA	Chelation	Absorption
Isoniazid/INH (Isoniazid)	Vitamin B_6	$\Downarrow$ Pyridoxal kinase	Metabolism
		$\Downarrow$ Hepatic/renal Vitamin D hydroxylation	
Trimethoprim/TMP	Folic acid	Folate antagonist	Metabolism
Anticoagulants			
Warfarin (Coumadin)	Vitamin K	$\Downarrow$ Reductase/carboxylation	Metabolism
Anticonvulsants			
Phenobarbital	Vitamin D, CA	Δ Vitamin D metabolites	Metabolism
	Folic acid	$\Uparrow$ Hepatic microsomal enzymes	
Phenytoin (Dilantin)	Vitamin D, CA	Δ Vitamin D metabolites	Metabolism
	Folic acid	$\Uparrow$ Hepatic microsomal enzymes	
Antihypertensives			
• Vasodilators Hydralazine (Apresoline)	Vitamin B_6	$\Downarrow$ Pyridoxal kinase	Metabolism
• Loop diuretics Furosemide (Lasix)	Na, K, CA, Cr, Mg, Zn, Vitamin B_1, B_6	$\Uparrow$ Renal excretion	Excretion
• Thiazide diuretics Hydrochlorothiazide (HydroDIURIL)	Na, K, Mg, Zn	$\Uparrow$ Renal excretion	Excretion
• Triamterene/ hydrochlorothiazide (Dyazide)	Na, CA	$\Uparrow$ Renal excretion	Excretion
	Folic acid	$\Downarrow$ Dihydrofolate reductase	Metabolism
Antihyperlipidemics			
Cholestyramine (Questran) Colestipol (Colestid)	Vitamin A, D, E, K, B_{12}, beta-carotene, folic acid, CA, Fe, Zn	Adsorption to anion exchange resin	Absorption
Anti-Inflammatory Agents			
Prednisone (Deltasone)	Vitamin D, CA	$\Downarrow$ Hepatic/renal Vitamin D hydroxylation	Metabolism
Colchicine	Vitamin B_{12}	Mucosal injury	Absorption
Sulfasalazine (Azulfidine)	Folic acid	$\Downarrow$ Dihydrofolate reductase	Metabolism
Indomethacin (Indocin)	Vitamin C, Fe	Mucosal injury	Absorption
Sulindac (Clinoril)	Folic acid	$\Downarrow$ Dihydrofolate	Metabolism
Naproxen (Naprosyn)			
Ibuprofen (Motrin)			
Aspirin	Vitamin C, Fe	Mucosal injury	Absorption
	Folic acid	Competition for binding sites	Excretion

TABLE 6.4 Mechanism of Drug Effects on Specific Nutrient Absorption, Metabolism, and Excretion (Continued)

Drug Group	Nutrient Influenced	Mechanism of Nutritional Alteration	Kinetic Alteration
Antineoplastics (general)	Most nutrients	Mucosal injury	Absorption
Methotrexate	Folic acid	Folate antagonist	Metabolism
Antiulcer Agents			
• H_2 receptor antagonists Cimetidine (Tagamet)	Vitamin B_{12}, folic acid, Fe, Zn	⇓ Gastric acid secretion	Absorption
Ranitidine (Zantac)			
Famotidine (Pepcid)	Vitamin D, Ca	⇓ Hepatic/renal vitamin D hydroxylation	Metabolism
Proton pump inhibitors	B_{12}, folic acid, Fe, Zn	⇓ Gastric acid secretion	Absorption
Omeprazole (Prilosec)			
Lansoprazole (Prevacid)	Vitamin D, CA	⇓ Hepatic/renal vitamin D hydroxylation	Metabolism
Antacids			
Aluminum and magnesium	Phosphate	Precipitation	Absorption
hydroxides (Amphogel, Maalox, Mylanta)	Vitamin B_{12}, folic acid, Fe, Zn	⇓ Gastric acid secretion	
Na bicarbonate (Alka-Seltzer)	Vitamin B_{12}, folic acid, Fe, Zn	⇓ Gastric acid secretion	Absorption
Laxatives			
• Lubricants			
Mineral oil (Haley's M-O)	Vitamins A, D, E, K, beta carotene	Solubilization	Absorption
• Stimulant cathartics			
Phenolphthalein (Ex-Lax)	CA, Vitamins D, K	⇑ GI motility	Absorption
Bisacodyl (Dulcolax)			
Psychotherapeutics			
• Tricyclic antidepressants			
Amitriptyline (Elavil)	Vitamin B_2	⇓ Flavin adenine dinucleotide	Metabolism
Nortriptyline (Pamelor)			
Imipramine (Tofranil)			
Desipramine (Norpramin)			
Doxepin (Sinequan)			
Neuroleptics			
Chlorpromazine (Thorazine)	Vitamin B_2	⇓ Flavin adenine dinucleotide	Metabolism
Thioridazine (Mellaril)			
Fluphenazine (Prolixin)			
Thiothixene (Navane)			

Key: ⇓ = *inhibit or decrease;* ⇑ = *induce or increase;* Δ = *change*

Alcohol's Effects on Nutrition

Alcohol is both a drug and a food which provides substantial amounts of energy. It is widely abused by individuals of all ages. Among the aged, its abuse is especially easy since the risks of intoxication from a given dose of alcohol are elevated because lean body mass and total body water decrease with age. The consequence is that the total volume of distribution of alcohol is smaller and peak blood alcohol levels are higher than in younger persons.[85] Greater physiological sensitivity to the effects of alcohol and greater psychological vulnerability to alcohol abuse due to depression, loneliness, and lack of meaningful roles combine to make alcohol abuse risks high in the aged. Alcohol use should be avoided entirely among the elderly with known dementia, chronic medication with psychoactive drugs, a previous history of alcohol abuse, or chronic and extreme depression.

Moderate alcohol use (one or two drinks per day) has been associated with some health benefits. Alcohol in moderation is an appetite stimulant, enhancing the taste of food. It increases HDL cholesterol levels, thereby lowering atherosclerotic risks. Moderate alcohol intake is also associated with lowered congestive heart failure rates.[86] Since elderly energy intakes are already low, however, care must be taken to ensure that calories from alcohol do not displace other items in the diet which provide not only energy but also protein, vitamins, and minerals.

Theories of Aging Related to Nutrition

Though the mechanisms of aging are not clearly understood, there is evidence suggesting that nutrition influences the aging process.[87] Aging, and related diseases, viewed from a nutritional perspective, results from the influence of different nutrients on immunological, genetic, neurological, and endocrinological functions. For example, oxidative mechanisms may play an important role in the aging process. It is important, therefore, to emphasize the relationship between health and nutrition in the elderly.

Since nutrients are obtained from the food we eat and utilized by the cells of the body, nutritional factors have been directly credited for their role in longevity. Malnutrition can contribute to chronic diseases. A combination of good nutrition and exercise leads to better health and energy levels and notably improves an individual's capability to withstand psychological and physical stresses.

For more information on theories of aging as they relate to nutrition, see CD.

Exercise, Nutrition, and Aging

Advancing age is associated with a remarkable number of changes in body composition, including reduction in lean body mass and increase in body fat. Decreased lean body mass occurs primarily as a result of losses in skeletal muscle mass. This age-related loss in muscle mass, or sarcopenia, accounts for the age-associated decrease in BMR, muscle strength, and activity levels, which, in turn, are the cause of decreased energy requirements of the elderly.[88] A reduction in the body's major protein pool requires that adequate dietary protein to replace obligatory nitrogen loss and to support protein turnover is essential for maintaining muscle mass. Sedentary lifestyle also contributes to this loss and exercise helps to preserve muscle fibers.[89] In sedentary persons, the main determinant of energy expenditure is fat-free mass.[88,90] It also appears that declining energy needs are not matched by an appropriate decline in energy intake in many older adults, with the ultimate result being increased body fat content. Increased body fat and increased abdominal obesity are linked to the greatly increased incidence of non-insulin-dependent diabetes and heart disease among the elderly. Regular exercise can affect nutrition needs and functional capacity in the elderly.[88,91] (Refer to Chapter 13, Cardiopulmonary and Cardiovascular Considerations, for a more extensive review of the benefits of exercise and nutrition, and exercise prescription.)

Supplementing Nutrients

It is well known by nutritionists that the best sources of vitamins and minerals are natural sources. A balanced diet, in moderate amounts, is more trustworthy than nutritional supplements. Nutrients from ingested foods, because of their biocompatability with the metabolic makeup of humans, are more readily absorbed, metabolized, and utilized than supplemental doses of vitamins and minerals. With the aging gastrointestinal tract, often vitamin pills are not actually broken down or utilized. Supplements are often taken ad lib without consideration of their interaction with other supplements. Table 6.5 provides a summary by this author of the importance of specific nutrients, where to find them naturally, and what nutrient supplements should concomitantly be taken to enhance in the metabolism of each vitamin or mineral. Rule of thumb: If you take vitamins, a multivitamin is the best recommendation. Mixing and matching supplements could lead to devastating consequences.

Despite the fact that the way to get an abundant supply of nutrients is through healthy eating (a variety of foods on a daily basis), many elderly individuals do not consume a balanced diet. There are conditions and illnesses that deplete vitamins from their systems and need to be replenished. Many elders are on chronic drug regimens that

TABLE 6.5   Nutrient Role, Natural Sources, and Complementary Vitamins and Minerals

Vitamins	Role of Nutrient	Natural Sources	More Effective With . . .
A	Need for normal growth/vision, for healthy teeth, nails, bones, glands; powerful antioxidant	Fish liver oils, dairy products, liver, dark-green and yellow vegetables	B-complex, C, D, E, calcium, phosphorus, zinc
Beta-carotene (Pro Vitamin A)	Converted into vitamin A only as the body needs it; antioxidant	Yellow and orange fruits and vegetables	B-complex, C, D, E, calcium, phosphorus, zinc
B_1 (Thiamine)	Needed for healthy nervous system, muscle tone, normal digestion, energy; processes carbohydrates, fat, protein	Brewer's yeast, wheat germ, liver, whole-grain cereals, nuts, pork, beef, peas/beans, fish, peanuts	B-complex, B_2, folic acid, niacin C, E, manganese, sulfur
B_2 (Riboflavin)	Necessary for good vision, skin, nails, hair; converts carbohydrates to ATP; processes amino acids and fats; folic acid and B_6 activation; antioxidant	Brewer's yeast, liver, leafy vegetables, whole-grain breads, milk	B-complex, B_6, niacin, C
B_3 (Niacin)	Helps release energy, necessary for healthy nervous and digestive systems; regulates cholesterol	Lean meats, poultry, fish, nuts	B-complex, B_1, B_2, C
B_5 (Pantothenic Acid)	Important for healthy skin/nerves, energy release, healthy digestive tract; activates adrenal gland; energy from fats; makes acetylcholine; synthesis of cholesterol	Organ meats, brewer's yeast, egg yolks, whole-grain cereals, salmon, dairy products, meat	B-complex, B_1, B_{12}, C, sulfur, biotin
B_6 (Pyridoxine)	Essential for production of antibodies, nerve tissue, red blood cells and for metabolism of fats. Helps regulate body fluids; building block for all proteins and some hormones; synthesis of neurotransmitters	Organ meats, whole-grain cereals, bananas, potatoes, raisin bran, lentils, turkey, tuna	B-complex, B_1, B_2, B_5, C, sodium, magnesium, potassium, linoleic acid
B_{12} (Cobalamin)	Essential for normal function all body cells including brain and nerve cells; DNA replication	Liver, kidney, muscle meats, fish, dairy products, eggs, poultry	B-complex, B_6, folic acid, C, potassium, sodium
Biotin	Essential to metabolism of fats, carbohydrates, and proteins	Organ meat, egg yolks, whole-grain cereals, brewer's yeast, milk, oatmeal, mushrooms, bananas, peanuts, soy	B-complex, B_{12}, folic acid, B_5, sulfur
C (Ascorbic Acid)	Essential for healthy teeth, bones, joints, red blood cells, immune system, muscle contraction	Citrus fruits/juices, tomatoes, green peppers, strawberries, all other fruits and vegetables	All vitamins/minerals, calcium, magnesium

(cont.)

TABLE 6.5   Nutrient Role, Natural Sources, and Complementary Vitamins and Minerals (Continued)

Vitamins	Role of Nutrient	Natural Sources	More Effective With . . .
D	Important for health of bones, teeth, collagen, cartilage, nervous system, heart, and aids blood-clotting	Fish liver oil, eggs, sunshine (reacts with skin to form D internally)	A, C, calcium, phosphorus
E (Trocopherol)	Helps protect unsaturated fats from abnormal breakdown and prolongs life of red blood cells, nerve/brain tissue	Vegetable oils, wheat germ, whole-grain cereals, green vegetables, seeds, nuts	A, B-complex, B_1, C, selenium, manganese
Folic Acid	Part of B-complex. Essential for normal metabolism of growing cells/tissues, red blood cells, heart health	Green leafy vegetables, liver, brewer's yeast	B-complex, B_{12}, biotin, B_5, C
Minerals			
Calcium	Essential for strong teeth/bones. Health and functioning of nerve, brain, heart tissue	Milk, dairy products, green leafy and green vegetables, soy products, dried peas, other beans, sardines	A, C, D, Fe, magnesium, boron, phosphorus, manganese
Copper	Needed to utilize iron and for health of bones, nerves and connective tissue	Liver, whole-grain cereals, almonds, green leafy vegetables, dried peas/beans, seafoods, kidney, egg yolk	Cobalt, iron, zinc
Iodine	Helps regulate metabolism. Normal functioning of thyroid gland	Seafood, iodized salt, kelp, sea-weed, vegetables grown in iodine-rich soil	Not established
Iron	Quality of blood, oxygenation, increases resistance to stress/disease, enhances immune system, important for proper muscle functioning	Liver, oysters, heart, lean meat, egg yolk, wheat germ, fish, leafy green vegetables	B_{12}, folic acid, C
Magnesium	Essential for healthy nerves/muscles and for producing energy. Healthy collagen, bones, and teeth; muscle relaxation; cell production; clotting of blood; formation of ATP; activates all B vitamins	Green vegetables, wheat germ, soy beans, figs, corn, apples, almonds, grains, nuts, beans, fish, meat	B_6, C, D, calcium, phosphorus, protein
Manganese	Activates enzymes in body. Important for health of reproductive organs; glucose tolerance; antioxidant	Whole-grain cereals, egg yolks, green vegetables, wheat germ, nuts, beans, bran, beet tops, pineapple, seeds	B_1, E, calcium, phosphorus
Phosphorus	Cell growth/maintenance, energy production, tooth/bone/muscle health, kidney function, nerve conduction	Meat, fish, poultry, eggs, whole grains, seeds, nuts, milk, cheese	A, D, calcium, iron, manganese, protein

TABLE 6.5 Nutrient Role, Natural Sources, and Complementary Vitamins and Minerals (Continued)

Vitamins	Role of Nutrient	Natural Sources	More Effective With . . .
Potassium	All tissue growth, muscle contraction; O_2 to brain; H_2O and pH balance; blood pressure regulation and neuromuscular function; metabolism of carbohydrates and protein	All fruits and vegetables, oranges, whole grains, sunflower seeds, nuts, meats, mint leaves, potatoes, bananas, melons, beans, milk	B_6, sodium, phosphorus
Selenium	A natural antioxidant regulates various metabolic processes; immune system function; activates hormones	Cereal bran/germ, broccoli, onions, tomatoes, tuna, brewer's yeast, corn oil, nuts, whole grains, seafood	Vitamin E
Zinc	Tissue growth, muscle contraction, bone health	Shellfish, nuts, liver, kidney, egg yolks	A, calcium, copper, phosphorus

increase the risk of progressive nutrient depletion. Appropriate levels of vitamin supplementation have been proposed for specific drug therapies in the elderly.[92] It is fairly common for drug-related depletion of nutrients in geriatric patients to be complicated by dietary inadequacy or by disease states that induce nutrient deficiencies.[71]

Notwithstanding such well-justified therapeutic needs for nutrient supplementation, it is important to recognize the extensive nature of self-prescribed supplement use among older adults. The estimated prevalence of nutrient supplementation in the elderly ranges from 30% to 70%.[71] While several of the factors discussed above suggest that there may be valid reasons to recommend nutrient supplementation for older adults, current trends indicate that their supplementation regimens are not always appropriate. Self-selected supplements are not often based on individual needs, but on something the person heard or read, along with his or her belief that the choice of supplements will have a beneficial effect.

NUTRITIONAL PROGRAMS
FOR THE ELDERLY

Federal food assistance programs were the result of the Surgeon General's 1979 report. Excellent references are available on community nutrition services for the aged.[93,94] They include food and nutrition services for the healthy aged, such as the elderly meals program, meals for maintaining the dependent aged at home, and food and nutrition services for the aged in group care and health care facilities.

Under the auspices of the Older Americans Act, the federal government's Administration on Aging provides congregate and home-delivered meals to over 2.5 million Americans 65 years of age and older. Those who participate in the "Meals on Wheels" program for the homebound aged are often economically poor and have multiple diseases, with a relatively high prevalence of nutritional deficiencies which are correctable by provision of adequate food and nutritional supplements.[95–102] The meals provide a minimum of a third of the RDA and, in this sense, are helpful in sustaining the nutrition of the aged.

In addition, the opportunity for social interaction provided by congregate dining or regular visits to deliver meals to the homebound elderly is important and may increase food intake as well as improve the quality of life. The elderly who attend congregate meals tend to be healthier than those receiving home-delivered services.[95] In addition to providing substantial amounts of daily nutrient intakes, the elderly who attend congregate meal sites can also be screened for referral to other preventive services.

The federal food stamp program, which provides coupons that increase food purchasing power, are available for the poor elderly. While only about 30% of the aged now participate in the program and the program benefits are only about $60 per month, the availability of this extra food money may be a great help in increasing diet quality. At present, many eligible elderly individuals fail to apply for or use this program.[96,103]

The aged who reside in group care or health care facilities are in especially fragile health and often have special nutritional needs or feeding requirements. Conditions of participation in the Medicare and Medicaid programs require that the institutions maintain certain standards with respect to food and nutrition services in order to obtain certification and licensure.[97] Dietary and institutional consultants can assure that these standards are met, and plan to implement more extensive nutrition services in these institutions, including appropriate menus which meet the RDA and therapeutic diet needs, dining rooms that are available and accessible for those who use them, feeding assistance where needed, and the attainment of food safety regulations.[94,97]

Unfortunately, undernutrition is prevalent in long-term care facilities.[98] It has been determined that a combination of behavioral, environmental, and disease-related factors greatly influence nutrition status. Our efforts as health care prefessionals must be directed toward influencing some of these factors to minimize undernutrition in the institutionalized elderly.

Scientific evidence increasingly supports that good nutrition is essential to the health, self-sufficiency, and quality of life of older adults.[12, 99–101] With the population of the United States living longer than ever before, the older adult population will be more diverse and heterogeneous as we move forward in the 21st century. The oldest-old and minority populations will grow more quickly than the young-old and non-Hispanic white populations, respectively. For the 34-plus million adults 65 years of age and older living in the United States, a broad array of culturally appropriate food and nutrition services, physical activities, and health and supportive care customized to accommodate the variations within this expanding population is needed. With changes and lack of coordination in health care and social support systems, health care professionals must be proactive and collaborate with existing services for the elderly to improve policies, interventions, and programs that support older adults throughout the continuum of care to ensure nutritional well-being and quality of life.

References

1. Saltzman JR, Russell RM. The aging gut. Nutritional issues. *Gastroenterol Clin North Am*. 1998; 27 (2):309–324.
2. Steen B. Preventive nutrition in old age—A review. *J Nutr Health Aging*. 2000; 4(2):114–119.
3. US Department of Health, Education, and Welfare. *Public Health Service. Healthy People: The Surgeon General's Report on Health Promotion and Disease Prevention 1979*. Washington, DC: US Government Printing Office; 1979.
4. Wartow NJ. The national initiative on health promotion for older persons: The role of the administration on aging. *Top Geriatr Rehabil*. 1990; 6(1):69–77.
5. de Jong N. Nutrition and senescence: Healthy aging for all in the new millennium? *Nutrition* 2000; 16(7–8):537–541.
6. Steen B. Body composition and aging. *Nutr Rev*. 1988; 46:45–51.
7. Ritz P. Physiology of aging with respect to gastrointestinal, circulatory, and immune system changes and their significance for energy and protein metabolism. *Eur J Clin Nutr*. 2000; 54(suppl 3):S21–S25.
8. Chernoff R. Aging and nutrition. *Nutrition Today*. 1987; 22(2):4–11.
9. McGee M, Jensen GL. Nutrition in the elderly. *J Clin Gastroenterol*. 2000; 30(4):372–380.
10. Bosch JP, Saccaggi A, Lauer A, et al. Renal functional reserve in humans, effect of protein intake on glomerular filtration rate. *Am J Med*. 1984; 75:943–950.
11. Uchida S, Tsutsumi O, Hise MK, et al. Role of epidermal factor in compensatory renal hypertrophy in mice. *Kidney Int*. 1988; 33:387–392.
12. American Dietetic Association. Position of the American Dietetic Association: Nutrition, aging, and the continuum of care. *J Am Diet Assoc*. 2000; 100(5):580–595.
13. Ivan L. Nutrition, aging, old age. *Orv Hetil*. 1998; 139(49):2951–2956.
14. Yancik R. Cancer burden in the aged: An epidemiologic and demographic overview. *Cancer*. 1997; 80(7):1273–1283.
15. Lesourd B, Mazari L. Nutrition and immunity in the elderly. *Proc Nutr Soc*. 1999; 58(3):685–695.
16. Chandra RK. Nutrition and immunology: From clinic to cellular biology and back again. *Proc Nutr Soc*. 1999; 58(3):681–683.
17. Proceeding of a conference on nutrition and immunity. Altlanta, Georgia, May 5–7, 1997. *Nutr Rev*. 56(1 pt 2):S1–S186.
18. Turczynowski W, Szczepanik AM, Klek S. Nutritional therapy and the immune system. *Przegl Lek*. 2000; 57(1):36–40.
19. Macallan DC. Nutrition and immune function in human immunodeficiency virus infection. *Proc Nutr Soc*. 1999; 58(3):743–748.
20. Wick G, Grubeck-Loebenstein B. Primary and secondary alterations of immune reactivity in the elderly: Impact of dietary factors and disease. *Immunol Rev*. 1997; 160(12):171–184.
21. Lesourd BM. Nutrition and immunity in the elderly: Modification of immune responses with nutritional treatments. *Am J Clin Nutr*. 1997; 66(2):478S–484S.
22. Chandra RK. Nutrition and the immune system: An introduction. *Am J Clin Nutr*. 1997; 66(2):460S–463S.

23. Stallone DD. The influence of obesity and its treatment on the immune system. *Nutr Rev.* 1994; 52(1): 37–50.

24. Sanchez A. Role of sugars in human neutrophilic phagocytosis. *Am J Clin Nutr.* 1973; 26(5):1180–184.

25. Nutter RL, Gridley DS, Kettering JD. Modification of a transplantable colon tumor and immune responses in mice fed different sources of protein, fat, and carbohydrate. *Cancer Lett.* 1983; 18(1): 49–62.

26. Szabo G. Monocytes, alcohol use, and altered immunity. *Alcohol Clin Exp Res.* 1998; 22(2):216S–219S.

27. MacGregor RR, Louria DB. Alcohol and infection. *Curr Clin Top Infect Dis.* 1997; 17(2):291–315.

28. Kelley DS, Daudu PA. Fat intake and immune response. *Prog Food Nutr Sci.* 1993; 17(1):41–63.

29. Yaqoob P. Monounsaturated fats and immune function. *Proc Nutr Soc.* 1998; 57(3):511–520.

30. Tashiro T, Yamamori H, Takagi K. n-3 versus n-6 polyunsaturated fatty acids in critical illness. *Nutrition.* 1998; 14(4):551–553.

31. Wu D, Meydani SN. n-3 polyunsaturated fatty acids and immune function. *Proc Nutr Soc.* 1998; 57(3): 503–509.

32. Fortes C, Forastiere F, Agabiti N. The effect of zinc and vitamin A supplementation on immune response in an older population. *J Am Geriatr Soc.* 1998; 46(1):19–26.

33. Girodon F, Lombard M, Galan P. Effect of micronutrient supplementation on infection in institutionalized elderly subjects: A controlled trial. *Ann Nutr Metab.* 1997; 41(1):98–107.

34. Macknin ML. Zinc lozenges for the common cold. *Cleveland Clin J Med.* 1999; 66(1):27–32.

35. Semba RD. Vitamin A, immunity, and infection. *Clin Infect Dis.* 1994; 19(3):489–499.

36. Santos MS, Meydani SN, Leka L. Natural killer cell activity in elderly men is enhanced by betacarotene supplementation. *Am J Clin Nutr.* 1996; 64(4): 772–777.

37. Gerber WF. Effect of ascorbic acid, sodium salicylate, and caffeine on the serum interferon level in response to viral infection. *Pharmacology.* 1975; 13(2): 228–232.

38. Anderson R. The immunostimulatory, anti-inflammatory and antiallergic properties of ascorbate. *Adv Nutr Res.* 1984; 9(1):19–45.

39. Meydani SN, Barklund MP, Liu S. Vitamin E supplementation enhances cell-mediated immunity in healthy elderly subjects. *Am J Clin Nutr.* 1990; 52(3): 557–563.

40. Penn ND, Purkins L, Kelleher J. The effect of dietary supplementation with vitamins A, C and E on cell-mediated immune function in elderly long-stay patients: A randomized controlled trial. *Age Ageing.* 1991; 20(2):169–174.

41. Pike J, Chandra RK. Effect of vitamin and trace element supplementation on immune indices in healthy elderly. *Int J Vitam Nutr Res.* 1995; 65(1):117–127.

42. Girodon F, Lombard M, Galan P. Effect of micronutrient supplementation on infection in institutionalized elderly subjects: A controlled trial. *Ann Nutr Metab.* 1997; 41(1):98–107.

43. Exton-Smith AN. The problem of subclinical malnutrition in the elderly. In: Exton-Smith AN, Scott DL, eds. *Vitamins in the Elderly.* Briston: Wright and Sons, Ltd.; 1968: 12–18.

44. Gambert SR, Guansing AR. Protein-calorie malnutrition in the elderly. *J Am Geriatr Soc.* 1980; 28: 272–275.

45. Foley CJ, Tideiksaar R. Nutritional problems in the elderly. In: Cambert SR, ed. *Contemporary Geriatric Medicine.* New York: Plenum Press; 1980: I.

46. Vellas B, Guigoz Y, Baumgartner M, Garry PJ, Lauque S, Albarede JL. Relationships between nutritional markers and the Mini-Nutritional Assessment in 155 older persons. *J Am Geriatr Soc.* 2000; 48(10):1300–1309.

47. Sacks GS, Dearman K, Replogle WH, Cora VL, Meeks M, Canada T. Use of subjective global assessment to identify nutrition-associated complications and death in geriatric long-term care facility residents. *J Am Coll Nutr.* 2000; 19(5):570–577.

48. Natlow AB, Heslin J. *Geriatric Nutrition.* Boston: CBI Publishing; 1980.

49. Dyer AR, Stamler J, Berkson DM, Lindberg HA. Relationship of relative weight and body mass index to 14-year mortality in the Chicago People Gas Co. study. *J Chronic Dis.* 1975; 28:109–123.

50. Master AM, Lasser RP, Beckman G. Tables of average weight and height of Americans aged 65–94 years. *JAMA.* 1960; 172:658–662.

51. Duerksen DR, Yeo TA, Siemens JL, O'Connor MP. The validity and reproducibility of clinical assessment of nutritional status in the elderly. *Nutrition,* 2000; 16(9):740–744.

52. Vellas B, Guigoz Y, Garry PJ, Nourhashemi F, Bennahum D, Lauque S, Albarede JL. The Mini Nutritional Assessment (MNA) and its use in grading the nutritional state of elderly patients. *Nutrition.* 1999; 15(2):116–122.

53. Wolinsky FD, Coe RM, Chavez MN, et al. Further assessment of the reliability and validity of a nutritional risk index: Analysis of a three wave panel to study elderly adults. *Health Services Res.* 1986; 20: 977–990.

54. Fillenbaum GG. *The Well-being of the Elderly: Approaches to Multidimensional Assessment.* Geneva: World Health Organization; 1984. WHO Offset Publication No. 34.

55. Sacks GS, Dearman K, Replogle WH, Cora VL, Meeks M, Canada T. Use of Subjective Global Assessment to identify nutrition-associated complications

and death in geriatric long-term care facility residents. *J Amer Coll Nutr.* 2001; 19(5):570–577.

56. Detsky AS, McLaughlin JR, Baker JP. What is subjective global assessment of nutritional status? *J Parenteral Enteral Nutr.* 1987; 11(1):8–13.

57. Hirsh S, de Obaldia N, Petermann M. Subjective global assessment of nutritional status: Further validation. *Nutrition.* 1991; 7(1):35–38.

58. Riogo SP, Sanchez-Vilar O, Gonzalez de Villar N. Geriatric nutrition: Studies about MNA. *Nutr Hosp.* 1999; 14(5)suppl 2:32S–42S.

59. Guigoz Y, Vallas B, Garry PJ. Mini Nutritional Assessment: A practical assessment tool for grading the nutritional state of elderly patients. *Facts and Research in Gerontology.* 1994; suppl 2:15–59.

60. Branch LG, Jette AM. Personal health practices and mortality among the elderly. *Am Public Health.* 1984; 74:1126–1129.

61. Steen B, Rothenberg E. Aspects of nutrition of the elderly at home—A review. *J Nutr Health Aging.* 1998; 2(1):28–33.

62. O'Hanlon P, Kohrs MB. Dietary studies of older Americans. *Am J Clin Nutr.* 1988; 31:1257–1269.

63. Russell RM. The aging process as a modifier of metabolism. *Am J Clin Nutr.* 2000; 72(2 suppl): 529S–532S.

64. Russell RM, Rasmussen H, Lichtenstein AH. Modified Food Guide Pyramid for people over seventy years of age. *J Nutr.* 1999; 129(3):751–753.

65. National Research Council. *Committee Report on Dietary Allowances of the Food and Nutrition Board.* Washington, DC: National Academy of Sciences; 1989.

66. Lowenstein FW. Nutritional requirements of the elderly. In: Young EA, ed. *Nutrition, Aging and Health.* New York: Alan Liss; 1986: 61–89.

67. Wolinsky FD, Coe RM, Miller DK, et al. Measurement of global and functional dimensions of health status in the elderly. *J Gerontol.* 1984; 39:88–92.

68. Korhs MB, Czajka-Narins D. Assessing nutrition of the elderly. In: Young EA, ed. *Nutrition, Aging and Health.* New York: Alan Liss; 1986: 25–59.

69. Roe DA. Therapeutic effects of drug-nutrient interactions in the elderly. *J Am Diet Assoc.* 1985; 85: 174–178.

70. Smith CH, Bidlack WR. Dietary concerns associated with the use of medications. *J Am Diet Assoc.* 1984; 84:901–908.

71. Blumberg J, Couris R. Pharmacology, nutrition, and the elderly: Interactions and implications. In: Chernoff R. *Geriatric Nutrition: The Health Professional's Handbook.* 2nd ed. Gaithersburg, MD: Aspen Publishers; 1999: 342–365.

72. Lotz M, Zisman E, Bartter C. Evidence for phosphorus depletion syndrome in man. *N Engl J Med.* 1968; 278:409–415.

73. Rud RK, Singer FR. Magnesium deficiency and excess. *Annual Rev Med.* 1981; 32(2):245–259.

74. Insogna KL, Bordley DR, Caro JF. Osteomalacia and weakness from excessive antacids. *JAMA.* 244: 2544–2546.

75. Benn A, Swan CJH, Cooke WT. Effect of intraluminal pH on the absorption of pteroylmonoglutamic acid. *Cr Med J.* 1971; 16(1):148–150.

76. Spencer H, Lender M. Adverse effects of aluminum-containing antacids on mineral metabolism. *Gastroenterol.* 1989; 76:603–606.

77. Wasnich R, Benfante R, Yanok-Heilbrun L, Vogel J. Thiazide effect on the mineral content of bone. *N Eng J Med.* 1983; 309:344–347.

78. Frame B, Guiang HL, Frost HN. Osteomalacia induced by laxative ingestion. *Arch Intern Med.* 1971; 128:794–796.

79. Lawrence VA, Lowenstein JE, Eichner ER. Aspirin and folate binding: In vivo and in vitro studies of serum binding and urinary excretion of exogenous folate. *J Lab Clin Med.* 1984; 103(6):944–948.

80. Welling P. Nutrient effects on drug metabolism and action in the elderly. *Drug Nutr Interact.* 1985; 4(1): 183–193.

81. Nutt JG, Woodward WR, Hammerstad JP. The "on-off" phenomenon in Parkinson's disease: Relation to levodopa absorption and transport. *N Engl J Med.* 1984; 310:483–488.

82. Hathcock JN. Metabolic mechanisms of drug-nutrient interactions. *Fed Proc.* 44(1):124–129.

83. Ciccone CD. Pharmacokinetics II: drug elimination. In: Ciccone CD. *Pharmacology in Rehabilitation.* 2nd ed. Contemporary Perspectives in Rehabilitation. Philadelphia, PA: FA Davis; 1996: 32–43.

84. Anderson KE. Nutrient regulation of chemical metabolism in humans. *Fed Proc.* 44(1):130–134.

85. Vestal RE, Norris AH, Tobin JD, et al. Antipyrin metabolism in man: Influence of age, alcohol, caffeine and smoking. *Clin Pharm Ther.* 1975; 18: 425–432.

86. Alderman E, Coltart D. Alcohol and the heart. *Brit Med Bull.* 1982; 38:77–81.

87. Richard MJ, Roussel AM. Micronutrients and ageing: Intakes and requirements. *Proc Nutr Soc.* 58(3): 573–578.

88. Evans WJ, Cyr-Campbell D. Nutrition, exercise, and health aging. *J Am Diet Assoc.* 1997; 97(6): 632–638.

89. Butler RN. Fighting frailty. Prescription for healthier aging includes exercise, nutrition, safety, and research. *Geriatrics.* 2000; 55(2):20.

90. Russell RM. The aging process as a modifier of metabolism. *Am J Clin Nutr.* 2000; 72(2 suppl): 529S–532S.

91. Sonn U, Rothenberg E, Steen B. Dietary intake and functional ability between 70 and 76 years of age. *Aging.* 1998; 10(4):324–331.

92. Roe DA. *Handbook: Interactions of Selected Drugs and Nutrients in Patients.* Chicago, IL: American Dietetic Association; 2001.

93. Smiciklas-Wright H, Fosmire GJ. Government nutrition programs for the aged. In: Watson RR, ed. *CRC Handbook of Nutrition in the Aged.* Boca Raton, FL: CRC Press; 1985: 323–334.

94. Fanelli MT, Kaufman M. Nutrition and older adults. In: Phillips HT, Gaylord SA, eds. *Aging and Public Health.* New York: Springer; 1985: 76–100.

95. Lipschitz DA, Mitchell CO, Steele RW, Milton KY. Nutritional evaluation and supplementation of elderly subjects participating in a "Meals on Wheels" program. *J Parent Ent Nutr.* 1985; 9:343–347.

96. Mayer J. Hunger and undernutrition in the United States. *J Nutr.* 1990; 120(8):919–923.

97. Martinez-Spencer A, Westley C. Nutrition for better aging in long-term care. *Lippincott's Prim Care Pract.* 1999; 3(2):174–178.

98. Keller HH. Malnutrition in institutionalized elderly: How and why? *J Am Geriatr Soc.* 1993; 41(11): 1212–1218.

99. Finn SC. Nutrition and healthy aging. *J Womens Health Gend Based Med.* 2000; 9(7):711–716.

100. Maaravi Y, Berry EM, Ginsberg G, Cohen A, Stessman J. Nutrition and quality of life in the aged. *Aging.* 2000; 12(5):402.

101. Visser M. Nutritional state and quality of life in old age. *Aging.* 2000; 12(4):320.

102. Butler RN. Fighting frailty. Prescription for healthier aging includes exercise, nutrition, safety, and research. [editorial] *Geriatrics.* 2000; 55(2):20.

103. Villers Foundation. *On the Other Side of Easy Street: Myths and Facts about the Economics of Old Age.* Washington, DC: Villers Foundation; 1986.

7

Geriatric Pharmacology

BY J. MARK TROTTER, MICHELLE E. MOFFA-TROTTER, WENDY K. ANEMAET

Pearls

- Medication use in the older population exceeds that in the younger population in part because of the increased prevalence of disease, clinical practice guidelines calling for combination drug therapy, direct consumer advertising, inappropriate prescribing practices, and unmonitored self-medication.

- Detecting unintended drug effects, sub- and supratherapeutic dosing, and medication adherence issues are all within the purview of quality rehabilitation care provision.

- Pharmacokinetics describes how the body handles and disposes of a drug. Age-related changes in drug absorption, distribution, metabolism, and excretion help explain alterations in drug actions and drug effects in the older population.

- Pharmacodynamics describes what the drug does to the body, and age-related changes in homeostatic mechanisms and receptors place the older adult at an increased risk for drug sub- and supratherapeutic effects.

- Drug-related problems, including underutilization, inappropriate prescribing practices, polypharmacy, drug interactions, adverse drug reactions, and nonadherence, are twice as likely in the geriatric population and cost in excess of $75 billion annually.

- Close monitoring of patient signs and symptoms, particularly with newly prescribed medications or dose changes, assists in early detection of adverse drug reactions.

- Medication nonadherence in the older population ranges from 40% to 76%; and common barriers cited by older patients include adverse drug reactions, knowledge deficit, sensory and language issues, cognitive impairment, dosing parameters, physical limitations, multiple pharmacy or prescribing physician source, and medication cost.

- Some medications have special rehabilitation considerations and may require adjustments in therapy scheduling and/or therapy provision.

INTRODUCTION

The number of drugs prescribed to older adults continues to increase worldwide.[1-7] While the geriatric population represents less than 15% of the United States population, this age group purchases over 30% of all prescription and 40% of all nonprescription medications nationally.[8] Indeed, medication prescription is the most frequent therapeutic intervention offered, with 75% of older adults leaving a physician's office with an order for a medication.[9] Community-dwelling older adults use an average of two to six prescription drugs regularly with most taking three agents daily.[10-15] The 2002 Slone Survey found that over 50% of older adults use five or more different medications weekly and 12% use ten or more different medications weekly.[16] Medication use in the institutionalized population is significantly higher than in the community-dwelling population, with an average of five to eight prescribed drugs used on a regular basis.[17-18]

In addition to prescription drugs, those over 65 consume an average of one to three over-the-counter medications[10,14] and the use of nonprescription agents is highest in this population.[19] Herbal supplement use is also rising, with nearly 25% of older adults estimated to use such alternative therapies.[20-22] Put together, 60% to 88% of the geriatric population takes at least one medication on a daily basis ([8,15,23]) and each older adult fills approximately fifteen to twenty prescriptions per year[24] (Box 1). Annual prescription drug sales in the United States exceed 3.2 billion prescriptions with total direct drug costs of over $204.2 billion.[25]

Most Common Drug Classes Prescribed to the Older Population

Analgesic agents
Anti-infective agents
Cardiovascular agents
Gastrointestinal agents
Hormones
Psychotherapeutic agents
Respiratory agents
Topical agents

Adapted from ref 15

Prevalence of Chronic Disease in the Older Population, 2003–2004

Coronary heart disease 21.4%
Hypertension 51.9%
Stroke 9.3%
Emphysema 5.2%
Asthma 8.9%
Chronic bronchitis 6.0%
Cancer 20.7%
Diabetes 16.9%
Ulcer 11.9%
Liver disease 1.4%
Chronic joint symptoms 46.0%
Doctor-diagnosed arthritis 50.0%

Adapted from ref 26

There are several reasons for the disproportionate use of medications in the older population. Most importantly, the prevalence of disease increases exponentially with age (Box 2). For example, prevalence rates for coronary heart disease and cancer exceed 20%, and the rates for hypertension and arthritis each exceed 50% in the older population.[26]

With advances in the medical understanding of disease pathophysiology and treatment, clinical practice guidelines increasingly call for combination drug therapy, or the use of two or more medications, to optimally manage the chronic conditions so common in the older population (Box 3).

Clinical Practice Guidelines Recommending Use of Combination Drug Therapy for the Older Population

Hypertension   The Seventh Report of the Joint National Committee on Prevention, Detection, Evaluation, and Treatment of High Blood Pressure. *J Am Med Assoc.* 2003; 289:2560–2572.
Access at: www.nhlbi.nih.gov

Coronary Artery Disease   ACC/AHA guidelines for secondary prevention for patients with coronary and other atherosclerotic vascular disease: 2006 update. *Circulation* 2006; 113:2363–2372.
Access at: www.acc.org

Angina   ACC/AHA guideline update for the management of patients with chronic stable angina. *J Am Coll Cardiol.* 2003; 41:159–168.
Access at: www.acc.org

ACC/AHA guideline update for the management of patients with unstable angina and non-ST segment elevation myocardial infarction. *J Am Coll Cardiol.* 2002; 40:1366–1374.
Access at: www.acc.org

Acute Coronary Syndrome   Management of acute coronary syndromes in patients presenting without persistent ST-segment elevation. *Eur Heart J.* 2002; 23:809–840.
Access at: www.escardio.org

Myocardial Infarction   ACC/AHA guidelines for the management of patients with ST-segment elevation myocardial infarction. *Circulation.* 2004; 110: 588–636.
Access at: www.acc.org

Management of acute myocardial infarction in patients presenting with ST-segment elevation. *Eur Heart J.* 2003; 24:28–66.
Access at: www.escardio.org

Heart Failure   ACC/AHA guidelines for the evaluation and management of chronic heart failure in the adult. *J Am Coll Cardiol.* 2001; 38:2101–2113.
Access at: www.acc.org

(cont.)

Guidelines for the diagnosis and treatment of chronic heart failure. *Eur Heart J.* 2001; 22:1527–1560.
Access at: www.escardio.org

Heart Failure Society of America (HFSA). 2006 comprehensive heart failure practice guideline. *J Cardiac Failure.* 2006; 12(1):10–38.
Access at: www.hfsa.org

Chronic Obstructive Pulmonary Disease   Standards for the diagnosis and treatment of patients with chronic obstructive pulmonary disease: A summary of the ATS/ERS position paper. *Eur Resp J.* 2004; 23:932–946.
Access at: www.thoracic.org

Renal Disease   National Kidney Foundation. *Kidney Disease Outcome Quality Initiative Clinical Practice: Guidelines for Chronic Kidney Disease: Evaluation, classification and stratification.* New York: National Kidney Foundation; 2002.
Access at: www.kidney.org

Diabetes   American Association of Clinical Endocrinologists medical guidelines for the management of diabetes mellitus: The AACE system of intensive diabetes self-Management—2002 update. *Endocr Pract.* 2002; 28(suppl): January–February:40–82.
Access at: www.aace.com

Gastroesophageal Reflux Disease   Updated guidelines for the diagnosis and treatment of gastroesophageal reflux disease. *Am J Gastrolenterol.* 2005; 100:190–200.
Access at: www.acg.gi.org

Canadian Consensus Conference on the management of gastroesophageal reflux disease in adults—Update 2004. *Can J Gastroenterol.* 2005; 19:15–35.
Access at: www.aan.org

Peptic Ulcer Disease   Management of helicobacter pylori infection. *Am Fam Phys.* 2002; 65(7): 1327–1339.
Access at: www.aafp.org

Canadian Helicobacter Study Group Consensus Conference: Update on the management of helicobacter pylori—An evidence-based evaluation of six topics relevant to clinical outcomes in patients evaluated for H pylori infection. *Can J Gastroenterol.* 2004; 18(9):547–554.
Access at www.cag-acg.org

Dementia   American Psychiatric Association. *Treating Alzheimer's disease and Other dementias of late life.* May 1997 *The Am. J Psychiatry* 154(5 Suppl):1–39.
Access at: www.appi.org

Practice parameter: Management of dementia: Report of the quality standards subcommittee of the American Academy of Neurology. *Neurol.* 2001; 56: 1154–1166.
Access at: www.aan.org

Parkinson's Disease   Practice parameter: Treatment of Parkinson's disease with motor fluctuations and dyskinesia: Report of the Quality Standards Subcommittee of the American Academy of Neurology. *Neurol.* 2006; 66:983–995.
Access at: www.aan.org

Pain   Advances in neuropathic pain. *Arch Neurol.* 2003; 60:1524–1534.
Access at: www.guidelines.gov or www.archneur.ama-assn.org

The management of persistent pain in older persons. *J Am Geriatr Soc.* 2002; 50:S205–S224.
Access at: www.ags.org

Practice parameter: Treatment of postherpatic neuralgia. *Neurol.* 2004; 63:959–965.
Access at www.aan.org

Another contributing factor to the rise in medication use with age is the result of consumer advertising by pharmaceutical companies.[27,28] Patients with symptoms often expect to receive prescriptions for their problems.[29] With direct advertising, patients may be more likely to request a specific medication from their physician, even in instances when no clear indication for that drug class exists. Inappropriate prescribing practices also compound the problem.[30] Finally, unmonitored self-medication with over-the-counter, herbal, and "left over" prescription drugs may contribute to the higher rate of medication use and drug-related complications in the older population.

With the high prevalence of chronic disease, functional impairment, and pain in the rehabilitation population, the typical geriatric rehabilitation patient is often on a complex medication regimen to address his or her multifactorial needs[15] (Box 4).

Medication Use and Expense According to Health Status in the Community-Dwelling Older Population

Health Status	N (%)	Mean Drug Expenses per Annum	Uses ≥ 3 Drugs (%)	Uses 3 Drugs Chronically (%)
No comorbidity and no ADL difficulty	13.1%	$ 345	14–22%	5%
1–2 comorbidities and no ADL difficulty	43.6%	$1099	51–54%	21–23%
≥ 3 comorbidities and/or ADL difficulty	43.3%	$2275	73–77%	43–46%

Comorbidity was defined as the presence of hypertension, coronary heart disease, acute myocardial infarction, angina, stroke, diabetes, arthritis, osteoporosis, emphysema/chronic obstructive pulmonary disease, Alzheimer's disease, Parkinson's disease. Adapted from ref 15

As part of the interdisciplinary team, therapists should gain competency in the drug regimen review and monitoring process. Discerning unintended drug effects, subtherapeutic dosing, and medication adherence issues are all within the purview of quality rehabilitation care provision. Competency begins with an understanding of the age-related changes that impact pharmacologic parameters in the older population.

PHARMACOKINETICS IN THE OLDER POPULATION

Pharmacokinetics describes how the body handles and disposes of a drug. Age-related changes in pharmacokinetics may partially explain why the older population responds differently to drugs than the younger population. Absorption, distribution, metabolism, and excretion are four aspects of pharmacokinetics impacted by the aging process (see Figure 7.1).[29–38]

Absorption

Absorption is the rate at which a drug leaves the administration site and the extent to which this occurs. Bioavailability is an index measure of the amount of drug that reaches the systemic circulation. Manufacturers use bioavailability data to determine the optimum drug dosage or strength that produces a desired therapeutic effect. For example, manufacturers compensate for low bioavailability with higher dose potency so that enough of the drug is successfully absorbed in the adult population. The largest determinant of bioavailability is the medication's administration route. Intravenous agents have 100% (e.g., ampicillin) bioavailability, while oral agents may have as little as 1% (e.g., alendronate) or as much as 100% (e.g., flucona-

zole) bioavailability. On the other hand, the bioavailability of topical agents is neglible, since topicals are designed to act locally, the drugs do not reach the systemic circulation to any large extent. Age-related changes that may impact absorption include changes in tissue perfusion, saliva production, and gastrointestinal function (Box 5).

Drug Administration Routes

Enteral: Directly to GI Tract	Parenteral: Bypass the GI Tract	Topical: Bypass the GI Tract
Oral	Injection	Inhalation
Sublingual	Intravenous	Transdermal
Buccal	Intra-arterial	
Nasogatsric	Subcutaneous	
Rectal	Intramuscular	
	Intrathecal	

Source: *Trotter, J.M., Moffa-Trotter, M.E., Anemaet, W.K.* Medication Profile in Pharmacology for Rehabilitation Professionals *course material. Clearwater, FL: A&T Rehabilitation Solutions; 2005: 8.*

Reduced tissue perfusion and muscle atrophy may impair absorption of intramuscular injections and, accordingly, they are less preferred in the older population.[33] Impaired tissue perfusion may also affect absorption of transdermal agents.[33] Thus, transdermal agents seen in the rehabilitation population such as nitrate and fentanyl

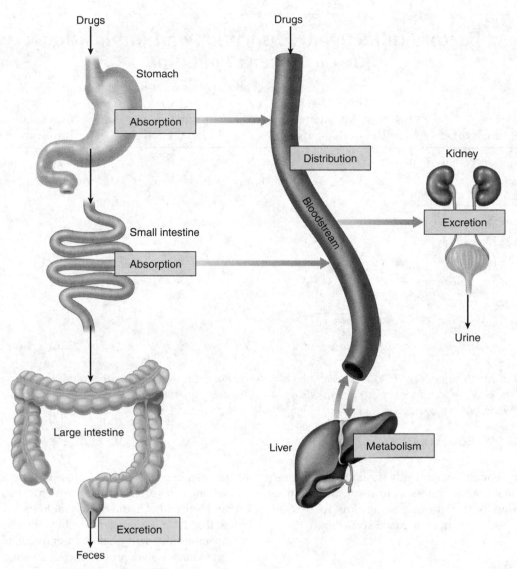

Figure 7.1   The Four Aspects of Pharmacokinetics

patches are dosed to therapeutic effect (i.e., control of angina or pain) rather than standard dosing guidelines, which are geared toward a largely young population. Impaired saliva production may retard absorption of buccal route agents,[32] but fortunately these are rarely encountered in the older population.

Because of cost and ease of administration, oral formulations are the most commonly used. Following administration, oral agents largely undergo passive diffusion within the gastrointestinal epithelium. Age-related changes to the gastrointestinal system include increased gastric acid pH and reduced secretion, 30% smaller surface area,

weaker peristalsis, delayed gastric emptying, 40% reduction in splanchnic blood flow, and slower intestinal motility[39] (Box 6). While these changes do not reduce drug absorption per se, they may delay the rate of absorption and the time required to attain peak drug effect. Some notable exceptions relevant to rehabilitation include levadopa and propanolol, which may each have upward of 50% higher bioavailability in the older population and require compensatory dose reductions. Also of note, a minority of drugs utilize active transport for absorption, but the function of this mechanism is equivocal across all age groups.

Factors Influencing Absorption and Implications for the Older Population

Age-Related Changes	Chronic Diseases that Attenuate Age-Related Changes	Drugs and Other Factors that Attenuate Age-Related Changes	Potential Implications
⇓ gastric acid secretion	Diarrhea	Antacids	⇓ absorption rate
⇓ gastric acidity	Malabsorption syndromes	Anticholinergics	⇑ time till peak effect
⇓ gastrointestinal surface area	Pancreatitis	Drug-food interactions	
⇓ gastric emptying		Laxatives	
⇓ splanchnic blood flow**			
⇓ intestinal motility			
⇓ active transport mechanism			
⇓ gastric dopa			
⇓ decarboxylase*			

* Levadopa is degraded by decarboxylase, and reduced decarboxylase levels with age cause higher levadopa concentrations in the older population.
** Propanolol is extensively (near 90%) metabolized on first pass through the liver in the general population. The diminished splanchnic blood flow with age allows greater absorption of the drug into the systemic circulation before reaching the liver, so bioavailability of propanolol is significantly higher in the older population.
Adapted from refs 36, 38

In the older population, clinically significant changes in drug absorption are not common. However, therapists assist the physician by monitoring symptoms so that any needed dose adjustments may be made accordingly.

Distribution

Distribution is the extent of drug dispersion in the systemic circulation to the site of action. Most of this occurs passively and the remainder occurs with active protein transport via albumin, alpha-1 glycoprotein, and corticosteroid-binding globulin. Changes in central and peripheral circulation, serum protein levels, and body composition may impact distribution with age.

Passive diffusion relies on the cardiovascular system to carry the drug from the administration site to the target site. The lowered cardiac output and increased peripheral vascular resistance seen in the geriatric population slow the rate of passive drug transport within the body. Drugs that rely on active transport, specifically through binding of albumin or alpha-1 glycoprotein, may also experience a change in distribution with age.

Overall, protein binding capacity diminishes 15% to 25% with age.[40] Albumin levels decline 10% to 12% in the older population,[41] and the prevalence of renal disease and malnourishment associated with low albumin is higher in this population. If less circulating albumin is available for drug binding, more of that drug remains in the circulation, causing a higher free-fraction drug level. Clinical significance is usually negligible, but it may cause an exaggerated or supratherapeutic effect in older patients with low serum albumin levels. This is most likely in high-risk patients using drugs that have a high affinity for albumin and a narrow therapeutic index like phenytoin and warfarin. Conversely, levels of alpha-1 glycoprotein increase with age. The net effect is a nearly 40% reduction in free-fraction drug levels in medications reliant on this transport mechanism,[42] such as lidocaine and phenytoin; however, this has not proven to be clinically significant in the older population.

The largest determinant of passive drug distribution in those over 65 is the change in body composition over time. Medications are largely water or fat soluble. Water-soluble agents like nonsteroidal anti-inflammatory agents, many antibiotics, and acetaminophen have decreased distribution with age because of the 10% to 25% reduction in total body water content[43-45] and the 12% to 19% loss of lean body mass.[44] As a result, more of the drug remains in circulation, causing a higher free-fraction drug level and attenuated drug effects. In this case, lower starting doses are often beneficial. On the other hand, total body fat increases 20% to 40% with age,[39,43,46] so fat-soluble drugs like many antiarrhythmics, diazepam, and lidocaine are more rapidly and extensively absorbed into adipose tissue reservoirs. Here, the drug requires more time and a higher loading dose to attain the desired therapeutic effect. Fat-soluble agents may also have a prolonged duration of action because of the large drug reserve available (See Box 7).

Factors Influencing Distribution and Implications for the Older Population

Age-Related Changes	Diseases that Attenuate Age-Related Changes	Drugs and Other Factors that Attenuate Age-Related Changes	Implications
⇓ cardiac output	Heart failure	Dehydration	⇓ volume of distribution for water-soluble drugs
⇑ peripheral vascular resistance	Edema	Drug-drug interactions	
⇓ body water content	Hepatic failure	Malnourishment	⇑ volume of distribution for fat-soluble drugs
⇓ lean body mass	Hypertension	Obesity	
⇑ fat mass	Renal failure	Protein binding displacement	
⇓ serum albumin			
⇑ serum alpha-1 glycoprotein		Sarcopenia	

Adapted from refs 36, 38

Clinically significant changes caused by altered drug distribution are more likely in high-risk patients such as those with low albumin (e.g., renal disease, malnourishment, heart failure) and/or marked body composition changes (e.g., dehydration, sarcopenia, obesity). These factors should be addressed by the physician when he or she formulates the drug prescription. The therapist assesses patient symptomology regularly to assist the physician in adjusting drug dosage and dosing intervals as needed to obtain a safe therapeutic effect despite any age-related change in distribution.

Metabolism

The biologic transformation of a drug into an inactive molecule, a more soluble compound, or a more potent metabolite is called metabolism, and it occurs primarily in the liver. With age, hepatic blood flow decreases 40%[47–51] and liver size declines 25% to 35%.[51] Nevertheless, liver function is compositely unaffected by old age in the well elderly population. In old age, medications dependent on hepatic metabolism, such as the 50% of agents metabolized by cytochrome P450 enzymes, may be prone to drug accumulation and prolonged drug effects because less of the drug is metabolized through the liver (Box 8). Indeed, these drugs, including warfarin, steroids, and ibuprofen, can have a 50% to 75% reduction in hepatic clearance compared to the younger population.[31,50,52,53] Physicians adjust for this by prescribing a lower initial dose and titrating slowly to the desired therapeutic effect. Therapists assist in this process by updating the physician about sub- or supratherapeutic effects that warrant further dose changes.

Factors Influencing Metabolism and Implications for the Older Population

Age-Related Changes	Diseases that Attenuate Age-Related Changes	Drugs and Other Factors that Attenuate Age-Related Changes	Implications
⇓ hepatic blood flow	Cancer	Alcohol consumption	⇑ half-life
⇓ liver size	Heart failure	Drug-drug interactions	⇓ drug clearance for hepatically cleared drugs
	Fever	Drug-food interactions	
	Hepatic insufficiency	Malnutrition	
	Thyroid disease	Tobacco use	
	Viral infection		

Adapted from refs 36, 38

Excretion

Excretion is the elimination of the drug from the body and it is the pharmacokinetic parameter most affected by age. Drug clearance describes the body's ability to eliminate a drug and is used to determine the steady-state concentration for a given dose. The kidney is the primary organ responsible for drug elimination. Renal function declines by 35% to 50% with age[54] and is marked by a 20% to 25% nephron loss[55], reduced tubular secretion, decreased renal blood flow, a 25% to 50% decline in glomular filtration rate[37], and fibrosis. Average renal clearance declines 50% to 75% with age[31], so renally cleared drugs experience a prolonged half-life in those over age 65. This means that circulating free-fraction drug levels are elevated and a prolonged drug effect may occur, particularly in patients with marked renal impairment (Box 9). Drugs dependent on renal clearance, such as gabapentin, multiple antibiotics, and antivirals, must be dose-adjusted by the physician to avoid these adverse consequences.

Factors Influencing Excretion and Implications for the Older Population

Age-Related Changes	Diseases that Attenuate Age-Related Changes	Drugs and Other Factors that Attenuate Age-Related Changes	Implications
⇓ renal blood flow	Hypovolemia	Drug-drug interactions	⇑ half-life
⇓ glomular filtration rate	Renal insufficiency		⇓ drug clearance for renally
⇓ tubular secretion			excreted drugs

Adapted from refs 36, 38

Pharmacokinetics assists in explaining drug actions and determining drug effects. For example, the processes of distribution, metabolism, and elimination all help determine the half-life, or time it takes for one half of the original drug dose to be removed from the body. Half-life may be reduced by 50% with age and is an important pharmacokinetic variable because it reflects the drug's duration of action. Half-life is used to determine therapeutic dosing intervals so that a steady-state concentration of the drug remains within a therapeutic range. This is important for chronic diseases such as seizures, hypertension, and diabetes in which symptom fluctuations may precipitate adverse events.

The volume of distribution is the relative portion of a drug in the body as a function of body mass. At-risk older adults (e.g., those with hypoalbuminuria, obesity, heart failure) may require a 10% to 20% loading dose adjustment to compensate for alterations in distribution. In practical terms, this is done when physicians follow the "start low, go slow" principle of drug loading and titration for the older population.

Drug clearance is a function of the volume of distribution, metabolism, and excretion (Box 10). Physicians use drug clearance to determine the drug dosage required at each dosing interval to achieve a consistent therapeutic effect.

Pharmacokinetics also help determine important time-based drug effects such as onset of action, peak effect, and duration of action (Box 11).

Implications of Age-Related Changes for Pharmacokinetic Variables

Drug Action	Pharmacokinetic Variable	Change with Age	Implication
Half-life	Distribution	⇑	⇑ dose interval
	Metabolism		
	Excretion		
Volume of distribution	Distribution	⇑ fat-soluble drug	First dose adjustment
		⇓ water-soluble drug	
Clearance	Distribution	⇓	⇓ dose of drug
	Metabolism		⇑ dose interval
	Excretion		

Implications of Age on Time-Based Drug Effects

Drug Effect	Description	Impact of Age
Onset of action	Time required for the drug to elicit a therapeutic effect	Delayed onset of action
Peak effect	Time required for the drug to attain its maximal effect	Delayed peak effect
Duration of action	Time that the drug concentration is sufficient to elicit a therapeutic effect	Prolonged duration of action

Source: *Trotter, J.M., Moffa-Trotter, M.E., Anemaet, W.K.* Medication Profile in Pharmacology for Rehabilitation Professionals *course material. Clearwater, FL: A & T Rehabilitation Solutions; 2006: 12.*

These pharmacokinetic variables may directly impact rehabilitation interventions. For example, a common area of disability among the rehabilitation population is pain. Physicians often prescribe analgesic agents to address this problem. To optimize pain management during rehabilitation, the therapist should consider specific analgesic drug effects to enhance patient tolerance of therapy and, ultimately, rehabilitation goal attainment. With a prescription for ibuprofen, the pharmacokinetics of this drug is such that the onset of action is one hour, peak effect occurs within one to two hours, and duration of action is four to eight hours. For ibuprofen, then, the ideal pretreatment window for analgesic effect is 60 to 90 minutes prior to the rehabilitation. Such drug-specific pharmacokinetic information could also be used in patients with gastrointestinal symptoms, respiratory impairments, and some neurologic disorders to optimize treatment scheduling and improve tolerance to the rehabilitation program.

PHARMACODYNAMICS IN THE OLDER POPULATION

Pharmacodynamics describes the response of the body to the effects of a drug at a given concentration. It explains what the drug does to the body. All medications elicit an intended or unintended response through their mechanisms of action. The ideal response is a therapeutic effect, but age-related changes in pharmacodynamics place the older adult at risk for sub- or supratherapeutic effects. Older adults exhibit altered drug pharmacodynamics and this is attributed to changes in homeostatic mechanisms and receptor alterations.[29,31–34,36–38]

Homeostatic Mechanisms

Homeostatic mechanisms decline with age. Older adults have a diminished functional reserve capacity and their ability to respond to physiologic challenges is reduced. Declines in orthostatic blood pressure maintenance, thermoregulation, postural and gait stability, and cognitive reserve all negatively affect the older adult's ability to preserve equilibrium, especially following a drug challenge (Box 12). Consequently, the introduction of drugs like antihypertensive agents and anticholinergic agents that act on compromised homeostatic mechanisms may precipitate unintended effects such as postural hypotension and cholinergic effects more readily in the older population.

Impaired Homeostatic Mechanisms with Age

Homeostatic Mechanism	Age-Related Changes
Thermoregulation	$\Downarrow$ basal temperature
	Blunted febrile response
Blood pressure maintenance	Hypertension
	Prone to orthostasis
Volemic maintenance	Prone to dehydration
Respiratory function	Blunted sensitivity to $\Uparrow$ carbon dioxide levels

(cont.)

Homeostatic Mechanism	Age-Related Changes
Clotting cascade	Clotting response
Insulin regulation	Insulin resistance
Bone homeostasis	Bone absorption > bone formation
Skeletal muscle maintenance	Muscle protein catabolism > muscle protein synthesis
Bladder function	Incontinence
Bowel function	Constipation
Gait and postural stability	Prone to falls
Cognitive reserve	⇓ cognitive function, memory

Receptor Alterations

Many drugs exert their effect by binding to specific receptors within the body. With advanced age, there is a reduction in the number of receptors, receptor competency (up- and down-regulation), and drug-receptor affinity (Box 13). This is of consequence because these receptor changes make the target tissue more or less responsive to drug binding. Therefore, receptor changes affect how the older patient responds to a drug.

Factors Influencing Receptor Response in the Older Population

Neurotransmitter	Receptor	Primary Locations	Responses	Age-Related Changes
Acetylcholine (cholinergic) "rest and digest" response	Muscarinic (M_1–M_5)	Heart	⇓ heart rate	⇓
			⇓ heart contraction	
		Vascular smooth muscle	Relaxation	
		Intestinal smooth muscle	Contraction ⇑	
Parasympathetic		Sweat glands	Glandular secretions	Unknown
	Nicotinic	Postganglionic neurons	Neurotransmitter release	
		Skeletal muscle	Contraction	
Norepinephrine (adrenergic) "fight or flight" response	Alpha-1	Vascular smooth muscle	Contraction	⇓
		Intestinal smooth muscle	Relaxation	
		Radial muscle iris	Contraction (pupil dilation)	
		Ureters	Contraction	
Sympathetic		Urinary sphincter	Contraction	
		Spleen capsule	Contraction	
	Alpha-2	CNS inhibitory synapses	⇓ sympathetic outflow	⇓
		Presynaptic terminal @ adrenergic synapses	⇓ norepinephrine release	
		Intestinal smooth muscle		
		Pancreas	Relaxation and ⇓ secretion	
			⇓ insulin release	
	Beta-1	Cardiac muscle	⇑ heart rate	⇓
		Kidneys	⇑ heart contractility	
		Fat cells	⇑ renin secretion	⇑
			⇑ lipolysis	

(cont.)

Neurotransmitter	Receptor	Primary Locations	Responses	Age-Related Changes
	Beta-2	Bronchiole smooth muscle	Relaxation	⇓
		Skeletal muscle and liver arterioles	Vasodilation	
		Gastrointestinal smooth muscle	Relaxation	
		Skeletal muscle and liver cells	⇑ cellular metabolism	
		Ureters	Relaxation	
		Gall bladder	Relaxation	
Dopamine	D_1 (D_5)	CNS synapses	Activates adenylyl cyclase	⇓
	D_2 (D_3, D_4)	Basal ganglia		
		Other CNS locations	Inhibits adenylyl cyclase	
Gamma-aminobutyric acid (GABA)	GABAa GABAb	CNS inhibitory synapses	Inhibition of neural pathways	Unknown
Seronergic	Serotonin	Brain stem	Mood modulation	⇓
		Hippocampus	Anxiety modulation	
		Limbic system	Sleep cycling between	
		Medulla	NREM and REM	
		Hypothalamus		
		Substantia nigra		
		Cranial blood vessels		
		Spinal cord	Vasoconstriction	
		Gastrointestinal tract	Pain perception	
			Appetite stimulation	
			Sexual function	

The central nervous system experiences a decline in the number of dopaminergic and cholinergic neurons and receptors with age.[56–58] As a result, the older patient requires a smaller dose of central nervous system agents, such as selective serotonin reuptake inhibitors, to elicit a therapeutic effect compared to the younger population. Alpha receptors experience down-regulation with age so that administration of alpha agonists like clonidine may generate a decreased effect. The down-regulation and reduced sensitivity of adenosine alpha-1 receptors, and heart muscarine receptors with age also cause impaired receptor stimulation, resulting in a subtherapeutic drug effect compared in the geriatric population. One well-studied change in pharmacodynamic receptors is the down-regulation of the beta adrenergic system. Nonselective beta-blockers like propranolol are known to have a smaller effect on hypertension in the older population because of reduced receptor sensitivity. The older population also has depressed blood pressure and respiratory homeostatic mechanisms. Consequently, beta-1 selective blockers like metoprolol are preferred because they selectively target the cardiac beta-1 receptors and avoid the respiratory consequences of bronchiole beta-2 blockade, which are more likely with nonselective agents in older adults.[59]

When coupled with pharmacokinetic alterations, the age-related pharmacodynamic changes cause the older patient to have a higher sensitivity to drugs. Because of impaired homeostatic mechanisms, the older population is less able to compensate for the higher physiologic challenge posed by medications and is at a greater risk for unintended drug effects (Box 14). Therapists use their frequent contact with patients to closely monitor for drug-related problems.

Pharmacodynamic Changes on Select Medications in the Older Population

Drug	Indications	Age-Related Pharmacodynamic Change
Albuterol	Chronic obstructive pulmonary disease	⇓ bronchodilatory effect
	Emphysema	
Diazepam	Anxiety	⇑ sedative response
Furosemide	Heart failure	⇓ peak diuretic effect and duration of action
	Hypertension	
	Renal disease	
Morphine	Pain	⇑ analgesic response

Glyburide and nitroglycerin evidence no pharmacodynamic change with age.
Adapted from ref 59

DRUG-RELATED PROBLEMS IN THE OLDER POPULATION

Drug-related problems are twice as likely in the geriatric population[60] and include underutilization, inappropriate prescribing practices, polypharmacy, drug interactions, adverse drug reactions, and nonadherence. In the United States, as much as 28% of hospitalizations are secondary to drug-related problems[61] and direct and indirect costs exceed $75 billion annually[62]. In many cases, these problems are preventable.[63] In addition to pharmacokinetic and pharmacodynamic changes, numerous factors increase the risk for drug-related problems in the geriatric population (Box 15).

Factors Associated with Drug-Related Problems in the Older Population

Drug-Related Problem	Associated Factors
Underutilization[64]	Lack of quality research on drug therapy in the older population to guide treatment decisions
	Physician fear of adverse drug reactions
	Patient financial barriers
Inappropriate Prescribing Practices[65,66]	Lack of quality research on drug therapy in the older population to guide treatment decisions
	Physician fear of adverse drug reactions
	Comorbidities, particularly atherosclerotic disease, chronic obstructive pulmonary disease, heat failure, hypertension, non-insulin diabetes mellitus, and pleural effusion
Polypharmacy[67,68]	Age
	Comorbidities, particularly asthma, cardiovascular disease, diabetes mellitus, gastrointestinal disorders, and psychiatric conditions
	Prescribing cascade*
	Failure to discontinue drugs with minimal therapeutic effect
	Multiple prescribing physicians
	Multiple filling pharmacies
	Self-medication

(cont.)

Drug-Related Problem	Associated Factors
Drug Interactions[69–71]	Age-related changes in pharmacokinetics
	Age-related changes in pharmacodynamics
	Inappropriate prescribing practices
	Polypharmacy
	Improper drug administration
	Nonadherence
Adverse Drug Reactions[10,29]	Age-related changes in pharmacokinetics
	Age-related changes in pharmacodynamics
	Comorbidities
	Inappropriate prescribing practices
	Polypharmacy
	Improper drug administration
	Nonadherence
Nonadherence[72–75]	Demographics, specifically income and race
	Polypharmacy
	Frequent dosing intervals
	Sensory impairment
	Cognitive impairment
	Adverse drug reactions
	Inadequate social support
	Patient knowledge
	Patient attitude and motivation
	Multiple providers

* Prescribing cascade: the deleterious prescription of additional drugs to treat the adverse drug reactions of other drugs.

Underutilization

Underutilization occurs when physicians refrain from prescribing medications for patients with indications known to benefit from drug therapy. Clinical treatment guidelines have been published for numerous conditions (Box 3) but have not been adopted as standards of care in routine clinical practice.[64] For example, medications such as warfarin,[76] HMG-CoA reductase inhibitors (statins),[77] angiotensin-converting enzyme (ACE) inhibitors, and beta-blockers[78,79] are underprescribed in the older population. Fifty-one percent of patients with osteoporosis are not taking calcium supplements[80] and only 24% are on drug therapy one year after fracture.[81] Of those with a history of stroke, over one-third are not on antiplatelet or anticoagulant therapy.[80] Hypertension is also largely undertreated, and among older adults with coronary artery disease, only 40% take aspirin and 34% take beta-blocker agents.[80,82] Just over two-thirds of older patients with heart failure are not on an ACE inhibitor despite its consideration as a first-line agent for this condition[80] and heart failure remains a largely undertreated condition in the geriatric population.[82]

Like other drug-related problems, underutilization must ultimately be addressed at the prescriber level. Nonetheless, therapists may offer assistance by screening for underutilization and directing patients to disease education sites such as those listed in Box 3. They may also encourage patients to discuss benefits and risks of drug therapy directly with their physician.

Inappropriate Prescribing Practices

Inappropriate prescribing practices are another drug-related problem encountered in the older population. Inappropriate prescribing generally refers to the prescription of a drug that has a greater potential to cause harm in the patient than to offer significant benefit. It may also include subtherapeutic dosing, overdosing, inappropriate drug selection, and adverse drug withdrawal events, which occur when select drugs (e.g., steroids, selective serotonin reuptake inhibitors, benzodiazepines) are withdrawn abruptly, precipitating potentially serious rebound symptoms. The sequelae of such inappropriate prescribing practices include polypharmacy, drug interactions, and adverse drug reactions.

The prevalence of inappropriate prescribing ranges from 12% to 40% in the institutionalized and community-dwelling population.[62,83–86] Determination of inappropriate prescribing is made through the application of standardized criteria to a drug regimen. The most widely used prescribing criteria for the geriatric population are Beer's Criteria. These were originally published in 1991 for nursing home residents, have been revised three times, and now include the community-dwelling population. Through literature review and expert consensus, they were most recently revised in 2003 and now include forty-eight drugs and/or medication classes to avoid in the elderly and twenty that should not be used in the presence of certain comorbidities[62] (Box 16).

Categories of Inappropriate Drugs in the Older Population

Category	Reason for Precaution	Affected Drugs
Drugs that should not be routinely used	Very likely to cause adverse drug reactions and/or toxicity	Barbiturates Chlorpropamide Long-acting benzodiazepines Meprobamate Meperidine
Potentially dangerous drugs that may be necessary to treat a specific condition	High adverse drug reaction profile; however, benefit may outweigh risk	Antiarrhythmics Nonsteroidal anti-inflammatories Warfarin
Drugs with limited efficacy and significant potential to harm	High adverse drug reaction, hypersensitivity, and/or interaction profile and risk usually outweighs benefit	Propoxyphene Quinine
Drugs with significant potential for benefit; however, alternative drugs with similar efficacy exist	Alternate drugs have similar benefit but improved safety profile	Antipsychotics Tricyclic antidepressants
Drugs often used at doses more suitable for the young population	Changes in hepatic metabolism and renal clearance with age necessitate dose reductions in the older population	Digoxin Hydrochlorothiazide Gabapentin

Adapted from refs 62, 66

Therapists may use explicit drug criteria as a crude initial screen in the drug regimen review process. While none of these medications are considered contraindications in the older population, their use serves as a "red flag" for the therapist, warranting more diligent monitoring for adverse drug reactions. Physicians may not know all of the medications a patient takes because patients do not volunteer this information and physicians may not ask.[87–89] Therapists in outpatient, home, and assisted living settings are in unique positions to assess for inappropriate prescribing practices such as self-medication, multiple prescribing physicians, and more than one filling pharmacy of which the referring physician may be unaware.

Polypharmacy

In past years, polypharmacy was defined as the use of two (to five) or more drugs. With the advancement of drug therapy and development of best practices for medication treatment often calling for combination drug therapy (Box 3), this definition has fallen out of favor. In the United States, polypharmacy is defined as the use of a medication for which no clear indication exists. There is a distinction between rational polypharmacy (drug prescription following clinical indications and best practice) and irrational polypharmacy (inappropriate drug prescribing, using more than one drug from the same class, prescribing drugs with similar pharmacologic action to treat different conditions, multiple providers, and self-medication).[90]

The frequency of polypharmacy varies from 5% to 78% depending on the definition of polypharmacy used.[12,52,91] One third of polypharmacy involves self-medication with over-the-counter and herbal drugs, most commonly acetaminophen, ibuprofen, and aspirin.[92] Fifty-four percent of older patients add medications like laxatives or tranquilizers to their prescribing regimen without health provider consultation.[93]

Polypharmacy is associated with numerous sequelae in the older population. A heightened risk for adverse drug reactions, medication administration errors from following a more complex regimen, nonadherence, and higher mortality rates have all been associated with polypharmacy.[86,90] As a result, *Healthy People 2010* includes the reduction of polypharmacy as an important goal for the older population.[94]

Therapists in the home, assisted living, and outpatient settings may comprehensively assess for polypharmacy since drug information must be collected directly from the patient or caregiver. Use of the "brown bag" technique,[95] in which the patient brings or shows all of his or her prescribed, over-the-counter, herbal, and vitamin and mineral supplements to the therapist for itemization (ostentatiously in a brown bag!), offers an important opportunity to provide the referring physician with a complete list of all the drugs a patient takes so that polypharmacy may be fully evaluated and addressed.[96–98]

Drug Interactions

There are four types of drug interactions that may occur in the older population (Box 17).

Categories of Drug Interactions in the Older Population

Interaction Type	Consequence	Common Examples
Drug-Drug	One drug alters the pharmacokinetics of the other	Beta-blockers and antiarrhythmics: cardiac decompensation
		Diuretics and steroids: hyperkalemia
	One drug potentiates or inhibits the effect of the other	Diuretics and nonsteroidal anti-inflammatories: renal impairment
		Methyldopa or clonidine with tricyclic antidepressants: hypertension
		Tricyclic antidepressants and antihistamines: anticholinergic effects
		Tramadol with selective serotonin reuptake inhibitors : ⇑ risk of serotonin syndrome
		Select antimicrobials (i.e. metronidazole) with warfarin: ⇑ hypoprothrombinemic response
Drug-Food	Food, alcohol, water, and beverages may increase or decrease drug absorption and/or metabolism	Fortified orange juice and antibiotics: ⇓ absorption
		Fortified cereal and antimicrobials: ⇓ absorption
		Food or beverage with bisphosphonates: almost full inhibition of absorption
		⇑ Vitamin K rich foods with warfarin: ⇓ hypoprothrombinemic response
Drug-Herbal	Herbal agents may alter drug metabolism	Warfarin and ginko, garlic, feverfew: ⇑ anticoagulant effect
		Warfarin and ginseng: ⇓ anticoagulant effect
		Nonsteroidal anti-inflammatories and gossypol or uva-ursi: ⇑ gastrointestinal symptoms
		Diuretics and dandelion or uva-ursi: ⇓ antihypertensive effect
		Digoxin and hawthorne: may potentiate digoxin effects
		Benzodiazepines and ginseng or kava kava or St. John's Wort: ⇑ sedation
Drug-Disease	Drug may precipitate physiologic effects that worsen disease symptoms	Benign prostrate hypertrophy and alpha agonists and/or anticholinergics: urinary retention
		Chronic obstructive pulmonary disease and beta-blockers: bronchoconstriction
		Dementia and anticholinergics: confusion
		Glaucoma and anticholinergics: exacerbation of glaucoma
		Hypertension and nonsteroidal anti-inflammatories: hypertension
		Parkinson's disease and antipsychotics: extrapyramidal symptoms

(cont.)

Interaction Type	Consequence	Common Examples
		Peripheral vascular disease and beta-blockers: intermittent claudication
		Constipation and anticholinergics or opiates or calcium channel blockers: constipation
		Osteoporosis and steroids: fracture
		Renal impairment and nonsteroidal anti-inflammatories: renal failure
		Diabetes and steroids: hyperglycemia
		Diabetes and quinolone or antimicrobial or steroids: either hyperglycemia and hypoglycemia

Adapted from refs 59, 96–98

Drug-drug interactions are the most common interaction in the older population. Over 47% of patients taking more than two drugs have a potential drug-drug interaction[99] and polypharmacy is an obvious risk factor for drug-drug interactions. The risk of an interaction is 13.2% with use of two drugs and escalates to 82% with use of seven or more drugs.[99] The risk of interactions approaches 100% with use of ten or more drugs in the elderly.[100] Drug-drug interactions are a contributing factor for hospitalization and significant morbidity.[101,102]

Drug-food interactions may occur in the digestive system, blood, or at cell receptor sites. Food and beverages have wide-ranging effects. For example, food may adversely affect drug solubility and absorption, or it may cause a drug to become more rapidly bioavailable. Alcohol may disrupt drug metabolism while high-fat content foods, fiber, and acidic juices may impair absorption. Most drug-food interactions are likely to produce treatment failure. In patients taking standard drug dosages who experience subtherapeutic effects, therapists should query the patient about how and when he or she takes the medications. Food precautions are included on the drug labels and should be followed exactly as prescribed.

When drug interactions occur, they are often "explained" as disease progression or attributed to nonadherence with the drug regimen.[102] Therapists may play a key role in bringing any new symptoms to the attention of the physician, particularly those whose onset can be tied to drug initiation or recent dose change of a prescribed, nonprescriptive, or herbal agent.

Adverse Drug Reactions

Adverse drug reactions (ADRs) are noxious, unintended reactions that occur at doses normally used for diagnosis, prophylaxis, or treatment. Common manifestations of ADRs include hypersensitivity (a true anaphylactic reaction), side effects, drug-induced disease, or drug-induced lab changes (Box 18).

Types of Adverse Drug Reactions

Type of Adverse Drug Reaction	Manifestation
Hypersensitivity	Contact dermatitis, eczema, urticaria, angioedema, thrombocytopenia, agranulocytosis, hemolytic anemia, acute asthma, anaphylaxis
Side Effects	Anticholinergic effects, confusional state/delirium, constipation, dehydration, depression, dizziness, extrapyramidal signs, fatigue/weakness, gastrointestinal upset, hypertension, hypocoagulation, postural hypotension, urinary incontinence, urinary retention
Drug-Induced Disease	Electrolyte imbalance, delirium, hypertension, hypotension, parkinsonism,
Drug-Induced Lab Test Change	Glucose level, hyperkalemia, hyponatremia, INR

In the older population, the ADR rate is two to three times higher than in the younger population,[103,104] and this becomes more disparate between specific age groups. For example, 70- to 79-year-olds have seven times the ADR rate as 20- to 29-year-olds.[104] Overall, prevalence rates average 20% to 35% in the geriatric setting[39,97,105–106] and at least 20% of ADRs occur from the use of over-the-counter and herbal agents.[107]

In the older population, ADRs are not only more frequent, but they have more adverse consequences associated with them. Those over 65 are four times more likely to require hospitalization for an ADR than the young population.[33] Indeed, ADRs are responsible for 17% to 28% of hospital admissions[9,61,104] and each year 106,000 to 140,000 individuals die from medications that were properly prescribed and administered.[108,109] If ADRs were ranked as a disease, they would be the fourth to sixth leading cause of death in the United States.[97,109,110]

Most ADRs occur within four days of drug initiation;[111] however, in older adults, ADRs are less likely to be recognized or reported.[112,113] Therapists assist in ADR detection by closely monitoring patient signs and symptoms, particularly with newly prescribed medications or dose changes. Because of the age-related changes in pharmacokinetics and pharmacodynamics and because numerous drugs exert their effects on receptors with wide-ranging locations and influence in the body (Box 13),

adverse drug reactions manifest themselves in unexpected ways. For example, anticholinergic agents such as antihistamines are used in the older population. Box 13 shows that cholinergic receptors are located in the heart, smooth muscle (intestinal and vascular), skeletal muscle, and sweat glands. Antihistamine agents competitively block the cholinergic response (i.e., diaphoresis, gastrointestinal motility, reduced cardiac output, etc.), not only at the desired location (respiratory tract) but also at all other cholinergic locations in the body (i.e., heart, vasculature, intestinal smooth muscle, sweat glands). This may cause a range of unanticipated anticholinergic effects (i.e., delirium, drowsiness, blurred vision, tachycardia, dry mouth, urinary retention, constipation, impaired diaphoretic response), particularly in the older adult with heightened sensitivity and impaired homeostatic mechanisms affected by the cholinergic system (i.e., thermoregulation). The most common drugs implicated with ADRs in geriatrics are listed in Box 19.

Common Adverse Drug Reactions in the Older Population

Adverse Drug Reaction	Implicated Drugs
Anticholinergic effects	Antiemetics, antihistamines, phenothiazine, tricyclic antidepressants
Confusional state/delirium	Antibiotics, antiparkinsonism agents, benzodiazepines, diphenhydramine, narcotics, tricyclic antidepressants,
Constipation	Anticholinergics, ferrous sulfate, narcotics, tricyclic antidepressants
Dehydration	Diuretics
Depression	Antiparkinsonism agents, beta-blockers, benzodiazepines, clonidine
Dizziness	Antihypertensives, benzodiazepines, tricyclic antidepressants
Extrapyramidal signs	Halperidol, metoclopramide, olanzopine, risperidone
Fatigue and weakness	Beta-blockers, digoxin, diuretics
Gastrointestinal upset	Antibiotics, metformin, narcotics, nonsteroidal anti-inflammatories, statins
Hypertension	Calcium channel blockers, glitazones, nonsteroidal anti-inflammatories
Hypocoagulation	Aspirin, heparin, nonsteroidal anti-inflammatories, warfarin
Postural hypotension	Alpha-blockers, antiarrhythmics, antipsychotics, dihydropyridines, nitrates, phenothiazines, tricyclic antidepressants
Urinary incontinence	Alpha-1 blockers (especially at drug initiation), benzodiazepines, diuretics
Urinary retention	Anticholinergics, diphenhydramine, tricyclic antidepressants

Nonadherence

Adherence is the extent to which a person's behavior coincides with medical or health advice.[114] It ranges from the failure to adopt a medication regimen to unintentional errors in drug administration (i.e., incorrect dose or frequency). Nonadherence in the older population ranges from 40% to 76%[92,115–117] and up to 11% of hospital admissions

and 58% of emergency room visits are attributed to medication nonadherence.[61,118–120] It is believed that 88% of these visits and admissions could have been prevented with adherence to the prescribed regimen.[121,122] Cost estimates for medication nonadherence exceed $100 billion[123–125] and it has been termed "America's other drug problem."[124,125]

Over fifty-one factors are associated with nonadherence and they can be categorized as follows: demographic, social support, physiology, cognitive, polypharmacy and dose frequency, patient consent, and motivation.[72] Drug adherence is measured in several ways, though no "gold standard" exists. Self-report, pill count, pharmacy refill records, biochemical testing, and electronic monitoring have all been used to assess adherence. Clinical judgment and therapeutic responses are not valid means of assessing carryover with a medication regimen, and patient self-report consistently underestimates adherence compared to third-party or electronic measurement methods.

If therapists suspect problems with medication adherence, an attempt should be made to determine the barriers to compliance (Box 20). Forgetfulness, impaired fine motor function, difficulty swallowing, knowledge deficits, and regimens that are too complex may all be potentially addressed and remedied by the patient's physician and/or pharmacist. Evidence of nonadherence with a drug regimen should be communicated to the physician in a very timely manner because of the associated adverse consequences that may result.

Barriers to Medication Adherence in the Older Population

Barriers to Medication Adherence

Adverse drug reactions	Patient may discontinue a drug because of perceived or actual side effects and allergies
Knowledge deficit	Patient has an asymptomatic condition and does not feel the need for medication
	Patient does not understand the purpose of the medications
	Patient does not understand proper administration and/or storage of the drug
Sensory and language impairment	Limited English literacy interferes with proper drug administration
	Impaired vision interferes with reading instructions, discriminating medications, and dosages
Cognitive impairment	Patient has a memory deficit and may forget to take medications as prescribed
	Patient cannot follow dosing instructions
Dosing parameters	Complex dosing schedule
	Inconvenient dosing schedule
Physical limitations	Impaired hand strength and dexterity to open medications, apply topical agents, or take medications as prescribed
	Impaired swallowing for oral formulations
Multiple pharmacy or prescribing physician source	Medications prescribed by > one physician or filled by > one pharmacy so potential for drug interactions may increase
Medication cost	Patient may not obtain medications because of perceived high costs and insufficient financial assistance

Source: *Trotter, J.M., Moffa-Trotter, M.E., Anemaet, W.K.* Medication Profile in Pharmacology for Rehabilitation Professionals *course material. Clearwater, FL: A & T Rehabilitation Solutions 2005: 24.*

DRUG REGIMEN MONITORING FOR REHABILITATION

Two broad responsibilities of the therapist are completing the medication profile and assisting the medical team in monitoring the patient's drug regimen.

Medication Profile

The medication profile is a record completed by the therapist that includes all of the prescriptions, over-the-counter drugs, herbals, vitamins, ointments, and drops taken by the patient either chronically or on an as-needed basis. The completed medication profile is then used to identify potential drug-related problems (Box 21).

Medication Profile

Drug Name	Strength	Route	Dose	Frequency	Status	Indication
Ramipril	5 mg	PO	1 tab	QD	R 101006	Hypertension
Atenolol	25 mg	PO	1 tab	QD	R 042306	Hypertension
Aspirin	325 mg	PO	1 tab	QD	R 062767	Secondary MI prevention
Simvastatin	40 mg	PO	1 tab	QD	R 091806	Hyperlipidemia
Vitamin E	400 iu	PO	1 cap	QD	—	Dietary supplement

Drug name: write exactly as listed on the medication label

Strength: expressed as metric weights (mg, gm), metric volume (ml) or concentration (mg/ml)

Route: PO by mouth; PR rectally; Top topically; SQ/SC subcutaneously; IV/IVB intravenous; IM intramuscular

Dose: the number of tablets, capsules, units, volume units to be taken at a single dosing interval

Frequency: QD once daily; BID twice daily; TID thrice daily; QID four times daily; 5XD five times daily; PRN as needed—include the "reason" for dose

Status: N new—include start date; C change—include change date; R reorder—include refill date; DC discontinued—include DC date

Indication: list the primary indication for which this drug is prescribed

Source: *Trotter, J.M., Moffa-Trotter, M.E., Anemaet, W.K.* Medication Profile in Pharmacology for Rehabilitation Professionals *course material. Clearwater, FL: A & T Rehabilitation Solutions 2005: 19.*

While many pharmaceutical print publications, periodicals, and personal data assistant (PDA)–based aids are available to assist in this process, Web-based drug information sites also offer convenient access to updated drug information that is useful for detecting potential adverse dug reactions, drug interactions, and inappropriate prescribing practices (Box 22).

Web-Based Sources for Updated Drug Information for Performing the Drug Regimen Review

Food and Drug Administration: www.fda.gov

Medscape Drug Reference: www.medscape.com/druginfo

Medlineplus: www.nln.nih.gov/medlineplus/medlineplus.html

WebMD Drug Index A to Z: www.webmd.com

RxList: www.rxlist.com

Drug Regimen Monitoring

Drug regimen monitoring is the process by which therapists identify drug-related problems during the patient's episode of care (Box 23). Just like pain assessment, compliance with a home program, and response to therapy, with practice, the drug regimen review becomes a seamless part of the therapist's routine assessment each treatment session.

Drug Regimen Monitoring Questions for Rehabilitation

Cues to Update Medication Profile
Does the patient report recently adding or stopping any drugs, over-the-counter pills, or herbals since last session?
Are these changes in the amount of medicine the patient takes or time(s) he/she takes the medicine?

Allergy
Does the patient report (or does he or she manifest) an allergic reaction?

Side Effects
Does the patient have (or manifest evidence of) any side effects?

Subtherapeutic Dosing
Does the patient believe the treatment is working?
Are the symptoms, disease, or condition adequately controlled?

Nonadherence (assessed by observation, preferably)
Does the patient store drugs as prescribed?
Is the patient taking the drugs exactly as prescribed?
Is the patient's drug consumption congruent with refill date for chronic medications?

Source: *Trotter, J.M., Moffa-Trotter, M.E., Anemaet, W.K.* Medication Profile in Pharmacology for Rehabilitation Professionals *course material. Clearwater, FL: A & T Rehabilitation Solutions 2005; 21.*

REHABILITATION-SPECIFIC CONSIDERATIONS

Rehabilitation involves the application of therapeutic exercises and modalities that may, in the presence of select medications, require special considerations in the older population. For example, because of time-based drug effects, optimal timing for rehabilitation may be affected. Alternately, some medications may call for changes in how therapists monitor tolerance to rehabilitation interventions. Box 24 provides a quick reference of commonly prescribed drugs that benefit from and/or require special considerations from the therapist.

Commonly Used Drugs with Specific Implications for Rehabilitation

Drug	Impact on Therapy Scheduling	Impact on Therapy Provision
Diuretics	Schedule therapy 2 hours after administration of loop diuretics to minimize polyuria-related disruptions	None
Beta-blockers	Immediate-release formulations may not offer sustained blood pressure control at dose end, so scheduling therapy within 1 to 2 hours after dosing administration optimizes antihypertensive effect	Beta-blockers lower heart rate and cardiac output so the normal rise in heart rate with exercise may be blunted. Tolerance to exercise should be assessed using a Perceived Rating of Exertion scale, blood pressure, and/or a physician-determined target exercise heart rate. Systemic thermal modalities such as whirlpool and aquatic therapy should be maintained at < 95° to minimize any additive hypotensive effect. Blood pressure assessment before and after treatment is also recommended.
Calcium Channel Blockers	Schedule therapy 2 to 6 hours after administration to optimize antihypertensive effect	Verapamil and dilitiazem lower heart rate and cardiac output; follow beta-blocker recommendations. Dihydropyridines may increase heart rate, so the normal rise in heart rate and blood pressure with exercise and thermal modalities may be exaggerated; follow beta-blocker recommendations.
Alpha-1 Blockers	Administer first or newly increased doses at bedtime; alternately schedule rehabilitation > 3 hours following drug administration to minimize potent first-dose effects (dizziness, hypotension, palpitations)	Alpha-1 blockers may increase heart rate so the normal rise in heart rate and blood pressure with exercise and thermal modalities may be exaggerated; follow beta-blocker recommendations.
Central Alpha-2 Adrenergics	Schedule therapy > 1 to 2 hours after dose administration to optimize antihypertensive effect	None
Anticoagulant Agents	None	Anticoagulants increase bleeding time so caution is needed with wound care and manual techniques to lower risk for hematoma formation.

(cont.)

Drug	Impact on Therapy Scheduling	Impact on Therapy Provision
Cardiac Glycosides	None	Cardiac glycosides lower heart rate; follow beta-blocker recommendations.
Hypoglycemics	None	Exercise and thermal modalities increase absorption of injectable insulin, so advise the patient to rotate injection sites on therapy days to body areas that will not be directly involved in rehabilitation interventions.
Levodopa	Schedule therapy within 2 to 3 hours of morning dose to optimize motor symptom control	None
Antacids	Schedule therapy 30 minutes after drug administration to optimize symptom control, particularly if therapy involves known aggravating activities such as supine or prone and/or takes place right after meals	None
Antipsychotic Agents	Schedule therapy 1 to 3 hours after dose administration to optimize behavioral effect	None
Opioids	Schedule therapy 30 to 90 minutes after oral drug administration to optimize analgesic effect	None
Nonsteroidal Anti-inflammatories	Schedule therapy 60 to 90 minutes after oral drug administration to optimize analgesic effect	None
Tricyclic antidepressants	Agents that cause sedation should be taken at bedtime to minimize impaired participation with rehabilitation	None
Topical and Transdermal Agents	Schedule therapy 1 hour after topical application to optimize analgesic effect	Because topicals are applied transdermally, removal of the agent is required prior to the application of modalities to the drug treatment site. Thermal modalities should not be applied over a trandermal or topical agent site, and reapplication of the agent should occur no sooner than 30 minutes after modality application.

When used at normal doses, some common medications without direct implications for rehabilitation include antidementia agents, angiotensin converting enzyme (ACE) inhibitors, angiotensin receptor blockers (ARB), aldosterone antagonists (AA), direct vasodilator agents, antiplatelet agents, nitrates, inotropes, anticonvulsants, bisphosphonates, selective estrogen receptor modulator (SERM) agents, parathyroid hormone (PTH), estrogen, testosterone replacement, calcitonin, mucosal protective agents; antisecretory agents, proton pump inhibitor (PPI) agents, prokinetic agents, antimicrobial agents, prostanoid agents.

References

1. National Center for Health Statistics. *Chartbook on Trends in the Health of Americans 2005.* Hyattsville, MD: National Center for Health Statistics; 2005.

2. Linjakumpu T, Hartikainen S, Kluukka T, et al. Use of medications and polypharmacy are increasing among the elderly. *J Clin Epidemiol.* 2002; 55: 809–817.

3. Veehof L, Stewart R, Haaijer-Ruskamp F, et al. The development of polypharmacy: A longitudinal study. *Fam Pract.* 2002; 17(3):261–267.

4. Williams BR, Nichol MB, Lowe B, et al. Medication use in residential care facilities in the elderly. *Ann Pharmacother.* 1999; 33(2):149–155.

5. Burt CW. National trends in use of medications in office-based practice. *Health Affairs.* 1985–1999; 21: 206–214.

6. Cherry DK, Burt CW, Woodwell DA. *National Ambulatory Medical Care Survey: 2000 Summary.* Hyattsville, MD: National Center for Health Statistics; Advance Data from Vital and Health Statistics, No. 328., 2002.

7. Hse RY, Lin MS, Chou MH, et al. Medication characteristics in an ambulatory elderly population in Taiwan. *Ann Pharmacother.* 1997; 31(3):308–314.

8. Williams C. Using medications appropriately in older adults. *Am Fam Phys.* 2002; 66(10):1917–1924.

9. Larsen P, Martin JL. Polypharmacy and elderly patients. *AORN J.* 1999; 69(3):625, 627–628.

10. Routledge PA, O'Mahony MS, Woodhouse KW. Adverse drug reactions in elderly patients. *Brit J Clin Pharmacol.* 2004; 57:121–126.

11. Kennerfalk A, Ruigomez A, Wallander MA, Wilhelmsen L, Johanddon S. Geriatric drug therapy and health care utilization in the United Kingdom. *Ann Pharmacother.* 2002; 36:797–803.

12. Jorgenson T, Johanssonn S, Kennerfalk A, Waalander MA, Svardsudd K. Prescription drug use, diagnoses and healthcare utilization among the elderly. *Ann Pharmacother.* 2001; 35:1004–1009.

13. Anderson G, Kerluke K. Distribution of prescription drug exposures in the elderly: Description and implications. *J Clin Epidemiol.* 1996; 49:929–935.

14. Stewart RB, Cooper JW. Polypharmacy in the aged. Practical solutions. *Drugs Aging.* 1994; 4:49–61.

15. Moxey ED, O'Conner JP, Novielli KD, Teutsch S, Nash DB. Prescription drug use in the elderly: A descriptive study. *Health Care Fin Rev.* 2003; 24(4): 127–141.

16. Kaufman DW, Kelly JP, Rosenberg L, Anderson TE, Mitchell AA. Recent patterns of medication use in the ambulatory adult population of the United States: The Slone Survey. *J Am Med Assoc.* 2002; 287:337–344.

17. Field TS, Gurwitz JH, Avorn, et al. Risk factors for adverse drug events among nursing home residents. *Arch Intern Med.* 2001; 161:1629–1634.

18. Sloane PD, Zimmerman S, Brown LC, Ives TJ, Walsh JF. Inappropriate medication prescribing in residential care/assisted living facilities. *J Am Geriatr Soc.* 2002; 50:1001–1011.

19. Conn V. Self management of over-the-counter medications by older adults. *Pub Health Nurs.* 1991; 96:29–35.

20. Foster DF, Phillips S, Hamel MD, Eisenberg DM. Alternative medicine use in older Americans. *J Am Geriatr Soc.* 2000; 49(12):1560–1565.

21. Astin JA, Pelletier KR, Marie A. Complementary and alternative medicine use among elderly persons: One year analysis of Blue Shield Medicare supplement. *J Gerontol Med Sci.* 2000; 55A(1):1548–1553.

22. Miller LG. Herbal medicinals: Selected clinical considerations. Focusing on known or potential drug-herb interactions. *Arch Intern Med.* 1998; 158(20): 2200–2211.

23. Ihara E, Summer L, Shirey L. Prescription drugs: A vital component of health care. In: *Challenges for the 21st Century: Chronic and Disabling Conditions.* Washington, DC: Center on an Aging Society, Georgetown University; 2002: 1–5.

24. Stagnitti MN. MEPS Medical Expenditure Panel Survey. Statistical Brief 21: Trends in outpatient prescription drug utilization and expenditures 1997–2000; Web-only publication Date: July 25, 2003. Access at: www.meps.ahrg.gov/mepsweb/data-files/publications/st21/stat21.pdf

25. National Association of Chain Drug Stores. *2004 Community Pharmacy Results.* Accessed May 20, 2006, at www.nacds.org

26. National Center for Health Statistics. *Data Warehouse on Trends in Health and Aging: Prevalence of selected chronic conditions by age, sex, and race 2003–2004.* Accessed May 20, 2006, at http://www.cdc.gov/nchs/agingact.htm

27. Bell RA, Kravitz RL, Wilkes MS. Direct-to-consumer prescription drug advertising and the public. *J Gen Intern Med.* 1999; 14:651–657.

28. Woloshin S, Schwartz LM, Tremmel J, Welch HG. Direct-to-consumer advertisements for prescription drugs: What are Americans being sold? *Lancet.* 2001; 358(9288): 1141–1146.

29. Merle L, Laroche ML, Dantoine T, Charmes JP. Predicting and preventing adverse drug reactions in the very old. *Drugs Aging.* 2005; 22(5):375–392.

30. Rochon PA, Gurwitz JH. Optimizing drug treatment for elderly people: The prescribing cascade. *Brit Med J.* 1997; 315:1096–1099.

31. Ginsberg G, Hattis D, Sonawane B. Pharmacokinetic and pharmacodynamic factors that can affect sensitivity to neurotoxic sequele in elderly individuals. *Env Health Persp.* 2005; 13(9):1243–1249.

32. Wright RM, Warpula DPM. Geriatric pharmacology: Safer prescribing for the elderly patient. *J Am Pod Med Assoc.* 2004; 94(2):90–97.

33. McLean AJ, LeCouteur. Aging biology and geriatric clinical pharmacology. *Pharmacol Rev.* 2004; 56(2): 163–184.

34. Turnheim K. Drug therapy in the elderly. *Exp Gerontol.* 2004; 39:1731–1738.

35. Kirirons MT, O'Mahony MS. Drug metabolism and ageing. *Brit J Clin Pharmacol.* 2004; 57(5):540–544.

36. Noble RE. Drug therapy in the elderly. *Metab.* 2003; 52(10):27–30.

37. Turnheim K. When drug therapy gets old: Pharmacokinetics and pharmacodynamics in the elderly. *Exp Gerontol.* 2003; 38:843–853.

38. Bressler R, Bahl JJ. Principles of drug therapy for the elderly patient. *Mayo Clin Proc.* 2003; 78(12): 1564–1577.

39. Chutka S, Evans JM, Fleming KC, et al. Drug prescribing in elderly patients. *Mayo Clin Proc.* 1995; 70:685.

40. Schmucher DL. Liver function and phase 1 drug metabolism in the elderly. *Drugs Aging.* 2001; 18:837–851.

41. Campion EW, deLabry LO, Glynn RJ. The effect of age on serum albumin in healthy males: Report from the Normative Aging Study. *J Gerontol.* 1988; 43:M18–M20.

42. Grandison MD, Boodinot FD. Age related changes in protein binding of drugs: Implications for therapy. *Clin Pharmacokinet.* 2000; 38:271–290.

43. Beaufrere B, Morio B. Fat and protein redistribution with aging: Metabolic considerations. *Eur J Clin Nutr.* 2000; Vol 54 Suppl 3:S48–S53.

44. Masoro EJ, Snyder D. Exploration of aging and toxic response issues. Peer Review Report prepared for the United States Environmental Protection Agency Contract 68-C-99-238. 2001

45. Steen B, Lundgren BK, Isaksson B. Body water in the elderly [letter] *Lancet.* 1985; 1:10.

46. Vestel RE. Aging and pharmacology. *Cancer.* 1997; 80:1302–1310.

47. Wynne HA, Cope E, Mutch E, Rawlins MD, et al. The effect of age upon liver volume and apparent liver blood flow in healthy man. *Hepatol.* 1989; 9(2):297–301.

48. Woodhouse KW, Wynne HA. Age-related changes in liver size and hepatic blood flow. The influence on drug metabolism in the elderly. *Clin Pharmacokinet.* 1988; 15:287–294.

49. Marchesini G, Bau V, Brunori, et al. Galactose elimination capacity and liver volume in man. *Hepatol.* 1988; 8:1079–1083.

50. LcCourteur DG, McLean AJ. The aging liver: Drug clearance and an oxygen diffusion barrier hypothesis. *Clin Pharmacokinet.* 1998; 34(5):359–373.

51. Zeeh J, Platt D. The aging liver: Structural and functional changes and their consequences for drug treatment in old age. *Gerontol.* 2002; 48(3): 121–127.

52. McLean AJ, LeCourteur DG. Aging biology and geriatric clinical pharmacology. *Pharmacol Rev.* 2004; 56:163–184.

53. LeCourteur DG, McLean AJ, Fraser R, Hilmer S, Rivory LP, McLean AJ. The hepatic sinusoid in aging and cirrhosis: Effects on hepatic substrate disposition and drug clearance. *Clin Pharmacokinet.* 2005; 44(2):187–200.

54. Yuen GJ. Altered pharmacokinetics in the elderly. *Clin Geriatr Med.* 1990; 6:257–267.

55. Beck LH. Changes in renal function with aging. *Clin Geriatr Med.* 1998; 14:199–209.

56. Hammerlein A, Derendorf H, Lowenthal DT. Pharmacokinetic and pharmacodynamic changes in the elderly. Clinical implications. *Clin Pharmacokinet.* 1998; 35:49–54.

57. Swift CG. Pharmacodynamic changes in homeostatic mechanisms, receptor and target organ sensitivity in the elderly. *Brit Med Bull.* 1990; 46:36–52.

58. Turnheim K. Drug dosage in the elderly: Is it rational? *Drugs Aging.* 1998; 13:357–379.

59. Beers M, Berkow R. *The Merck Manual of Geriatrics: Clinical Pharmacology.* 3rd ed. Whitehouse Station, NJ: Merck Research Laboratory; 2000–2006.

60. Rothschild JM, Bates DW, Leape LL. Preventable medical injuries in older patients. *Arch Intern Med.* 2000; 160:2717–2728.

61. Col N, Fanale JE, Keonholm P. The role of medication in noncompliance and adverse drug reactions in hospitalization of the elderly. *Arch Intern Med.* 1990; 150:841–845.

62. Fick DM, Cooper JW, Wade WE, et al. Updating the Beer's criterion for potentially inappropriate medication use in older adults: Results of the US Consensus Panel of Experts. *Arch Intern Med.* 2003; 163(22):2716–2724.

63. Gurwitz JH, Field TS, Harrold LR, Rothschild J, et al. Incidence and preventability of adverse drug events among older persons in the ambulatory setting. *J Am Med Assoc.* 2003; 289:1107–1116.

64. Gurwitz JH. Polypharmacy: A new paradigm for quality drug therapy in the elderly? *Arch Intern Med.* 2004; 164(18):1957–1969.

65. Chutka DS, Takahashi PY, Hoel RW. Inappropriate medications for elderly patients. *Mayo Clin Proc.* 2004; 79(1):122–139.

66. Chutka DS, Takahashi PY, Hoel RW. Inappropriate medication use in the elderly. *Essent Psychopharmacol.* 2005; 6:331–340.

67. Fulton MM, Allen ER. Polypharmacy in the elderly: A literature review. *J Am Acad Nurs Pract.* 2005; 17(4):123–132.

68. Frazier SC. Health outcomes and polypharmacy in elderly individuals. *J Gerontol Nurs.* 2005; 31(9): 4–11.

69. Leibovitch ER, Deamer RL, Sanderson LA. Food-drug interactions: Careful dose selection and patient counseling can reduce the risk in older patients. *Geriatr.* 2004; 59(3):32–33.

70. Delafuente JC. Understanding and preventing drug interactions in elderly patients. *Crit Rev Oncol Hematol.* 2003; 48:133–143.

71. McCabe BJ. Prevention of food-drug interactions with special emphasis on older adults. *Crit Opin Clin Nutr Metab Care.* 2004; 7:21–26.

72. vanVliet MJ, Schuurmans MJ, Grypdonk MHF, Duijnstee MS. Improper intake of medication by elders—Insights on contributing factors: A review of the literature. *Res Theor Nurs Pract.* 2006; 20(1): 79–93.

73. Hughes CM. Medication non-adherence in the elderly: How big is the problem? *Drugs Aging.* 2004; 21(12):793–811.

74. Vik SA, Maxwell CJ, Hogan DB. Measurement, correlates, and health outcomes of medication adherence among seniors. *Ann Pharmacother.* 2004; 38: 303–312.

75. Schlenk EA, Dunbar-Jacob J, Engberg S. Medication non-adherence among older adults: A review of strategies and interventions for improvement. *J Gerontol Nurs.* 2004; 30(70):33–43.

76. McCormick D, Gurwitz JH, Goldberg RJ, et al. Prevalence and quality of warfarin use for patients with atrial fibrillation in the long-term care setting. *Arch Intern Med.* 2001; 161:2458–2463.

77. Lemaitre RN, Psaty BM, Heckbert SR, et al. Therapy with hydromethylgutaryl coenzyme a reductase inhibitor (statins) and associated risk of incident cardiovascular events in older adults: Evidence from the Cardiovascular Health Study. *Arch Intern Med.* 2002; 162:1395–1400.

78. Gattis WA, Larsen RL, Hasselblad V, Bart BA, O'Conner CM. Is optimal angiotensin-converting enzyme inhibitor dosing neglected in elderly patients with heart failure? *Am Heart J.* 1998; 136:43–48.

79. Knight EL, Avorn J. Quality indicators for appropriate medication use in vulnerable elders. *Ann Intern Med.* 2001; 135:703–710.

80. Sloane PD, Gruber-Balding A, Zimmerman S, et al. Medication under treatment in assisted living settings. *Arch Intern Med.* 2004; 164(18):2031–2037.

81. Andrade SE, Maunder SR, Chan KE, et al. Low frequency of treatment of osteoporosis among postmenopausal women following a fracture. *Arch Intern Med.* 2003; 163(17):2052–2057.

82. Bunged T, McAlister F, Johnson J. Underutilization of ACE inhibitors in patients with congestive heart failure. *Drugs.* 2001; 61(14):2021–2033.

83. Goodling MR. Inappropriate medication prescribing for elderly ambulatory care patients. *Arch Int Med.* 2004; 164(3):305–312.

84. Zhan C, Sang J, Bierman AS, et al. Potentially inappropriate medication use in the community dwelling elderly: Findings from the 1996 Medical Expenditure Panel Survey. *J Am Med Assoc.* 2001; 286: 2823–2829.

85. Spore DL, Mor V, Larrat P, Hawes C, Hiris J. Inappropriate drug prescriptions for elderly residents of board and care facilities. *Am J Pub Health.* 1997; 87:404–409.

86. Hanlon JT, Schmader KE, Boult C, et al. Use of inappropriate prescription drugs by older people. *J Am Geriatr Soc.* 2002; 40:26–34.

87. Bull SA, Hu XH, Hunkeler EM, et al. Discontinuation of use and switching of antidepressants: Influence of patient-physician communication. *J Am Med Assoc.* 2002; 288:1403–1409.

88. Bell RA, Kravitz RL, Thom D, Krupat E, Azari R. Unmet expectations for care and the patient-physician relationship. *J General Intern. Med.* 2002; 17: 817–824.

89. Bikowski RM, Ripsin CM, Lorraine VL. Physician-patient congruence regarding medication regimens. *J Am Geriatr Soc.* 2001; 49:1353–1357.

90. Brager R, Sloand E. The spectrum of polypharmacy. *Nurs Pract.* 2005; 30(6):44–50.

91. Woodward MC. Deprescribing: Achieving better health outcomes for older people through reducing medications. *J Pharm Pract Res.* 2003; 33:323–328.

92. Bedell S, Jabour S, Goldberg R, et al. Discrepancies in the use of medications: Their extent and predictors in an outpatient practice. *Arch Intern Med.* 2000; 160(14):2129–2134.

93. Hasan M, Woodhouse K. The accuracy of information on current drug therapy in geriatric out-patients' records. *Arch Gerontol Geriatr.* 1996; 22: 21–25.

94. US Department of Health and Human Services. 2001b. *Healthy People 2010.* Section 17: Medical product safety. Accessed May 20, 2006, at www .healthypeople.gov/

95. Prybys K, Melville K, Hanna J, Gee A, Chyka P. Polypharmacy in the elderly: Clinical challenges in emergency practice: Part 1: Overview, etiology, and drug interactions. *Em Med Rep.* 2002; 23(11): 145–153.

96. Ewing AB. Altered drug response in the elderly. In Armour D, Cairns C, eds. *Medicines in the Elderly.* London: Pharmaceutical Press; 2002:17, 23.

97. Petrone K, Katz P. Approaches to appropriate drug prescribing for the older adult. *Prim Care Clin Office Pract.* 2005; 32:755–775.

98. Miller LG. Herbal medicinals: Selected clinical considerations. Focusing on known or potential drug-herb interactions. *Arch Intern Med.* 1998; 158(20): 2200–2211.

99. Goldberg RM, Mabee J, Chan L, Wong S. Drug-drug and drug-disease interactions in the ED: Analysis of a high-risk population. *Am J Emerg Med.* 1996; 14:447–450.

100. Flaherty JH, Perry HM, Lynchard GS, Morley JE. Polypharmacy and hospitalization among older home care patients. *J Gerontol: Ser A Biol Sci Med Sci.* 2000; 55(10):M554–M559.

101. Hanlon JT, Fillenbaum GG, Kuchibhatla M, et al. Impact of inappropriate drug use on mortality and functional status in representative community dwelling elders. *Med Care.* 2002; 40:166–176.

102. Seymour RM, Routledge PA. Important drug-drug interactions in the elderly. *Drugs Aging.* 998; 12: 485–494.

103. Carbonin P, Pahor M, Bernebei R, Sgadari A. Is an age an independent risk factor for adverse drug reactions in hospitalized medical patients? *J Am Geriatr Soc.* 1991; 39:1093–1099.

104. Beard K. Adverse reactions as a cause of hospital admission in the aged. *Drugs Aging.* 1992; 2:356–367.

105. Giron MST, Wang HX, Bernsten C, et al. The appropriateness of drug use in an older nondemented and demented population. *J Am Geriatr Soc.* 2001; 49:277.

106. Bordet R, Gautier S, Lelouet H, Dupuis B, Caron J. Analysis of the direct cost of adverse drug reactions in hospitalized patients. *Eur J Clin Pharmacol.* 2001; 56:935–941.

107. Stewart RB, Cluff LE. Studies on the epidemiology of adverse drug reactions, VI: Utilization and interactions of prescription and nonprescription drugs in outpatients. *John Hopkins Med J.* 1971; 129:319–331.

108. Classen DC, Pestotnik SL, Evans RS, Lloyd JF, Burke JP. Adverse drug events in hospitalized patients: Excess length of stay, extra costs, and attributable mortality. *J Am Med Assoc.* 1997; 277:301–306.

109. Lazarou J, Pomeranz B, Corey P. Incidence of adverse drug reactions in hospitalized patients. A meta analysis of prospective studies. *J Am Med Assoc.* 1998; 279(15):1200–1205.

110. Sorensen JM. Herb-drug, food-drug, nutrient-drug, and drug-drug interactions: Mechanisms involved and their medical implications. *J Altern Complement Med.* 2002; 8:293–308.

111. Veehof LJG, Stewart RE, Meyboom-deJong B, Haaijer-Ruskamp FM. Adverse drug reactions and polypharmacy in the elderly in general practice. *Eur J Clin Pharmacol.* 1999; 55(7):533–536.

112. Klein LE, German PS, Levine DM, Feroli ER, Ardery J. Medication problems among outpatients. A study with emphasis on the elderly. *Arch Intern Med.* 1984; 144:1185–1188.

113. Mannesse CK, Derkx FH, deRidder MA. Do older hospital patients recognize adverse drug reactions? *Age Ageing.* 2000b; 29:79–81.

114. Sackett DL, Haynes RB. *Compliance with Therapeutic Regimens.* Baltimore: John Hopkins University Press; 1976.

115. Nichol M, Venturini F, Sung J. A critical evaluation of the methodology of the literature on medication compliance. *Ann Pharmacother.* 1999; 33:531–539.

116. Gray SL, Mahoney JE, Blough DK. Medication adherence in elderly patients receiving home health services following hospital discharge. *Ann Pharmacother.* 2001; 35:539–545.

117. Donnan PT, MacDonald M, Morris AD. Adherence to prescribed oral hypoglycemic medication in a population of patients with type 2 diabetes: A retrospective cohort study. *Diabetic Med.* 2002; 19: 279–284.

118. Toh SL, Low CL, Goh SH. Drug related visits of geriatrics to the emergency department. ASHP Annual Meeting. 1998; 55:pINTL-3.

119. Grymonpre RE, Mitenko PA, Sitar DS, Aoki FY, Montgomery PR. Drug-associated hospital admissions in older medical patients. *J Am Geriatr Soc.* 1988; 36:1092–1098.

120. McKenney JM, Harrison WL. Drug-related hospital admissions. *Am J Hosp Pharm.* 1976; 33:792–795.

121. Mannesse CK, Derkx FH, deRidder MA. Contribution of adverse drug reactions to hospital admissions of older patients. *Age Ageing.* 2000b; 29:35–39.

122. Beijer HJM, Blaey CJD. Hospitalisations caused by adverse drug reactions (ADR): A meta analysis of observational studies. *Pharm World Sci.* 2002; 24: 46–54.

123. Lewis A. Non-compliance: A $100 billion problem. *Remington Rep.* 1997; 5(4):14–15.

124. Bond WS, Hussar DA. Detection methods and strategies for improving medication compliance. *Am J Hosp Pharm.* 1991; 48:1978–1988.

125. Wright EC. Non-compliance or how many aunts has Matilda? *Lancet.* 1993; 342:909–913.

8

Principles and Practice of Geriatric Rehabilitation

Pearls

- The purpose of geriatric rehabilitation is to assist the disabled aged in recovering lost physical, psychological, or social skills so that they may become more independent.

- Forty percent of all disabled persons are over age 65; the oldest-old (over 85) compose the highest percentage of disabled persons.

- The decline in muscle strength and mass, respiratory reserve and cardiovascular functioning, kyphotic postural changes, poorer eyesight, poor hydration and marginal nutritional intake, and many other physiological and physical changes associated with inactivity and aging, lead to frailty.

- Three major principles influence geriatric rehabilitation. These are variability, hypokinetics, and optimal health. The influence of these can be seen in the systems of the body and should be differentiated from normal versus pathological aging.

- CMS (previously HCFA) interpretive guidelines define a physical restraint as "any manual method or physical or mechanical device, material or equipment attached to or adjacent to the resident's body, which the individual cannot remove easily, that restricts freedom of movement or normal access to one's body."

- Managing falls in the aged requires recognizing that falls are not a normal part of aging and may be due to medication, fear of falling, inactivity, chronic illness, postural instability, the use of restraints, or a combination of these.

- The goals for adapting an environment for the older person are to ensure safety, increase mobility, and enhance comfort and communication.

INTRODUCTION

Normal aging is not necessarily burdened with disability; however, almost all conditions that cause disability are more frequently seen in the older population. As a result, the aged are more likely to require assessment for rehabilitative services. The mutual exclusion of geriatrics and rehabilitation is unjustified, and functional assessment for needed rehabilitative services should be an essential part of routine evaluation by all health care disciplines working with the aged population. Geriatrics teaches that maximal functional capabilities be attained; therefore, it can be argued that rehabilitation is the foundation of geriatric care. The purpose of this chapter is to provide clinicians with

knowledge of rehabilitation principles and practices in working with the aged individual and to help them apply interventions to provide high-quality care.

The basis of geriatric rehabilitation is to assist the disabled aged in recovering lost physical, psychological, or social skills so that they may become more independent, live in personally satisfying environments, and maintain meaningful social interactions. This may be done in any number of settings including acute and subacute care settings, rehabilitation centers, home and office settings, or in long-term care facilities such as nursing homes.

Because of the complexity of the interventions needed in dealing with the aged, an interdisciplinary team approach may be required. The rehabilitation process also requires that patients and their families be educated. Finally, rehabilitation is more than a medical intervention: it is a philosophical approach that recognizes that diagnoses and chronological age are poor predictors of functional abilities, that interventions directed at enhancing function are important, and that the "team" should always include patients and their families.

DISABILITY: A DEFINITION

The meaning of disability is key to an understanding of rehabilitation. When referring to alterations in an individual's function, three terms are often used interchangeably: "impairment," "disability," and "handicap." A more distinct understanding of these concepts is useful in geriatric rehabilitation, and a "systems approach" is most useful. In the systems approach, a problem at the organ level (e.g., an infarct in the right hemisphere) must be viewed in terms of not only its effects on the brain but also its effects on the person, the family, the society, and, ultimately, the nation. It goes beyond the pure "medical model," in which only the current medical problem is assessed to determine rehabilitative goals. From this perspective "impairment" refers to a loss of physical or physiologic function at the organ level. This could include alterations in heart function, nerve conduction velocity, or muscle strength. Impairments usually do not affect the ability to function. However, if impairment is so severe that it inhibits the ability to function "normally," then it becomes a "disability." Rehabilitation interventions are most often oriented toward adaptation to or recovery from disabilities. Given the proper training or adaptive equipment, people with disabilities can pursue independent lives. Obstructions in the pursuit of independence can arise, however, when people with disabilities confront inaccessible buildings or situations that limit rehabilitation interventions, such as low toilet seats, buttons on an elevator that are too high, or signs that are not legible. In these cases a disability becomes a "handicap." Society's environment creates the handicap.

In this chapter we will be primarily concerned with rehabilitative approaches employed to reduce disabilities.

DEMOGRAPHICS OF DISABILITY IN THE ELDERLY

The elderly are disproportionately affected by disabling conditions when compared with younger cohorts. According to Wedgewood,[1] the old-old age group (85 plus years of age) comprises the highest percentage of disabled persons; indeed, 40% of all disabled persons are over the age of 65. Three-fourths of all cerebrovascular accidents

occur in persons over the age of 65;[2-4] the highest incidence of amputations has been reported in the aged;[5,6] and hip fractures occur most frequently between the ages of 70 to 78, on average.[6,7] The Federal Council on the Aging has reported that, of all those persons studied over the age of 65, 86% have at least one chronic condition, and 52% have limitations in their activities of daily living (ADLs).[8] It is the impact of these disabilities on the level of independence that needs to be considered, rather than the presence of an impairment or disability.

Disabilities in old age are associated with a higher mortality rate, a decreased life span, greater chronic health problems (e.g., cardiovascular, musculoskeletal, or neurological), and an increased expenditure for health care. Disabilities resulting in an inability to ambulate, feed oneself, or manage basic ADLs, such as toileting or self-hygiene (e.g., bathing), are very strong predictors of loss of functional independence and an increased burden on caregivers.[9] The greater the disability, the greater the risk of institutionalization. Rehabilitative measures can be cost-effective when they enhance the patient's functional ability and help him or her attain greater levels of independence. Higher functional capabilities and greater levels of independence have been associated with fewer hospitalizations and a lower mortality rate among the aged.[10-12]

Geriatric rehabilitation includes both institutional and noninstitutional services for aged with chronic medical conditions that are marked by deviation from the normal state of health and manifested in physical impairment. Unless treated, these conditions have the potential for causing substantial, and frequently cumulative, disability. The aged with disabilities need assistance with such daily functions as bathing, dressing, and walking. This increased need for help is often compounded when there is no spouse, nearby family, or friends able to assist the patient. With this social isolation, which is common in the elderly, continuing professional medical care is required to ward off the debilitating effects of inactivity and depression.

It is difficult for 32% of people over the age of 75 who live at home to climb ten steps; 40% have difficulty walking a mile; and 22% are unable to lift ten pounds. These percentages translate into millions of older people with some limitation in ADLs.[12,13] While dramatic gains have been made, we need to seek ways to prevent frailty and to help the frail elderly cope with ADLs. The impact of frailty is enormous in terms of costs of care in long-term care settings. Disability in the elderly is not inevitable. In fact, disability rates fell during the 1980s, according to the National Institute on Aging's National Long-Term Care Survey.[13] While the general population of people aged 65 and older grew by 14.7% between 1982 and 1989, the number of people with chronic disabilities or in nursing homes increased by 9.2%. This means that the proportion of people with disabilities fell, and there were hundreds of thousands fewer people with disabilities than expected.[14] Figure 8.1 provides a graphic representation of the number of projected and the number of actual chronically disabled persons aged 65 and over.

FRAILTY: MEDICALLY COMPLEX ELDERLY

Though it is difficult to concisely define the term "frailty," the concept of frailty is well understood in geriatric rehabilitation. The use of the word "frail" conjures up a clear mental image for most clinicians. Compromises in cognition, sensorimotor input and integration,[15] polypharmacy, dehydration, and malnutrition are components of frailty. Decline in muscle strength and mass,[16] respiratory reserve and cardiovascular functioning, kyphotic postural changes, poorer eyesight, poor hydration and marginal nutritional intake, and many other physiological and physical changes associated with inactivity and aging, lead to frailty. Any of these conditions, in isolation or in combination, can create frailty. The presence of multidiagnostic situations in the elderly leads to multiple drug and nutrient interactions and complex medical management with the resulting side effects of progressive loss in functional reserve and physiological homeostasis. Concomitant diseases such as congestive heart failure, renal disease, osteoporosis, diabetes, chronic lung disease, and arthritis (to name a few), add to the level of frailty.

Impaired physical functioning has been documented in one-third of older hospitalized patients.[17] With any admission for acute illnesses or injury in an older person, there is significant short-term deterioration in mobility and other functional domains.[18] Decline in physical function, while a negative outcome in itself, has also been associated with a number of adverse consequences such as falls, disability, and mortality.[12,18,19]

Functional dependence develops in approximately 10% of nondisabled community-dwelling persons over the age of 75 each year.[12] Increasing levels of disability are associated with substantial mortality leading to the adverse outcomes of hospitalization, nursing home placement, and greater use of home care services.[19] It is estimated that it costs $9,600 for each disabled, community-living older person annually and at least $15 billion is spent each year on long-term care.[14,20] Functional dependence leads to increasing levels of frailty, especially in the medically complex, multisystem-involved elder. With each medical insult and hospitalization, there is a decreasing level of physiologic capacity associated with difficulty in recovery to premorbid functional abilities.[20,21] Movement of frail older people through the health care system is relevant for clinicians. Cost-containment strategies that encourage providers to substitute less costly care in the community for the more expensive care in hospitals and nursing homes may have implications for the patient's functioning, ability to remain at home, or other treatment outcomes.[19,21] An understanding of this issue is essential to assure that frail older patients receive the services they need and are treated appropriately.

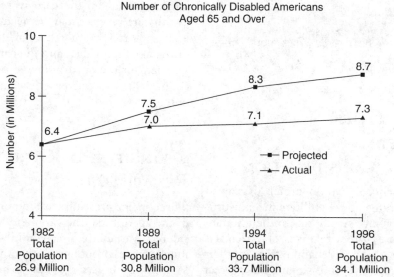

Figure 8.1   Number of Chronically Disabled Older Americans. (Created from data: Manton, K.G., Corder, L., Stallard, E. Chronic disability trends in elderly United States populations: 1982–1994. *Proc Natl Acad Sci USA*. 1997; 94:2593–2598.)

Mrs. K, 78 years of age, who lived alone and independently, became frail because of the complacency of preventive and medical interventions and because of the limitations in the reimbursement system. Diagnosed with worsening arthritis and osteoporosis, she fell and broke her hip. Following surgery, rehabilitation was only partially successful when she was discharged from this service due to lack of insurance coverage and sent home. After a second fall, she entered a nursing home and became depressed. Antidepressant drugs made her lightheaded and dizzy. She fell again, breaking her other hip. She was unable to participate in rehabilitation due to confusion and medical complications, and she became bedridden. Unfortunately, this is not an atypical rehabilitation scenario. Mrs. K's progressive frailty might have been prevented or reversed at several points. One such point might have been from a preventive perspective, before she developed osteoporosis, which can be prevented or at least alleviated through exercise, nutrition, and, in some cases, hormone replacement therapy. Mrs. K's first fall could have been prevented with simple and practical measures, such as muscle-strengthening exercises, balance training, protective ambulatory devices, and environmental assessment and modification for safety.

FUNCTIONAL ASSESSMENT OF THE ELDERLY

The assessment of functional capabilities is the cornerstone of geriatric rehabilitation. The ability to walk, to transfer (e.g., from bed to chair or chair to toilet), and to manage basic ADLs independently is often the determinant of whether hospitalized aged patients will be discharged home or to an extended-care facility. Functional assessment tools, which are practical, reliable, and valid, are necessary to assist all interdisciplinary team members in determining the need for rehabilitation or long-term care services. In the home care setting, precise assessment of a patient's function can detect early deterioration and allow for immediate intervention. (See Chapter 10 for specific information on functional assessment tools.)

For more information on functional assessment background, see CD.

FUNCTIONAL ABILITIES OF THE CAREGIVER: A REHABILITATIVE CONSIDERATION

Aged patients, given a choice, would prefer to stay at home rather than recuperate and rehabilitate in an institutional setting. The elderly have strong ties to their homes; and the help of their spouses, other relatives, and friends is a crucial component in making rehabilitation in their homes possible. Home care by professionals can protect the health of informal caregivers and maximize the patient's ability to perform ADLs by including a systematic assessment of the living environment as a key part of care planning. Provision of such assistance openly acknowledges that caregivers (often aged themselves) have some

decrease in physical ability which needs to be considered as it relates to caring for disabled relatives. It has been demonstrated that over 90% of persons 75 to 84 years of age can manage, without help, to perform such tasks as grooming, bathing, dressing, and eating.[22] The more complicated skills of transferring and ambulation are more compromised, with over 50% of persons aged 75 to 84 years of age presenting with limitations in their capabilities of performing these activities without assistance. These ADLs require greater assistive skills on the part of the caregiver. Assessment of the home environment needs to incorporate the abilities (or disabilities) of the individual(s) providing care. Adaptive equipment, such as a sliding board for transfers or a rolling walker for ambulation, is available to assist the caregiver in caring for his or her spouse, relative, or friend. Attention to the abilities of the caregiver can facilitate the ease of care and decrease the burden placed on the caregiver. The provision of home health care services may be necessitated when safety is an issue. Thorough evaluation of the functional capabilities of the aged individual and the caregiver, in addition to assessment of the environmental obstacles that may be encountered, will increase the likelihood of a positive outcome.

PRINCIPLES OF GERIATRIC REHABILITATION

Three major principles are important in the rehabilitation of the aged. First, the variability of the aged must be considered. Variability of capabilities within an aged group is much more pronounced than within younger cohorts. What one 80-year-old can do physically, cognitively, or motivationally, another may not be able to accomplish. Second, the concept of activity is key in rehabilitation of the aged. Many of the changes over time are attributable to disuse. Finally, optimum health is directly related to optimum functional ability. In acute situations, rehabilitation must be directed toward (1) stabilizing the primary problem(s); (2) preventing secondary complications such as bedsores, pneumonias, and contractures; and (3) restoring lost functions. In chronic situations, rehabilitation is directed primarily toward restoring lost functions. This can best be accomplished by promoting maximum health so that the aged are best able to adapt to their care environment and to their disabilities. Each of these principles—variability, inactivity, and optimum health—will be discussed in greater detail in the following sections.

Variability of the Elderly

Unlike any other age group, the aged are more variable in their level of functional capabilities. In the clinic, we often see 65-year-old individuals who are severely physically disabled, yet, sitting right alongside of that individual is a 65-year-old who is still building houses and felling trees. Even in the old-old, variability in physical and cognitive functioning is remarkable. For example, at one end of the spectrum is John Kelly, who, at the age of 87, was still running the Boston Marathon, while at the other end of the spectrum is a frail bedridden 87-year-old person in a nursing home who is not responsive to his or her environment. The differences can also be identified cognitively and are just as remarkable. The spectrum moves from the demented, institutionalized aged to those aged who are presidents and Supreme Court justices. Chronological age is a poor indicator of physical or cognitive function.

The impact of this variability is an important consideration in defining rehabilitation principles and practices of the aged. A wide range of rehabilitative services must be provided to address the varying needs of the aged population in different care settings. Awareness of this heterogeneity helps to combat the myths and stereotypes of aging and presents a foundation for developing creative rehabilitation programs for the aged. Older persons tend to be more different from themselves (as a collective group) than other segments of the population. Given this fact, interdisciplinary team members, policy makers, and planners in rehabilitation settings need to be prepared to design a wide range of services and treatment interventions. This becomes more difficult as the number of aged increases and the budget decreases; however, creating new and innovative rehabilitation programs could ultimately improve the functional capabilities and the resulting quality of life for many aged individuals.

For examples of variability in aging, see CD.

Activity versus Inactivity

The most common reason for losses in functional capabilities in the aged is inactivity or immobility. There are numerous reasons for immobilizing the aged. "Acute immobilization" is often considered to be accidental immobilization. Acute catastrophic illnesses include severe blood loss, trauma, head injury, cerebral vascular accidents, burns, and hip fractures, to name only a few. The patient's activity level is often severely curtailed until acute illnesses become medically stable. "Chronic immobilization" may result from long-standing problems that are undertreated or left untreated. Examples of chronic problems include cerebral vascular accidents (strokes), amputations, arthritis, Parkinson's disease, cardiac disease, pulmonary disease, and low back pain. Environmental barriers are a major cause of "accidental immobilization" in both the acute and chronic care settings. These include bed rails, the height of the bed, physical restraints, an inappropriate chair, no physical assistance available, fall precautions imposed by medical staff, no orders in the chart for mobilization, social isolation, and environmental obstacles (stairs or doorway thresholds are examples). Cognitive impairments, central nervous system (CNS) disorders (such as cerebral vascular accidents, Parkinson's disease, and multiple sclerosis), peripheral neuropathies resulting from diabetes, and pain with movement can also severely reduce mobility. Affective disorders such as depression, anxiety, or fear of falling may also lead to accidental immobilization. In addition, sensory changes, terminal illnesses (such as cancer or cirrhosis of the liver), acute episodes of illness like pneumonia or cellulitis, or an attitude of "I'm too sick to get up" can negatively affect mobility.

The process of deconditioning involves changes in multiple organ systems, including the neurological, cardiovascular, and musculoskeletal systems to varying degrees. Deconditioning is probably best defined as the multiple changes in organ system physiology that are induced by inactivity and reversed by activity (e.g., exercise).[16,23] The degree of deconditioning depends on the degree of superimposed inactivity and the prior level of physical fitness. The term "hypokinetics" has been coined to describe the physiology of inactivity.[24] Deconditioning can occur at many levels of inactivity. For simplicity and clarity, two major categories of inactivity or hypokinetics will be examined: the acute hypokinetic effects of bed rest and the chronic inactivity induced by a sedentary lifestyle or chronic disease.

Looking at the aging process with one eye on the adverse effects of bed rest or hypokinetics as a possible concomitant of deconditioning and disability can lead to discovering more about the potential use of exercise as one of our primary rehabilitation modalities. The phrase "use it or lose it" is a concept with tremendous ramifications for aging, especially in geriatric rehabilitation. Exercise has not been viewed as an important factor in health until recently. Until the 1950s the rate-of-living theory was promoted. According to this theory, the body would be worn out faster and life shortened by expending energy during exercise.[25] Conversely, studies in the past decade have shown that regular exercise does not shorten life span and may in fact increase it.[26] Exercise is increasingly viewed as beneficial for both the primary and secondary prevention of disease.[27]

There are several challenges to understanding the interaction between inactivity and health in older persons. The first is that the process of aging itself causes some changes that parallel the consequences of hypokinetics or inactivity. Several studies have provided strong evidence which separates the aging process from the sedentary lifestyle.[28–43] It has been found that older individuals can improve their flexibility, strength, and aerobic capacity to the same extent as younger individuals. The second challenge in studying inactivity is separating the effects of inactivity from those of disease.[36,37] It is obvious that some effects of aging can be directly related to inactivity. Many aged individuals who are deconditioned may also have superimposition of acute or chronic disease. Studies on younger subjects have helped to clarify some of the effects of inactivity alone (e.g., bed rest on physiological changes and functional performance).

Another challenge exists: the challenge of understanding the relationship between physiologic decline and functional loss. Is the inability to climb stairs in an 85-year-old primarily from cardiovascular deconditioning, muscle weakness, impaired balance secondary to sensory losses, or a sedentary lifestyle? Is there a new disease process beginning? Is this normal aging? An important concept in geriatric rehabilitation is that threshold values of physiologic functioning may exist.[27,31] An aged person who is below these thresholds may suddenly lose an essential functional skill. An understanding of the consequences of inactivity is particularly important in addressing rehabilitation needs of the aged individual. Table 8.1 summarizes the complications of bed rest.

For additional information on the effects of bed rest on the organ systems, see CD.

TABLE 8.1 Systemic Complications of Bed Rest

Neurosensory	Sensory deprivation	Musculoskeletal	Muscle atrophy
	↓ EEG activity		↓ muscle strength
	↓ thermoregulation		↓ muscle oxidative capacity
	↓ cognition		↓ aerobic capacity
	↓ in reaction time		Bone loss (osteoporosis)
	↓ balance		↓ hyaluronic acid
	↑ postural sway		↓ glycoproteins
Cardiovascular	↓ cardiac output		Joint contractures
	↑ resting heart rate (HR)		Osteoarthritis
	↓ oxygen uptake	Gastrointestinal	Constipation
	↓ total blood volume	Genitourinary	Urinary tract infection
	↓ aerobic capacity		Urinary incontinence
	↑ HR and BP with activity		Renal calculi
	Delayed postactivity recovery time	Skin	Pressure sores
	Orthostatic hypotension	Functional	Impaired ambulation
	Venous thrombophlebitis		↓ Activities of daily living
Respiratory	Atelectasis		↑ Risk of falls
	Relative hypoxemia	Psychological	Sensory deprivation
	↑ risk of pneumonia		Anxiety, fear, depression
	↓ chest wall compliance		Mood changes
	↓ intercostal muscle strength		Hallucinations
	↓ vital capacity		Perceptual disturbances
	Impaired gas exchange		Sleep disturbances
	↓ resting arterial oxygen tension		
	↑ alveolar-artial oxygen gradient		
	↓ peripheral perfusion		

The evaluation and treatment of hypokinetics is crucial in the total care of the elderly. Passive range of motion (PROM) or active-assistive range of motion (A-AROM) is appropriate even in the most immobilized patients to prevent the consequences of immobilization. Aging and inactivity are both associated with a loss of lean body mass and a gain in body fat.[31,34] Some degree of changes associated with aging are directly related to inactivity. Active aged individuals show lesser degrees of these changes, and exercise programs in sedentary aged persons have been shown to positively modify those changes associated with aging. Exercise has been shown to reverse the physiological changes of inactivity including a return of cardiovascular and cardiopulmonary response to pre–bed rest base lines, and a return of muscle strength and flexibility.[27] A mnemonic representation of the effects of bed rest is helpful in remembering the overall effects of inactivity on functional capabilities:

B—Bladder and bowel incontinence and retention; bedsores

E—Emotional trauma; electrolyte imbalances

D—Deconditioning of muscles and nerves; depression; demineralization of bones

R—ROM loss and contractures; restlessness; renal dysfunction

E—Energy depletion; EEG activity decreases

S—Sensory deprivation; sleep disorders; skin problems

T—Trouble

The elderly are especially susceptible to the complications of bed rest. Aging changes and common chronic diseases result in a decrease in physiologic reserve and a decreased ability to tolerate the changes which occur with bed rest. The physiology of aging and bed rest have many features in common and may be additive in their effects. The changes that commonly occur with aging and prolonged bed rest independently lead to osteoporosis, decreased endurance, and impaired mobility, and increase the predisposition to falls, deep venous thrombosis, sensory deprivation, and pressure sores.

With the numerous adverse effects of bed rest it should be prescribed judiciously and with full awareness of its potential complications and the need for preventive exercise prescription. Any elderly patient on bed rest should be on a physical or occupational therapy program. When full activity is not possible, limited activity such as movement in bed, activities of daily living, and intermittent sitting and standing will reduce the frequency of some complications of bed rest. Prolonged bed rest causes significant cardiovascular, respiratory, musculoskeletal, and neuropsychological changes. Complications are often irreversible. Complete bed rest should be avoided at all costs.

Optimal Health

The last principle in geriatric rehabilitation is the principle of "optimal health." The great English statesman Benjamin Disraeli said, "The health of people is really the foundation upon which all their happiness and their powers as a state depend." The World Health Organization defines health as a state of complete physical, mental, and social well-being, not merely the absence of disease or infirmity.[44] The existence of complete physical health refers to the absence of pathology, impairment, or disability. Physical health is quite achievable. Mental and social well-being are closely related and possibly less obtainable in this day and age. Mental health as defined by the World Health Organization would include cognitive and intellectual intactness as well as emotional well-being. The social components of health would include living situation, social roles (i.e., mother, daughter, vocation, etc.), and economic status.

There are some cumulative effects—biological, physiological, and anatomical—that may eventually lead to clinical symptoms. It has also been noted in the chapter that some of these changes are associated with inactivity and not purely a result of progressive aging effects. In light of this, a preventive approach to physical health needs to be in the foreground when addressing the needs of the aged.

Preventing impairment and disability is a key principle in geriatric rehabilitation. It is reasonable to assume that the health status of individuals in their 70s and subsequent decades of life is in a suboptimal range. Thus, the scope of health status for the aged should be focused toward preventing the complications that could result from suboptimal health. When considering suboptimal health then, the goal of geriatric rehabilitation should be to strive for relative optimal health (i.e., the maximal functional and physical capabilities of the aged individual considering his or her current health status).

In reviewing the importance of promoting relative optimal health in terms of the musculoskeletal, sensory, or cardiopulmonary systems, an example of an aged woman with a hip fracture may help.

The patient may be in suboptimal health and suffering from osteoporosis; however, she is not treated until she fractures her hip. The resulting complications could include pneumonia, decubiti from bed rest, all of the changes previously noted in relation to inactivity, and possibility of death. Intervention at the suboptimal level was needed here rather than waiting for an illness or disability to occur. This intervention could include weight-bearing exercises to enhance the strength of the bone, strengthening exercises of the lower extremities to provide adequate stability and endurance, balance and postural exercises to facilitate effective balance reactions and safety, education in nutrition, and modification of her living environment to ensure added safety in hopes of avoiding the kind of fall that results in a hip fracture.

Another excellent example of preventive intervention to maintain optimal health would be in the case of the diabetic aged individual. It is known that sensory loss in the lower extremities resulting from diabetes mellitus often predisposes diabetic individuals to ulceration of the foot. An ill-fitting shoe or a wrinkle in the sock may go unnoticed and lead to friction, skin breakdown, and a resulting foot ulcer. If undetected, even the smallest ulcer may lead to amputation of a lower extremity. Screening of the foot during evaluation can prevent this devastating loss. Intervention could include education of the aged individual in foot inspection (or education of a family member or friend if the diabetic aged individual's eyesight is compromised), proper shoe fitting, and techniques for dealing with sensory loss (e.g., as temperature sensation diminishes, the individual needs to test bath water temperature with a thermometer, or have one's spouse test the water before putting his or her insensitive feet into a steamy bath). With proper skin care and professional (podiatric) care of the nails and calluses, there is less likelihood that injury will occur. The cost of a therapeutic diabetic shoe (the P.W. Minor Thermold shoe, for example) is $130 to $160 per pair, and this shoe provides protection and ample room for the forefoot. Compare this to the cost of ulcer care, which averages $6,000, and the cost of hospitalization and rehabilitation for amputation, which averages $30,000.[45]

The principle of obtaining relative optimal health in geriatric rehabilitation not only is cost-effective but also would clearly lead to an overall improvement in the quality of life. Encouraging healthy behaviors, such as decreasing obesity, stress, and smoking, and increasing activity, could be the element necessary in maintaining health and striving for optimal health as defined by the World Health Organization.[44]

Health care professionals involved in geriatric rehabilitation need to be good *evaluators* and *screeners*. Good investigative skills could detect a minor problem with the potential of developing into a major problem. Thorough assessment of physical, cognitive, and social needs could help us to modify rehabilitation programs accordingly to truly improve the health and functional ability of our aged clients.

REHABILITATIVE MEASURES

Rehabilitation should be directed at preventing premature disability. A deconditioned aged individual is less capable of performing activities than a conditioned aged individual. For example, the speed of walking is positively correlated to the level of physical fitness in an aged person.[46] When cardiovascular capabilities are diminished (i.e., maximum aerobic capacity), walking speeds are adjusted by the aged person to levels of comfort. Himann[46] found that exercise programs geared for improving cardiovascular fitness improved the speed of walking. The more conditioned the individual, the faster the walking pace. The faster the walking pace, the smoother the momentum, decreasing the likelihood of falling. The better-conditioned elder is also more agile and has improved reaction times to balance perturbation when compared to an unfit older individual.

If disease and physical disability are superimposed on a hypokinetic sequelae, the functional consequences can be disastrous, because pain often prevents mobility. For instance, the pain experienced by an aged individual with an acute exacerbation of osteoarthritic knee pain accompanied by inflammation of the knee capsule may reflexively inhibit quadriceps contraction. While strength of the quadriceps may have been poor in the first place due to inactivity, the absence of pain still permitted this individual to rise from a chair or ascend shallow steps. Now, with the presence of acute pain, these activities cause severe discomfort and threaten the capability of maintaining an independent lifestyle. In this situation, rehabilitation efforts should focus medically on

- Reducing the inflammation through drugs or ice (physician, nurse);
- Maintaining joint mobility during the acute phases by joint mobilization techniques of oscillation and low-grade passive range in addition to modalities, such as interferential current, to assist in reducing the edema, and decreasing the discomfort (physical therapy);
- Joint protection techniques and prescription of adaptive equipment such as a walker to protect the joint (occupational and physical therapy);
- Provision for proper nutrition in light of medications/nutrient (pharmacist/dietician) effects and evidence that vitamin C is a crucial component in health of the synovium;[47]
- Social and psychological support (social worker, psychologist, religious personnel) to provide emotional and motivational support.

These interventions to prevent the debilitating effects of bed rest highlight the need for an interdisciplinary approach when addressing geriatric rehabilitation.

Rehabilitation of the aged individual should emphasize functional activity to maintain functional mobility and capability, improvement of balance through exercise and functional activity programs (e.g., weight shifting exercises, ambulation with direction and elevation changes, reaching activities), good nutrition and good general care (including hygiene, hydration, bowel and bladder considerations, appropriate rest and sleep), as well as social and emotional support.

It is important to optimize overall health status by implementing the concept of independence. The more an individual does for him- or herself, the more he or she is capable of doing independently. The more that is done for an aged individual, the less capable that person becomes of functioning on an optimal independent level and the more likely the progression of a disability.

Health Awareness and Beliefs

The advancing stages of disabilities increase an individual's vulnerability to illness, emotional stress, and injury. An older person's subjective appraisal of personal health status influences how he or she reacts to the symptoms, perceives his or her vulnerability, and perceives his or her abilities to perform a given activity. Often an aged person's self-appraisal of health is a good predictor to the rehabilitation clinician's evaluation of health and functional status, but such assessments may also differ in many ways. In older persons, perceptions of one's health may be determined in large part by one's level of psychological well-being and by whether or not one continues in rewarding roles and activities.[48]

Because an aged individual's perception of his or her health status is an important motivator in compliance with a rehabilitation program, it is important to discuss this further. One interesting study showed that even when age, sex, and health status (as evaluated by physicians) were controlled for, perceived health and mortality from heart disease were strongly related.[49] Those who rated their health as poor were two to three times as likely to die as those who rated their health as excellent. A Canadian longitudinal study of persons over 65 produced similar results.[50] Over three years, the mortality of those who described their health as poor at the beginning of the study was about three times that of those who initially described their health as good.

Yet, despite this apparent awareness among older persons of their actual state of health, the elderly are known to fail to report serious symptoms and wait longer than younger persons to seek help. Rehabilitation professionals need to listen carefully to their aged clients with this in mind. It appears that, contrary to the popular view that older individuals are somewhat hypochondriacal, aged persons generally deserve serious attention when they bring complaints to their caregivers.

The perceived level of health will greatly impact the outcomes of functional goals in the geriatric rehabilitation setting, whether it is acute, rehabilitative, home, or chronic care. Rosillo and Fagel[51] found that improvement in rehabilitation tasks correlated well with patients' appraisal of their potential for recovery, but not very well with others' appraisal. Stoedefalke[52] reported that positive reinforcement (frequent positive feedback) for older persons in rehabilitation greatly improved their performance and feelings of success. This indicates that aged persons can improve in their physical functioning when modifications in therapeutic interventions provide feedback more often. Some research indicates that older persons with chronic illness have low initial aspirations with regard to

their ability to perform various tasks.[53] As situations in which they succeeded or failed occurred, their aspirations changed to more closely reflect their abilities.

Older persons may have different beliefs about their abilities compared to younger persons.[54] When subjects were given an unsolvable problem, younger subjects ascribed their failure to not trying hard enough, while older subjects ascribed their failure to inability. On subsequent tests, younger individuals tried harder and older subjects gave up. This holds extreme importance in the rehabilitation potential of an aged person. If the person sees the cause of failure as an immutable characteristic, then little effort in the future can be expected.

Aged individuals may have a higher anxiety level in rehabilitation situations because they fear failure or are afraid of "looking bad" to their family or therapist.[55] Eisdorfer[55] found that if anxiety is high enough, then the behavior is redirected toward reducing the anxiety rather than accomplishing the task. Weinberg[56] found that subjects set their own goals for task achievement, even if they are directed to adopt the therapist's goals. In another study, Mento, Steele, and Karren[57] found that the best performance at difficult tasks, as many rehabilitation tasks are, occurs when the aged person sets a very specific goal, such as walking ten feet with a walker. If the person simply tries to "do better," then performance is not improved as much. These are important motivational components to keep in mind when working with an aged client. Perhaps the therapeutic approach of the clinician may have the greatest impact on the successful functional outcomes in a geriatric rehabilitation setting.

Exercise Programming

Exercise programs have potential for improving physical fitness, agility, and speed of response.[31] They also serve to improve muscle strength, flexibility, bone health, cardiovascular and respiratory response, and tolerance to activity.[58] Evidence suggests that reaction time is better in elders who engage in physical exercise than in those who are sedentary.[59] Stelmach and Worringham[59] showed a positive correlation between individuals' ability to maintain their balance when stressed and their level of fitness. Initial test scores on reaction time were significantly improved following a six-week stretching and calisthenics program in individuals 65 years of age and older. This has great clinical significance when considering the increasing incidence of falls with age (an area to be discussed in more detail in a subsequent section of this chapter).

In addition, exercise has been shown to provide social and psychological benefits affecting the quality of life and the sense of well-being in the elderly.[60] Intuitively, it would appear plausible that an aged individual who is in better physical condition will experience less functional decline and maintain a higher level of independence and a resulting improvement in his or her perceived quality of life. The risks of encouraging physical activity are small and can be minimized through careful evaluation. While all the exercise and activity programs that constitute therapeutic exercise cannot be described in detail in this chapter, Table 8.2 summarizes therapies for various conditions seen most frequently in geriatric rehabilitation settings.

Specialized exercise techniques, such as proprioceptive neuromuscular facilitation (PNF), Bobath, and sensory integration techniques, are very useful in regaining and maintaining functional mobility and strength and improving sensory awareness in elderly individuals.[61] Though these therapeutic exercises vary in application techniques, the concept of integrating sensory and motor function is consistent in each.

These exercise techniques are methods of placing specific demands on the sensory motor system in order to obtain a desired response. Facilitation, by definition, implies the promotion or hastening of any natural process—the reverse of inhibition; specifically, the effect produced in nerve cells by the introduction of an impulse. Thus, these techniques, though highly complex and requiring specialized training to employ, may simply be defined as methods of promoting or hastening the response of the neuromuscular mechanism through stimulation of the proprioceptors.[62]

The normal neuromuscular mechanism is capable of a wide range of motor activities within the limits of the anatomical structure, the developmental level, and inherent and previously learned neuromuscular responses. The normal neuromuscular mechanism becomes integrated and efficient without awareness of individual muscle action, reflex activity, and a multitude of other neurophysiological reactions. Variations occur in relation to coordination, strength, rate of movement, and endurance, but these variations do not prevent adequate response to the ordinary demands of life.

The deficient neuromuscular mechanism is inadequate to meet the demands of life in proportion to the degree of the deficiency. Responses may be limited in aged persons by the faulty neuromuscular response previously discussed as sequelae of the aging process, inactivity, trauma, or disease of the nervous or the musculoskeletal system.

Deficiencies present themselves in terms of limitation of movement as evidenced by weakness, incoordination, adaptive muscle or connective tissue shortening, or immobility of joints, muscle spasm, or spasticity. It is the deficient neuromuscular mechanism that becomes the concern of the rehabilitation team in a geriatric setting. These techniques are very useful in successfully retraining the neuromuscular system in the aged person. Specific demands placed on the patient by a physical or occupational therapist have a facilitating effect on the individual's neuromuscular mechanism. The facilitating effects of these therapeutic exercises are the means used in physical and occupational therapy to reverse limitations of the aged person.[62]

A general measure to ensure the highest functional capacity should encourage early resumption of daily activities following trauma or acute illness. Safety measures to prevent falls and avoid accidents should include reinforcing the use of properly fitted shoes with good soles, low broad heels, and heel cups or orthotics to stabilize the foot during ambulation. The importance of wearing prescription eyeglasses needs to be stressed, and the staff and family should be educated in reducing potential hazards within the patient's living environment (decreasing the amount of furniture, securing all loose rugs and carpeting, obtaining a commode, installing handrails around the toilet and tub areas and railings in the hallways as needed). These are just a few examples of safety proofing the environment in which the elder lives so that individuals may function at their maximum level. Adaptive equipment to enhance the ease of activities of daily living is often a useful adjunct for gaining independence. Adapting the environment to improve safety is essential in geriatric rehabilitation and will be discussed more thoroughly in a subsequent section of this chapter.

Pain Management

Pain management is a very important factor in geriatric rehabilitation, but it is one of the most difficult pathophysiologic phenomena to define. Pain is human perception or recognition of a noxious stimulus. In geriatric rehabilitation two basic types of pain—acute and chronic—are dealt with. Chronic pain can be broken down even further into two subcategories—acute-chronic and chronic-chronic.

Treatment of acute pain may include medications to reduce inflammation, ice, heat, or compression (also to reduce edema when warranted), rest, and gentle mobility exercises (low-grade oscillation techniques of joint mobilization are very helpful in pain relief and maintenance of joint mobility). Rarely are modalities such as ultrasound or electrical currents (high galvanic current reduces edema; interferential current neutralizes the tissue and assists in fluid removal) used in the acute pain situation in the aged individual, although they are widely used in acute sports-related injuries in younger populations. The reasons for this are not documented, though the clinical experience of the authors of this book teaches that the more conservative approaches of rest, ice, compression, or elevation, and gentle exercise in combination with nonnarcotic analgesics seem to be quite effective in treating acute pain in the older person.

Chronic pain is more frequently observed in the aged and is more difficult to control. Chronic pain may not always correspond with objective findings. It is well recognized that emotional and socioeconomic factors play a role in chronic pain. Tension and anxiety often lead to muscle tension and decreased activity, and this can be a viscious cycle. Situational depression may exacerbate this type of pain. In management of acute-chronic pain, such as the example of an acute osteoarthritic condition, treatment is similar to the acute pain management with the exception

TABLE 8.2   Rehabilitation Therapies for Common Conditions

Cerebral Vascular Accident (Stroke)

Physical Therapy
- Pregait activities (if individual is not ambulatory)
- Gait/balance training (if individual is ambulatory)
- Provision of assistive ambulatory devices (quad cane, hemi-walker)
- Ambulation on different types of surfaces (stairs, ramps)
- Provision of appropriate shoe gear and orthotics
- Education and provision of appropriate bracing
- Range-of-motion, strengthening, coordination exercises
- Proprioceptive neuromuscular facilitation
- Bobath techniques to modify tone
- Sensory integration
- Joint mobilization techniques (when appropriate)
- Functional electrical stimulation (when appropriate)
- Positioning and posturing (chair, feeding needs)
- Family and patient education for home management
- Alternative interventions—Qi Gong, T'ai Chi, Yoga, Feldenkrais

Occupational Therapy
- Training in activities of daily living (grooming, dressing, cooking, etc.)
- Transfer training (toilet, bathtub, car, etc.)
- Activities and exercise to enhance function of upper extremities
- Training to compensate for visual-perceptual problems
- Provision of adaptive devices (reachers, special eating utensils)

Speech Therapy
- Language production work
- Reading, writing, and math retraining
- Functional skills practive (checkbook balancing, making change)
- Therapy for swallowing disorders
- Oral muscular strengthening

Parkinson's Disease

Physical Therapy
- Gait training
- Provision for appropriate shoe gear and orthotics
- Training in position changes
- General conditioning, strengthening, coordination, and range-of-motion exercises
- Breathing exercises
- Training in functional instrumental activities of daily living
- Proprioceptive neuromuscular facilitation/sensory integration
- Alternative interventions—T'ai Chi, aquatic therapy, Qi Gong, Feldenkrais

(cont.)

TABLE 8.2   Rehabilitation Therapies for Common Conditions (Continued)

Occupational Therapy
- Fine/gross motor coordination of upper extremities
- Provision of adaptive equipment
- Basic self-care activity training
- Transfer training

Speech Therapy
- Improving respiratory control
- Improving coordination between speech and respiration
- Improving control of rate of speech
- Use of voice amplifiers and/or alternate communication devices

Arthritis

Physical Therapy
- Joint protection techniques
- Joint mobilization for pain control and mobility
- Conditioning, strengthening, and range-of-motion exercises
- Gait training
- Provision of proper shoe gear and orthotics
- Modalities to decrease pain and edema, and break up adhesions
- Provision of assistive ambulatory devices (when appropriate)
- Alternative interventions—T'ai Chi, Qi Gong, Feldenkrais, Yoga, aquatics
- Refer for nutritional counseling

Occupational Therapy
- Range-of-motion and strengthening exercise of upper extremities
- Splinting to protect involved joints, decrease inflammation, and prevent deformity
- Joint protection techniques
- Provision of adaptive devices to promote independence and avoid undue stress on involved joints

Amputees

Physical Therapy
- Fitting and provision of temporary and permanent prosthetic devices
- Teaching donning and doffing of prostheses
- Progressive ambulation
- Provision of assistive ambulatory devices
- Training in stump care
- Wound care (when appropriate)
- Provision of shoe gear and protective orthotic for uninvolved extremity
- Instruction in range-of-motion, strengthening, and endurance activites for both involved and uninvolved extremities
- Balance activities
- Transfer training
- Patient education in skin care and monitoring
- Alternative therapies—Qi Gong, Yoga, Feldenkrais
- Refer for nutritional counseling

TABLE 8.2   Rehabilitation Therapies for Common Conditions (Continued)

Occupational Therapy
- Teaching donning and doffing of prostheses
- Training in stump care
- Transfer training
- Training in activities of daily living

Cardiac Disease

Physical Therapy
- Patient education
- Conditioning and endurance exercises (walking, biking, etc.)
- Breathing and relaxation exercises
- Strengthening and flexibility exercises
- Monitoring of patients' vital signs during exercise
- Stress management techniques
- Alternative interventions—Qi Gong, T'ai Chi, Yoga
- Refer for nutritional counseling

Occupational Therapy
- Labor-saving techniques
- Improving overall endurance for participation in activities of daily living
- Monitoring patients' participation in activities of daily living

Pulmonary Disease

Physical Therapy
- Patient education
- Breathing control exercises
- Chest physical therapy
- Conditioning exercises
- Joint mobilization of rib cage
- Relaxation and stress management techniques
- Alternative interventions that incorporate controlled breathing patterns—Yoga, Qi Gong, T'ai Chi, Feldenkrais

Occupational Therapy
- Training in labor-saving techniques
- Monitoring of participation in activities of daily living
- Improving endurance of upper extremities

Low Back Pain

Physical Therapy
- Joint mobilization/stabilization
- Modalities to decrease pain and improve tissue mobility
- Strengthening and flexibility exercises
- Instruction in proper body mechanics for lifting, sitting, and sleeping
- Provision of proper shoe gear and shock-absorbing orthotics
- Correction of leg length discrepancy (when appropriate)

(cont.)

TABLE 8.2   Rehabilitation Therapies for Common Conditions (Continued)

Low Back Pain (cont.)

Physical Therapy(cont.)

- Postural training for positioning
- Relaxation and stress management techniques
- Alternative approaches to encourage posture—Qi Gong, T'ai Chi, Yoga, Feldenkrais

Occupational Therapy

- Training in ergonomic techniques
- Training in energy conservation and positioning at rest

Alzheimer's Disease

Physical Therapy

- Sensory integration techniques
- Gait training (when appropriate)
- Balance activities
- Provision of proper shoe gear and orthotics
- General conditioning exercises
- Reality orientation activities/validation techniques
- Alternative interventions—dancing, hammock, T'ai Chi, Qi Gong

Occupational Therapy

- Sensory integration techniques
- Activities of daily living (grooming, feeding, etc.)
- Reality orientation activities/validation techniques

Hip Fractures

Physical Therapy

- Range-of-motion, strengthening, and conditioning exercises
- Positioning
- Progressive weight bearing and gait training
- Provision of assistive ambulation devices
- Provision of proper shoe gear, lift on the involved side, and orthotics for shock absorption
- Balance activities
- Transfer training
- Referral to nutritionist if presence of osteoporosis

of the inclusion of various modalities. For instance, ultrasound may be used to break up a tissue adhesion; interferential or high galvanic electrical stimulation may be used to break up adhesions, reduce swelling, and enhance circulation to the painful area. Joint mobilization techniques are often employed to improve and maintain mobility. Nonnarcotic analgesics can be prescribed, but the aged are more susceptible to the cumulative effects, as well as side effects, of the long-term use of these drugs.

Foot pain and/or discomfort from bony changes, such as those induced by lifelong use of ill-fitting shoes,

arthritic changes, or age-related shifting of the fat pads under the heel and the metatarsal heads, can severely curtail the ambulatory abilities of the aged. Proper shoe gear and shock-absorbing orthotics that place the foot in a neutral position have been clinically observed to facilitate ambulation and prevent disability.

Though few studies have documented this effect of reducing plantar foot pressures or altering the weight-bearing pattern of the foot during gait in aged individuals, this author has completed one study (currently unpublished) that clearly demonstrates a decrease in discomfort as a result of reduced pressure and alteration in the weight-bearing pattern and an increase in walking distance and functional capabilities. This has important ramifications in the area of geriatric rehabilitation.

Assistive Devices

Assistive devices, such as a cane, a quad cane (a more stable, four-legged cane), or a walker, can also be prescribed to improve stability during ambulation and reduce the stresses on painful joint.

Wheelchair prescription may be necessary for longer distances (usually recommended for use outside the home) or when ambulation is no longer possible (e.g., in the case of a bilateral amputation or severe diabetic neuropathy). Wheelchairs should be prescribed to meet the specific needs of the aged individual. For instance, removable arms may be needed to enhance the ease of transfers, or elevating leg rests may be prescribed for lower extremity elevation when severe cardiac disease results in lower extremity edema.

Likewise, if advanced rheumatoid arthritis or quadriplegia limits upper extremity capabilities, an electric wheelchair will greatly improve an individual's capabilities of locomotion. Other considerations may be a one-arm manual drive chair for a hemiplegic or a "weighted" chair to shift the center of gravity and improve the stability of the chair in transfers for the bilateral amputee. This author often prescribes the use of golf-like carts or other motorized carts for community-dwelling elders to enhance their ability to move around town or long corridors in assisted living or senior housing environments. Though the older individual may be an independent ambulator within his or her home, the use of such a cart is a means of energy conservation when longer distances of locomotion are required. All of these considerations necessitate a team approach in obtaining the equipment that best suits the individual's needs.

Proper positioning and seating for the aged individual who must sit for extended periods is required to decrease discomfort and keep pressures off of bony prominences, provide adequate postural support, facilitate feeding, and prevent progression of joint contractures and deformities. Many specialized chairs and adaptive positioning pads are on the market and address specific positioning needs. Armchairs which assist in rising from a seated position include higher chairs that decrease the work of the lower extremities for standing, or electric "ejection" chairs that actually extend to bring the individual to a near standing position. Functional assessment of the aged person is vital in the prescription of these specialized devices.

Understanding and managing the patient's sensation of fatigue is essential in any exercise program. Fatigue, a word understood by everyone, lacks precise definition. Darling[63] likened the concept of fatigue to the concept of pain. Both must be considered from physiologic and psychologic points of view. Physiologic types of fatigue include "muscle" fatigue from prolonged use of a muscle group, "circulatory" fatigue associated with elevated blood lactate levels during prolonged activity, and "metabolic" fatigue in which exercise depletes glycogen (energy) stores. General fatigue is related to more subtle factors like interest, reward, and motivation.

Given these definitions, it is easy to understand why a deconditioned person can experience fatigue. From a treatment perspective it is essential to determine what sensation the aged individual is describing as fatigue. Elevated vital signs and progressively weak muscle contractions suggest that rest is needed. A vaguer complaint of fatigue in the absence of these changes would not necessarily be a basis for reducing exercise. In fact, poor aerobic fitness may be related to an otherwise healthy aged person's complaint of fatigue.[64]

One therapeutic principle we often use successfully in motivating elderly individuals is to not give them instructions that include specific times or numbers of repetitions. For instance, "do this exercise for as long as you feel comfortable and then stop and rest." Or, "lift this weight as many times as you feel comfortable lifting it and then stop and rest." This omits the potential for failing by not making it to the prescribed time or number of repetitions. The authors of this book find that once a specific "number" is not looming in front of the older exercisers, fatigue does not set in as readily. They no longer have markers (i.e., "I'm halfway there") by which to measure, so the task becomes less ominous and never results in failure.

Another principle that works well with the older adult exerciser is the communication rule of exercise. Rather than having the patient focus on vital sign monitoring (which the clinician can do during assessment and evaluation), the level of exercise is based on the ability to speak. Mild exercise that is not aerobic results in the individual's ability to carry on a fluid conversation without shortness of breath. Moderate exercise, or exercise in the submaximal aerobic range, results in more staccato sentences with frequent pauses for breath. In other words, the individual can speak but would rather not. The maximal exercise range, which you rarely want to take an individual into, results in the inability to speak. This is the range that mountain climbers in low oxygen environments find themselves in. In the maximal range, all air inhaled is needed for the provision of oxygen to the working muscles.

What should be the prescribed level of exercise in an older adult? This will be based on the elder's overall physical, physiological, emotional, and cognitive condition. However, a good rule of thumb in activity and exercise in the elderly is *anything above rest works*.

In providing activity and exercise programs for the aged, normal aging changes in the musculoskeletal, neuromuscular, cardiovascular, and pulmonary systems will affect functional capacity. In addition, confusion, decreased sensory awareness, postural changes, cardiovascular limitations resulting from deconditioning, motivation, and perceived level of fatigue all affect the potential for rehabilitation and need to be assessed prior to implementing activity or exercise programs. Specific exercise recommendations are included in the chapters specific to each system (e.g., Chapters 11 through 14).

For information on nutritional considerations, see CD.

RESTRAINTS

The use of physical restraints, in an attempt to keep patients safe, continues to be practiced despite evidence that restraints often increase the incidence of falls.[65] Decreasing the use of physical restraints continues to be a challenge for the health care team. It is important to understand the law regarding restraints as well as the risks, benefits, and implications for their use. This section of the chapter addresses regulations, types of restraints, documentation, and alternatives to the use of restraints.

The Omnibus Budget Reconciliation Act (OBRA) states that "a patient has the right to be free from any physical or chemical restraints imposed for purposes of discipline or convenience, and not required to treat the resident's medical symptoms."[66] By this statement, OBRA did not mandate an environment free of restraints but placed restrictions on the use of physical or mechanical devices that are not medically necessary. Despite OBRA guidelines, restraints still rank in the top ten of the Center for Medicare and Medicaid's Service's (CMS—formerly Health Care Finance Administration [HCFA]) list of most commonly cited deficiencies in long-term care facilities.

The reasons given by long-term care team members for the use of physical restraints are numerous: to prevent injury to self and other residents; control of agitated or restless behavior; management of a resident's cognitive deficit and poor judgment; mobility impairments placing the resident at risk for falls; and resistance to medical treatment. Although these may seem to be noble support statements, there are a number of risks associated with physical restraints. A list of benefits and risks associated with the use of restraints is provided in Table 8.3.

Physical restraints affect a number of aspects of the elderly person's life in the institutional setting. A great deal of research has investigated the association of restraint use with other parameters such as falls, cognition, and activities of daily living impairment. Phillips[67] found that residents in long-term care facilities with the poorest ADL function were more likely to be restrained. A balance problem further increased this likelihood. Ejaz and colleagues[65] compared a restrained group who underwent restraint reduction to a nonrestrained group. They found that serious falls, resulting in hematoma, fracture, or loss of consciousness, did not increase in the restraint reduction group although nonserious falls did (i.e., those re-

TABLE 8.3   Benefits and Risks of Physical Restraints

Benefits of Restraints
• Prevention/protection from falls and other accidents or injuries (questionable)
• Allows medical treatment to proceed without patient interference
• Maintenance of body alignment
• Increases patient's feeling of security and safety
• Protects other patients and staff from physical harm
Risks of Restraints
• Injury from falls
• Accidental death by strangulation
• Skin abrasions and breakdown
• Immobilization sequelae (deconditioning, muscle atrophy, contractures, osteoporosis, orthostatic hypotention, deep vein thrombosis, pneumonia, incontinence)
• Decline in ADLs, functional mobility
• Cardiac stress
• Increased mortality
• Dehydration, reduced appetite
• Disorganized behavior
• Social/emotional isolation

quiring first aid, cuts, bruises). Rate of falls in the experimental group, however, matched but did not exceed the rate of falls in the control group. This provides some evidence to dispel the myth that untying the elderly would increase serious falls.

In order for the long-term care team to reduce restraints, it is important to understand which devices are considered restraints and the implications of their use. CMS interpretive guidelines define a physical restraint as "any manual method or physical or mechanical device, material or equipment attached to or adjacent to the resident's body, which the individual cannot remove easily, that restricts freedom of movement or normal access to one's body."[68] Further, the guidelines state that physical restraints include leg, arm, and vest restraints; hand mitts; soft ties; binding a resident who is bedbound by tucking sheets in tightly; bed rails; and chairs that prevent rising.

"Devices on clothing that trigger electronic alarms to warn staff that a resident is leaving a room"[68] are not necessarily considered restraints, according to the guidelines. This definition, although helpful, often leaves the long-term care team with questions regarding the proper use of restraints. The following is information and recommended practice for a number of physical restraints.

Side rails are often utilized to keep an individual from falling out of bed and to deter attempts to get out of the bed. A number of deleterious effects have been cited due to the use of side rails. These negative consequences include increasing the distance one falls from the bed, obstruction of vision, creating noise, trauma if the body strikes the side rails, creating a sense of being trapped, and dislodging/pulling tubes during raising and lowering.[69] Donius and Radr[69] recommend a thorough risk level assessment to determine necessity of side rail use. Table 8.4 is an example of a risk level assessment for the use of side rails.

Vest, waist, pelvic, and extremity tie-on devices are generally considered to be restraints. These types of restraints should rarely be used and only if alternatives have failed. Further, they should be used for only brief periods of time.

Position change and body alarm devices in and of themselves are not considered restraints; however, if the staff responds to the sound of the alarm by restricting the resident's mobility (i.e., making the resident sit back down when attempting to stand up rather than addressing needs), then the facility's response would be considered restrictive.

Reclining wheelchairs and geri chairs are considered restraints when they restrict a resident's normal mobility and require a physician's order for use. Lap cushions or trays, wheelchair bars, and seat belts can be restraints if the resident is unable to remove these devices independently. Lap cushions and trays particularly are not restraints if they are used to provide support for residents who do not attempt to stand or lean forward. Wedge cushions that raise residents' feet off the floor if they propel a wheelchair or that limit their ability to stand would be considered a restraint.

A number of restraint alternatives have been proposed for various resident impairments. Cohen[70] found the most common restraint-reducing alternatives to include wedge cushions, wheelchair modifications (e.g., lowering seats, footrests, etc.), and physical and occupational therapy consultation to improve functional mobility and safety through exercise and activity. This author has successfully employed a seated hammock in cognitively compromised patients who are at risk for falls because of sundowning, pacing, or both. Placed in a calming environment (e.g., paying attention to noise, activity, and colors) the hammock serves to soothe the typically confused and anxious patient. Hung so that the front edge of the hammock is eighteen inches from the floor, an elderly individual with fair or better quadriceps strength can easily arise from the hammock. The seated hammock has been used on Alzheimer's units for well over a decade, and anecdotal experience reveals a high level of success in calming and protecting these patients from falls without restraining them.

Regardless of whether a device considered a restraint is used or a restraint alternative is found, appropriate documentation is necessary. The Food and Drug Administration (FDA) recommends that each facility define and communicate an institutional policy for restraints and that restraints are removed at least every two hours for ADLs. Further, documentation in the chart for use of restraints should include the medical reason for the restraint; the type of restraint selected; and the time frame for use.[71] When a restraint is used, a physician's order is necessary.

A responsible party should sign a consent form that explains the benefits and risks of the restraint. Restraints and restraint alternatives can be determined and documented in the context of a team restraint committee consisting of social services, physical and occupational therapy, appropriate nursing staff, the administrator, and the physician if available. Consultants to the team may include the pharmacist and nutritionist.

The use of physical restraints has become a concern for nursing home caregivers due to the OBRA guidelines and accusations of elderly abuse. The most common definition of a physical restraint is "any device placed on or near one's body to limit freedom of voluntary movement or normal access to one's own purpose." It is easy to say "no restraints"; however, there are circumstances for use and emergency procedures. A fundamental ethical dilemma occurs as well as a caregiver's responsibility to protect the patient. Initiation of a restraint should be a team effort, and the removal of restraints should also be a team process

TABLE 8.4 Risk Level Assessment for use of Side Rails on Bed

Level I: Low Risk
Side rails are not necessary for residents in this group. They may be used because of the person's preference but are not considered restraints. Residents at this level are able to get into and out of bed without assistance and safely, or do not move without staff assistance.
Level II: Moderate Risk
These residents have the desire to get into and out of bed unassisted but lack the ability to do so safely. These residents need side rails or an alternative if side rails are not used. Side rails are then considered restraints and need a physician's order.
Level III: High Risk
Side rails are used to restrict movement of these residents because there are no alternatives, alternatives have failed, or the benefit of using side rails outweighs the burden. Side rails are then considered restraints and need a physician's order.

Donius and Rader (see ref 69)

to give the resident the least restrictive device. Finding appropriate options to maintain safety and mobility for the residents of long-term care institutions continues to be a challenge. Only through a coordinated team approach can we decrease the use of restraints in the institutional setting. A guiding principle is to "use restraint before using restraints" and to be creative in finding alternatives.

FALLS IN THE ELDERLY

Falls are not part of the normal aging process, but are due to an interaction of underlying physical dysfunction, medications, and environmental hazards.[72] Poor health status, impaired mobility from inactivity or chronic illness, postural instability, and a history of previous falls are observable risk factors. The ultimate goals of rehabilitation are to combat the inactivity and loss of mobility that predisposes to falls.

Some of the ad hoc measures currently used to prevent falls, such as physical restraints and medications to reduce activity, are now suspected of increasing the risk of falling.[72]

Medical conditions are often a cause of falling. A pathological fracture secondary to severe osteoporosis may result in a fall (rather than the fracture resulting from the fall), or an arrhythmia may induce dizziness. Certain drugs, such as digoxin used in treating an arrhythmia, may also induce dizziness or fatigue (see Chapter 7 for tables listing drugs that cause adverse side effects that may result in falls in the elderly).

The fear of falling is often a cause for inactivity and is commonly seen in an individual who has sustained a previous fall. It must be noted here that older individuals may not have experienced a fall themselves, but may limit their activity because their neighbor fell. Their observation of the sequelae of events experienced by their neighbor makes them fearful of having the same thing happen in their life. As a result, they limit their activities and the activities they do are guarded. The guarding patterns that aged individuals use as a result of this fear (e.g., grabbing furniture that may not be stable or supportive) may in fact lead to further danger. Intervention by a psychiatrist or psychologist is often necessitated to diminish this fear.

Functionally, limitations of range of motion, decreased muscle strength and joint mobility, coordination problems, or gait deviations can predispose an elderly individual to falling. Specific strengthening and gait training programs assist in preventing falls by improving overall strength and coordination, balance responses and reaction time, and awareness of safe ambulation practices (for example, freeing one hand for use of a handrail when carrying packages up the stairs). Some individuals will have inadequate strength and balance to ambulate without an assistive device, or assistive ambulatory devices may also provide a safer mode for locomotion. Walking aids, such as canes and walkers, are beneficial for prevention of falls

in some cases,[73] whereas, in other cases, they actually contribute to the cause of the fall.[74] Assess the appropriateness of the assistive device, and ensure that the aged individual is using it properly. With proper instruction, patients can usually function safely within their environment without falling.

Gait evaluation is one of the most important components in fall prevention. The "Get-up and Go" test is a method used often to test functional strength, balance, coordination, and safety during gait. See Appendix 1 for administration and a copy of the Get-up and Go tool. The aged individual is asked to get up out of the chair without using his or her hands, walk approximately ten feet down the hall, turn around, come back to the chair, and then stand still. What follows are ways the therapist can glean information once the Get-up and Go is completed. While the patient is standing still, the rehabilitation therapist can give a gentle push on the sternum to test the patient's righting reflexes. The individual can be directed to sit down without the use of his or her hands. Each component of the test can be analyzed. For instance, the inability to arise from the chair without the assistance of the hands is indicative of hip extensor, quadriceps weakness, or both. If step symmetry is absent (i.e., if the individual is taking irregular steps), the cause can often be pinpointed just by observation. A leg length discrepancy may be present or the hip abductors may be weak. These alterations in anatomical structure or muscle status can easily be determined by close evaluation of the gait pattern. Lower extremity pain may also result in nonrhythmical steps as the individual attempts to avoid the painful extremity. Tendencies to veer, lose balance, or hold on to surrounding objects may be indicative of dizziness, muscle weakness, or poor vision. A loss of balance while turning or a stiff, disjointed turn may alert the clinician to the possibility of neurological disorder, such as Parkinson's disease or drug-induced muscle rigidity (often seen in aged individuals on haloperidol or other psychotropic medications).

With good basic education for the patient and the family and modification of the environment to reduce hazards, it is possible to prevent falls through methods that do not undermine mobility or autonomy. It is important to identify and treat reversible medical conditions, as well as physical impairments in gait and balance. Many falls can be prevented through: proper exercise to maintain strength; sensory integration techniques to promote all functional activities by improving balance and coordination; good shoes and orthotics to provide a proper base of support and gait training activities; and modifications to safety proof the living environment.

Rehabilitation specialists have an important role in recommending interventions to prevent falls. When disease states and medication responses are stable, an individualized program of safety education, environmental adaptations, lower extremity strengthening exercises, balance exercises, and gait training should be implemented.

Safety education is an important first step in the prevention of falls. Many older individuals are not aware that they are at risk for falling. Often, simple instructions about environmental adaptations and encouraging a person to allow plenty of time for functional activities are all that is needed to facilitate safety. Many aged people feel the need to rush to answer a phone or doorbell. They should be discouraged from rushing, because that could result in a fall. Caregivers and visitors should also be a part of the safety education process. They are often able to remind the person who is at risk for falling of the need for added precaution.

Aged persons who complain of dizziness during changes of position should be evaluated for postural hypotension. These individuals should be taught to change positions slowly and to wait before moving to another position in order to allow the blood pressure to accommodate to the change.

Any individual who has fallen is at risk for falling again. In fact, clustering of falls has been seen in some older individuals during the months preceding death.[75] Inability to rise or lack of assistance after a fall can produce devastating consequences. In one study, half of the aged persons who lay on the floor for longer than six hours after a fall died within six months.[76] Having a phone in every room or obtaining a cellular phone may be a necessity for aged persons who live alone. A "buddy system" in which older persons call each other regularly during the day is a means of "checking up" and early detection of a fall. Individuals at risk can also be provided with a device such as the "lifeline," which summons emergency personnel by pushing a button.

Eighty-five percent of all falls occur at home,[77] most commonly on stairs,[78] on the way to and from the bathroom,[79,80] and in the bedroom.[81] Environmental evaluation and adaptation is needed for those aged individuals who have fallen or are at risk for falling. See Chapter 9 for environmental evaluation forms.

Safety evaluation should address such questions as "Are the carpets tacked down?" "Is the pathway from the bed to the bathroom obstacle free?" and "Is there nighttime lighting?" Additional environmental suggestions include adaptive equipment for the shower or bathtub (i.e., using a tub seat and a handheld showerhead can improve safety and independence while bathing). Adaptations may also be necessary in order to avoid falls on route to the bathroom. Individuals with urinary urgency, evening fatigue, or disorientation in the middle of the night should be encouraged to use a bedside commode.

The purpose of strengthening exercises to prevent falls is to provide adequate force production of the lower extremities and trunk muscles for support of posture and control of balance. Strengthening can be done in a standard fashion or in a closed-chain functional fashion. For example, practicing sit-to-stand movements and the reverse is a functional means of strengthening extensors and flexors of the lower extremity. Going up and down stairs one stair at a time requires less strength, range of motion, and balance than walking step over step. A functional way to progress this activity, then, is to begin with one stair at a time and progress to step over step.

No matter which approach is selected for strengthening, the following precautions are recommended:

- Many aged individuals suffer from osteoporosis. Resistance and unilateral weight bearing may be excessive for them.
- Many aged individuals have osteoarthritis. Isometric exercise may be less painful for them. Prolonging the amount of time that the contraction is held may be an effective way to increase strength without adding external resistance.[82] Don't be afraid to attempt strength training, and explain to the patient that muscle pain may occur but significantly increased joint pain is not expected. Be flexible and try different approaches.
- It is especially important for aged individuals to avoid holding their breath (Valsalva maneuver) during exercise. Counting out loud helps to avoid this problem.
- Aged individuals should be taught to monitor their heart rate during exercise.

Therapeutic exercises designed to improve balance are an important part of fall prevention. Balance exercises can be organized to address three areas: posture control or response to perturbation, weight shifting, and anticipatory adjustments to limb movements.[83] It is somewhat helpful for older individuals to be able to respond to an external perturbation, such as a push to the shoulder or sternum, with a postural adjustment that brings the center of gravity back over the base of support. The usual response to a lateral perturbation will be extension of the weight-bearing leg along with elongation of the trunk on the weight-bearing side. Flexion and abduction of the non-weight-bearing leg will also be seen.[84] A small backward force should stimulate the reaction of the dorsiflexors at the ankles and flexion at the hips, whereas a small forward push should be followed by plantar flexion at the ankles and extension at the hips.[85]

Weight shifting of the entire body during standing involves muscular activity similar to that used in response to a perturbation; however, during weight shifting, the muscle activation occurs voluntarily. Balance must also be controlled when a limb movement occurs, such as reaching with the upper extremity or swinging with the lower extremity. In this case, the postural adjustment actually occurs in anticipation of the limb movement, in order to prevent the center of gravity from moving outside of the base of support. This mode of training is more useful for older persons as it more closely parallels functional activities. For example, a forward movement of the arm should be preceded by ankle plantarflexion and hip extension. In this way, a small backward movement of the center of gravity counteracts the forward displacement caused by the moving arm. Practicing each of these activities in anticipation of limb movement in standing, will help prepare the aged individual to use postural adjustment effectively during functional standing activities, such as cooking, transfers, and ambulation. These activities are directed toward improvement of the motor component of balance.

Altering the sensory conditions during balance activities encourages the aged person to attend to support surface or visual information selectively. Balancing in bare feet with eyes open or closed helps maximize the amount of somatosensory information that is available from the soles of the feet. On the other hand, balancing while standing on a piece of foam[86] disrupts information from the sole of the foot and from stretch receptors in the ankle muscles and forces the individual to practice using visual input to stabilize posture. Maintaining balance while turning the head from side to side or nodding the head is also important. Many aged people report falling during head movements,[87] while looking up to hang curtains, while getting the cereal off the second shelf in the cabinet, or while changing a lightbulb. Aged individuals should be instructed to use caution during upward head movements.

When an individual is unable to control standing balance and is about to fall, the normal response is protective extension of the arms or legs. Protective reactions, such as arm extension and the stepping response, should also be practiced. Upper extremity protective extension can be practiced both forward and sideways against the wall in the standing position.[88] Lower extremity protective reactions should be practiced in standing in forward, sideways, and backward directions. Brisk and accurately directed limb extension is the goal.

Balance exercises can be incorporated into functional activities for the aged. Moving from sit to stand and from stand to sit are examples of controlled voluntary weight shifting. Shifting the trunk forward and back and from side to side while sitting are also examples of voluntary weight shifting. Voluntary weight shifting while standing with the back to a wall is a safe way to facilitate control of balance. Dancing has also been recommended as a functional activity to improve balance for prevention of falls.[89] T'ai Chi and Qi Gong exercise, because of the slow, controlled movements beyond the center of gravity, have also been shown to substantially improve balance and postural stability in the elderly.[90,91] Postural adjustments in anticipation of arm movements can be practiced during functional activities by standing and reaching for objects on the kitchen or closet shelves. Reaching should be practiced in a variety of directions.

Ambulation requires weight shifting. Manual guidance during ambulation helps organize the time and direction of weight shifting.[31,88] Functional ambulation requires interaction with a variety of different support surfaces; therefore, it should be practiced on smooth as well as uneven surfaces and on level ground as well as inclines, curbs, and stairs. Varying the amount of available light and background noise also stimulates realistic environmental conditions. If step lengths are irregular, footprints on the floor make good targets for foot placement.[92]

Manual guidance is also useful for improving ambulation speed. A variety of ambulation speeds is necessary for function. Challenging activities, like crossing a busy street, can be made less threatening if the aged individual practices with the therapist or caregiver.

An area of intervention which is commonly overlooked (or avoided) in working on balance and falls in the elderly, is teaching an elder *how* to fall and, more importantly, *how* to get back up from the floor. It is helpful to use the thick track and field mats used for the high bar and pole vault jumps. These mats are at least eighteen inches thick and provide sufficient protection during a fall. Aquatic falling is also helpful. In both instances, the elderly individual can practice falling knowing they will land on a soft and forgiving medium. The key to falling is *relaxation*. As many readers have learned in ski school, if an individual tries to stop a fall, he or she is more likely to be rigid when meeting the ground, and much more likely to sustain an injury. Conversely, if the individual relaxes into the fall, he or she will more likely roll with impact and sustain the least amount of injury.

Difficulty rising from the floor after a fall is common in older adults and is associated with substantial morbidity.[93] This tends to be an underappreciated problem, one which is rarely addressed when working with the elderly. In a study by Tinetti and colleagues[93] only 49% of community-dwelling fallers were able to get up after a fall without assistance. Interestingly, most of the falls associated with the inability to get up without help (85%) were not associated with serious injury.[93] Thus, the inability to get up after a fall is common and not simply a consequence of a fall-related injury. Up to 20% of fallers remain on the floor for one hour or more;[94] and dehydration, pressure sores, muscle injury, and renal failure may be associated with long periods of time spent on the floor following a fall. Fear of falling appears to be increased in previous fallers, particularly those with a history of difficulty rising alone after a fall.[95] Despite the high risk of difficulty in rising from the floor after a fall, few therapists teach older adults how to rise from the floor.[96]

Some researchers have analyzed the motions used to rise from a supine position on the floor to a standing position,[97,98] finding that movement patterns differ somewhat as age increases[99] and when comparing sedentary to physically active adults.[100] Few studies have included healthy or frail older adults; however, Alexander and associates[94] investigated the ability of older adults in rising from the floor and explored how rising ability might differ based on initial body position and with or without the use of an assistive device. The findings from this study were that older adults (in their sixth and seventh decades of life) have more difficulty rising from the floor regardless of initial body position compared to younger adults, and it takes two to three times longer to accomplish this task with or without support (e.g., assistance using furniture). There were no significant advantages to using support to assist with rising. Data from this study and others may serve as the foundation for future interventions to improve the ability to rise from the floor. The Section on Geriatrics of the American Physical Therapy Association has developed a poster that provides a nine-step protocol for getting up from the floor. This is a helpful tool for teaching an older adult a step-by-step way of rising after a fall. Figure 8.2 provides this poster as an example for how to teach this strategy to older adults.

Risk factors for falling among the aged suggest that falling should not be considered a normal concomitant of aging; rather, it should alert the health care professional to the possibility of underlying disease or accelerated sensory or neuromuscular degeneration secondary to disuse. Secondary or multiple diagnoses, use of multiple medications, especially diuretics and barbiturates, decreased vision and lower extremity somatosensation, and decreased lower extremity strength all appear to contribute to balance and gait deficits, which in turn result in falling. Prevention of falls depends on addressing the specific problem area for each individual at risk. A team approach will be the most effective means to prevent falling by the aged.

Adapting the Environment

The process of adapting to the environment, or of adapting the environment to the aged person, is especially important in geriatric rehabilitation. With decreased physiologic reserves, the aged person may not be able to continue an activity that is extremely demanding. For instance, an older person with a stroke and underlying cardiac insufficiency may need to learn wheelchair mobility skills. Therefore, the environment will need significant modification. Doors may need to be widened, ramps installed, and counters lowered. Financial concerns and personal preferences may restrict opportunities for obtaining new housing or adapting the present home.

The interaction between the aged person and his or her environment becomes potentially precarious as one ages. These interactions are affected by the aged person's underlying physical status, living surroundings, and social support system. Of course, all persons interact with their environment. As one ages, however, the physiologic reserves, underlying medical problems, affective states, and a host of other factors, complicate the relationship between the aged individual and the environment.

The purpose of rehabilitation providers is to manipulate the environment to make it safer. Assistive walking devices or modifications of the home may be recommended. But even these interventions are subject to differences when dealing with aging persons. The aged person with a disability may view such aids as unattractive or demeaning. The individual has a choice in selecting eyeglasses, which may enhance his or her appearance, but walkers or chrome-plated grab bars seem to project an image of illness and disability, which the aged person may try to avoid. The older person may have difficulty finding someone who can install home modifications. Some retired senior volunteer programs (RSVPs) have carpenters available for this purpose, but many communities are without such support services. As a result, often needed modifications are not affordable for the older individual.

Tasks are carried out within a physical and social context, which has the potential for facilitating or hindering the use of functional capabilities. Push-button controls placed at the front of a range assist aged individuals with low vision, whereas dials situated at the back of the range handicap them. Similarly, caregivers can enhance functional independence by providing aged individuals with adaptive equipment, such as plate guards, bath brushes with elongated handles, and sock aids, or they can promote dependence by feeding, bathing, and dressing the individual.

Evaluation of the environment is more difficult than task analysis because the environment of concern is the one in which the individual actually lives and has to function, rather than a hospital or nursing home. Evaluation of physical space aims at ascertaining architectural barriers, safety and functional features, and the extent to which available equipment can be operated by the aged individual. Evaluation of the social context probes the availability of caregivers, their skills in rendering care and their need for training, their attitudes toward functional independence, and their experience of caregiver burden.

Those with disabilities or physiological or anatomical changes resulting from inactivity and aging may experience memory loss, disorientation, decreased ability to perform normal physical activity, a deteriorating ability to remember details, difficulty in verbal expression, and impairment in judgment. Each of these factors is important when modifying the physical and social environment to meet the rehabilitation needs of the aged. Recent US government hearings and reports suggest that social and organizational characteristics of institutions and the home setting could postpone the time when aged people become bedridden and require skilled nursing care.[101,102]

It is reasonable for the direct caregiver to seek advice about practical strategies that could reduce confusion or injury on the part of the disabled aged to prolong care at home. Environmental designs for aged patients have been studied, and several factors are consistently identified as environmental hazards: poor illumination; inadequate color differentiation; cluttered furnishings; confusing layout, such as a table in a dimly lit hallway; bland, nondistinct textiles; architectural features, such as split level rooms; and climate control.[103] Certain environmental features are a threat to

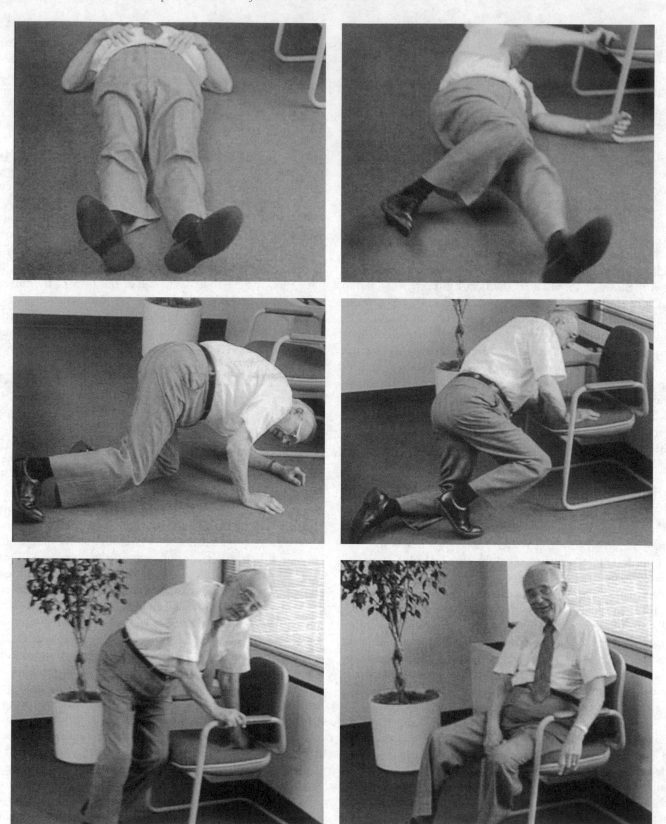

Figure 8.2   Falls: What to do if you fall at home.
1.   Remain calm and assess your situation.
2.   Roll over slowly. Locate the nearest sturdy chair.
3.   Crawl or shuffle to the chair.
4.   Kneel, then stand up using the chair.
5.   Then turn and sit down.
6.   Call or wait for help.

safety, can produce anxiety, and amplify cognitive deficits.[104] Cohen[105] found that behavioral approaches (e.g., using environmental cues like color coding or labeling objects) had advantages over drugs in the treatment of cognitive impairments. Additional studies emphasized that encouragement of independence, self-sufficiency, and social interaction is critical to prolonging cognitive functions.[106]

The aged individual's environment may have some negative effects on his or her communication. Older people living alone are often isolated in home or community settings; that is, an environment in which few opportunities for successful, meaningful communication are available.[107] This can result in impairment in their communication skills. An aged person needs an environment that stimulates and reinforces communication. Geriatric rehabilitation should encourage participation in a variety of activities that can serve as a basis for conversation and interaction. Providing socially stimulating environments within a hospital, rehabilitation, or long-term care setting can be provided by organized recreational and social therapies. This becomes more difficult in the home setting; although often resources, such as church, community groups, or senior centers, can facilitate social interaction. Meaningful conversation is a crucial component in enhancing and reinforcing cognitive functioning and a sense of well-being for the aged individual.[106,107]

Visual limitations, such as farsightedness, decreased ability to adapt to changes in lighting conditions requiring increased illumination to see, and an increased sensitivity to glare, are not uncommon in the elderly patient.

Several changes normally occur within the aging eye that affect safety and need to be considered when adapting an older person's environment. The lens of the eye begins to thicken and yellow, and the muscles that control dilation of the pupil weaken. The thickening of the lens and delayed pupil dilation mean that the glare and reflections often encountered in the environment cannot be tolerated.[108] In fact, the older eye needs approximately three times the amount of light to function adequately. The older person also has difficulty with depth perception and color differentiation, which can interfere with ambulation (poor judgment in distance), ADLs, and driving an automobile. Color vision deficiencies in the aged have been described by Andreasen.[108] IIc found that the aged individual has difficulty distinguishing between shades of blue-green, blue, and violet and is unable to distinguish between two shades of a similar color. The elderly maintain their ability to differentiate between brighter colors, such as orange and red.[108] Several authors suggest the need for large pattern designs or solid bright colors in upholstery and textiles to enhance visibility, interest, and appeal (reducing the likelihood of bumping into or falling over furniture). Small patterns can produce blurring of vision, eye fatigue, and dizziness.[109]

Independence can be facilitated by bright and sharply contrasting colors. Considering the poorer differentiation of similar colors, if an aged individual is in a poorly lit living room with a blue carpet, light blue walls, and lavender and blue flowered furniture and draperies, it could be trouble. Contrasting colors or better lighting, which even is economically more feasible, could positively facilitate safety in that room. Color coding of walls and corridors in hospitals and nursing homes using bright colors can help aged persons find their own rooms, bathrooms, sitting rooms, and so on. Contrasting colors are extremely important, because they can eliminate the difficulty of independently managing a stairwell or a poorly lit hall where shadows can be hazards. Often this contrast can be accomplished through the use of fluorescent colors of tape (orange, lime green, or red).

Different colors have differing effects on an individual's emotional state.[109] The colors red, yellow, and orange have been associated with excitement, stimulation, and aggression.[109] Red increases muscular tension and increases blood pressure. It could be used as a visual stimulant with the elderly to alert them of environmental changes or hazards, such as stairs or level changes. It must be noted, however, that individuals with cataracts lose the shorter frequencies in the spectrum. This includes red, orange, and in extreme cases yellow.

Although elderly persons often need to be stimulated, aged individuals with dementia require soothing and warm colors, such as light oranges and blues in their living quarters to enhance relaxation and comfort.

Higher, reasonably firm, supportive, comfortable chairs with high backs allow rising from a sitting position with minimal assistance. Wide armrests, either wooden or metal, allow identification by touch when eyesight is poor or trunk rotation is limited. An aged individual should always be instructed to feel the chair seat with the back of his or her legs before attempting to sit down.

Human beings have a great propensity for adapting to less than ideal conditions. The aged, particularly those with a severe disability, have much more difficulty. Sensory stimulation should be incorporated into every aspect of rehabilitation. Repetitive visual cues using graphics, color, and lighting encourage independence, thereby increasing pride and self-esteem.

Hellebrandt[110] proposes a focus on the maintenance of good health and residual mental function, the latter through socialization, physical, and recreational activities. The relationship between physical condition and behavior is particularly important in patients with dementia.[111] Changes in environmental design can accommodate the normal physiological changes of aging and prevent the effects of disuse. If the older person cannot manage the environment safely, her or his independence, socialization, and ADLs are hindered.

Appendix A

Mathias S, Nayak USL, Isaacs B. Balance in elderly patients: The "Get-up and Go" test. *Arch Phys Med Rehabil.* 1986; 67:387–389.

Get-up and Go.

Population:	Elderly population
Description:	The Get-up and Go test measures the sense of balance that the patient has. It was designed for the patient to perform a series of tasks in which any deviation from a normal performance would be noted.
Mode of Administration:	The Get-up and Go is a task performance exam.
Completion:	
Time to Complete:	About five minutes
Time to Score:	Scoring is accomplished while the test is administered.
Scoring:	Balance function is scored on a five point ordinal scale, which is as follows:

    1 normal
    2 very slightly normal
    3 mildly abnormal
    4 moderately abnormal
    5 severely abnormal

Interpretation:	A score of normal may be interpreted that the patient did not appear to be at risk for a fall. A score of very slightly normal or mildly abnormal or moderately abnormal reflects the patient's movement and possibility of stumbling. A score of severely abnormal meant that the subject appeared to be at a serious risk of falling during the exam.
Reliability:	40 elderly patients, at all levels of disability, took the Get-up and Go exam and were video-taped for observation and testing
	Interrater reliability was tested by showing the video-tapes to different groups of observers. The Kendall coefficient of concordance test was computed and it was found that the agreement within each group was higher than could have occurred by chance.
	When comparing this test with a measure of sway, some inconsistencies were found. However, these were explained by the observation that the observers were basing their score more heavily on gait than on balance and when this is accounted for the measure is fairly reliable.
Validity:	not reported
Reference:	Mathias S, Nayak USL, Isaacs B. Balance in elderly patients: The "Get-up and Go" test. *Arch Phys Med Rehabil.* 1986; 67:387–389.

Get-up and Go

Instructions: The patient is instructed to perform the following tasks while a trained observer watches and evaluates. The observer then gives the patient a score based on the following criteria:

    1 normal
    2 very slightly normal
    3 mildly abnormal
    4 moderately abnormal
    5 severely abnormal

Tasks:
   Patient is asked to sit comfortably in a chair.
   Patient is then asked to rise.
   Patient is asked to stand still.
   Patient is asked to walk towards a wall.
   Before they reach the wall the patient is asked to turn without touching the wall and return to the chair.
   Patient is asked to turn around and sit down.

Mathias, S., Nayak, U.S.L., Isaacs, B. Balance in elderly patients: The "Get-up and Go" test. *Arch Phys Med Rehabil.* 1986; 67:387.

References

1. Wedgewood J. The place of rehabilitation in geriatric medicine: An overview. *Int Rehabil Med.* 1985; 7(1):107.

2. Warshaw GA, Moore JT, Friedman SW, et al. Functional disability in the hospitalized elderly. *JAMA.* 1982; 248(7):847–850.

3. National Center for Health Statistics. *Health, United States, 1999, with Health and Aging Chartbook.* Hyattsville, MD: National Center for Health Statistics; 1999: 36–37.

4. National Center for Health Statistics. *Health, United States, 1999, with Health and Aging Chartbook.* Hyattsville, MD: National Center for Health Statistics; 1999: 34–35.

5. Clark G, Blue B, Bearer J. Rehabilitation of the elderly amputee. *J Am Geriatr Soc.* 1983; 31:439.

6. Centers for Disease Control and Prevention. *Unrealized Prevention Opportunities: Reducing the Health and Economic Burden of Chronic Disease.* Atlanta, GA: Centers for Disease Control and Prevention, National Center for Chronic Disease Prevention and Health Promotion; 1997.

7. Kumar VN, Redford JB. Rehabilitation of hip fractures in the elderly. *Am Fam Physician.* 1984; 29:173.

8. Federal Council on the Aging. *The Need for Long-Term Care. A Chartbook of the Federal Council on Aging.* Washington, DC: US Government Printing Office; 2000. US Department of Health and Human Services Publication No. (OHDS) 81-20704, 29.

9. Enright RB, Friss L. Employed care-givers of brain-damaged adults: An assessment of the dual role. Unpublished thesis, University of Arizona; 1997.

10. Lehman JF, Guy AW, Stonebridge JB, et al. Stroke: Does rehabilitation affect outcome? *Arch Phys Med Rehabil.* 1975; 56:375.

11. Rubenstein LZ, Josephson KR, Guriand B. Effectiveness of a geriatric evaluation unit: A randomized trial. *N Engl J Med.* 1984; 311:1664.

12. Fried LP, Guralnik JM. Disability in older adults: Evidence regarding significance, etiology, and risk. *J Am Geriatr Soc.* 1997; 45(1):92–100.

13. Ferrucci L, Gauralnik JM, Pahor M, Corti MC, Havlik RJ. Hospital diagnoses, Medicare charges, and nursing home admissions in the year when older persons become severely disabled. *JAMA.* 1997; 277:728–734.

14. Manton KG, Corder L, Stallard E. Chronic disability trends in elderly United States populations: 1982–1994. *Proc Natl Acad Sci USA.* 1997; 94: 2593–2598.

15. Lundin-Olsson L, Nyberg L, Gustafson Y. Attention, frailty, and falls: The effect of a manual task on basic mobility. *J Am Geriatr Soc.* 1998; 46(6): 758–761.

16. Fiatarone MA, O'Neill EF, Ryan ND, Clements KM, Solares GR, Nelson ME, Roberts SB, Kehayias JJ, Lipsitz LA, Evans WJ. Exercise training and nutritional supplementation for physical frailty in very elderly people. *N Engl J Med.* 1994; 330(25): 1769–1775.

17. Inouye SK, Wagner DR, Acampora D. A predictive index for functional decline in hospitalized elderly medical patients. *J Intern Med.* 1993; 8(7):645–652.

18. Winograd CH, Lindenberger EC, Chavez CM, Mauricio MP, Shi H, Bloch DA. Identifying hospitalized older patients at varying risk for physical performance decline: A new approach. *J Am Geriatr Soc.* 1997; 45(5):604–609.

19. Fried TR, Mor V. Frailty and hospitalization of long-term stay nursing home residents. *J Am Geriatr Soc.* 1997; 45(3):265–269.

20. Buchner DM, Wagner EH. Preventing frail health. *Clin Geriatr Med.* 1992; 8(1):1–17.

21. Pearlman DN, Branch LG, Ozminkowski RJ, Experton B, Li Z. Transitions in health care use and expenditures among frail older adults by payor/ provider type. *J Am Geriatr Soc.* 1997; 45(5): 550–557.

22. Branch LG, Jette A. The Framingham Disability Study: Social disability among the aging. *Am J Public Health.* 1981; 71:1202.

23. Siebens AW, Schmedt JF, Eckberg DL, et al. Homodynamic consequences of cardiovascular deconditioning—Functional effects. *Circulation.* 1990; 82(4): 694.

24. Lewis CB. *Aging: The Health Care Challenge.* Philadelphia: FA Davis; 1990.

25. Holloszy JO. Exercise, health, and aging: A need for more information. *Med Sci Sports Exerc.* 1983; 15:1.

26. Schneider El, Reed JD. Modulations of aging processes. In: Finch CE, Schneider EL, eds. *Handbook of the Biology of Aging.* New York: Academic Press; 1985.

27. Astrand PO. Exercise physiology and its role in disease prevention and in rehabilitation. *Arch Phys Med Rehabil.* 1987; 68:305.

28. Greenleaf JE, Reese RD. Exercise thermoregulation after 14 days of bed rest. *J Appl Physiol.* 1980; 48: 72–77.

29. Haines RF. Effect of bed rest and exercise on body balance. *J Appl Physiol.* 1974; 36:323.

30. Taylor HL, Henschel JB, Keys A. Effects of bed rest on cardiovascular function and work performance. *J Am Physiol.* 1949; 2:223.

31. Shepard RJ. *Physical Activity and Aging.* 2nd ed. Rockland, MD: Aspen Publishers; 1987.

32. Rikli R, Busch S. Motor performance of women as a function of age and physical activity level. *J Gerontol.* 1986; 41:645.

33. Ernes CG. The effects of a regular program of light exercise on seniors. *J Sports Med.* 1979; 19:185.

34. Buskirk ER. Health maintenance and longevity; exercise. In: Finch CE, Schneider EL, eds. *Handbook of the Biology of Aging.* New York: Academic Press; 1985.

35. Spiraduso WW. Physical fitness, aging, and psychomotor speed: A review. *J Gerontol.* 1980; 35:850.

36. Dietrick JE, Whedon GD, Shorr E. Effects of immobilization upon various metabolic and physiologic functions of normal men. *Am J Med.* 1948; 4:3–9.

37. Saltin B, Astrand PO, Grover RF, et al. Response to exercise after bed rest and after training. *Circulation.* 1968; 38(Suppl 7):1.

38. Miller PB, Johnson RL, Lamb LE. Effects of four weeks of absolute bed rest on circulatory functions in man. *Aerospace Med.* 1964; 35:1194.

39. Lamb LE, Stevens PM, Johnson RL. Hypokinesia secondary to chair rest from 4 to 10 days. *Aerospace Med.* 1965; 36, 755.

40. DeBusk RF, Convertino VA, Hung J, Goldwater D. Exercise conditioning in middle-aged men after 10 days of bed rest. *Circulation.* 1983; 68:245.

41. Buller AJ, Eccles JC, Eccles RM. Interaction between motor neurons and muscles in respect of the characteristic speeds of their responses. *J Physiol.* 1960; 150:417–419.

42. Ryback RS, Lewis OF, Sewab RS, Blum K. Psychobiologic effects of prolonged weightlessness (bed rest) in young healthy volunteers. *Aerospace Med.* 1971; 42:408–411.

43. Ryback RS, Lewis OF, Lessard CS. Psychobiologic effects of prolonged bed rest (weightless) in young, healthy volunteers (study II). *Aerospace Med.* 1971; 42:529–534.

44. World Health Organization. *Constitution of the World Health Organization.* Geneva: World Health Organization; 1964.

45. American Diabetes Association. *Direct and Indirect Costs of Diabetes in the United States in 1997.* Alexandria, VA: American Diabetes Association Report; 1998.

46. Himann JE. Age-related changes in speed of walking. *Med Sci Sports Exerc.* 1998; 44:161–165.

47. Palmoski MJ, Colyer RA, Brandt KD. Joint motion in the absence of normal loading does not maintain normal articular cartilage. *Arthritis Rheum.* 1985; 23:325.

48. Siegler IC, Costa PT, Jr. Health behavior relationships. In: Birren JE, Schaie KW, eds. *Handbook of the Psychology of Aging.* 2nd ed. New York: Van Nostrand Reinhold; 1985.

49. Kaplan E. Psychological factors and ischemic heart disease mortality: A focal role for perceived health. Paper presented at the annual meeting of the American Psychological Association, Washington, DC; 1999.

50. Mossey JM, Shapiro E. Self-rated health: A predictor of mortality among the elderly. *Am J Public Health.* 1982; 72:800–808.

51. Rosillo RA, Fagel ML. Correlation of psychologic variables and progress in physical therapy: I. Degree of disability and denial of illness. *Arch Phys Med Rehabil.* 1970; 51:227.

52. Stoedefalke KG. Motivating and sustaining the older adult in an exercise program. *Top Geriatr Rehabil.* 1985; 1:78.

53. Nader IM, et al. Level of aspiration and performance of chronic psychiatric patients on a simple motor task. *Percept Mot Skills.* 1985; 60:767.

54. Prohaska T, Pontiam IA, Teitleman J. Age differences in attributions to causality: Implications for intellection assessment. *Exp Aging Res.* 1984; 10: 1–11.

55. Eisdorfer L. Arousal and performance: Experiments in verbal learning and a tentative theory. In: Talland GA, ed. *Human Aging and Behavior.* New York: Academic Press; 1968.

56. Weinberg R, Bruya L, Jackson A. The effects of goal proximity and goal specificity on endurance performance. *J Soc Psychol.* 1985; 7:296.

57. Mento A, Steele RP, Karren RJ. A meta-analytic study of the effects of goal setting on task performance: 1966–1984. *Organ Behav Hum Decis Process.* 1987; 39:52.

58. Smith E, Serfass R. *Exercise and Aging: The Scientific Basis.* Hillside, NJ; Enslow Publishers; 1981.

59. Stelmach CE, Worringham CJ. Sensorimotor deficits related to postural stability: Implications for falling in the elderly. In: Radebaugh TS, et al., eds. *Clinics of Geriatric Medicine.* Philadelphia: WB Saunders; 1985: 1(3).

60. McPherson BD, ed. *Sport and Aging: The 1984 Olympic Scientific Congress Proceedings.* Champaign, IL: Human Kinetics Publishers; 1986: 5.

61. Seltzer B, Rheaume Y, Volicer L, et al. The short-term effects of in-hospital respite on the patient with Alzheimer's disease. *Gerontologist.* 1988; 28(1): 121–124.

62. Knott M, Voss DE. *Proprioceptive Neuromuscular Facilitation: Patterns of Techniques.* 2nd ed. New York: Harper and Row Publishers; 1968.

63. Darling RC. Fatigue. In: Downey JA, Darling RC, eds. *Physiological Basis of Rehabilitation Medicine.* Philadelphia: WB Saunders; 1971.

64. Kohl HW, Moorefield DL, Blair SN. Is cardiorespiratory fitness associated with general chronic fatigue in apparently healthy men and women? *Med Sci Sports Exerc.* 1987; 19(S6).

65. Ejaz F, Jones J, Rose M. Falls among nursing home residents: An examination of incident reports before

and after restraint reduction programs. *J Am Geriatr Soc.* 1994; 42(7):960–964.

66. OBRA '87. Omnibus Budget Reconciliation Act of 1987, Public Law 100-203. Washington DC: US Government Printing Office; 1987: 172.

67. Phillips C. Use of physical restraints. *Med Care.* 1996; 34(11).

68. HCFA. *State Operations Manual, Part II: Guidance to Surveyors for Long Term Care Facilities, Interpretive Guidelines.* 483.13(a); 2000.

69. Donius M, Rader J. Use of side rails: Rethinking a standard of practice. *J Gerontol Nurs.* 1994; 20(11): 23–27.

70. Cohen C. Old problem, different approach: Alternatives to physical restraints. *J Gerontol Nurs.* 1996; 22(2):23–29.

71. Stolley JM. Freeing your patients from restraints. *Am J Nursing.* 1995; 43(2):27–31.

72. Christiansen J, Juhl E, eds. The prevention of falls in later life. *Danish Med Bull.* 1987; 34(suppl)(4): 1–24.

73. Kalchthaler T, Bascon RA, Quintos V. Falls in the institutionalized elderly. *J Am Geriatr Soc.* 1978; 26:424.

74. Tinetti ME. Factors associated with serious injury during falls by ambulatory nursing home residents. *J Am Geriatr Soc.* 1987; 35:644.

75. Gryfe CI, Amies A, Ashley MJ. A longitudinal study of falls in an elderly population: I. Incidence and morbidity. *Age Ageing.* 1977; 6:201.

76. Wild D, Nayak US, Isaacs B. How dangerous are falls in old people at home? *Brit Med J.* 1981; 282:266.

77. Tideiksaar R. Fall prevention in the home. *Top Geriatr Rehabil.* 1987; 3(1):57–64.

78. Droller H. Falls among elderly people living at home. *Geriatrics.* 1955; 10:239–244.

79. Archea JC. Environmental factors associated with stair accidents by the elderly. *Clin Geriatr Med.* 1985; 1:555.

80. Ashley MJ, Gryfe CT, Aimes A. A longitudinal study of falls in an elderly population. II. Some circumstances of falling. *Age Ageing.* 1997; 30:211–217.

81. Louis M. Falls and their causes. *J Gerontol Nurs.* 1993; 33:142–148.

82. Lawrence MS. Strengthening the quadriceps: Progressively prolonged isometric tension method. *Phys Ther Rev.* 1956; 36:658.

83. Horak FB. Clinical measurement of posture control in adults. *Phys Ther.* 1987; 67(12):1881.

84. Bobath B. *Adult Hemiplegia: Evaluation and Treatment.* 2nd ed. London: Heineman Medical Books; 1978.

85. Woollacott MJ, Shumway-Cook A, Nashner L. Aging and posture control. *Int J Aging Hum Devel.* 1986; 23:97.

86. Shumway-Cook A, Horak FB. Assessing the influence of sensory interaction on balance. *Phys Ther.* 1986; 66(10):1548.

87. Stout RW. Falls and disorders of postural balance. *Age Ageing.* 1978; 7:134.

88. Carr JH, Shepard RB. *A Motor Relearning Program for Stroke.* 2nd ed. Rockville, MD: Aspen Publishers; 1987.

89. Gabell A. Falls in the elderly: Will dance reduce their incidence? *Human Movement Studies.* 1986; 12:119.

90. Bottomley JM. The use of T'ai Chi as a movement modality in orthopaedics. *Ortho Phys Ther Clinics North Am.* 2000; 9(3):361–373.

91. Wolf SL, Coogler C, Xu T. Exploring the basis for Tai Chi Chuan as a therapeutic exercise approach. *Arch Phys Med Rehabil.* 1997; 79:886–892.

92. Bottomley JM. Gait in later life. *Ortho Phys Ther Clinics North Am.* 2001; 10(1):131–149.

93. Tinetti ME, Liu WL, Claus EB. Predictors and prognosis of inability to get up after falls among elderly persons. *JAMA.* 1993; 269(1):65–70.

94. Alexander NB, Ulbrich J, Raheja A, Channer D. Rising from the floor in older adults. *J Am Geriatr Soc.* 1997; 45(5):564–569.

95. Tinetti ME, Richman D, Powell L. Falls efficacy as a measure of fear of falling. *J Gerontol.* 1993; 45(3): P239–P243.

96. Simpson JM, Salkin S. Are elderly people at risk of falling taught how to get up again? *Age Ageing.* 1993; 22(3):294–296.

97. Van Sant AF. Rising from a supine to erect stance: Description of adult movement and a developmental hypothesis. *Phys Ther.* 1988; 68(2):185–192.

98. Unrau K, Hanrahan SM, Pitetti KH. An exploratory study of righting reactions from a supine to standing position in adults with Down syndrome. *Phys Ther.* 1994; 74(12):1116–1124.

99. Ford-Smith CD, Van Sant AF. Age differences in movement patterns used to rise from a bed in subjects in the third through fifth decades of age. *Phys Ther.* 1993; 73(5):300–309.

100. Green L, Williams K. Differences in developmental movement patterns used by active versus sedentary middle-aged adults coming from a supine position to erect stance. *Phys Ther.* 1992; 72(8):560–568.

101. Government Document. *Alzheimer's Disease: Report of the Secretaries Task Force on Alzheimer's Disease.* Washington, DC: US Government Printing Office; 1999. Rockville, MD: US Department of Health and Human Services, Public Health Service, Alcohol, Drug Abuse, and Mental Health Administration. DHHS Pub. No. (ADM) 84–1323.

102. Government Document. *Alzheimer's Disease.* Washington, DC: US Government Printing Office; 1999. Joint hearing before the Subcommittee on Health

and Long-Term Care of the Select Committee on Aging and the Subcommittee on Energy and Commerce. House of Representatives, 105th Congress, first session.

103. Liebowitz B, Lawton MP, Waldman A. Evaluation: Designing for confused elderly people. *AIA Journal.* 1979; 2:59–61.

104. Weldon S, Yesavage JA. Behavioral improvement with relaxation training in senile dementia. *Clin Gerontol.* 1982; 1(1):45–49.

105. Cohen GD. The mental health professional and Alzheimer's patient. *Hosp Community Psychiatry.* 1984; 35(2):115–116, 122.

106. Reifler BV, Wu S. Managing families of the demented elderly. *J Fam Pract.* 1982; 14(6):1051–1056.

107. Lubinski R. Speech, language, and audiology programs in home health care agencies and nursing homes. In: Beasley DS, Davis GA, eds. *Aging: Communication Processes and Disorders.* New York: Grune & Stratton; 1981.

108. Andreasen MK. Making a safe environment by design. *J Gerontol Nurs.* 1985; 11(6):18–22.

109. Sharpe DT. *The Psychology of Color and Design.* Chicago: Nelson-Hall; 1974.

110. Hellebrandt FA. The senile dement in our midst: A look at the other side of the coin. *Gerontologist.* 1978; 18:67–70.

111. Lawton MP. Assessing the competence of older people. In: Kent D, Kastenbaum R, Sherwood S, eds. *Research Planning and Action for the Elderly.* New York: Behavioral Publications; 1972.

9

Patient Evaluation

Pearls

- The essential setting for evaluating an older person is a noncompeting environment that is well lit, has nonglare surfaces, is wheelchair accessible, and is color contrasted with low pile carpet or nonslip floors.
- The initial interview should focus on functional decrements and include questions on history, social support, and subjective findings.
- When physically assessing the aged, consider breaking up the initial evaluation into several visits.

- When assessing pain in the elderly, use additional pain tools, such as pain diagram, pain diaries, pain language tools, and general pain evaluations.
- The environment should be assessed for safety and optimal functioning because as older persons becomes frailer, they become more dependent on the environment.
- Psychosocial aspects of an older person may be awkward for the physical therapist to assess; however, using the straightforward approach will be easiest.

INTRODUCTION

Of all the elements of patient care, evaluation is the most crucial. A comprehensive evaluation provides the practitioner with all the necessary information for designing an appropriate program. Since older patients often present with complex problems because of multiple pathologies and the effects of aging, a thorough evaluation may be more difficult. Nevertheless, it is even more important to determine the exact nature of the problem. This chapter divides evaluation into seven main components: preparation, expectations, the interview, physical assessment, environmental assessment, psychosocial assessment, and functional assessment. Assessment will be covered briefly here in terms of the initial evaluation. For a more detailed account, please refer to Chapter 10.

PREPARATION

Setting

What background is essential for a good evaluation of older patients? A quiet noncompeting environment is important because there is a high probability that the patient will have some hearing loss,[1] and background noise will make it difficult for the patient to hear questions. In addition, many older persons suffer from vision loss. Therefore, examination areas should be well lit and nonglare. Therapists should provide enough room for movement, and doorways and room space should be large enough to be wheelchair accessible. The room should have a comfortable, sturdy, 18-inch (or higher) chair available.[1] Optimally, the bed or treatment table should be automatically adjustable for height. The floor should have a low pile carpet or a low gloss nonslippery floor. Finally, the colors in the room should be those that make the older person most at ease, such as reds, oranges, gold, and beige. These colors should also be contrasted to avoid visual misinterpretation.[2] This scenario is for a clinical setting; however, many evaluations are done in the home. In the home setting try to imitate this background as closely as possible.

Tools

Any general evaluation form can be sufficient for the initial evaluation visit; however, specific forms for functional, physical (orthopedic, neurological, and cardiopulmonary), environmental, and psychosocial assessment are helpful and often cue the clinician to ask appropriate questions. It should be noted that many of the functional evaluation forms listed in Chapter 10 can be given to the patient prior to the evaluation. Forms for different diagnoses can be used by the clinician to look for specific problems.

See CD for orthopedic, neurological, and cardiopulmonary forms.

Timing

When is the best time to do an evaluation? There are times during the day when people perform better. It would be impossible to schedule evaluations to fit each patient's peak performance; however, a thorough clinician should ask the patient when he or she performs the best and note it. Only one time is contraindicated for an initial evaluation, and that is immediately following a large meal.[3] This is due to the decrease in blood flow to the brain for one hour after a large meal, which is most apparent in older patients.[3] Therefore, it is not good to overtax the system by doing an evaluation immediately after a large meal.

EXPECTATIONS

A clinician unfamiliar with treating geriatric patients can expect different levels of performance from an older person in an initial evaluation as compared to a younger person. Clinical experience shows that the older patient cannot tolerate a similar history taking session as that of younger patients. Initial evaluation may need some modification, especially in the physical performance area. Robin McKenzie, for example, requests that his patients both extend and flex the trunk approximately ten times.[4] This type of repetition is too rigorous for most older persons. Physically, most older persons can tolerate one or two repetitions of a movement, and can tolerate rolling into different positions one to two times. For these reasons, a clinician may need to anticipate two sessions to complete a thorough evaluation.

INTERVIEW

Though a great deal of information can be collected from the interview process, much of it is not useful. Limiting responses and directing questions is the key to a successful interview.

A good way to start an interview is to ask the patient, "Why are you here to see me?" A good follow-up to this question is "What do you expect from physical therapy?" These two questions give the interviewer the main problem (usually in functional terms) and the patient's goals (again, in functional terms).

The next important piece of information is the relevant history. One way to get this information is to ask, "How did this happen?" Follow-up questions along this line are "Have you had anything similar to this before?" and "What do you think contributed to this?" To obtain additional medical history information that could impact the rehabili-

tation progress ask, "What other medical problems do you have that I need to know about?" or, "What other medical problems do you have that may affect your progress?"

Other important information that can easily be gathered in the initial interview is the patient's social support system. For example, a question like "Do you live alone?" followed by "Who is the main person that helps you when you are ill or having difficulties with any of your daily activities?" will give the clinician important insight into the patient's social support. Age, weight, and medication usage can all be asked in the initial interview.

The initial interview session can also be used to gather information on subjective areas. Pain assessments are the major subjective tests used by the geriatric therapist. When assessing pain in the elderly person the clinician should be aware of two different presentations of symptoms in the older patient from the younger. First, older people tend to underreport pain, and second, they are less sensitive to pain.[5,6] There are several pain ratings available for assessing pain in the elderly; some are better than others.

PHYSICAL ASSESSMENT

Physical assessment is probably the most important aspect of the physical therapist's time with a patient. Physical assessment will provide the therapist with both subjective and objective data from which to develop and monitor a treatment program.

See CD for sample forms for the orthopedic, neurological, and cardiopulmonary assessment.

The application of physical assessment tools in the geriatric patient is similar to younger patients except for the variables listed in the beginning of the chapter as well as the following:

1. The therapist should relate physical findings to function. For example, what is the patient unable to do with shoulder flexion limited to 90°?
2. An entire assessment may need to be broken up and conducted in several sessions. The older person may not have the endurance to complete an entire physical assessment.
3. Psychosocial components must be considered along with physical parameters (see subsequent section).
4. Pain can be a major component and should be assessed thoroughly in an older person (see next section).

Pain Assessment

Pain evaluation tools can be divided into four categories. The first includes general pain evaluation tools. (For example, asking a patient to rate his or her pain as severe, moderate, or mild.) Pain diagrams are the second type of pain evaluation tools. An example of a pain diagram is the visual analog scale, which is simply a 100 mm line with a label at top and bottom.[7] Figure 9.1 is an example of a visual analog scale. To use this scale, the older person simply marks the place that corresponds to his or her pain. The clinician then measures the distance from no pain to the mark. For example, on an initial evaluation a patient may have 67 mm of pain on the visual analog scale and two weeks later she marks her pain as 23 mm. However, pain diagrams pose potential problems for older patients. The tests require abstract thinking, and older persons do not tend to perform as well on tests of this nature.[6]

The third group of pain assessment tools are pain language tools. A good example of a pain language tool is the McGill-Melzak Pain Questionnaire.[8] This one-page questionnaire uses different pain descriptors to rank the person's pain. This particular test has been used with older populations; however, specific reliability and validity for this test and the older population has not been demonstrated.

The final type of pain tool is a pain diary, which is a running record of the person's pain. There are pros and cons for this tool. A pain diary can be useful, because it helps the patient focus and become aware of how pain affects is or her life.[9] A major drawback of it is that the patient often becomes too focused on his or her pain as a result.[10]

The interview process can provide a wealth of information for the clinician. According to Rothstein and associates, the information synthesizing process begins in the interview process, even before the clinician lays hands on the patient.[11]

Physical Assessment—How To

Once the interview session is over, the physical process begins. If a treatment session could be extended to four hours, it would be possible to evaluate every aspect of the person during the physical assessment session. In reality, though, treatment sessions often last less than an hour, and it becomes crucial that the clinician choose to assess the areas that may affect the problem. The other reason for focusing on the major problem area is that the older person may have limited stamina.[12]

Table 9.1 lists the more common problems among older people that a clinician should be aware of during an initial evaluation.[13]

ENVIRONMENTAL ASSESSMENT

Because there are so many changes that are common among the older population, environmental assessments may be necessary for the institution or the home.

> See CD for an environmental assessment form for the home and the institution. These forms can be used by the clinician, family, or patient.

Assessing the environment should not be taken lightly. Lawton's "environmental docility hypothesis" states that the proportion of the behavior attributable to the environment increases as the person's competence decreases.[14] In addition, the older person has diminished senses and, therefore, reacts less to the environment. This results in a cascade of internalization and a decrease in reality and function.[15] Some evidence shows that enriched environments can favorably affect older persons.[16,17]

The assessment of color and lighting is an extremely important aspect of the environmental evaluation. The use of appropriate color can minimize the adverse effects of sensory deprivation, enhance mood, and improve function.[18] Color usage follows several simple rules:

1. Increase lighting as much as possible (up to three times as much as for younger persons).[19]
2. Use matte surfaces. Avoid glare on any surface.

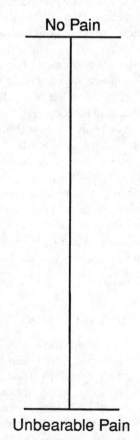

No Pain

Unbearable Pain

Figure 9.1   Visual analog scale.

3. Use contrasting colors as much as possible (that is, light and dark, different hues, cold and warm colors).

4. Use cues; however, make sure they are of adequate size and are clear and visible.

5. Use daylight fluorescent light. This light offers a broader distribution of light.[20]

TABLE 9.1   Problems more common or severe in the elderly

1. Falls
2. Syncope
3. Hip fracture
4. Urinary incontinence
5. Fecal incontinence
6. Fecal impaction
7. Pressure sores
8. Hearing and vision impairment
9. Stroke
10. Dementia syndrome
11. Parkinsonism
12. Normal pressure hydrocephalus
13. Polymyalgia rheumatica/giant cell arteritis
14. Osteoporosis
15. Osteoarthritis
16. Paget's disease
17. Carpal tunnel syndrome
18. Spinal stenosis
19. Diabetic hyperosmolar nonketotic coma
20. Inappropriate antidiuretic hormone secretion
21. Accidental hypothermia
22. Chronic lymphatic leukemia
23. Basal cell carcinoma
24. Angioimmunoblastic lymphadenopathy with dysproteinemia
25. Solid tumors
26. Tuberculosis
27. Herpes zoster
28. Arteriosclerosis
29. Amyloidosis
30. Colonic angiodysplasia
31. Isolated systolic hypertension
32. Postural hypotension

Reprinted with permission from Besdine, R.W. Clinical approach to the elderly. In: Rowe, J.W., Besdine, R.W. Geriatric Medicine. 2nd ed. Boston: Little Brown; 1988: Table 3–5:30.

PSYCHOSOCIAL ASSESSMENT

Specific psychosocial assessment forms are described in Chapters 4 and 10; therefore, this section will discuss when a psychosocial assessment is appropriate. The areas most important to the outcome of rehabilitation are depression and dementia. Depression is important because it will affect the participant's assessment and expectation of the rehabilitation program. The depressed client will have lower expectations and tend to underassess progress. In addition, depression can cause lethargy, which may discourage the client from participating in an exercise program.[21] Therefore, if the astute clinician senses depression from the global signs (e.g., pessimism, low self-esteem, loss of interest, and preoccupation with body aches), administering a depression test may be beneficial. The Geriatric Depression Scale is a good tool for assessing the older population. (See Chapters 4 and 10 for further discussion.) Once the clinician has determined that depression is a major problem, he or she should be aware that complaints of lethargy may only be a manifestation of depression. In addition, the clinician can also be on guard for subjective ratings of improvement or lack thereof.

Dementia, or brain syndromes, may also require special considerations in the rehabilitation program. If the clinician notices that the client has difficulty remembering during the initial questioning, then dementia may be the cause. Any of the brain syndrome screening tools may be administered at this time. If a patient does have a dementia, then the clinician must modify and simplify the treatment program so that the patient will derive the most benefit. Making the program more familiar, shorter, simpler, and more dependent on automatic responses will assist the patient with dementia. In addition, providing instruction to the care giver is crucial.

The final aspect of applying a psychological assessment is implementation. Many patients will resent being asked psychosocial questions in a physical therapy setting. A good approach is to say, "I am going to ask you a few questions that will measure mental processes. The questions may seem silly, but if we begin an exercise program that is too stressful for you, one of the first areas to show a change is your mental processing. Therefore, I need to get an initial assessment." Finally, as stated above, psychological assessments can be used to measure exercise tolerance.

FUNCTIONAL ASSESSMENT

Functional assessment is the most important part of the patient evaluation. Functional tools can be used in an initial evaluation (see Chapter 10 for various tools). Following the initial evaluation, an additional visit can be conducted for an in-depth functional evaluation. Medicare has a code (97750) for physical performance tests in the area of geriatrics, and these tests usually take more time than the initial evaluation.

- Walk 900 to 1000 feet
- While walking can carry a package averaging 6.7 pounds
- Walk two flights of stairs, across grass, and over obstacles (i.e., sticks)
- Achieve postural transitions
  - stop three times
  - reach forward, up, and down at least once
  - change directions four times
  - back up

Figure 9.2   Tasks that differentiated community-dwelling older adults with and without disability.

What should go into a comprehensive functional evaluation such as this? The answer to this question is limitless. Unlike the test for younger persons, there are a myriad of tests for older persons. Below is an example of what a functional capacity evaluation of an older person could look like and how it could be conducted, written up, and submitted. There is no one definitive test for function. What makes us the true functional experts is our professional judgment in choosing the best tests.

Shumway-Cook in 2002 identified tasks that are necessary to be independent as a community-dwelling older person.[22] See Figure 9.2. These are the goals that can be pursued in our rehabilitation efforts.

Is there one test that will pick up this information? The answer is no. However, a combination of tests and measures could provide this information. Even with this combination of tests, not all these variables can be addressed. The following functional tests measure most of these variables in a standardized fashion.

One combination could be as follows:

The Physical Performance Test[23]
The Multi-directional Reach Test[24]
The Two Minute Walk Test[25]
The Fukada Step Test[26]
A Balance test (choose one)
  Berg Balance Scale[27]
  Tinetti Balance Scale[28]
  Gait Abnormality Rating Scale[29]
  One Legged Stand Test[30]

Each of these tests takes 5 to 15 minutes to perform, which would require one hour of time. What would follow is a write-up of the results and copies of each of the tests with the interpretation. Suggestions for treatments and goals would be identified in the report.

This would be submitted to the payer within 48 hours of testing. In addition, persons could pay out of pocket. For example, a 50-year-old daughter might be concerned about her mother's independence and safety at home. She would be willing to pay for this test. This test could then be taken to the family physician to show the need for a rehabilitation intervention. Another avenue for reimbursement would be to submit four units of code 97750 to Medicare. In some areas of the country this test cannot be submitted with an initial evaluation or reevaluation code. A therapist may want to conduct this evaluation after two or three visits. A reassessment billed the same can be conducted and submitted one month later as the patient progresses.

Here is a sample test write-up. It is time for professionals to become the functional experts by using and packaging standard functional tools for patients.

Comprehensive Functional Assessment (CFA)   Date _____

Mrs. _____ was evaluated initially on _____. At that time she revealed deficits in many areas ranging from motion to strength to balance and gait. She was advised that a more comprehensive test of these areas could be conducted for additional comprehensive assessment of her problems. She agreed to these extensive tests.

Mrs. _____ received the following tests for her CFA:

1. The Timed Up and Go Test
2. The Physical Performance Test
3. The Berg Balance Scale
4. Dynamometry Testing of selective muscle groups

The Timed Up and Go Test
This test is used to evaluate mobility skills in older persons. This test incorporates functional components of sitting to standing, ambulation, turning, and standing to sitting. Three practice tests are done and averaged. Mrs. _____ average score was _____. Scoring for this test is as follows:

>30 seconds identifies people who are more dependent;
<10 seconds identifies people who are considered freely mobile; and 10 is the cutoff between fallers and nonfallers.

As you can see from Mrs. _____ score, she is _____.

The Physical Performance Test

This test measures several aspects of physical functioning of older people. There are nine items on this test unless the person will never need to encounter stairs. If stairs will never be an issue, then there are seven items that are scored on this test. The patient performs all the items while being observed and timed by the examiner. The total score is then calculated. There are several interpretations to this test. The total possible score on this test is 36 for the nine-item test and 28 for the seven-item test.

1. <15 is predictive of recurrent falls on the nine-item test.
2. On the nine-item test
   a. 32–36 not frail
   b. 25–32 mild frailty
   c. 17–24 moderate frailty
   d. <17 dependent
3. On the seven-item test
   a. Independence = 21–28
   b. Dependence = 3–15

As you can see from Mrs. _____ score of _____, she is _____.

The Berg Balance Scale (BBS)

This test is designed to measure balance in older adults and predict fallers. The test has 14 distinctive performance tasks that are evaluated as they are performed by the patient. The tasks are rated by the examiner on a 0 to 4 scale with a score of 4 equating to the highest level of performance. Scores below 45 indicate a risk of falling, and scores less than 36 bring the fall risk up to 100%.

Mrs. _____ scored _____ on the BBS. This indicates that she _____.

Comprehensive Muscle Dynamometry

In the past five years normative data have been published that provide comparative information on expected values for strength in representative muscle groups. This test is conducted by the examiner on one muscle representative of each muscle group. Below are the test results next to the normative values. There are no normative values for trunk stability, so a manual test is done.

1. Triceps L_____R_____ norms for age _____
2. Quadriceps L_____R_____ norms for age _____
3. Hip abduction L_____R_____ norms for age _____
4. Ankle Dorsiflexion L_____R_____ norms for age _____
5. Shoulder Flexion L_____R_____ Norms for age _____
6. Trunk Stability _____ Normal _____

From the information noted above, Mrs. _____ has the following deficits:
1. _____
2. _____
3. _____

Suggested

Plan _____

_____

_____

Attached are the copies of her tests.

Signed,

References

1. Cooper BA. Model of implementing color contrast in the environment of the elderly. *Am J Occup Ther.* 1985; 39:253–258.

2. Cristarella M. Visual functions of the elderly. *Am J Occup Ther.* 1977; 31:432–440.

3. Lipsitz L, Fullerton R. Post prandial blood pressure reduction in healthy elderly. *J Am Geriatr Soc.* 1986; 34(4):267–270.

4. McKenzie R. *The Lumbar Spine: Mechanical Diagnosis and Therapy.* Waikanee, New Zealand: Spinal Public; 1981.

5. Harkins S, Kiventis J, Price D. Pain and the elderly. In: Benedette C, et al., eds. *Advances in Pain Management in the Elderly.* New York: Raven Press; 1984.

6. Ferrel B. Pain management in the elderly. *J Am Geriatr Soc.* 1991; 36:64–73.

7. Lewis C. *Documentation: Physical Therapists Course in Successful Reimbursement.* Bethesda, MD: Professional Health Educators; 1987.

8. Melzak R. *The Puzzle of Pain.* New York: Basic Books; 1973.

9. Mannheimer J. *Clinical Transculaneous Nerve Stimulation.* Philadelphia: FA Davis; 1984.

10. Woodruff L. Pain and Aging. Paper presented at APTA June Conference; 1990.

11. Echternach J, Rothstein J. Hypothesis-oriented algorithms. *Phys Ther.* 1989; 69:559–564.

12. Haines RF. Effect of bed rest and exercise on body balance. *J Appl Physiol.* 1974; 36:323.

13. Besdine RW. Clinical approach to the elderly. In: Rowe JW, Besdine RW. *Geriatric Medicine.* 2nd ed. Boston: Little Brown; 1988.

14. Lawton MP. Assessment, integration and environments for older people. *Gerontologist.* 1970; 10: 38–46.

15. Kraus A, Spasoff R, Beattie E. Elderly applicants to long-term care institutions: Their characteristics, health problems and state of mind. *J Am Geriatr Soc.* 1976; 24(3):117–125.

16. Birren F. Human response to color and light. *Hospitals.* 1979; 53(14):93–96.

17. Whelihan W. Geriatric centers environment fosters interaction. *Hosp Prog.* 1980; 61:50–55.

18. Hiatt L. Care and design for color and use of color in environments for older persons. *Nursing Homes.* 1981; 30:18–22.

19. Corso J. Sensory processes and age effects in normal adults. *J Gerontol.* 1971; 26:90–105.

20. Sylvania GTE. Engineering Bulletin 0-341. Fluorescent Lamps. Montreal, Canada.

21. Zarit S. Aging and mental disorders. In: *A Psychological Approach to Assessment and Treatment.* New York: Free Press; 1980.

22. Shumway-Cook A Patla AE, Stewart A, Ferrucci L, Ciol MA, Guralnik JM. Environmental demands associated with community mobility in older adults with and without mobility disabilities. *Phys Ther.* 2002; 82(7):670–681.

23. Reuben DB, Siu AL. An objective measure of physical function of elderly outpatients: The physical performance test. *JAGS.* 1990; 38:1105–1112.

24. Newton RA. Validity of the multi-directional reach test: A practical measure for limits of stability in older adults. *Med Sci.* 2001; 56A(4):M248–M252.

25. Butland RJA, Pang J, Gross ER, Woodcock AA, Geddes DM. Two-, six-, and twelve-minute walking tests in respiratory disease. *Brit Med J.* 1982; 284: 1607–1608.

26. Fukuda T. *Statokinetic Reflexes in Equilibrium and Movement.* Tokyo: University of Tokyo Press; 1984.

27. Berg K, Wood-Dauphinee S, Williams JI, Gayton D. Measuring balance in the elderly: Preliminary development of an instrument. *Physiother Can.* 1989; 41(6):304–311.

28. Tinetti ME. Performance-oriented assessment of mobility problems in elderly patients. *J Am Geriatr Soc.* 1986; 34:119–126.

29. VanSwearingen JM, Paschal KA, Bonino P, Yang JF. The modified gait abnormality rating scale for recognizing the risk of recurrent falls in community-dwelling elderly adults. *Phys-Ther.* 1996; 76(9): 994–1001.

30. Vellas BJ, Wayne SJ, Romero L, Baumgartner RN, Garry PJ. One-leg balance is an important predictor of injurious falls in older persons. *J Am Geriatr Soc.* 1997; 45:735–738.

10

Functional Assessment

Pearls

- A sample tool for assessing cognitive changes in mental status of the elderly is the Mini-Mental State Examination (MMSE).
- The Geriatric Depression Scale is a useful tool for assessing depression in the elderly.
- The Holmes and Rahe Life Events Scale is one of the best known tools for assessing stress levels.
- Functional assessment is a method of measuring an individual's performance.
- Numerous functional assessment tools are available for evaluating older persons. Choose the tool best suited to the setting, clientele, mode of administration, and domain to be evaluated.

- Standard physical therapy measures, such as strength, range of motion, posture, and gait, change with age and may be better assessed with specific tools and norms designed for the elderly.
- Cardiopulmonary parameters, as well as nerve conduction velocity, change with age and require different normative values for assessment comparison.
- Assessing ethnicity of the elderly will help health professionals recognize bias and differences that may obstruct care.

INTRODUCTION

The demands in health care for cost-effective care are pushing rehabilitation and medical professionals to prove the efficacy and efficiency of the care provided. The obvious place for caregivers to begin this process is in the area of assessment. The evolution of medicine and rehabilitation has been a mixture of science, philosophy, sociology, and intuition. Some of the finest practitioners may be some of the worst scientists. However, they may have an extraordinary intuitive sense. Because of this fine mixture, it is difficult to quantify assessments, treatments, and outcomes. Nevertheless, this needs to be done. The work in health care assessment has grown exponentially in the last thirty years, and more tools are being developed and more scrutiny is being applied to treatment interventions and outcomes.

This chapter will discuss three important components of the physical therapist's assessment of the elderly. The first section will discuss mental status measures for older persons; the second will discuss the most common functional assessment tools for the elderly; and the third will discuss the modifications needed when assessing the older

person using accepted physical measures, such as goniometry, manual muscle tests, and nerve conduction velocity.

Each section will provide a detailed example tool and a CD reference for further information.

MENTAL STATUS MEASURES

Mini-Mental State Examination

The Mini-Mental State Examination (MMSE) was published in 1975 by Folstein[1] and it has been widely used since then to assess cognitive changes in older patients. The MMSE was developed to assess patients who have deficits in memory, language, or both. These deficits correlate to intellectual impairment that may indicate Alzheimer's disease. The test indicates impairment, though it does not make a diagnosis.[2] The MMSE correlates with Wechsler Intelligence Scales and the Wechsler Memory Test, as well as to cerebral lesions detected by CAT scan.[1,2]

The test is relatively easy to administer and takes between five and ten minutes. The test and its instructions for administration can be found in Figure 10.1.

Mini-Mental State Exam

Orientation:	Maximum Score	Score	Instructions
What is the (year) (season) (date) (day) (month)?	5	____	Ask for the date. Then proceed to ask other parts of the question. One point for each correct segment of the question.
Where are we: (state) (county) (town) (hospital) (floor)?	5	____	Ask for the facility then proceed to parts of the question. One point for each correct segment of the question.

Registration:			
Name three objects (bed, apple, shoe). Ask the patient to repeat them.	3	____	Name the objects slowly, one second for each. Ask him to repeat. Score by the number he is able to recall. Take time here for him to learn the series of objects, up to 6 trials, to use later for the memory test.

Attention and Calculation:			
Count backwards by 7s. Start with 100. Stop after 5 calculations.	5	____	Score the total number correct. (93, 86, 79, 72, 65)

Alternate question:			
Spell the word "world" backwards.	5	____	Score the number of letters in correct order. (dlrow = 5. dlorw = 3)

Recall:	Maximum Score	Score	Instructions
Ask for the three objects used in question 2 to be repeated.	3	____	Score one point for each correct answer. (bed, apple, shoe)

Language:			
1. Naming: Name this object. (watch, pencil)	2	____	Hold the object. Ask patient to name it. Score one point for each correct answer.
2. Repetition: Repeat the following– "No ifs, ands or buts."	1	____	Allow one trial only. Score one point for correct answer.
3. Follow a 3-stage command: "Take the paper in your right hand, fold it in half, and put it on the floor."	3	____	Use a blank sheet of paper. Score one point for each part correctly executed.
4. Reading: Read and obey the following: Close your eyes.	1	____	Instruction should be printed on a page. Allow patient to read it. Score by a correct response.
5. Writing: Write a sentence.	1	____	Provide paper and pencil. Allow patient to write any sentence. It must contain a noun, verb, and be sensible.
6. Copying: Copy this design.	1	____	All 10 angles must be present. Figures must intersect. Tremor and rotation are ignored.
	Total Score	____	(Max. 30) Test is not timed.

Figure 10.1   (Reprinted with permission from Folstein, M.F., Folstein, S.E., McHugh, P.R. Mini-mental state. A practical method for grading the cognitive state of patients for the clinician. *J Psychiatr Res.* 1975; 12:189–198.)

The maximum score possible on this test is 30. A score below 24 indicates cognitive impairment and is not considered normal for older persons. A score of 21 to 24 is considered mild intellectual impairment, a score of 16 to 20 reflects moderate impairment, and a score below 15 is considered severely impaired.[1] The MMSE also relates to depression and is indicative of depression at a score of 19. Patients show improvement on the MMSE scores as the depression is ameliorated.[3]

For Additional Tools on Mental Status, See CD.

Depression Scales

Despite the high prevalence of depression in the older population, the diagnosis of depression may be missed.[4] However, when screening instruments are used, the recognition of depression is increased.[5]

The Geriatric Depression Scale (GDS). One of the most used tools for depression is the GDS. This 30-item, yes-or-no questionnaire determines that a score of over 8 has a 90% sensitivity and an 80% specificity in detecting depression in the older population.[6] There is also a short version consisting of the following 15 questions: 1–4, 7, 9, 10, 12, 14, 15, 17, and 21–23. A score of over 5 on this form may indicate depression.[7] The test and the method of scoring are shown in Figure 10.2.

For more Tools on Depression, See CD.

Stress Measures

A final area of psychosocial assessment is stress.

The Holmes and Rahe Life Events Scale. The most widely used tool for evaluating stress is the Holmes and Rahe Life Events Scale.[8] This scale is shown in Figure 10.3. In administering this tool, the therapist asks the patient to circle the events that have occurred in the last year or will occur in the coming year. The therapist adds up the scores, and the total score is compared to the following scale. A score of below 180 points indicates mild stress or less than a 40% chance of a serious illness in the next year; a score of 180 to 300 indicates moderate stress or a 40% chance of developing a serious illness in the next year; and a score above 300 indicates severe stress or an 80% chance of a serious illness in the next year.[8]

Functional Assessment

The word "function" is repeated eighty-eight times in the current Center for Medicare and Medicaid Services (CMS) regulations on rehabilitation.[9] This fact should encourage rehabilitation professionals to think about and use functional measures, because CMS uses these regulations as requirements for payment.

Functional measurement is also important because it differs from the current methods physical therapists and occupational therapists use to assess patient status, and they may not truly reflect a patient's functional level. These measures, such as range of motion, strength, and other musculoskeletal parameters, may be important to assessment, but they do not always relate to function. If rehabilitation professionals are to show efficacy in what they do, it is important that they assess function in conjunction with musculoskeletal parameters. Combining these two assessments will make a truly comprehensive rehabilitation evaluation possible.

A recent study by Mary Tinetti scrutinizes the use of musculoskeletal measures.[10] Her study showed very little relationship between musculoskeletal measures and functional outcomes of older patients.[10]

A third factor contributing to the importance of functional evaluation is the ability to give a beginning and end point based on a functional outcome, as well as a relationship of this outcome to a patient's independence. For example, the Barthel Index (see Figure 10.4) can rate a patient's difficulty with bathing or walking. The patient's ability to perform these tasks is assigned a level that is indicated by a number. As the person progresses with treatment, he or she is moved to higher levels. If patients regress, they are ranked at a lower level. In addition, the total scoring on this index indicates to the assessor when the patient is able to go home or is in need of assistance.

These numbers translate to a patient's specific ability to function and can be very helpful in making decisions related to disposition and the need for continued care. On the other hand, a muscle strength measure indicating normal (5/5) muscle strength means nothing if the person cannot get in and out of a tub or eat independently. The combination of strength and function measures is extremely helpful, however, when assessing cause and outcome.

The purpose of this section is to encourage the health professional to avoid doing unnecessary and time-consuming tests. Many of these functional tests can be done by the patient with paper and pencil prior to the treatment program and on discharge without unnecessarily monopolizing the health professional's time.

A final justification of functional evaluation comes from an article written by Robert Kane, Dean of the School of Public Health at the University of Minnesota.[11] Dr Kane is a well-respected researcher in gerontology and health care and an advocate for functional assessment for geriatricians. In his article, he states that a specialty is not truly a specialty until it has its own instrument. He gave radiology as an example. This discipline would not have its current credibility or base if it were not for x-rays. Also, cardiology would not have evolved into a specialty if it

Geriatric Depression Scale

1. Are you basically satisfied with your life? (no)

2. Have you dropped many of your activities and interests? (yes)

3. Do you feel that your life is empty? (yes)

4. Do you often get bored? (yes)

5. Are you hopeful about the future? (no)

6. Are you bothered by thoughts that you just cannot get out of your head? (yes)

7. Are you in good spirits most of the time? (no)

8. Are you afraid that something bad is going to happen to you? (yes)

9. Do you feel happy most of the time? (no)

10. Do you often feel helpless? (yes)

11. Do you often get restless and fidgety? (yes)

12. Do you prefer to stay home at night, rather than go out and do new things? (yes)

13. Do you frequently worry about the future? (yes)

14. Do you feel that you have more problems with memory than most? (yes)

15. Do you think it is wonderful to be alive now? (no)

16. Do you often feel downhearted and blue? (yes)

17. Do you feel pretty worthless the way you are now? (yes)

18. Do you worry a lot about the past? (yes)

19. Do you find life very exciting? (no)

20. Is it hard for you to get started on new projects? (yes)

21. Do you feel full of energy? (no)

22. Do you feel that your situation is hopeless? (yes)

23. Do you think that most persons are better off than you are? (yes)

24. Do you frequently get upset over little things? (yes)

25. Do you frequently feel like crying? (yes)

26. Do you have trouble concentrating? (yes)

27. Do you enjoy getting up in the morning? (no)

28. Do you prefer to avoid social gatherings? (yes)

29. Is it easy for you to make decisions? (no)

30. Is your mind as clear as it used to be? (no)

Score one point for each response that matches the yes or no answer after the question.

Figure 10.2   Geriatric Depression Scale. (Adapted and reprinted with permission from Yesavage, J.A., Brink, T.L. Development and validation of a geriatric depression screening scale: A preliminary report. *J Psych Res.* 1983; 17:41.)

The Holmes and Rahe Social Adjustment Scale

Rank	Life Event	Mean Value
1	Death of spouse	100
2	Divorce	73
3	Marital separation	65
4	Jail term	63
5	Death of close family member	63
6	Personal injury or illness	53
7	Marriage	50
8	Fired at work	47
9	Marital reconciliation	45
10	Retirement	45
11	Change in health of family member	44
12	Pregnancy	40
13	Sex difficulties	39
14	Gain of new family member	39
15	Business readjustment	39
16	Change in financial state	38
17	Death of close friend	37
18	Change to different line of work	36
19	Change in number of arguments with spouse	35
20	Mortgage over $10,000	31
21	Foreclosure of mortgage or loan	30
22	Change in responsibilities at work	29
23	Son or daughter leaving home	29
24	Trouble with in-laws	29
25	Outstanding personal achievement	28
26	Wife begin or stop work	26
27	Begin or end school	26
28	Change in living conditions	25
29	Revision of personal habits	24
30	Trouble with boss	23
31	Change in work hours or conditions	20
32	Change in residence	20
33	Change in schools	20
34	Change in recreation	19
35	Change in church activities	19
36	Change in social activities	18
37	Mortgage or loan less than $10,000	17
38	Change in sleeping habits	16
39	Change in number of family get-togethers	15
40	Change in eating habits	15
41	Vacation	13
42	Christmas	12
43	Minor violations of the law	11

Figure 10.3   The Holmes and Rahe Social Adjustment Scale. (Reprinted with permission from Holmes, T., Rahe, R. The social readjustment rating scale. *J Psychosom Res.* 1967; 11:213–218.)

Barthel Index

The following presents the items or tasks scored in the Barthel Index with the corresponding values for independent performance of the tasks:

	"Can do by myself"	"Can do with help of someone else"	"Cannot do at all"
Self-Care Index			
1. Drinking from a cup	4	0	0
2. Eating	6	0	0
3. Dressing upper body	5	4	0
4. Dressing lower body	7	4	0
5. Putting on brace or artificial limb	0	2	0 (Not applicable)
6. Grooming	5	0	0
7. Washing or bathing	6	0	0
8. Controlling urination	10	5 (Accidents)	0 (Incontinent)
9. Controlling bowel movements	10	5 (Accidents)	0 (Incontinent)
Mobility Index			
10. Getting in and out of chair	15	7	0
11. Getting on and off toilet	6	3	0
12. Getting in and out of tub or shower	1	0	0
13. Walking 50 yards on the level	15	10	0
14. Walking up/down 1 flight of stairs	10	5	0
15. If not walking: propelling or pushing wheelchair	5	0	0 (Not applicable)

Barthel Total: Best score is 100; worst score is 0.

NOTE: Tasks 1–9, the Self-Care Index (including control of bladder and bowel sphincters), have a total possible score of 53. Tasks 10–15, the Mobility Index, have a total possible score of 47. The 2 groups of tasks combined make up the total Barthel Index with a total possible score of 100.

Figure 10.4   Barthel Index. (Reprinted with permission from Mahoney, F.I., Barthel, D.W. Functional evaluation: The Barthel Index. *Md Med J.* 1965; 14(2):61–65.)

were not for heart catheterization. He then asserts that geriatrics will truly not be accepted as a specialty until the professionals in that area have a similar tool. He believes that the tool for geriatrics is functional assessment.[11]

By extrapolating on his thoughts, it can be seen that rehabilitation is an area where functional assessment is a tool, especially for rehabilitation professionals in the area of geriatrics. The following sections follow this argument and advocate functional assessment for rehabilitation professionals, particularly for those working in geriatrics.

What Is Functional Assessment?

Functional assessment differs from traditional assessment in several ways. For example, it targets specific behaviors and tasks a patient wishes to accomplish. If a therapist were to ask a patient, "What do you want from physical therapy?" the patient would not say, "I want my muscles to test normal or 5/5." Rather, he or she would answer, "I want to increase the strength in my legs," or "I want to run 10 miles pain free." These responses are rarely indicated in rehabilitation notes or incorporated into work goals. Instead, many notes state that the goal of treatment is to increase strength or function. This is not enough. A goal stated in slightly more specific functional terms is, "Increase strength so that the patient is able to run a marathon without pain," or "the patient is able to walk from bed to bathroom unassisted, without falling or losing balance." An even better functional statement would be a quantified response, such as "The patient scores 80 on the Barthel and can return home independently."

Richard Bohannon and colleagues, in an article in the *International Journal of Rehabilitation Research*, showed that the number-one priority when rehabilitating stroke patients is the patient walking independently.[12] Physical therapists may forget this when implementing various measures and techniques. Therefore, if the focus is on function, therapists will not lose sight of patients' needs.

The goal of rehabilitation is to assist people in achieving their highest level of function, but confusion often interferes with this. Instead of focusing on the goal, therapists focus on the signs and symptoms. When measuring and treating range of motion, strength, or endurance, the goal of function must be maintained. The second area of confusion and poor implementation of function is the use of function to mean different things (for example, the function of a knee or a hip). Instead, function must be examined in terms of the whole individual[13] and, more specifically, how that person functions versus how his or her shoulder functions.

If function is defined as the normal or characteristic performance of the individual,[14] the individual is the unit of analysis rather than the body part or organ system. It is not just a shoulder or a kidney that is being studied, it is a whole person. Can the patient reach up into the cabinet even if she has a rotator cuff tear, and does she need to? Is

there some modification that she should be taught to adapt to her environment?

Understanding function includes more than understanding physical function, because there are four components of function.[15] The first is physical function, which is the component that physical therapists work with the most. This subsection of function includes sensory motor performance, walking, climbing stairs, and other activities of daily living. The second component is mental function, including intelligence, cognitive ability, and memory. The third is emotional function defined as coping with life's stressors, anxieties, and satisfactions. The fourth is social function. This area looks at a person's interaction with family members and the community, and any economic considerations. A good reference for functional assessment tools in older persons is Kane and Kane's *Assessing the Elderly*.[13] The next section will give an example of a functional tool.

Other functional assessment tools can be found on the CD.

Functional Assessment Tools

The Barthel Index.   The Barthel Index is one of the most widely known and well-established physical functional parameters assessment tools.[16] It measures toileting, bathing, and ambulation (Figure 10.4).[16] On the Barthel Index, the best score is 100 and the worst is 0. Tasks 1 through 9 have a possible score of 53, and tasks 10 through 15 have a possible score of 47, for a total possible score of 100.

Exploring a few items on this index will demonstrate how it is scored. If a patient can drink from a cup independently, the patient gets 4 points. If, however, the patient needs someone's help or cannot do it at all, he or she gets 0. The reason this scoring mechanism seems strange is because it is a weighted scale. Weighted scales were developed to correlate with other measures. In a weighted scale, the accomplishment of one item may be more important to a specific measure and is, therefore, scored higher than others. Because of this weighing, it is imperative to use the numbers shown on the tool.

To administer this test, give a patient the form without the numbers, and allow the patient to check the appropriate column. Later, the scorer can add up the numbers. This test is more reliable, however, if a health professional assesses and grades each task as the patient performs it.[16]

What do the numbers mean? The test reflects the patient's ability to perform activities of daily living (ADLs) without an attendant.[16] It correlates well with clinical judgment and mortality, as well as with discharge to a less restrictive environment.[16] A score of 60 or above means that a person can be discharged home but will require at least two hours of assistance in ADLs. If the person scores

TABLE 10.1 Procedure for Functional Assessment Screening in the Elderly

Target Area	Assessment Procedure	Abnormal Result	Suggested Intervention
Vision	Test each eye with Jaeger card while patient wears corrective lenses (if applicable)	Inability to read greater than 20/40	Refer to ophthalmologist
Hearing	Whisper a short, easily answered question, such as "What is your name?" in each ear while the examiner's face is out of direct view	Inability to answer question	Examine auditory canals for cerumen and clean if necessary. Repeat test; if still abnormal in either ear, refer for audiometry and possible prosthesis
Arm	Proximal: "Touch the back of your head with both hands" Distal: "Pick up the spoon"	Inability to do task	Examine the arm fully (muscle, joint, and nerve), paying attention to pain, weakness, limited range of motion. Consider referral for physical therapy
Leg	Observe the patient after asking: "Rise from your chair, walk ten feet, return, sit down"	Inability to walk or transfer out of chair	Do full neurologic and musculoskeletal evaluation, paying attention to strength, pain, range of motion, balance, and traditional assessment of gait. Consider referral for physical therapy
Urinary incontinence	Ask: "Do you ever lose your urine and get wet?"	Yes	Ascertain frequency and amount. Search for remediable causes including local irritations, polyuric states, and medications. Consider urologic referral
Nutrition	Weigh the patient. Measure height	Weight is below acceptable range for height	Do appropriate medical evaluation
Mental status	Instruct: "I am going to name three objects (pencil, truck, book). I will ask you to repeat their names now and then again a few minutes from now." [See text discussion.]	Inability to recall all three objects after 1 minute	Administer Folstein Mini-Mental Status Examination. If score is <24, search for causes of cognitive impairment. Ascertain onset, duration, and fluctuation of overt symptoms. Review medications. Assess consciousness and affect. Do appropriate laboratory tests
Depression	Ask: "Do you often feel sad or depressed?"	Yes	Administer Geriatric Depression Scale. If positive (normal score, 0 to 10), check for antihypertensive, psychotropic, or other pertinent medications. Consider appropriate pharmaceutical or psychiatric treatment
ADL-IADL[a]	Ask: "Can you get out of bed yourself?"; "Can you dress yourself?"; "Can you make your own meals?"; "Can you do your own shopping?"	No to any question	Corroborate responses with patient's appearance; question family members if accuracy is uncertain. Determine reasons for the inability (motivation compared withphysical limitation). Institute appropriate medical, social, or environmental interventions
Home environment	Ask: "Do you have trouble with stairs inside or outside of your home?"; ask about potential hazards inside the home with bathtubs, rugs, or lighting	Yes	Evaluate home safety and institute appropriate countermeasures
Social support	Ask: "Who would be able to help you in case of illness or emergency?"	. . .	List identified persons in the medical record. Become familiar with available resources for the elderly in the community

[a]ADL-IADL: activities of daily living-instrumental activities of daily living.
Reproduced with permission from Lachs, M., Feinstein, A., Cooney, L., et al. A simple procedure for general screening for functional disability in elderly patients. Ann Intern Med. 1990; 112:699–704.

80 or above, it means that he or she can be discharged home but will require assistance of up to two hours in self-care. When working with a patient who has been assessed as independent in self-care and scores a 50 on the Barthel Index, this would indicate the contrary.

The final question to be answered is when should various tools be used. The most efficient way to use these tools is to have a goal in mind for its use, such as to establish a baseline to show improvement, to screen for problems, to set rehabilitation goals, or to monitor the patient's progress.[17]

The medical community in general is developing a keen interest in functional assessment. Lachs and Williams, in the *Annals of Internal Medicine*, urge general practitioners to use functional assessments.[17,18] In addition, this article specifically delineates physical therapy as an appropriate referral once functional deficits are noted. Table 10.1 is a procedural chart on functional assessment from Lachs work.[18]

Therapists in geriatrics must get involved in functionally assessing patients not only for the efficacious assessment potential but also for continuity of care from medical peers.

MODIFIED PHYSICAL THERAPY MEASURES

Musculoskeletal Parameters

Strength. It is widely accepted that strength decreases with age. However, no studies exist to date that show a difference in the strength decline with age using simple

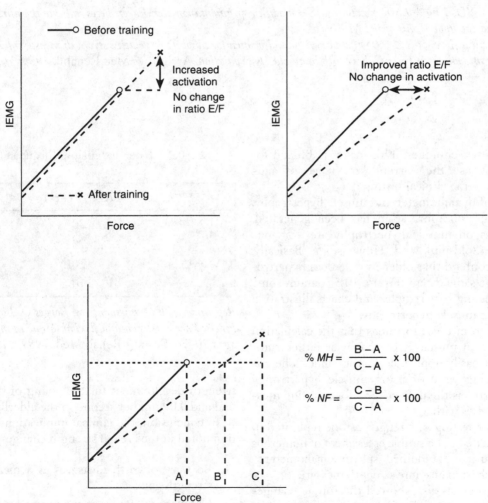

$$\% \ MH = \frac{B - A}{C - A} \times 100$$

$$\% \ NF = \frac{C - B}{C - A} \times 100$$

Figure 10.5   Hypertrophy in older men. **A.** Strength gain due to neural factors. **B.** Strength gain due to hypertrophy. **C.** Evaluation of percentage contributions of neural factors (NF) vs. hypertrophy (MH). (Reprinted with permission from Moritani, T., Devries, H.A. Potential for gross muscle hypertrophy in older men. *J Gerontology.* 1980; 35(5):673.)

TABLE 10.2   Absolute and Relative Strength Measurements

Muscle Groups	Men Strength (kg)	Men Strength/Body Weight (kg/kg)	n	Women Strength (kg)	Women Strength/Body Weight (kg/kg)	n
Shoulder abductors	12.4 ± 5.0[a]	0.17 ± 0.07	37	9.3 ± 3.3	0.15 ± 0.05	81
Shoulder flexors	12.7 ± 5.0[a]	0.17 ± 0.07	37	9.3 ± 3.4	0.14 ± 0.05	81
Elbow extensors	14.9 ± 4.6[a]	0.20 ± 0.06	37	11.2 ± 3.3	0.19 ± 0.06	81
Elbow flexors	15.2 ± 5.1[a]	0.21 ± 0.07	37	10.9 ± 3.9	0.18 ± 0.06	81
Hip extensors	14.4 ± 5.8[a]	0.19 ± 0.08	31 (2)	11.6 ± 4.0	0.19 ± 0.06	69 (1)
Hip flexors	16.2 ± 6.7[a]	0.23 ± 0.09	31 (2)	10.8 ± 3.3	0.18 ± 0.06	74 (1)
Knee extensors	19.1 ± 5.7[a]	0.27 ± 0.09	31 (5)	16.7 ± 4.8	0.28 ± 0.08	77 (2)
Dorsiflexors	15.1 ± 4.5[a]	0.21 ± 0.07	37	12.6 ± 4.1	0.21 ± 0.06	79
MS grip	23.2 ± 4.4	0.33 ± 0.08	20 (17)	20.1 ± 5.7	0.31 ± 0.09	74 (7)
Dynamometer grip	30.8 ± 6.6[a]	0.43 ± 0.1[a]	37	21.6 ± 6.1	0.36 ± 0.08	64

Values are means ± SD, 1 kg = 9.806 newtons. MS = modified spygmomanometer. Parentheses indicate the number of measurements that exceeded the upper limit of the MS.
[a] *Indicates significant difference (p ≤ 0.05) between men and women for absolute or relative strength measurements.*
Reprinted with permission from Rice, C. Strength in an elderly population. Arch Phys Med Rehabil. 1989; 70:391–397.

manual muscle test techniques. This makes it difficult for a practitioner to use the current knowledge of age's strength changes in the clinical setting.

In the realm of dynamometer and muscle hypertrophy, some clinically useful information has been generated. The best sources on muscle hypertrophy are Tomanek and Woo, and Goldspink and Howells.[19,20] Basically, these resources contend that older muscle does hypertrophy but not to the same extent. Figure 10.5 contains some formulas for assessing hypertrophy and charts illustrating the comparison in muscle hypertrophy.[21]

It is apparent from these formulas that the calculation for the difference in muscle hypertrophy is rather cumbersome and not easily applicable in the clinic. The authors suggest being wary of using muscle hypertrophy measures (i.e., girth) as the only criteria for assessing muscle strength increases with age.

Dynanomomter testing of strength can be replicated in the clinic. Rice carried out a simple assessment of numerous joints' strength using a modified sphygmomanometer.[22] Table 10.2 is his chart of absolute strength measures.[22]

Borges and associates also showed the torque changes with age in the knee using the Cybex dynamometer (see Table 10.3).[23]

Finally, Vandervoort and Hayes found a 71% decrease in plantarflexor muscle isometric strength in the elderly as compared with the young.[24] This study was done on both young and old healthy women.[25] Their findings revealed

TABLE 10.3   Knee Extension Torque at 90 Degrees Per Second

	Age (Years)	Torque
MEN	20	122
	70	78
WOMEN	20	68
	70	38

Reprinted with permission from Borges O. Isometric and isokinetic knee extension and flexion torque in men and women aged 20–70. Scand J Rehab Med. 1989; 21:45–53.

strength development for the young of 0.16 nm per second and 0.09 nm per second in the elderly group.

In conclusion, the clinical implications of the information noted in the area of strength changes with age are

1. Be wary of girth measures as a means of reflecting strength gains.
2. Compare outcomes to the norms noted. For example, compare knee extension torques to Borges's measures versus measures of torque on younger persons.
3. Compare strength measures to Rice's norms versus the classic manual muscle test for more comparable findings.

TABLE 10.4   Upper and Lower Limb Range of Motion Mean Values and Standard Deviations for Age Groups Combined by Sex and for Sexes Combined[a] (Ages 60–84)

Upper Limb Motion	Men (age groups combined)		Women (age groups combined)		Diff. Between		Sexes Combined	
	$\overline{X}$	s	$\overline{X}$	s	M/W	p^b	$\overline{X}$	s
Shoulder abduction	155	22	175	16	−20[c]	<0.001	165	21
flexion	160	11	169	9	−9	<0.001	165	11
extension	38	11	49	13	−11[c]	<0.001	44	13
medial rotation	59	16	66	13	−7	NS	62	15
lateral rotation	76	13	85	16	−9	0.02	81	15
Elbow beginning flexion	6	5[d]	1	3	−5[d]	<0.001	4	5
flexion	139	14	148	5	−9	0.002	143	11
Radioulnar pronation	68	9	73	12	−5	NS	71	11
supination	83	11	65	11	+18	<0.001	74	14
Wrist flexion	62	12	65	8	−3	NS	64	10
extension	61	6	65	10	−4	0.05	63	9
radial deviation	20	6	17	6	+3	NS	19	6
ulnar deviation	28	7	23	7	+5	0.01	26	7
Hip beginning flexion	11	3	11	5	0	NS	11	4
flexion	110	11	111	12	−1	NS	111	11
abduction	23	9	24	6	−1	NS	23	7
adduction	18	4	11	4	+7	<0.001	14	5
medial rotation	22	6	36	7	−14[c]	<0.001	29	10
lateral rotation	32	6	30	7	+2	NS	31	7
Knee beginning flexion	2	2	0	1	+2	<0.001	1	2
flexion	131	4	135	7	−4	0.01	133	6
Ankle plantar flexion	29	7	40	6	−11[c]	<0.001	34	8
dorsiflexion	9	5	10	5	−1	NS	10	5
Subtalar inversion	31	11	29	10	+2	NS	30	10
eversion	13	6	12	5	+1	NS	12	6
First metatarsophalangeal								
beginning flexion	3	7	1	4	+2	NS	2	5
extension	62	17	59	8	+3	NS	61	17
flexion	5	7	8	16	−3	NS	6	8

[a]*All values reported in integers.*
[b]*Univariate* t *tests,* df *= 1, 58 (*t *values can be obtained from any statistical text with table of critical values for* t *distribution).*
[c]*Difference > intertester error.*
[d]*One man deleted because of the presence of pathologically restricted ROM,* n *= 29.*
Reprinted with permission from Walker, J., Sue, D., Miles-Elkousy, N., Ford, G., Trevelyan, H.: Active mobility of the extremities in older subjects. Phys Ther. 1984; 64(6):919–923. Reprinted with permission of the American Physical Therapy Association.

Range of Motion. The literature on range-of-motion norms is still somewhat controversial. For example, Walker et al. showed no significant differences in range of motion in 28 joints of young and old subjects[25] (Table 10.4).

Frekany and Leslie showed that even if an older group did have motion limitation, it could be normalized with appropriate stretching exercises.[26] James and Parker give probably the most comprehensive and recent reference on joint range-of-motion norms of the lower extremity[27] (Figure 10.6).

Information also exists on upper extremity and spinal norms for range of motion. These are listed in chart form in Tables 10.5 through 10.8. These findings, even though controversial, can assist the therapist to set more appropriate goals. If, for example, as was stated in Bassey's chart, the norms for shoulder flexion are 129, then a goal of 170 is inappropriate. Keeping these charts for review can help to design appropriate programs.

Postural Changes with Age. Posture changes with age. Perfect posture demonstrates a plumb line that bisects the ear, just anterior to the acromion process, through the greater trochanter, just posterior to the patella and just anterior to the lateral malleolus (see Figure 10.7).[28]

Changes in posture with age include[28]

1. Forward head.
2. Rounded shoulders.
3. Change in lordotic curve (either flatter or more curved).
4. Increased hip flexion.
5. Increased knee flexion.

Standard means of assessing posture are acceptable for older persons. The clinician must be sure to align the plumb line from the malleoli and up; otherwise a false alignment will be noted.

A good tool for rating and screening posture is the REEDCO Posture Score Sheet (see Figure 10.8). This evaluation tool is self-explanatory, and it is not singular to older persons. It can be used on young and old to provide

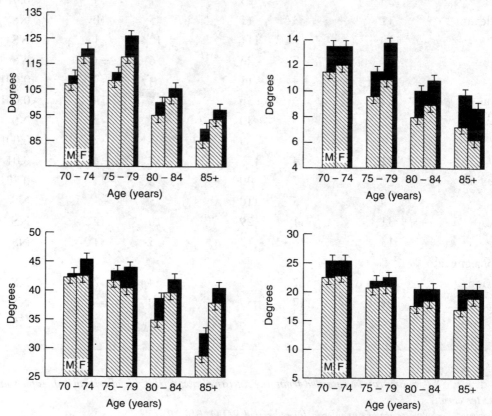

Figure 10.6 Lower extremity range of motion. **A.** Knee flexion. **B.** Ankle dorsi-
flexion (knee extended). **C.** Ankle plantar flexion (knee extended).
D. Ankle dorsiflexion (knee flexed). (Reprinted with permission from
James, B., Parker, A. Active and passive mobility of lower limb joints in
elderly men and women. Lower extremity range of motion. *Am J Phys
Med Rehabil.* 1989; 68(4):162–167.)

TABLE 10.5   Spinal Range of Motion: Means and Standard Deviations in 10-Year Intervals for Lumbar Range of Motion

	Shöber (cm)				Extension (°)				R Lat Flexion (°)				L Lat Flexion (°)			
	$\overline{X}$	s	CV	n^a	$\overline{X}$	s	CV	n	$\overline{X}$	s	CV	n	$\overline{X}$	s	CV	n
20–29	3.7	0.72	19.5	31	41.2	9.6	23.3	31	37.8	5.8	15.4	31	38.7	5.7	14.7	31
30–39	3.9	1.00	25.6	42	40.0	8.8	22.0	44	35.3	6.5	18.4	44	36.5	6.0	16.4	44
40–49	3.1	0.81	26.1	16	31.1	8.9	28.6	16	27.1	6.5	24.0	16	28.5	5.2	18.2	16
50–59	3.0	1.10	36.7	43	27.4	8.0	29.2	43	25.3	6.2	24.5	44	26.8	6.4	23.9	44
60–69	2.4	0.74	30.8	26	17.4	7.5	43.1	27	20.2	4.8	23.8	27	20.3	5.3	26.1	27
70–79	2.2	0.69	31.4	9	16.6	8.8	53.0	10	18.0	4.7	26.1	10	18.9	6.0	31.7	10

[a]Different "n's" appear in some age groups because of the difficulty in measuring patients with various medical conditions (e.g., rash).
Reprinted with permission from Fitzgerald, G.K., Wynveen, K.J., Rheault, W., Rothschild, B. Objective assessment with establishment of normal values for lumbar spinal range of motion. Phys Ther. *November 1983; 63(11):1778. Reprinted with permission of the American Physical Therapy Association.*

a quantitative approach to posture analysis. Since posture can be an important variable in movement, balance, and gait of older persons, it is imperative that the clinician assess it as objectively as possible.[29]

Gait Assessment

Gait changes with age are as variable as many of the other characteristics listed in this section are. What will be given here are norms or averages.

To begin the examination of the gait cycle, motion will be discussed. The first place that a change is noted in the old versus the young is in the preswing phase. Older persons show 5° less motion in plantarflexion when compared to young (i.e., 15° as compared to 20°).[30] The knee range of motion shows no difference. However, the hip exhibits 5° more flexion (i.e., 35° versus 30° in the younger population).[31] Gait velocity is also less in older persons. Average velocity in the young is 82.6 m/min, and it is 78.6 m/min in the 60 to 87 age range.[32] Stride length is also shorter in the older population. Healthy older persons have a stride length of 1.39 m and younger persons have an average stride length of 1.5 m.[33]

All of the changes noted are the only significant differences noted in healthy older persons. If other pathological factors are taken into consideration, then other gait abnormalities will be noted.

Gait Assessment.   Two tools are particularly good for assessing gait in older persons. The first tool is the Tinetti Gait and Balance Tests. Here are pages directly taken from the Functional Toolbox (Figure 10.9).[38] These pages show the tools parameters (population, description, mode of administration, time considerations, scoring mechanism, interpretation, reliability, validity, and additional references).

TABLE 10.6   Spinal/Neck Range of Motion

	Age		
	10	*30*	*80*
Flexion	35°	30°	27°
Lateral Flexion	63°	50°	30°
Extension	60°	50°	35°
Rotation	165°	150°	130°

Reprinted with permission from Lind, B., et al. Normal range of motion of the cervical spine. Arch Phys Med Rehab. *September 1989; 70:692–695.*

TABLE 10.7   Shoulder Flexion Range of Motion

Age	Male	Female
65–74 years old	129°	124°
75+ years old	121°	114°

Reprinted with permission from Bassey, E., et al. Flexibility of the shoulder joint measured as range of abduction in a large representative sample of men and women over 65 years of age. Eur J Appl Physiology. *1989; 58:353–360.*

TABLE 10.8   Shoulder Range of Motion

60–74 years old
Flexion: 159°
Abduction: 159°
75+ years old
Flexion: 159°
Abduction: 154°

Reprinted with permission from Boyle, S. Geriatric shoulder range of motion. Master's thesis. Philadelphia: University of Pennsylvania, February 1989.

Gait Abnormality Scale   Another excellent tool is the Gait Abnormality Rating Scale (GARS) by Wolfson and associates.[34] This tool was developed to detect fallers. It is, however, an excellent tool for quantifying aspects of gait patterns for older persons (see Table 10.9).

The GARS is quite easy to score. The patient is given the corresponding numerical value to each item listed, and the scores are added to get the individual's GARS score. Wolfson and co-workers found that persons scoring higher than 18 were more likely to fall. Not only is this a good tool for assessing gait, it also can be used to predict patients who are more vulnerable to falling.[34]

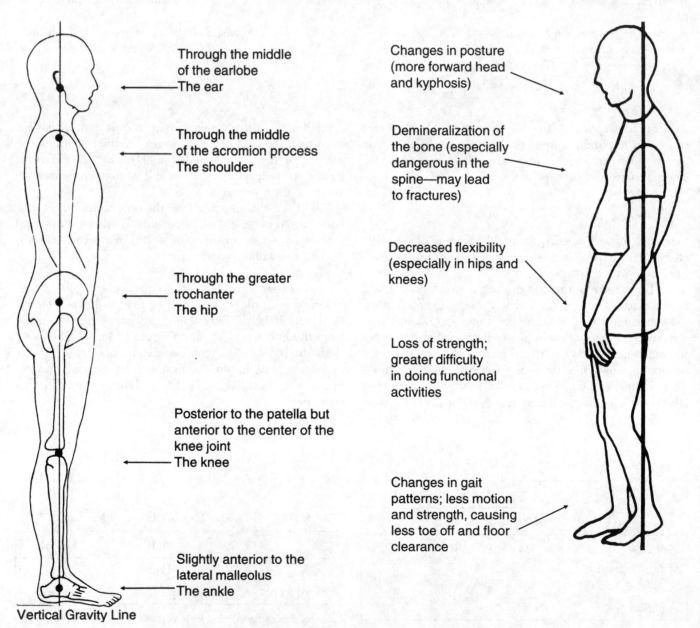

Figure 10.7   Posture changes with age. (Reprinted with permission from Lewis, C., Musculoskeletal changes with age. In: Lewis, C., ed. *Aging: The Health Care Challenge.* Philadelphia: FA Davis; 1990.)

POSTURE SCORE SHEET	Name _____			SCORING DATES			
	GOOD - 10	FAIR - 5	POOR - 0				
HEAD LEFT RIGHT	HEAD ERECT GRAVITY LINE PASSES DIRECTLY THROUGH CENTER	HEAD TWISTED OR TURNED TO ONE SIDE SLIGHTLY	HEAD TWISTED OR TURNED TO ONE SIDE MARKEDLY				
SHOULDERS LEFT RIGHT	SHOULDERS LEVEL (HORIZONTALLY)	ONE SHOULDER SLIGHTLY HIGHER THAN OTHER	ONE SHOULDER MARKEDLY HIGHER THAN OTHER				
SPINE LEFT RIGHT	SPINE STRAIGHT	SPINE SLIGHTLY CURVED LATERALLY	SPINE MARKEDLY CURVED LATERALLY				
HIPS LEFT RIGHT	HIPS LEVEL (HORIZONTALLY)	ONE HIP SLIGHTLY HIGHER	ONE HIP MARKEDLY HIGHER				
ANKLES	FEET POINTED STRAIGHT AHEAD	FEET POINTED OUT	FEET POINTED OUT MARKEDLY ANKLES SAG IN (PRONATION)				
NECK	NECK ERECT, CHIN IN, HEAD IN BALANCE DIRECTLY ABOVE SHOULDERS	NECK SLIGHTLY FORWARD, CHIN SLIGHTLY OUT	NECK MARKEDLY FORWARD, CHIN MARKEDLY OUT				
UPPER BACK	UPPER BACK NORMALLY ROUNDED	UPPER BACK SLIGHTLY MORE ROUNDED	UPPER BACK MARKEDLY ROUNDED				
TRUNK	TRUNK ERECT	TRUNK INCLINED TO REAR SLIGHTLY	TRUNK INCLINED TO REAR MARKEDLY				
ABDOMEN	ABDOMEN FLAT	ABDOMEN PROTRUDING	ABDOMEN PROTRUDING AND SAGGING				
LOWER BACK	LOWER BACK NORMALLY CURVED	LOWER BACK SLIGHTLY HOLLOW	LOWER BACK MARKEDLY HOLLOW				
			TOTAL SCORES				

Figure 10.8   Posture score sheet. (From REEDCO, Auburn, NY. Copyright 1974. Reprinted with permission.)

TINETTI ASSESSMENT TOOL

Balance Tests

Initial Instructions: Subject is seated in hard, armless chair. The following maneuvers are tested.

1. Sitting balance

Leans or slides in chair	= 0
Steady, safe	= 1 _____

2. Arises

Unable without help	= 0
Able, uses arms to help	= 1
Able without using arms	= 2 _____

3. Attempts to arise

Unable without help	= 0
Able, requires > I attempt	= 1
Able to arise, I attempt	= 2 _____

4. Immediate standing balance (first five seconds)

Unsteady (swaggers, moves feet, trunk sway)	= 0
Steady but uses walker or other support	= 1
Steady without walker or other support	= 2 _____

5. Standing balance

Unsteady	= 0
Steady but wide stance (medial heels > 4 in.	= 1
apart) and uses cane or other support	= 2 _____
Narrow stance without support	

6. Nudged (subject at max. position with feet as close together as possible, examiner pushes lightly on subject's sternum with palm of hand 3 times)

Begins to fall	= 0
Staggers, grabs, catches self	= 1
Steady	= 2 _____

7. Eyes closed (at maximum position No. 6)

Unsteady	= 0
Steady	= 1

8. Turning 360 degrees

Discontinuous steps	= 0
Continuous	= 1
Unsteady (grabs, staggers)	= 0
Steady	= 1 _____

9. Sitting down

Unsafe (misjudged distance, falls into chair)	= 0
Uses arms or not a smooth motion	= 1
Safe, smooth motion	= 2 _____

Balance score: _____

Figure 10.9

(Reprinted with permission. Tinetti, M.E. Performance Oriented Assessment of Mobility Problems in Elderly Patients. *J Am Geriatr Soc.* 1986; 34(2):119–126.)

Gait Tests

Initial Instructions: Subject stands with examiner, walks down hallway or across room, first at "usual" pace, then back at "rapid, but safe" pace (using usual walking aids)

10. Initiation of gait (immediately after told to "go")

Any hesitancy or multiple attempts to start	= 0	_____
No hesitancy	= 1	_____

11. Step length and height

a. Right swing foot

Does not pass left stance foot	= 0	_____
Passes left stance foot with step	= 1	_____
Right foot does not clear floor completely with step	= 0	_____
Right foot completely clears floor	= 1	_____

b. Left swing foot

Does not pass right stance foot	= 0	_____
Passes right stance foot with step	= 1	_____
Left foot does not clear floor completely with step	= 0	_____
Left foot completely clears floor	= 1	_____

12. Step Symmetry

Right and left step length not equal (estimate)	= 0	_____
Right and left step appear continuous	= 1	_____

13. Step Continuity

Stopping or discontinuity between steps	= 0	_____
Steps appear continuous	= 1	_____

14. Path (estimated in relation to floor tiles, 12-inch diameter; observe excursion of 1 foot over about 10 ft. of the course)

Marked deviation	= 0	_____
Mild/moderate deviation or uses walking aid	= 1	_____
Straight without walking aid	= 2	_____

15. Trunk

Marked sway or uses walking aid	= 0	_____
No sway but flexion of knees or back or spread arms out while walking	= 1	_____
No sway, no flexion, no use of arms, and no use of walking aid	= 2	_____

16. Walking Stance

Heels apart	= 0	_____
Heels almost touching while walking	= 1	_____

Gait Score: _____ : 12
Balance + Gait Score _____ : 28

Figure 10.9   (Continued)

TABLE 10.9   Components of the Gait Assessment Rating Score (GARS)

A. General Categories

1. Variability—a measure of inconsistency and arrhythmicity in stepping and arm movements.

   0 = fluid and predictably paced limb movements.

   1 = occasional interruptions (changes in velocity), approximately <25% of time.

   2 = unpredictability of rhythm approximately 25–27% of time.

   3 = random timing of limb movements.

2. Guardedness—hesitancy, slowness, diminished propulsion and lack of commitment in stepping and arm swing.

   0 = good forward momentum and lack of apprehension in propulsion.

   1 = center of gravity of head, arms, and trunk (HAT) projects only slightly in front of push-off, but still good arm-leg coordination.

   2 = HAT held over anterior aspect of foot, and some moderate loss of smooth reciprocation.

   3 = HAT held over rear aspect of stance-phase foot, and great tentativity in stepping.

3. Weaving—an irregular and wavering line of progression.

   0 = straight line of progression on frontal viewing.

   1 = a single deviation from straight (line of best fit) line of progression.

   2 = two to three deviations from line of progression.

   3 = four or more deviations from line of progression.

4. Waddling—a broad-based gait characterized by excessive truncal crossing of the midline and side-bending.

   0 = narrow base of support and body held nearly vertically over feet.

   1 = slight separation of medial aspects of feet and just perceptible lateral movement of head and trunk.

   2 = 3–4″ separation feet and obvious bending of trunk to side so that cog of head lies well over ipsilateral stance foot.

   3 = extreme pendular deviations of head and trunk (head passes lateral to ipsilateral stance foot), and further widening of base of support.

5. Staggering—sudden and unexpected laterally directed partial losses of balance.

   0 = no losses of balance to side.

   1 = a single lurch to side.

   2 = two lurches to side.

   3 = three or more lurches to side.

B. Lower Extremity Categories

1. % Time in Swing—a loss in the percentage of the gait cycle constituted by the swing phase.

   0 = approximately 3:2 ratio of duration of stance to swing phase.

   1 = a 1:1 or slightly less ratio of stance to swing.

   2 = markedly prolonged stance phase but with some obvious swing time remaining.

   3 = barely perceptible portion of cycle spent in swing.

2. Foot Contact—the degree to which heel strikes the ground before the forefoot.

   0 = very obvious angle of impact of heel on ground.

   1 = barely visible contact of heel before forefoot.

   2 = entire foot lands flat on ground.

   3 = anterior aspect of foot strikes ground before heel.

TABLE 10.9 Components of the Gait Assessment Rating Score (GARS) (Continued)

3. Hip ROM—the degree of loss of hip range of motion seen during a gait cycle.

  0 = obvious angulation of thigh backwards during double support (10°).

  1 = just barely visible angulation backwards from vertical.

  2 = thigh in line with vertical projection from ground.

  3 = thigh angled forward from vertical at maximum posterior excursion.

4. Knee Range of Motion—the degree of loss of knee range of motion seen during a gait cycle.

  0 = knee moves from complete extension at heel-strike (and late-stance) to almost 90° (@ 70°) during swing phase.

  1 = slight bend in knee seen at heel-strike and late-stance and maximal flexion at midswing is closer to 45° than 90°.

  2 = knee flexion at late stance more obvious than at heel-strike, very little clearance seen for toe during swing.

  3 = toe appears to touch ground during swing, knee flexion appears constant during stance, and knee angle during stance, and knee angle during swing appears 45° or less.

C. Trunk, Head, and Upper Extremity Categories

1. Elbow Extension—a measure of the decrease of elbow range of motion.

  0 = large peak-to-peak excursion of forearm (approximately 20°), with distinct maximal flexion at end of anterior trajectory.

  1 = 25% decrement of extension during maximal posterior excursion of upper extremity.

  2 = almost no change in elbow angle.

  3 = no apparent change in elbow angle (held in flexion).

2. Shoulder Extension—a measure of the decrease of shoulder range of motion.

  0 = clearly seen movement of upper arm anterior (15°) and posterior (20°) to vertical axis of trunk.

  1 = shoulder flexes slightly anterior to vertical axis.

  2 = shoulder comes only to vertical axis or slightly posterior to it during flexion.

  3 = shoulder stays well behind vertical axis during entire excursion.

3. Shoulder Abduction—a measure of pathological increase in shoulder range of motion laterally.

  0 = shoulders held almost parallel to trunk.

  1 = shoulders held 5–10° to side.

  2 = shoulders held 10–20° to side.

  3 = shoulders held greater than 20° to side.

4. Arm-Heel Strike Synchrony—the extent to which the contralateral movements of an arm and leg are out of phase.

  0 = good temporal conjunction of arm and contralateral leg at apex of shoulder and hip excursions all of the time.

  1 = arm and leg slightly out of phase 25% of the time.

  2 = arm and leg moderately out of phase 25–50% of time.

  3 = little or no temporal coherence of arm and leg.

5. Head Held Forward—a measure of the pathological forward projection of the head relative to the trunk.

  0 = earlobe vertically aligned with shoulder tip.

  1 = earlobe vertical projection falls 1″ anterior to shoulder tip.

  2 = earlobe vertical projection falls 2″ anterior to shoulder tip.

  3 = earlobe vertical projection falls 3″ or more anterior to shoulder tip.

(continued)

TABLE 10.9   Components of the Gait Assessment Rating Score (GARS) (Continued)

> 6. Shoulders Held Elevated—the degree to which the scapular girdle is held higher than normal.
>
>   0 = tip of shoulder (acromion) markedly below level of chin (1–2″)
>
>   1 = tip of shoulder slightly below level of chin.
>
>   2 = tip of shoulder at level of chin.
>
>   3 = tip of shoulder above level of chin.
>
> 7. Upper Trunk Flexed Forward—a measure of kyphotic involvement of the trunk.
>
>   0 = very gentle thoracic convexity, cervical spine flat, or almost flat.
>
>   1 = emerging cervical curve, more distant thoracic convexity.
>
>   2 = anterior concavity at mid-chest level apparent.
>
>   3 = anterior concavity at mid-chest level very obvious.

Reprinted with permission from Wolfson, L., Whipple, R., Amerman, P. Gait assessment in the elderly. A gait abnormality rating scale and its relation to falls. J Gerontol Med Sci. *1990; 45(1):M14. © The Gerontological Society of America.*

Figure 10.10   Normal changes seen with aging. (Reprinted with permission from Irwin, S., Zadai, C. Cardiopulmonary rehabilitation of the geriatric patient. In: Lewis, C., ed. *Aging: The Health Care Challenge. 2nd ed.* Philadelphia: FA Davis; 1990.)

TABLE 10.10   Assessment Process for Patient Interview and Physical Examination

Patient Interview

Patient perception of problem/disease process

   Specific didactic knowledge

   Emotional reaction

      embarrassment

      anxiety

      preoccupation

      denial

   Family perception of problem/disease process

   Patient description of disease progress and physical

      performance ability

   Patient history of dyspnea/orthopnea

Chart Review

Medical history

   Previous admissions and diagnosis

   Present medical problems: active/inactive

      present medications

      admitting diagnosis/objectives/care plan

Laboratory studies

   pulmonary function tests/ABGs

   metabolic studies/blood work

   recent EKG

   significant radiographic findings

Work/Social History

Present and past jobs/working environment

Present and past living locations

Social habits

   smoking

   alcohol

   physical activity

Observation

Patient position

   use of upper extremities

   use of musculature

Thoracic cage

   symmetry

   ratio of AP to Lat diameter

Breathing

   rate and depth

   rhythm

   pattern

Palpation

   subcostal angle/AP to Lat diameter

   localized expansion/symmetry

   excursion/mobility

   locate painful areas

Auscultation

   normal breath sounds

   abnormal breath sounds

   adventitious breath sounds

Reprinted with permission from Irwin, S., Zadai, C. Cardiopulmonary rehabilitation of the geriatric patient. In: Lewis, C., ed. Aging: The Health Care Challenge. *2nd ed. Philadelphia: FA Davis; 1990.*

TABLE 10.11   Exercise Testing Protocols

12-Minute Walk[a]	Level walking for 12 min distance recorded.	No equipment necessary yet correlates well with study results of more complex tests; can be used for patients who cannot accomplish either treadmill walking or bike riding because of dyspnea.
Low Level Functional	See Table 10.12.	Intermittent walk test for use with moderate to severely impaired patients. Allows flexibility of workload assignment and establishes an accurate baseline.
Balke Test[b]	Treadmill: speed constant at 3.0 mph; grade initially 10% increased by 3.5% every 2 min.	Slight increase in speed for patient with less impairment allows pulmonary and cardiovascular stress to come before leg fatigue.
Bruce[b]	Treadmill: speed initially 1.7 mph; grade initially 10%; both are increased every 3 min in a specified manner.	Can be used with relatively fit individuals to stress accurately all systems' response to exercise. Good to assess exercise-induced bronchospasm in fit individuals.
Bicycle Test[c]	Specific workload (i.e., watts or Kg/min) patient rides for a preset time, next work-load determined by patient response.	Intermittent subjective test based on patient response. Requires lower extremity strength and endurance to reach high metabolic response level.

[a]*McGavin, C.R., Cupta, S.P., McHardy, G.J.R. Twelve-minute walking test for assessing disability in chronic bronchitis.* Brit Med J. *1976; 1:822.*

[b]*From Physician's handbook for evaluation of cardiovascular and physical fitness, Tennessee Heart Association, 1972.*

[c]*Ellestad NH.* Stress Testing: Principles and Practice. *Philadelphia: FA Davis; 1979.*

Reprinted with permission from Irwin, S., Zadai, C. Cardiopulmonary rehabilitation of the geriatric patient. In: Lewis, C., ed. Aging: The Health Care Challenge. *2nd ed. Philadelphia: FA Davis; 1990.*

TABLE 10.12   Low-Level Functional Protocol

Collect resting data supine and sitting	ECG, BP, RR, HR, O_2sat, PFTs
Stage I	Objective assessment of dyspnea/1.5–2 mph, 0% grade
	Walk 6 min = 4 min stabilization + 2 min gas collection
	Rest: Patient returns to baseline HR, RR, and O_2sat
Stage II	Functional ambulation assessment/treadmill set at speed and incline equal to functional work capacity based on physiologic and symptomatic response to Stage I
	Walk 6 min = 4 min stabilization + 2 min gas collection
	Rest: Patient returns to baseline HR, RR, and ABGs
Stage III	Maximum exercise tolerance/treadmill set to produce HR of 70–85% max or predicted ventilatory max ($35 \times FeV_1$)
	Walk 6 min = 4 min stabilization + 2 min gas collection
	Rest: Patient returns to baseline HR, RR, and ABGs
Criteria to terminate test	85% predicted or HR_{max}, desaturation to 85% or lower SaO_2, reaching a ventilatory maximum ($35 \times FEV_1$), development of significant cardiac arrhythmias, or development of significant symptoms

Reprinted with permission from Irwin, S., Zadai, C. Cardiopulmonary rehabilitation of the geriatric patient. In: Lewis, C., ed. Aging: The Health Care Challenge. *2nd ed. Philadelphia: FA Davis; 1990.*

Chair Step Test

		HR/BP	HR/BP	HR/BP
6″	2 min	_____	_____	_____
12″	2 min	_____	_____	_____
18″	2 min	_____	_____	_____
18″	2 min	_____	_____	_____

Figure 10.11
(Adapted from Serfass, R.C., Agre, J.C., Smith, E.L. Exercise testing for the elderly.
Top Geriatr Rehab. October 1985; 1(1):58–67, with permission.)

In addition, the classic methods of assessing gait, such as the evaluation of shoe wear and standard gait analysis, are still applicable to the older population. The tools that have just been presented are extra ways of assessing gait that are specific to the older population.

Cardiopulmonary Tests

Chapters 5 and 13 provided background information on the complex array of physiological changes in the cardiopulmonary system with age. This section will discuss modifica-

tions in the assessment parameters that will be needed to account for these changes. The chart of normal changes found in Figure 10.10 offers an explanation for the parametric change seen in a typical cardiopulmonary assessment.[35] Table 10.10 is an outline of the typical assessment process for a patient interview and physical examination.[35]

In these assessments several changes can be noted for the average older person. These are

1. There may be an increase in the anterior-posterior diameter of the chest with age. This should be very

TABLE 10.13   Electrophysiologic Measurements in the Young and Old Subgroups and in the Combined Normal Control Population. Figures Represent Mean ± 1 SD

	Unit	Young Adults	Old Adults	Combined Population
Number of measurements		30	30	60
Age	years	31.6 ± 14.1	74.1 ± 7.5	52.8 ± 24.2
Height	cm	171.4 ± 9.2	163.4 ± 9.9	167.4 ± 10.3
Median motor CV	m/sec	59.4 ± 2.6	52.6 ± 4.0	56.0 ± 4.8
Median sensory CV	m/sec	64.3 ± 3.2	56.9 ± 5.0	60.6 ± 5.6
Median F-wave latency (F)	m/sec	26.7 ± 2.0	28.4 ± 2.3	27.5 ± 2.3
Tibial F-wave latency (F)	m/sec	48.5 ± 4.2	55.8 ± 6.7	52.1 ± 6.4
Median SEP latency (SEP)	m/sec	16.0 ± 1.4	16.2 ± 1.1	16.1 ± 1.3
Tibial SEP latency (SEP)	m/sec	34.4 ± 4.2	38.2 ± 3.8	36.3 ± 3.8
Spinal conduction (CV)	m/sec	55.8 ± 12.1	42.4 ± 13.1	48.4 ± 12.4

Reprinted with permission from Dorfman, L., Bosley, T. Age-related changes in peripheral and central nerve conduction in man. Neurology. *1979; 29:40.*

TABLE 10.14　Conduction Velocity and Latency (Normalized By Height) Changes With Age Corresponding to the Linear Regression Equation $y = a \times \text{Age} + b$[40]

Variable	Change with age (a)	y Intercept (b)	SD[a] $\dfrac{y/x}{y}$	SD[b] $\dfrac{y/x_{19}x_2}{y}$
Median motor CV	−0.15 m/sec/yr	63.9 m/sec		
Median sensory CV	−0.16 m/sec/yr	69.2 m/sec		
Spinal conduction (CV)	−0.24 m/sec/yr	60.8 m/sec		
Median F-wave latency (F)	+0.04 msec/m/yr	14.4 msec/m	0.056	0.054
Tibial F-wave latency (F)	+0.12 msec/m/yr	24.9 msec/m	0.076	0.067
Median SEP latency (SEP)	+0.015 msec/m/yr	8.8 msec/m	0.050	0.045
Tibial SEP latency (SEP)	+0.08 msec/m/yr	17.6 msec/m	0.078	0.071

[a]*Normalized average standard error of y corrected for* x *in the single linear regression analysis* y = ax + b.
[b]*Normalized average standard error of y corrected for* x_1 *and* x_2 *in the multiple linear regression analysis.*
$y - a_1 x_1 + a_2 x_2 + a_3 x_1 x_2 = b.$ (x_1 = age, x_2 = height.)
Reprinted with permission from Dorfman, L., Bosley, T. Age-related changes in peripheral and central nerve conduction in man. Neurology. *1979; 29:40.*

slight. If it is excessive, then it may indicate pathology (e.g., emphysema).

2. There may be a slight use of accessory muscles for breathing. Again, a slight use of these muscles is acceptable; however, as noted previously, more than that is indicative of pathology

3. Note that the following are signs of abnormal pathology or deconditioning: an elevated heart rate over 84 BPM prior to start of the exam,[36] a rise of over 20 BPM with the initial evaluation,[36] orthostatic hypotension, anxiety, arrhythmias, or fatigue during or later in the day.[36]

Exercising testing of the cardiovascular system was developed for younger populations, however, the tests can be modified for older persons. Table 10.11 lists five of the more common exercising-testing protocols.

The tests, even with modification and slowing for the older person, may be too vigorous. Table 10.12 gives low-level functional protocol.[35]

One more exercise test protocol was developed by Everett Smith.[37] This test is useful for the very low-level patient that either is unable to get out of a chair or performs better in a chair. This is the Chair Step Test shown in Figure 10.11. This test was developed by Smith and attempts to tax the cardiovascular system while controlling for those patients who may be unsafe on other cardiopulmonary exercise tests.[37] To perform this test, the patient sits in a chair and extends to touch, with alternating feet, boxes of various heights (as listed in Figure 10.11). Each stage lasts 5 minutes, with the last stage involving alternately raising the arms on the same side of the body to

shoulder level. The therapist monitors the patient at 2 minutes and 5 minutes. This test progresses the patient from 2.3 to 3.9 metabolic equivalents (METS).[36]

As noted in the previous sections, classic measures of cardiopulmonary functions are still appropriate for the older person. However, the clinician must be aware of changes that will affect those tests and choose to use more age-suitable ones.

Nerve Conduction Velocity

This section will discuss the manifestation of these systems in terms of nerve conduction velocities. (Again Chapters 5 and 12 describe the normal and pathological changes in the nervous system with age.) In all of the extremities, sensory nerve action potentials proprogate at a slower velocity and decrease in amplitude.[39] This decrement begins in the third decade and progresses in to the eighth decade. The amplitude of sensory potentials drops from 43 to 21 µv, and sensory velocity in digital nerves steadily declines from 57 to 48 m/sec.[40] Despite these changes, the refractory period is relatively unaffected in the older person.[39] Conduction velocity in the dorsal column shows little change before the age of 60; however, it declines sharply after 60 at a rate of ± 0.78 m/sec each year.[41] Tables 10.13 and 10.14 compare young and old conduction velocities.[40]

Motor conduction velocities slow at an even greater rate as do sensory nerves. The rate of decline of these nerves is 1 m/sec per decade after 15 to 24 years of age.[39] Several tables (see Tables 10.13 through 10.16) show the motor nerve conduction velocity changes with age.[41] Nerve conduction velocity can be assessed only by a therapist or physician specifically trained in this area.

TABLE 10.15   Maximum Sensory Conduction Velocity in Distal and Proximal Segments of Superficial Peroneal, Sural, and Posterior Tibial Nerve in 34 Subjects 15 to 33 Years Old, and 37 Subjects 40 to 65 Years Old (Temperature On Skin 35° to 37°C)[84]

Age Segment	(yr)	n[a]	A Conduction Velocity (m/sec)			n[a]	B Conduction Velocity (m/sec)		
			Mean	95%	SD		Mean	95%	SD
N, peroneus superficialis									
Bit toe—	15–25	19	46.1	39.0	4Ã1				
sup. ext. retinac.	40–65	17	42.2	36.0	6.3				
Sup. ext. retinac.	15–33	24	55.9	50.0	3.8	12	55.9	47.0	5.0
-capitul. fibul	40–65	23	52.9	47.0	3.7				
Sup. ext. retinac.	15–30	15	56.3	50.0	3.7				
-poplit. fossa	40–65	11	53.0	48.0	2.9				
Capitul. fibul.	15–25					13	55.8	47.0	4.7
-poplit. fossa	40–65					11	53.5	46.0	5.2
N. suralis									
Dors. ped.-	15–30	16	51.2	42.0	4.5				
lat. malleol.	40–65	15	48.3	40.0	5.3				
Lat. malleol.	15–30	21	56.5	51.0	3.4	16	55.9	49.0	4.2
-sura	40–65	16	54.8	46.5	4.5	12	56.3	47.0	5.5
Lat. malleol.	15–30	19	57.3	52.0	3.5				
-poplit. fossa	40–65	12	53.3	47.5	4.1				
Sura-	15–30					18	57.6	52.0	3.0
poplit. fossa	40–65					10	54.3	47.0	4.8
N. tibialis posterior									
Bit toe—	15–30	23	46.1	39.0	3.5				
med. malleol.	40–65	10	43.4	37.0	3.8				
Med. malleol.	15–30	17	58.6[b]	52.5	3.8	22	56.4	51.0	4.0
-poplit. fossa	40–52	7	57.4[b]	51.5	4.5	6	54.0	47.0	4.4

A: calculated from the latency measured between onset of the stimulus and the initial peak of the sensory potential.
B: calculated from the difference of latencies, measured at two sites of recording.
[a]Number of nerves.
[b]Conduction velocity in fibers of mixed nerve.
Reprinted with permission from Behse, F., Buchtal, F. Normal sensory conduction in the nerves of leg in man. J Neurol Neurosurg Psychiatry. *1971; 34:408.*

Nevertheless, all clinicians should be aware of changes with age that will affect the results of those tests.

Assessing Ethnicity

This final section on assessment deals with the concept of assessing ethnicity.[42] Rempusheski makes a strong plea to health professionals to recognize bias and differences in ethnic views of health care providers and recipients. Table 10.17 is a copy of her assessment categories.[43] These categories can be used by the practitioner interested in evaluating and planning programs most relevant and acceptable to the older person.

TABLE 10.16   Maximum Conduction Velocities of Ulnar Nerve Fibers to Muscles of the Hypothenar Eminence at Various Ages[85]

Age in Years	N[a]	Average Conduction Velocity	Standard Deviation
		m/sec	
3.5–10	8	61.5	6.30
10–20	8	57.1	6.19
20–30	35	58.4	4.28
30–40	7	57.4	6.45
40–50	2	56.8	—
50–60	3	49.7	—
60–70	10	51.3	5.26
70–82[b]	10	51.5	7.26

[a]*If more than one measurement was made on a single individual, the average only was used.*
[b]*Includes only one case above 80 years of age.*
Reprinted with permission from Wagman, I., Lesse, H. Conduction velocity of ulnar nerve in human subjects of different ages and sizes. Fed. Proc. 1950; 9:130.

TABLE 10.17   Assessment Categories with Which to Elicit Rituals, Beliefs, and Symbols of Care Activities

Sleep

Condition of room/environment: occupancy of room and bed/sleeping surface, kind of bed/sleeping surface and other furniture, condition of room (temperature, lights, doors and windows open or closed, other artifacts/symbols in room).

Kinds of covering, comforting materials: pillow/head support (height/number of supports used, type, positioning), covering (blanket type, sheet type, other).

Sleepwear: covering on head, body, legs, feet (type and variation by season or event).

Care of bed linen: kind of cleaning, frequency, how, by whom.

Bedtime ritual: time, tasks, others involved, food or liquid consumed, sensory stimulation, symbols/icons used.

Rules for sleeping: when, with whom, how, in what positions, where, beliefs related to rules.

Rules for awakening: by whom/what, how, mechanisms used.

Awakening rituals: time, tasks, others involved, food or liquid consumed, sensory stimulation, symbols/icons used.

Personal Hygiene

Tending one's body: rituals for mouth care (tools and substances used, time, who can assist); rituals for body and hair care (how, when, where, how often, substances used, taboos, gender rules, symbols, beliefs associated with aspects of ritual).

Associations with health/illness: care associated with body fluids/excretions, symbolism, body temperature, activities of tending one's body, substances used in rituals, seasonal/climate taboos, kinds of activities, time of day/year, gender rules, beliefs.

Eating

Kinds of foods: preferences, dislikes, specific to an event, ritual, specific to time of day/week/month/year, seasonal, rules or taboos for hot foods, cold foods, rules for amount, type, composition, beliefs, and symbolism associated with specific foods.

Schedule of foods: rules for when/when not to eat; amount related to time of day; healthy/ill status; associated with certain rituals, beliefs, symbols; before/after meal rituals, symbols/icons used/present.

Environment for eating: place, people, position, taboos/rules, symbols/icons used/present.

Implements/utensils: kind, number, rules for use of each, taboos, utensils as symbols.

Reprinted with permission from Rempusheski, V. The role of ethnicity in elder care. Nurs Clin N Am. September 1989; 24(3):717–724.

References

1. Folstein M. Mini-mental state: A practice of method for grading the cognitive state of patients for the clinician. *J Psychiatr Res.* 1975; 12:189–198.
2. Folstein M, Rabins P. Psychiatric evaluation of the elderly patients. *Primary Care.* September 1979; 6(3):609–619.
3. Kane R, Kane R. Measuring mental status. In: Kane R, Kane R. *Assessing the Elderly.* Lexington, MA: Lexington Books; 1981.
4. Prestidge B, Lalle C. Prevalence and recognition of depression among primary care outpatients. *J Family Pract.* 1987; 25:67–72.
5. German P, Shapiro S, Skinner EA. Use of health and mental health services. *J Am Ger Soc.* 1985; 33: 246–252.
6. Brink T, Yesavage J, Lum D, et al. Screening tests for geriatric depression. *Clin Gerontologist.* 1982; 1:37–42.
7. Yesavage J. The use of self-rating depression scales in the elderly. In: Poon E, ed. *Clinical Memory Assessment of Older Adults.* Washington, DC: American Psychological Association; 1986.
8. Holmes T, Rahe R. The social readjustment rating scale. *J Psychosom Res.* 1967; 11:213–218.
9. Intermediary Manual Part 3—Claims Process. Section 3904 Medical Review (MR) of Part 3 Intermediary Outpatient Physical Therapy (OPT) Bills [Edit], HCFA; 1988.
10. Tinetti M. Performance oriented assessment of mobility problems in elderly patients. *J Am Geriatr Soc.* 1986; 34(2):119–126.
11. Kane RL. Beyond caring: The challenge to geriatrics. *J Am Geriatr Soc.* 1988; 36(5):467–472.
12. Bohannon R, Andrews A, Smith M. Rehabilitation goals of patient with hemiplegia. *Int J Rehabil Res.* 1988; 11(2):181–183.
13. Kane RL, Kane RA. *Assessing the Elderly.* Lexington, MA: Lexington Books; 1981.
14. *Dorland's Medical Dictionary.* 26th ed. Philadelphia: WB Saunders; 1981.
15. Jette AM. State of the art of functional status assessment. In: Nothstein J, ed. *Measurement in Physical Therapy.* New York: Churchill Livingstone; 1988.
16. Mahoney FI, Barthel DW. Functional evaluation: The Barthel Index. *Md Med J.* 1965; 14(2):61–65.
17. Lachs M, Feinstein AR, Cooney LM, et al. A simple procedure for general screening for functional disability in elderly patients. *Ann Intern Med.* May 1990; 112(9):699–704.
18. Williams M. Why screen for functional disability in elderly persons? *Ann Intern Med.* May 1990; 112 (9):639.
19. Tomanek R, Woo Y. Compensatory hypertrophy of the plantare muscle in relation to age. *J Gerontol.* 1970; 25(1):23–29.
20. Goldspink G, Howells K. Work induced hypertrophy in exercised normal muscles of different ages and the reversibility of hypertrophy after cessation of exercise. *Am J Physiol.* 1974; 239:179–193.
21. Moritani T, Devries HA. Potential for gross muscle hypertrophy in older men. *J Gerontol.* 1980; 35 (5):673.
22. Rice C. Strength in an elderly population. *Arch Phys Med Rehabil.* 1989; 70(5):391–397.
23. Borges O. Isometric and isokinetic knee extension and flexion torque in men and women aged 20–70. *Scand J Rehab Med.* 1989; 21:45–53.
24. Vandervoort A, Hayes K. Plantarflexor muscle function in young and elderly women. *Eur J Appl Physiol.* 1989; 58:389–394.
25. Walker JSD, Walker JM, Sue D, et al. Active mobility of the extremities in older subjects. *Phys Ther.* 1984; 64(6):914–923.
26. Frekany G, Leslie D. Effects of an exercise program on selected flexibility measurements of senior citizens. *Gerontologist.* 1975; 182–183.
27. James B, Parker A. Active and passive mobility of lower limb joints in elderly men and women. *Am J Phys Med Rehab.* August 1989; 68(4):162–167.
28. Lewis C. Musculoskeletal changes with age. In: Lewis C, ed. *Aging: The Health Care Challenge.* Philadelphia: FA Davis; 2002: 135–160.
29. REEDCO Research. *REEDCO Posture Score Sheet.* Auburn, NY; 1978.
30. Murray MP. Gait as a total pattern of movement. *Am J Phys Med.* 1976; 46:290.
31. Murray MP, Kory RC, Clarkson BH. Walking patterns in healthy old men. *J Gerontol.* 1969; 24:169.
32. Andriacchi TP, Ogle JA, Galante JO. Walking speed as a basis of normal and abnormal gait measurements. *J Biomech.* 1977; 10:261.
33. Findley FR, Cody KA, Finizie RV. Locomotion patterns in elderly women. *Arch Phys Med Rehabil.* 1967; 50:140.
34. Wolfson L, Whipple R, Amerman P. Gait assessment in the elderly. A gait abnormality rating scale and its relation to falls. *J Gerontol Med Sci.* 1990; 45(1):M14–M15.
35. Irwin S, Zadai C. Cardiopulmonary rehabilitation of the geriatric patient. In Lewis C, ed. *Aging: The Health Care Challenge.* 2nd ed. Philadelphia: FA Davis; 1990; 181–210.
36. Siebens H, Deconditioning. In: Kemp B, Brummel-Smith K, Ramsdell JD, eds. *Geriatric Rehabilitation.* Boston, Little, Brown; 1990: 177–191.

37. Serfass RC, Agre JC, Smith E. Exercise testing for the elderly. *Top Geriatric Rehab*. October 1985; 1(1): 58–67.

38. Lewis, C. Functional Toolbox I Great Seminars and Books, 2000 Akron, Ohio.

39. Schaumburg H, Spencher P, Ochoa T. The aging human peripheral nervous system. In Katzman R, Terry R, eds. *The Neurology of Aging*. Philadelphia: FA Davis: 1975; 442–444.

40. Buchtal F, Rosenflack A, Behse F. Sensory potentials of normal and diseased nerves. In Dyck P, Thomas P, Lambert E. *Peripheral Neuropathy*. Philadelphia: WB Saunders; 1975: 433–446.

41. Dorfman L, Bosley T. Age-related changes in peripheral and central nerve conduction in man. *Neurology*. 1979; 29:38–44.

42. Rempusheski V. The role of ethnicity in elder care. *Nurs Clin N Am*. September 1989; 24(3):717–724.

43. Fitzgerald GK, Wynveen KJ, Rheult W, Rothschild B. Objective assessment with establishment of normal values for lumbar spine range of motion. *Phys Ther*. November 1983; 63(11):1778.

11

Orthopaedic Considerations

Pearls

- Thirty percent of all geriatric patients/clients consult their physicians because of musculoskeletal problems.
- Therapists need to assess the cause of strength declines (e.g., neuromuscular, cardiovascular, joint swelling, or joint changes) and treat the strength decrease accordingly.
- Treatment suggestions for flexibility decrements in the aged are to heat the muscle, gently stretch the muscle, reinforce the stretch by doing functional activities, and cool the muscle down in the lengthened position.
- Normal changes of the spine include less flexibility in the soft tissues, decreased mineralization of bones, osteophyte formation, and disc space narrowing.

- Osteoporosis is no longer considered an inevitable consequence of aging.
- Osteopenia refers to metabolic bone diseases that are characterized by x-ray findings of a subnormal amount of mineralized bone mass.
- Aging causes a decrease in motion of almost all of the body joints. Nevertheless, the older person can maintain independence. Osteoporosis, arthritis, fractures, as well as many other pathologies, respond favorably to exercise and rehabilitation programs.

INTRODUCTION

The principles of geriatric rehabilitation, posed in *Archives of Physical Medicine and Rehabilitation*, state that approximately 30% of all geriatric patients consult their physicians because of musculoskeletal problems.[1] Therefore, it appears that orthopaedics are a primary concern to therapists working with the elderly. This chapter will explore the changes with age in the musculoskeletal system. Pathologies specific to an older population will be discussed. Then a joint-by-joint approach will be taken that will examine evaluation and treatment of orthopaedic conditions in the elderly.

STRENGTH

Numerous studies cite the loss of strength with age.[2–4] The greatest loss of strength appears to be related to the selective loss of type II muscle fibers, which is thoroughly discussed in Chapter 3 of this text. Other variables can lead to strength loss. Lower levels of physical activity certainly heads the top of this list. A decrease in cardiovascu-

lar endurance results in less stamina even during activities of daily living. This sets the stage for progressive loss in overall strength. Poor nutrition can change the metabolic efficiency of energy exchange at the level of the sarcolema. A decrease in activity also leads to a diminished neuromuscular connection whereby transmission of nerve impulses to the muscle is slowed and the strength of the impulse lessened. Inhibition of muscle contraction is the consequence of the presence of edema, often seen in older adults with arthritic changes in the joints.[5] All of these variables will lead to a loss in overall muscular contraction strength. The clinical implications of these changes are that increasing activity could potentially reverse these strength changes. Some hypothetical examples might be:

1. If the decrease in strength is due to cardiovascular inefficiency leading to poor nutrient exchange, then an increase in activity level above rest would increase blood flow to the muscle and positively affect the health of the muscle tissue.
2. If the loss of strength is due to a decrease in the efficiency of the neuromuscular junction contact, exercise has been shown to improve nerve conduction

velocities, reaction times, and strength of muscle contraction.[4]

3. If the decrease in strength is due to swelling (i.e., reflex inhibition due to joint distention), then the swelling and subsequent strength loss can be alleviated by using modalities and anti-inflammatory medication prior to joint strength training.[5]

Other major reasons for the decline in strength with age are pathological in nature, all of which appear to be more prevalent in the elderly. An example of this is polymyalgia rheumatica, a systemic inflammatory disease of multiple joints that causes swelling, pain, and weakness.[6] Systemic rheumatological problems such as rheumatoid arthritis and lupus, like polymyalgia rheumatica, will diminish activities level secondary to pain and inflexibility and lead to a progressive loss in muscular strength. Parkinson's disease and cerebral vascular accidents, as well as other neurological pathologies, can result in strength loss owing to tone changes and the quality of muscle contraction. The presence of underlying pathology in addition to normal changes in muscle strength with age should be considered in the evaluation and intervention of elderly individuals. See Appendix 1 for evidence-based evaluation and treatment ideas.

FLEXIBILITY

Another major area of function change with age is flexibility. As a person ages, the muscles become more rigid and tend to become less flexible. There is a higher proportion of type I muscle fibers, making the muscle a stabilizer instead of the fast-reacting muscle.[7] There is also a decrease in elastin and an increase in collagen of the muscle tissue, further affecting the flexibility of muscle tissue (see Chapter 3).

In addition to these changes in muscle tissue, all connective tissues are affected by changes in elastin and collagen as described in detail in Chapter 3. The cartilage breaks down, restricting joint mobility. Tendons and ligaments become more rigid and less resilient to length changes often resulting in injury. Flexibility into extension is most often lost in the elderly.[8,9] Postural changes from kyphosis of the thoracic spine lead to flexed positions of all of the lower extremity joints, which may result in irreversible soft tissue contractures if not attended to by the therapist. The presence of contractures requires special consideration in older persons. To get the best results, prolonged static stretching—preceded by a heat modality—is often needed to restore flexibility of collagenous tissue. Functional activities that incorporate elongated muscle positions are also helpful in regaining flexibility.[9]

It must be recognized that once a contracture occurs in older adults, it takes longer to achieve the benefits of a stretching program. Prevention of contractures in the first place is the best mode of intervention. Encouraging ex-

tension-strengthening exercises, positioning to facilitate extension, postural and balance exercises, proper nutrition, and hydration will help to establish healthy and flexible muscle tissue in the older adult. The key phrase here is *"Extension Equals Function."*[8] See Appendix 2 for evidence-based evaluation and treatment ideas.

Posture

The third area of orthopaedic functional change is posture. The classic "senile posture," which is flexed, is certainly not an inevitable consequence of aging. However, in the presence of osteoporosis, compression wedge fractures of the thoracic vertebrae and compression fractures in the lumbar vertebrae result in characteristic postural changes. As noted in Figure 11.1, normal posture, absected with a plumb line running from the ear to the ankle, should fall through:

1. The middle of the earlobe.
2. The middle of the acromion process.
3. The middle of the greater trochanter.
4. Posterior to the patella but anterior to the center of the knee joint.
5. Slightly anterior to the lateral malleolus.

The most common posture changes with age, as depicted in Figure 11.2, include a forward head, rounded shoulders, decreased lumbar lordosis, and increased flexion in the hips and knees.[9] There are some variations in the way in which posture is evaluated; as discussed in Chapter 9 with progressive postual changes, modification of postual status is often more easily assessed using the middle of the lateral malleolus as the starting point and going up the kinetic chain. Treatment for postural changes in the elderly is to concentrate on extension throughout the kinetic chain. Stretching and flexibility exercises should be employed for any of the body parts that have deviated from the norm. Strengthening of extensors and work on balance activities are very important components to a postural intervention program. The key to maintaining posture is prevention, prevention, prevention. The key to any exercise program is extension, extension, extension.[8–10]

After reviewing strength, flexibility, and posture changes with age, it is important to note that there are several musculoskeletal orthopaedic pathologies that are extremely prevalent in the elderly.

OSTEOPOROSIS

Distinguishing "Normal" Aging of Bone from Osteoporosis

Osteoporosis is no longer considered an inevitable consequence of aging. Many of the sequelae associated with the development of osteoporosis can be prevented by

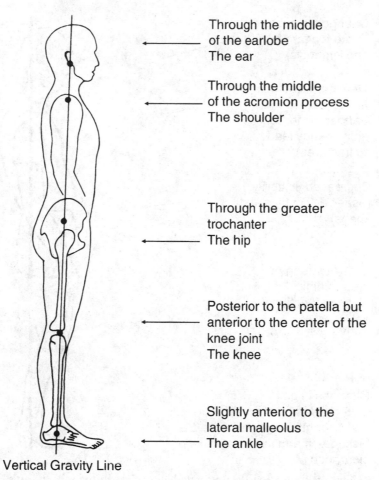

Through the middle
of the earlobe
The ear

Through the middle
of the acromion process
The shoulder

Through the greater
trochanter
The hip

Posterior to the patella but
anterior to the center of the
knee joint
The knee

Slightly anterior to the
lateral malleolus
The ankle

Vertical Gravity Line

Figure 11.1   Proper posture shown with a vertical gravity line. (Reprinted with permission from Lewis, C.B., Bottomley, J.M. Musculoskeletal changes with age. In: Lewis CB, ed. *Aging: The Health Care Challenge.* Philadelphia: FA Davis; 1990.)

development of a healthy peak bone mineral density during childhood with a maximum density at the time of physiological maturity and by utilizing sound nutritional and exercise practices throughout the lifetime to maintain mineralization of the bone.[10] Understanding the controlling mechanisms of bone cell response to nutritional and biochemical interventions and mechanical loading is important in preventing the development of osteoporosis (see also Chapter 3).

Mechanical Stress

Physical stress on bone stimulates increased bone deposition. Exercise can apply compressive and tensile stress; and in addition, simply overcoming the forces of gravity on the musculoskeletal system, or resisting impact, can stimulate bone deposition. Because of the large number of muscles (more than 600) that originate and insert on the

numerous bones of the skeletal system (around 206), muscle contraction, especially against resistance (gravity or external loads), can place large forces on the muscle tendon-bone joints, and these forces are relayed to the bone matrix. These facts are being revealed in tests with astronauts in the US space shuttle program; in addition, efforts are being made to use exercise in zero gravity as a means to retard increased bone resorption during space flights.

There is a clear age-related loss in bone mineral content. This loss occurs first in cancellous bone, which begins to decline before the third decade of life. Compact bone is retained for another decade before resorption increases[11-13] (Figure 11.3). The decline in trabecular bone mineral content is greater for women than men and greater again for postmenopausal women.[14-18] After menopause, the rate of trabecular bone mineral loss in women can increase to 7% per year, with the greatest loss in the first five years. This rate of loss is large compared

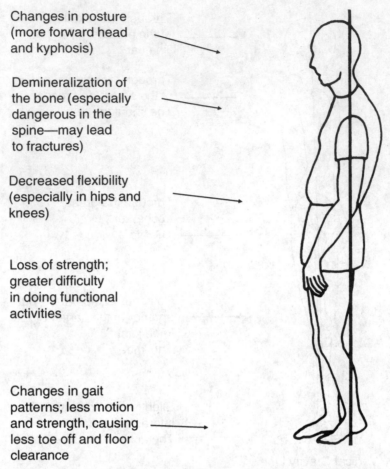

Changes in posture
(more forward head
and kyphosis)

Demineralization of
the bone (especially
dangerous in the
spine—may lead
to fractures)

Decreased flexibility
(especially in hips and
knees)

Loss of strength;
greater difficulty
in doing functional
activities

Changes in gait
patterns; less motion
and strength, causing
less toe off and floor
clearance

Figure 11.2   Postural changes with age. (Reprinted with permission from Lewis, C.B. What's so different about rehabilitating the older person? *Clinical Management.* May–June 1984; 4(3):12.)

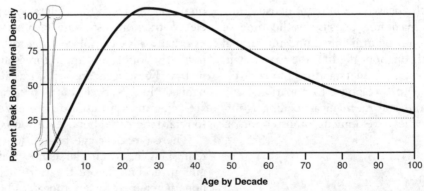

Figure 11.3   Life cycle changes in bone mineral content. Peaking at maturity and showing a gradual decline throughout the remainder of the life cycle. (Reprinted with permission from Bottomley, J.M. Age-related bone health and pathophysiology of osteoporosis. *Ortho Phys Ther Clinics of No. America.* 1998: 7(2):117–132. Artist: J.M. Bottomley.)

with the average loss before menopause of less than 1% per year.[14]

Conditions That Influence Age-Related Decrease in Bone Mineral Content

With aging there is a loss of bone mineral content as depicted in Figure 11.3. Several conditions can exaggerate this loss including nutrition, endocrinologic factors, and exercise-related factors. The two main determinants in the development and severity of osteoporosis are peak bone mineral content and the rate of bone mineral loss.[19] Thus it is important to understand the factors that increase peak bone mineral content, as well as how to retard bone mineral loss.

Effects of Exercise on Bone Remodeling

Exercise was reported to influence bone mineral content in a 1991 study that used a cross-sectional design.[20] Bone density was higher in athletes compared with sedentary controls, and athletes involved in weight bearing activities had the highest bone mineral content. The finding of increased bone mineral density in individuals involved in weight bearing activities has been shown repeatedly in similar cross-sectional studies.[20,21] Furthermore, it is believed that the amount of muscle mass is proportional to bone mineral content.[19,22] In other words: the stronger the muscle, the stronger the bone.

Exercise can affect the retention of bone mineral even in amenorrheic athletes involved in weight bearing activities. Exercise involving weight-bearing retains more bone mineral than nonweight bearing. For individuals who have been involved in exercise throughout their lives, there is evidence that they maintain a higher bone mineral density (decreased resorption) compared to sedentary controls.[23] The effects of exercise on the bone are discussed more extensively in a subsequent section of this chapter.

Risk Factors for Osteoporosis

Risk factors are not the cause, but they are contributing factors to the development of osteoporosis. The number of risk factors that predispose an individual to osteoporosis is not cumulative. That is to say, if you have three risk factors you are not three times more likely to develop osteoporosis. Rather, the more risk factors identified, the greater the predisposition toward the development of osteoporosis. Factors such as age, gender, genetic makeup, race, body type, and complexion may initiate the process. Other factors such as poor nutrition, inactivity, and smoking may serve to accelerate bony loss.

Age is by far the most important empirical determinant of bone mass. From the fourth decade on, less bone is formed than is resorbed at individual remodeling foci, and this imbalance increases with advancing age.[24] Although this imbalance in bone remodeling could be caused by osteoblast senescence, the observation that healing of fractures in the elderly is not delayed suggests that aging does not impair the response of osteoblasts to appropriate stimuli. Serum levels of both growth hormone and insulin-like growth factor 1, (which mediates the effect of growth hormone on bone and cartilage) have been shown to decrease with aging.[25]

There may be impaired regulation of osteoblast activity caused by abnormalities in either systemic or local growth factors which are genetically influenced. Therefore, genetic factors may predispose an individual to the development of osteoporosis. At least twelve local regulators of growth produced by bone, cartilage, or marrow cells have been identified.[26] Either age-related or genetic defects in the synthesis of one or more of these regulators may explain the uncoupling of bone formation from resorption that allows age-related bone loss. These factors include: skeletal growth factor, bone-derived growth factor, macrophage-derived growth factor, a factor resembling b-transforming growth factor, and prostaglandin E_2.

Table 11.1 summarizes the relative risk factors in the development of osteoporosis.

Gender clearly influences the development of osteoporosis. Females have a higher incidence of osteoporosis related to lower levels of estrogen.

Race also appears to have an impact on the development of osteoporosis. White women, particularly of northwestern European background, and Asians are more at risk than black women, in whom osteoporosis is actually very rare.[27] Family history also plays a part in the development of osteoporosis. Slight build, fair complexioned individuals with freckles and blond hair, all of which are genetically regulated, have a higher incidence of osteoporosis. Environmental factors, such as customary dietary habits developed within family structures, could play a role in increasing the risk for osteoporosis.

Mechanisms of the Benefits of Exercise

The effects of gravity and mechanical stress on the bone have been associated with functional adaptation of the bone.[28] In other words, there is a continual remodeling of bone in response to functional demands placed on the bone. According to Wolff's law, the internal architecture of the bone responds to stress by laying down more bone wherever the muscles are exerting their greatest force. Additionally, stress on the bone creates a negative potential within the bone according to the piezoelectric effect, thereby attracting positive ions, such as calcium.[28]

When force is applied to bone, bone bends and there is an inherent moment of inertia applied to the bone. These mechanical stresses or loads are crucial in keeping bone healthy. Mechanical loads stimulate bone cells within the

TABLE 11.1 Risk Factors for Osteoporosis

Age (postmenopausal)

Genetic Factors

Genders (females at risk)

Race (Caucasians, Asians more at risk)

Family history

Body build/small frame

Fair complexion

Nutritional Factors

Low body weight

Low dietary calcium intake

High alcohol consumption

Eating disorders (anorexic, bulimic, chronic crash dieting patterns)

High caffeine consumption (leaches calcium)

High vitamin A, D intake

High protein intake

High soft drink consumption (phosphorus binding with calcium)

Lifestyle Factors

Inactive/sedentary lifestyle (immobilization, bed rest, no gravity)

Cigarette smoking

Medical Factors

Early menopause (natural or surgically induced)

• Bilateral oophorectomy

Medication use: corticosteroids, anticoagulants, anticonvulsants, antacids

Menstrual cycle disorders (amenorrhea, dysmenorrhea)

No pregnancies

Contraceptive use

Safety Issues and Falls

Diseases causing secondary osteoporosis

Endocrine diseases (hyperparathyroidism)

Gastrointestinal diseases (IBS, malabsorption syndromes)

Bone marrow disorders (myeloma, carcinoma)

Connective tissue disorders (Marfan's, osteogenesis)

ment.[28] A minimum amount of strain is required to be effective for increased bone remodeling.

The major impact of activity on bone mass is localized. Bone mineral density is increased only in the areas that are stressed.[29–31] Weight-bearing and bone-site-specific forces are the key factors in the relationship of bone development and muscle pull.[30,31]

Muscle mass and strength bear an interesting relationship to bone mass. There is a positive correlation between muscle strength and muscle mass with the bone mineral density.[32,33] It appears that overall strength is the key factor as strength in one area typically reflects strength in other regions of the body. To effect change in bone mass, the training stimulus must exceed the normal loading of the muscle.

The type of exercise is very important. Sinaki's landmark studies[34,35] clearly demonstrated that in postmenopausal women who had sustained osteoporotic vertebral fractures, extension exercises significantly reduced the incidence of fracture reoccurrence, whereas flexion exercises increased the risk of fracture.

Based on current research it is important to consider the following factors when prescribing exercise to enhance bone mass: (1) Weight-bearing physical activity is essential for the normal development and maintenance of a healthy bone mass. (2) Sedentary elderly individuals may increase bone mass by becoming more active, but the primary benefit of the increased activity may be in avoiding the further loss of bone that occurs with inactivity. (3) The optimal program for older adults would include activities that improve strength, flexibility, and coordination that may indirectly, but effectively, decrease the incidence of osteoporotic fractures by lessening the likelihood of falling.[28–33]

Table 11.2 shows the World Health Organization's (WHO) recommended classification of osteoporosis based on bone mass measurements. Categories are defined by comparing an individual's bone mass to that of the average young adult. By WHO's definitions, osteopenia is described as a state of low bone mass. Individuals in this range are at an increased risk for fracture, and steps need to be taken to address diet modification and weight bearing exercise to prevent further bone loss. Individuals with greater loss in bone mass with no history of fracture are defined as having osteoporosis. These individuals are at an increased risk for fracture with minimal or no trauma. The most severe category are those people with marked loss in bone mass in addition to a history of fracture. These individuals are defined as having severe osteoporosis.[36] (See Appendix 3 for evidence-based evaluation and treatment ideas.

loaded region to deform and increase their synthesis of prostacyclin (PGI_2), prostaglandin E_2 (PGE_2), and other growth hormones, and increase their synthesis of RNA. This causes the cascade of events within the osteoblasts and osteoclasts in response to changes in bone strain, reflecting an adaptation to the imposed loading environ-

For Additional information on osteoporosis, see CD.

TABLE 11.2   World Health Organization Classification of Osteoporosis

Normal	Bone mineral density that is not more than one standard deviation below the young adult mean value
Osteopenia or low bone mass	Bone mineral density that lies between 1.0 and 2.5 standard deviations below the young adult mean value
Osteoporosis	Bone mineral density that is more than 2.5 standard deviations below the young adult mean value without a history of fracture
Severe osteoporosis	Bone mineral density more than 2.5 standard deviations below the young adult mean value with history of one or more fractures

World Health Organization as per Kanis, J.A., Melton, L.F. III, Christiansen, C., Johnson, C.C., Khalte, N. The diagnosis of osteoporosis. J. Bone Miner Res. *1994; 9:1137–1141.*

OSTEOPENIA

Osteopenia refers to metabolic bone diseases that are characterized by x-ray findings of a subnormal amount of mineralized bone mass. The most common osteopenia is osteoporosis, generally defined as a decrease in the quantity of bone, with an increased incidence of fractures from minimal trauma. One of the first signs of osteoporosis is alveolar bone loss, called dental osteopenia, followed by bone loss in vertebrae and long bones. Indeed there appears to be a strong correlation between skeletal osteopenia and density of alveolar bone.[37] Dental osteopenia leads to an inadequate amount of bone mass in the mandible, loss or mobility of teeth, edentulousness, and inability to wear dentures.[38]

It has been found that calcium deficiencies and calcium-phosphorus imbalances contribute to the development of osteopenia and the subsequent pathogenesis of osteoporosis.[39] Prevention and management include not only increased calcium intake but also estrogen therapy, dietary vitamin D, and exercise.

Osteopenia commonly is present in hyperthyroidism, and the development of hyperthyroidism aggravates normal age-related bone loss. Mild hypercalcemia is commonly seen in hyperthyroidism due to the endocrine imbalance of the thyroid hormone. Estrogen acts on the thyroid gland to produce calcitonin. In a condition in which there is too much thyroid hormone and too little estrogen, calcium absorption is decreased and calcium excretion is increased. In hypothyroidism, there is a mild decrease in the rate of calcium deposition in bone related to the imbalance between the decreased amount of thyroid hormone and a surplus of PTH.

OSTEOMALACIA

Osteomalacia is a bone disorder caused by a failure of normal calcification of the bone matrix. The most common causes of osteomalacia are vitamin D deficiency, a calcium deficiency, abnormal metabolism of vitamin D, and low serum calcium-phosporus levels. In contrast to osteoporosis, where there is a loss of bone mass and resulting brittleness of the bones, osteomalacia causes the bones to soften due to poor mineralization and an inability to absorb vitamin D, calcium, and phosphate.[40]

The primary etiology is a vitamin D deficiency, which results in poor absorption of calcium in the intestines and increased excretion of phosphate from the kidneys. Vitamin D is obtained from the diet (D_2 and D_3) and from biosynthesis following exposure to sunlight (D_3). Its metabolite, $1,25(OH)_2D$, enhances the gastrointestinal absorption of calcium and phosphate, and thus has a direct effect on the bone calcification process. Vitamin D deficiency may result from dietary restriction of food (e.g., too little fish, whole grain flour, and dairy products), malabsorption of vitamin D, or insufficient exposure to ultraviolet radiation.[40,41]

Vitamin D from the diet is absorbed in the upper small bowel via fat-dependent absorption. Derangement in upper intestinal function or fat malabsorption can result in vitamin D deficiency. Diagnoses such as pancreatic insufficiency, irritable bowel syndrome, biliary obstruction, or sprue can lead to poor absorption of this essential nutrient.

Once absorbed, vitamins D_2 and D_3 are hydroxylated in the liver to 25-hydroxyvitamin D and subsequently in the kidneys to $1,25(OH)_2D$. Interference with the metabolism of vitamin D may contribute to the development of osteomalacia. Liver disease, particularly cirrhosis of any etiology, may interfere with hepatic 25-hydroxylation of vitamin D. In renal failure, the deficiency of renal 25-OH-D 1-a-hydroxylase activity is the primary cause of osteomalacia, because it produces a deficiency of $1,25(OH)_2D$.

Certain drugs may also impede the absorption of vitamin D by causing an increase in vitamin D excretion or catabolism. Drugs that increase the hepatic degradation of 25-hydroxyvitamin D, such as phenytoin and phenobarbital, are known to predispose individuals to osteomalacia. In nephrotic pathologies, there may be an increase in vitamin D clearance and excretion, which results in a deficiency of vitamin D.[40,41]

Phosphorus is also essential for the calcification of bone. Hypophosphatemia may result from gastrointestinal or renal loss of phosphate, which is independent of parathyroid or vitamin D metabolism. Malabsorption and subsequent gastric and intestinal tract wasting of phosphates may be compounded by vitamin D deficiency and hyperparathyroidism. This malabsorption also may be exacerbated by phosphate-binding antacids. Renal wasting of phosphorus is a prominent feature of proximal renal tubular disorders. These disorders range from defects that limit phosphate absorption and increase phosphate clearance to renal failure which results in defects involving absorption of phosphorus, glucose, amino acid, uric acid, and vitamin K. In renal tubular acidosis, the acidotic state will repel positive ions, such as calcium and phosphorus, and contribute to the development of osteomalacia.[41]

The classic symptom of osteomalacia is generalized or localized bone pain. The pain is often exaggerated by movement, and bony tenderness is common. A complaint of general fatigue and achiness is often heard. Proximal myopathy and sensory polyneuropathy may accompany these complaints. Initially the progression of osteomalacia is insidious and deformity is unusual, though pathologic fractures ultimately may occur as bone strength declines and result in vertebral wedge fractures, bowing of the femur and tibia, and postural changes similar to those seen in osteoporosis. Gait and functional declines are associated with the overall loss in muscle strength.[40]

Treatment must address the nutritional-malabsorption component of this metabolic disorder. Dietary supplementation of vitamin D may be required to restore positive calcium balance and normal bone mineralization. The gastrointestinal, hepatic, or renal disorder underlying osteomalacia must be treated. Research indicates that exercise has a positive effect on osteomalacia only when adequate dietary vitamin D is provided and the metabolic disorder corrected. Then exercise has a positive effect on bone mass, similar to that described in osteoporosis.[40,41]

AVASCULAR NECROSIS

Death of bone and the cellular components of bone in the absence of infection is referred to as osteonecrosis or avascular necrosis. Avascular necrosis is the result of a disrupted arterial supply and most commonly affects the femoral head following an intracapsular or femoral neck fracture in which the circumflex arteries are injured as a result of the fracture. Avascular necrosis also can be the end result of a thrombosis of an artery supplying bone. The bone tissue becomes ischemic and permanent loss of bone occurs.[42]

Osteonecrosis, a process of "creeping substitution" where there is resorption of "dead" trabeculae and woven bone is laid down on dead trabeculae, results in the collapse of bone. Osteonecrosis can result from a number of etiologies, but most commonly it is associated with fracture, alcoholism, pancreatitis, diabetes mellitus, obesity, or gout. Other conditions that may lead to avascular necrosis include systemic lupus erythematosus, Cushing's disease, caisson disease, Gaucher's disease, idiopathic Chandlers disease, sickle cell anemia, and long-term corticosteroid use.[43]

Although the talus, scaphoid, and proximal humerus are susceptible to osteonecrosis, the femoral head is the most common site associated with this pathology. The femoral head and neck receive their circulatory supply from the medial and lateral femoral circumflex artery, which travel in a distal to proximal direction in the femoral neck and head. Fracture or displacement secondary to fracture of the neck of the femur can compromise the circulation to the head of the femur and lead to death of the bone. Following trauma or with insidious conditions, pain is reported in the groin, medial thigh, and knee, which is intermittent and associated with weight-bearing activities. Internal rotation, flexion, and adduction of the hip exacerbate the pain, and the patient will present with an antalgic gait. Radiographic examination will show the source of arterial disruption if a fracture is present but not for conditions like thrombosis. A more sensitive evaluation of bony status—a bone scan, magnetic resonance imaging (MRI), or CT scan—is required to detect earlier and subclinical stages of bone loss.

In the elderly, the treatment of choice is a total joint replacement.

PAGET'S DISEASE

Also known as osteitis deformans, Paget's disease of bone is an example of an imbalance in which bone formation overtakes bone resorption. Paget's disease is a progressive disorder associated with a marked increase in osteoblastic activity. At first there is a softening and later an overgrowth and hardening of bone. The disease progresses in three distinct stages: (1) osteoclastic, (2) osteoblastic, and (3) sclerotic. In the early stages, blood flow increases to the affected bone: primarily the skull, vertebrae, pelvis, and bones of the lower extremities. There is an initial osteoclastic, resorptive stage where abnormal proliferation of osteoclasts occurs. During this period of softening, characteristic deformities develop. The skull thickens and the forehead becomes prominent, the lower extremities bow, and the individual experiences the development of kyphosis in the thoracic vertebrae and a loss of the lumbar curve in the lumbar area with posterior prominence of the vertebrae. The initial resorption is followed by abnormal regeneration of bone through an overactive osteoblastic phase followed by sclerosis. The serum alkaline phosphatase levels are extremely high (over 100 units), indicating overactivity of the osteoblasts. The normal cancellous architecture is replaced by coarse, thickened layers of trabecular bone, and the cortical bone becomes thickened, irregular, eroded, and uneven. One would think that with the increased calcification of bone that the bone would be stronger; however, the converse is true: the bone is enlarged, eroded, and weakened by irregular alignment of trabeculae.[41,44]

The postural deformities seen in Paget's disease result in a progressively increased thoracic kyphosis and bowing of the femur and tibia. If the femoral neck softens to the point of collapse, a reduced femoral neck angle (coxa vara) results in a waddling gait pattern. These postural changes increase local mechanical stress and are associated with increasing fatigue and bone pain.[41]

On radiographs the vertebrae appear to be flattened and broadened. The cortical bone and end plates become exaggerated and the cancellous bone develops a coarse yet almost transparent appearance. Primarily affecting the axial skeleton, the progressive stages of Paget's disease weaken the bony structures resulting in significant postural deformities. If the femur and tibia are involved, they, in addition to the vertebrae, are common sites of pathological or stress fractures in individuals with Paget's disease.[41]

Symptoms are initially nonexistent and the disease begins insidiously and progresses slowly. Often the disease is first detected by an abnormal radiograph or an incidentally elevated serum alkaline phosphatate level. Pain that develops is deep, aching bone pain often associated with stress fractures, hypervascularity, and mechanical stress of the excessively weakened bones. If the skull is involved, headaches, tinnitus, vertigo, and hearing loss are frequent complaints. Hearing loss is associated with the involvement of the ossicles of the inner ear or foraminal collapse and encroachment of the eighth cranial nerve. As the disease progresses, individuals usually complain of extreme fatigue, lightheadedness, and overall "stiffness." If pain occurs acutely, it is usually indicative of a pathological fracture.

Cardiovascular involvement is often associated with Paget's disease as well. Due to vasodilatation of blood vessels in the bones, skin, and subcutaneous tissues overlying the affected bones, the individual may present with peripheral vascular involvement and an increase in cardiac output severe enough to result in congestive heart failure. In fact, it is the cardiac involvement that is the most common cause of death in the Paget's disease patient.[44]

Other clinical manifestations of Paget's disease include nerve palsy syndromes and dementia. Nerve palsy syndromes occur as a result of entrapment of the nerves due to bony collapse. With bony impingement on the structures at the base of the skull, slurred speech, incontinence, diplopia, and impaired swallowing can occur.

Osteosarcoma is reported in less than 1% of individuals with pagetic bone and may be heralded by a rapid enlargement of bone, increased bone mass, or an elevation in serum alkaline phosphate levels.

Two classes of drugs are approved by the FDA for the treatment of Paget's disease. Both classes of drugs suppress the abnormal bone remodeling that is associated with this disease. (1) Bisphosphonates, such as alendronate sodium (Fosamax), etidronate disodium (Didronel), and pamidronate disodium (Aredia), are drugs that inhibit abnormal bone resorption. (2) Calcitonin is a hormone secreted by the thyroid gland that also inhibits abnormal bone resorption (e.g., Calcimar, Miacalcin, and Osteocalcin). Other forms of treatment may include: chemotherapy in the presence of osteosarcoma, limb sparing resection, total joint replacement, or amputation.[44]

OSTEOARTHRITIS

The most prevalent orthopaedic joint pathology is osteoarthritis. It occurs in 50% of individuals aged 65 to 75 years old, and 70% of people over the age of 75.[44] Osteoarthritis is termed the wear-and-tear arthritis. The cause of primary osteoarthritis is unknown. It is defined as a noninflammatory progressive pathology of a movable articulation, especially a weight-bearing joint, and is characterized by deterioration of articular cartilage and formation of new bone at joint margins and remodeling of subchondral bone.[45] Osteoarthritis most commonly occurs in the carpometacarpal joint, the knees, and the hips. Patients will complain of pain during weight bearing in the joints, and the pain tends to be relieved by rest.

Classic treatment consists of nonsteroidal anti-inflammatory drugs (NSAIDs). However, NSAIDs for older persons have received a somewhat negative review in the medical literature due to side effects associated with long-term use.[46] Lia and Fortin[46] have encouraged physicians to use more local and specific approach modalities, such as exercises that are specific to improve a person's functioning in the osteoarthritic joints. It has been demonstrated that strengthening around an osteoarthritic joint can alleviate some of the pain, as well as increase the strength and improve the functional mobility of arthritic patients.[47,48] The clinical implication of these studies is that therapists should work with these patients on stretching and strengthening exercises frequently throughout the day. Specific techniques for the various joints of the body will be given in subsequent sections of this chapter.

In addition to pharmacological agents and exercise, typical interventions for osteoarthritis include education, rest, and possibly surgery. Patients should be instructed in joint protection and energy-conservation techniques that can help prevent acute flare-ups and help to minimize joint stress and pain.

Rehabilitation should include appropriate weight-bearing and non-weight-bearing exercises. An individually designed program of strengthening, range-of-motion, and cardiovascular fitness exercises should be implemented. The design of the strengthening program should include low weight and much repetition so as to minimize stress on the joints. Exercise that produces pain indicates that the joint is being overstressed through too much resistance or incorrect performance of the exercise. Exercises incorporating low-load, prolonged stretching performed several times a day will help to gain a more appropriate, length-tension relationship for the muscles surrounding the affected joint and may lead to decreased stress in the intra-articular and periarticular joint structures. Heat modalities may assist in decreasing pain and stiffness, and cold modalities may decrease pain and inflammation. Splints, braces, and walking aids may also be warranted to decrease the joint stresses.

Surgical interventions such as arthroscopy, arthroplasty, and osteotomy are often employed to provide symptomatic relief, improved joint mobility, and improved joint mechanics. Over 70% of hip and knee joint replacements are performed in older adults with osteoarthritis.[49] Rehabilitation following total hip or total knee replacement will be discussed in a subsequent section of this chapter. See Appendix 4 for evidence-based evaluation and treatment ideas.

RHEUMATOID ARTHRITIS

Rheumatoid arthritis (RA), a chronic, systemic inflammatory autoimmune disease, is the second major orthopaedic pathology affecting the joints in the elderly. Over 10% of people over the age of 65 are affected by rheumatoid arthritis and the prevalence of this disease increases with advancing age.[50] Rheumatoid arthritis classically affects younger women three times more than men, although this predominance is less evident beyond the age of 60.[50] The major differences between late-onset and early onset RA are that the exacerbations tend to be severe and the remissions tend to be much better. Therefore, the therapist must be cautious during the exacerbation phases and limit therapy to active assistive and active exercises. During the remission phases, the therapist can be much more aggressive when designing a strengthening and stretching program for an older patient than one for a younger person.

The characteristic feature of RA is chronic inflammation of the synovium, peripheral articular cartilage, and subchondral marrow spaces. Due to chronic inflammatory states, granulation tissue called pannus is laid down and the resulting friction erodes the articular cartilage.[50] Inflammation of the tendon sheaths also occurs, resulting in the fraying and eventual rupture of the tendons. The resultant deformities of the hands, with dislocation and lateral migration of the fingers, and the same deformities of the toes, are examples of the typical extremity deformities seen in patients with RA. Knee valgus is another example of deformities seen in this pathology.

Though the cause of RA is not specifically known, recent literature suggests that there is evidence of a genetic predisposition for the disease that is triggered by bacteria or viral infection. A definitive diagnosis is based on a combination of clinical manifestations and laboratory results. An individual with RA will often have a decreased red blood cell count, increased erythrocyte sedimentation rates, and a positive rheumatoid factor (RF).

Clinically, RA manifests itself bilaterally, primarily affecting the small joints of the hands and feet, ankles, knees, hips, shoulders, elbows, and wrists. Table 11.3 describes the typical joint deformities seen in RA. The other area commonly involved is the cervical spine. Tenosynovitis of the transverse ligament of the first and second

TABLE 11.3   Common Joint Deformities of Extremities in Rheumatoid Arthritis

Joint	Typical Deformity or Contracture
Hands (MCP/PIP/DIP)	MCP ulnar drift, swan-neck deformity, boutonnière deformity, mallet deformity, rheumatoid thumb deformity
Wrist (Carpal joints)	Volar subluxation, radial deviation
Elbow	Nodular enlargement, flexion and pronation contracture and/or deformity
Shoulder	Adduction and internal rotation contracture and/or deformity, may have subluxation
Toes (MTP/PIP/DIP)	Hallux valgus, hallux rigidus, hammer toes, claw toes, mallet toes, overlapping toes, lateral subluxation with lateral deviation
Subtalar/Midtarsal	Pronation, pes planus, instability
Ankle	Plantar equinus contracture and/or deformity
Knee	Genu valgus or genu varus, flexion contractures and/or deformity, subluxation of patella
Hip	Leg length discrepancy, flexion and adduction contractures and/or deformity

Key: *MCP—Metacarpal phalangeal joint*
     PIP—Proximal interphalangeal joint
     DIP—Distal interphalangeal joint
     MTP—Metatarsal phalangeal joint

cervical vertebra and erosion of the facet joints may lead to cervical instability with the risk of neurological damage from compression.[50] See Appendix 5 for evidence-based evaluation and treatment ideas.

THE AGING SPINE

Pain in the neck and back is not uncommon in the older population. Although there is a higher prevalence of this problem in the population aged 35 to 55, older persons do have a relatively high incidence of back and neck dysfunction.[51,52] Some of the major changes that are considered to be part of the normal aging process affect the cervical spine and back.

Muscles are less flexible, resilient, and strong.[51,52] Nevertheless, Rider and Daly found that older adults respond well to flexibility and strength training.[53] In their study, a group of older women whose average age was 72 were put on a spinal mobility program consisting of strengthening and stretching activities. The finding of this study was that functional mobility improved significantly.[53] The loss of flexibility of all soft tissues will affect mobility of the spine.

The bone tends to become less dense or be affected by osteoporosis, and as a result the older person will tend to lose height. Approximately 20% of height is lost by the thinning of the intervertebral discs, but the majority of the height loss is caused by the collapse of the cartilaginous end plates secondary to a decrease in bone density and ballooning in the disc area.[54]

Joints are more prone to osteophytes. Twomey[54] states that the layer of fat pads in older joints acts as cushions against osteophytes, and that these vascular systems are more highly innervated, which may cause more pain and sensitivity. If joint congruity is not maintained by the tone of the multifidus, there is a chance that torn portions of the cartilage would be displaced, particularly with sudden rotatory movement. Manipulative techniques, therefore, would be particularly successful in freeing the torn pieces of cartilage; however, if the techniques are too aggressive, they may gap the joints and conceivably exacerbate the damage due to shearing of articular cartilage in the joint capsules.[55] Aging changes in the cervical spine mean that older patients suffer from osteophyte formations and decreased range of motion with age. This was shown in an excellent study by Hayashi and associates.[52] In addition, older patients experience a higher incidence of vertebral anterolisthesis and retrolisthesis, and a slight decrease in the diameter of the spinal cord, which may or may not cause neurological symptomology.[54]

The implication of these changes is that the therapist needs to work on strengthening, flexibility, and the appropriate manual therapy techniques to alleviate the elderly patient's symptoms. Alternative exercise forms such as T'ai Chi and Qi Gong have also been shown to be effective in enhancing spinal mobility.[56]

SPINAL PATHOLOGY OF THE ELDERLY

Lumbar Stenosis

There are many pathologies that can affect the spine of an older person. The first spinal pathology to be discussed is lumbar stenosis, which is a multilevel impingement on structures in the lumbar spine ligaments, usually by osteophytes.[55] Pain may be in the back, hips, or lower extremities and worsens when the person walks or extends the lumbar spine.[55] It is usually partially or completely relieved with flexion. Lumbar stenosis rarely affects anyone under the age of 60.[57] Treatment for lumbar stenosis consists of:

- Rest for one to two hours in the afternoon with knees higher than the hips.
- Flexion exercises of the trunk.
- Heat and massage to decrease muscle spasm.
- Teaching and enforcing posterior pelvic tilting in all positions and activities. See Appendix 6 for evidence-based evaluation and treatment ideas.

Vertebral Compression Fractures

Vertebral compression fractures usually affect the spinal areas of the thoracic and upper lumbar spine for older persons. Fractures can occur during any kind of routine activity, such as bending, lifting, or rising from a chair. The patient often complains of immediate, severe local back pain. The pain may subside in several months, but in some cases, may continue for years. Other vertebral compression fractures, however, may cause no pain at all. The fracture may be gradual and asymptomatic, and diagnosed only by radiographs.[58] Multiple vertebral compression fractures will cause shortening of the spine and lead to the classic kyphotic position described earlier in this chapter. Progression of thoracic kyphosis can result in alveolar hyperventilation and retention of bronchial secretions with poor respiratory reserve. Eventually, the person may develop repeated episodes of pneumonia. Because all of the organs are compressed into a smaller space, often there are additional problems with abdominal symptoms, bloating, and constipation.[58]

Treatment for acute compression fractures is bed rest, but the patient must get out of bed every hour for ten minutes to work on stabilization of the back.[58] Pain relief modalities may be helpful, such as heat, ice, TENS, or electrical stimulation, to relieve some of the symptoms.[59] The authors of this book have found that the use of a six-inch Ace wrap or the binders used with rib fracture is very helpful in providing support and comfort in the area of the compression fracture. Once the person can tolerate exercise, extension exercises should be used extensively.[59] Any type of extension exercises to the thoracolumbar spine is helpful.[34,59] See Appendix 7 for evidence-based evaluation and treatment ideas.

Cervical Spondylosis

One of the pathologies affecting the neck of an older person is cervical spondylosis, which is defined as degenerative changes in the cervical spine. Symptoms of this are pain in the cervical spine with possible radiculitis into the shoulder, arms, or fingers.[60] The treatment for cervical spondylosis includes anti-inflammatories, keeping the neck in neutral or a slightly flexed position, manual traction, heat, active range of motion, and progressive resistive exercises that the patient can tolerate.[61]

Vertebral Artery Syndrome

A second pathology of the cervical spine is vertebral artery syndrome (VAS). An encroachment on the vertebral foramina results in VAS, and this can be caused by a multitude of things. The most likely cause is the combination of a narrowing of the disc, osteophyte formation from osteoarthritis, and a forward head positon.[62] The symptoms of VAS are dizziness, tinnitus, and blurred vision that occur in conjunction with a combination neck rotation and extension. The treatment for VAS is wearing a cervical collar to prevent extension, axial extension exercises, and cervical isometric exercises.[62]

The standard test for VAS is to rotate and fully extend the cervical spine while evaluating for dizziness, nausea, and nystagmus of the eyes. Caution when evaluating an elderly individual with suspected vertebral artery syndrome needs to be applied. Utilizing the standard vertebral artery test is not advisable and could actually be dangerous.[63–68] Performing the vertebral artery test may decrease blood flow in the vertebrobasilar circulation enough to result in infarction.[67,68] Arterial diagnostic testing would confirm the therapist's suspicions of the presence of VAS. The Dix-Hallpike maneuver[69] is the typical test performed in 45° of cervical rotation and 30° of extension to diagnose benign paroxysmal positional vertigo (BPPV). This maneuver does not place the older adult in as much risk as the vertebral artery test because the patient is not placed in end-range rotation or extension. Often nystagmus can be seen in older adults by placing them in supine with their head turned, although the supine position may not be comfortable for the severely kyphotic individual. An alternative is to perform the Dix-Hallpike test on the person with kyphosis using a tilt table with pillows to support the spine and head. By lowering the person's entire body, the person's alignment remains the same, yet there is stimulation to the semicircular canal. If the patient becomes vertiginous in the Trendelenburg position and complains of vertigo with head rotation and extension, this is indicative of the possibility that the individual has VAS.[70,71]

Rheumatoid Arthritis

A third pathology causing problems in the neck in the elderly is rheumatoid arthritis. Patients/clients with RA with subsequent neck pain will tend to experience the pain in the middle area and the posterior aspect of the cervical spine. Therapists should check the x-rays for atlanto-occipital subluxation. If present, the therapist should not use any manual techniques that could further exacerbate dislocation (e.g., mobilization, traction, or occipital release).[62] Proper treatment includes supporting the neck with a cervical collar, heat, ultrasound, gentle massage, and range-of-motion and progressive resistive exercises.[62]

Ossification of the Posterior Longitudinal Ligament

The fourth pathology of the neck is ossification of the posterior longitudinal ligament (OPLL). In OPLL, the ligament tends to ossify, usually over several segments of the cervical spine. This causes limitation in neck flexion and radiculopathy.[72] The treatment for OPLL consists of heat, cervical traction, and rest from sedentary static activities such as knitting, reading, computer, or desk work. In addition, stretching and range-of-motion or progressive resistive exercises are helpful.

In all of these pathologies, the therapist must first check the person's environment. Frequently, adding pillows between the knees while the person sleeps in the side-lying position can provide relief for low back pain. Putting a lumbar pillow in the wheelchair or changing the level of the footrests can provide relief for the entire spine. Since older patients spend so much time sitting, and wheelchair patients are so often bound to their chairs, the therapist must check their environments to make sure they are not exacerbating any spinal symptoms. Often a simple modification of the environment can provide tremendous relief from spinal pain. See Appendix 8 for evidence-based evaluation and treatment ideas.

The Upper Extremity

The Shoulder

Range of motion in the shoulder does decline with age. Despite the fact that studies have documented age changes,[73,74] clinically there is evidence to show that if a person uses the shoulder more frequently, the range of motion decrease will be less. The aging shoulder is more prone to certain pathologies, such as the ones discussed here: osteoarthritis, bursitis, and rotator cuff tears.

Osteoarthritis The first pathology, osteoarthritis, is very rare and may be overdiagnosed. Only 2% of shoulder problems in the elderly are truly osteoarthritis.[75] The symptoms of true osteoarthritis are a constant ache, crepitus, difficulty sleeping, and weakness. When the therapist moves the shoulder, there is a hard-end felt with joint movement. In addition, there will be a grinding and a dryness with shoulder movement.[76,77]

Treatment of osteoarthritis, when the patient has severe joint pain, is rest, gentle pain-free range-of-motion exercises, and anti-inflammatories.[76] Once the patient can move through range with less pain, however, heat or ice, functional adaptation, joint mobility, gentle weight-bearing isometrics, and range-of-motion exercises can be helpful. In addition, thermal modalities, such as ultrasound and ice, can be very helpful in alleviating pain.

Bursitis The second shoulder problem, which is more commonly seen than osteoarthritis in the elderly population, is bursitis. The symptoms of bursitis are:

1. A palpable tenderness in the area of the inflamed bursa;
2. Pain with movement of the muscle affected by the temporary bursa;
3. Symptom relief with rest.[77]

The patient will usually have a recent history of overuse of the shoulder prior to the initial onset of symptoms.[78]

Treatment for bursitis is heat or ice, ultrasound, and energy conservation. Painful movements should be avoided, and the patient should begin pain-free isometrics when he or she can tolerate them. No exercise should be done that exacerbates the pain, but having the patient exercise below and above a painful arc will be useful.

Rotator Cuff The third shoulder pathology, and the one most commonly seen in the elderly, is rotator cuff problems. The rotator cuff is composed of the infraspinous, the supraspinatus, subscapularis, and teres minor. X-ray of the subacrominal space of less than 5 mm is diagnostic of a rotator cuff tear.[78]

With the rotator cuff, the patient will complain of pain when sleeping on the shoulder. He or she will be positive on the impingement sign when the arm is brought to full passive flexion, and pain will be present for the last 10 to 20 degrees. Crepitus and catching sensations due to fibrosis and scarring may also be present. If the problem progresses, the patient/client may even have atrophy of the rotator cuff muscles and definite weakness in the shoulder abductors and flexors.[79]

Treatment for impingement, tears, and tendonitis of the rotator cuff is symptomological management. If the person has pain throughout an arc, the therapist should avoid range-of-motion exercises that use the arc and irritate the rotator cuff. The patient can be instructed to passively move the shoulder through that range and to do some end-range stretching and strengthening exercises. Heat, ultrasound, and electric stimulation may help decrease the inflammation. Passive-active assistive stretching

exercises can also be helpful, as will isometrics that do not encourage tightness in the shoulder musculature. The person must exercise the arm at least twice a day to see significant improvement.

Adhesive Capsulitis Rotator cuff dysfunctions can become more irritating problems if the person develops a frozen shoulder. Although frozen shoulders are not always preceded by rotator cuff problems, it is a common occurrence in the aged. With frozen shoulders or adhesive capsulitis, a person may or may not experience pain. A capsular pattern, where external rotation is most limited and abduction, flexion, and internal rotation of the shoulder are also limited, is a symptom of adhesive capsulitis. The person may display a protracted scapula and atrophy of the deltoid, rotator cuff,[78] biceps, and triceps. Tenderness of the anterior joint may also be present.

Treatment for a frozen shoulder is heat or ice, depending on how painful the joint is and how well the person tolerates ice. Extremely painful joints may need the numbing effect of ice. Ultrasound can also be used to relieve some inflammation. Joint mobilization must be done in all limited directions, followed by active assistive or passive range of motion and contract-relaxed stretching. Posture work and scapular retraction exercises are also helpful.

Humeral Fracture Humeral fractures are the final pathology to be discussed here. Classically, they will be either displaced or nondisplaced. Slightly more nondisplaced fractures occur, and they usually require pinning or wires. A fractured humerus usually requires that the patient use a sling for one week. After that time, the patient can remove the sling to work on general pendulum exercises, shoulder shrugs and circles, protraction and retraction, and any active motion exercises for the hand or wrist. At this point, the person should be doing no passive range of motion. For the first week, the patient should also learn ways of writing, eating, and performing daily ADLs without stressing the shoulder.[77]

By the third week the patient can begin gentle isometrics, either against the wall or using Theraband™. Active range of motion in the pain-free ranges can begin at this point as well, and the person should begin doing scapular humeral rhythm motion in front of the mirror; that is, elevating the arms without raising the shoulders. This type of activity can also be used for all the previously noted shoulder pathologies. One of the most prevalent problems is that patients with shoulder pathologies have poor scapular humeral rhythm. Normally, they do not achieve full range of motion, because they are never taught how to properly move the shoulder. Simply working with patients in front of a mirror and encouraging them not to lift the shoulders as the arm is lifted is adequate for attaining the desired results.

By the sixth or eighth week, if the patient is healed, joint mobilization can begin. Passive range of motion can also begin, but scapular humeral rhythm should be stressed.

See Appendix 9 for evidence-based evaluation and treatment ideas.

THE LOWER JOINTS OF THE UPPER EXTREMITY

The joints of the upper extremity (the elbows, wrists, and hands) show minimal changes in the range of motion with age. However, strength does decline.[80,81] The practitioner should be careful when looking at grip strength measures in the elderly, because studies have shown that the older patient's grip and pinch strength may be influenced by extraneous variables. These variables range from mental status to gait and balance problems. Therefore, grip strength may not be a true indicator of strength in the older population.[82,83]

The Elbow

Almost one-quarter of all elbow traumas and one-third of elbow fractures are fractures of the radial head,[84] which usually are stabilized with an internal fixation device. For the first three weeks, the patient is immobilized in a hinged splint with the forearm held neutral. The patient can do range-of-motion exercises with the hand and shoulder, and to control swelling, cold packs can be applied for ten minutes every hour. At day twenty-one, active range-of-motion exercises can be started and passive range and progressive resistive exercises (PRE) can be increased gently as the patient/client tolerates. This regimen is followed slowly until twelve to fifteen weeks.[84]

It is important to note that since this is such a painful fracture, practice and skill acquisition on a visual level may be beneficial. According to Maring,[85] the experimental group who visualized a forearm activity did much better than the control group who did not.

The Wrist

The most common pathology of the wrist is Colles' fracture, which is a fracture of the distal radius as a result of a fall on the hand. It can be treated by closed reduction, or it can be reduced by screws.[86] The therapist will usually see the patient once while the extremity is in a cast for instruction in edema control and for range-of-motion exercises for the uncasted upper extremity joints. After four weeks, the cast is usually removed, and at that time the therapist can use modalities as needed, such as heat, ice, and electrical stimulation to control swelling and increase circulation. Gentle joint mobilizations to the carpal joints, active range of motion, and gentle passive and resistive exercises can be started at this time. By six weeks, when the person is completely healed, the therapist can begin work on more vigorous passive resistive, contract-relax stretch-

ing exercises, or both. The therapist should be sure to reinforce the exercises with daily, functional activities at home.

Rheumatoid arthritis or osteoarthritis often affects the wrist. Marked limitation in joint mobility can severely impede functional capabilities. Often splints are advised to protect the wrist during activity. Joint protection techniques should be a part of therapy intervention. Teaching an individual how to manage activities of daily living without stressing the joints of the wrist will decrease the amount of pain and inflammation.

The Hand

The most common pathologies in the aging hand are (1) rheumatoid arthritis, (2) osteoarthritis, and (3) Dupuytren's contracture. In rheumatoid arthritis, the synovial fluid in the joints of the hand becomes particularly painful, and the person may develop ulnar drifting and significant deformities of the hand. The patient may undergo surgery or arthroplasty for severe deformities; nevertheless, the therapist can work on light exercises and splinting to help alleviate pain symptoms, as well as focusing on range-of-motion deficits.[87]

Arthritis Osteoarthritis of the hand is more common than RA. It most commonly involves the interphalangeal joints and the carpometacarpal joint of the thumb. Since the thumb is so important for functioning, this particular problem can be devastating. The patient will present with pain, swelling, and weakness, possibly due to overuse of the hand. The treatment involves joint protection, splinting to stabilize the thumb, joint mobilization, and strengthening exercises. Heat, ice, paraffin, and ultrasound can also give relief from pain and inflammation.[87,88]

Dupuytren's Contracture The final pathology involving the hand is Dupuytren's contracture, which is relatively uncommon in people under 50. It is caused by excessive collagen formation around tendons, nerves, and blood vessels in the palm of the hand, and it can cause minimal or permanent flexion of the fingers, usually of the proximal interphalangeal joints. Figure 11.4 demonstrates a typical Dupuytren's contracture. It is usually not painful, and, therefore, people often delay treatment. However, treating the problem early can be extremely effective. Heat and ultrasound to the fascia of the hand followed by unidirectional transverse friction massage, stretching, and splinting in a stretched position can be extremely helpful. Patients are encouraged to continue the friction massage, range-of-motion exercises, and heating at home to enhance the benefits of the therapeutic regimen.[87]

See Appendix 10 for evidence-based evaluation and treatment ideas.

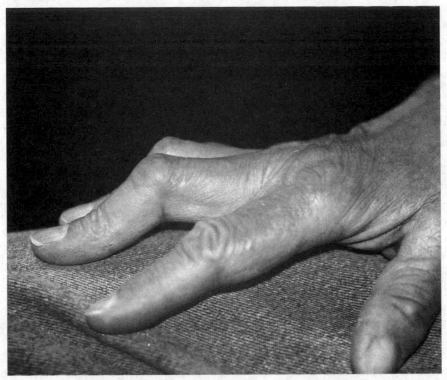

Figure 11.4   Typical Dupuytren's contracture in an elderly homeless male. (Photo by: J.M. Bottomley.)

THE LOWER EXTREMITY

The Hip

The hip shows a decrease in range of motion similar to the other joints of the body, as demonstrated in the work of James and Parker.[89] In addition, Kramer and co-workers[90] found that older women have 61% less force in their hip abductors than younger women.

The normal changes with age of decreased range of motion and strength will have a significant impact on an older person's gait, stability, and balance and may lead to a downward spiral for some of the pathologies that are commonly seen by therapists. The three major pathologies to be discussed in this section are osteoarthritis, hip fracture, and total hip replacement.

Hip Osteoarthritis

Patients with hip osteoarthritis may constantly complain of pain around or over the hip area. Even if a patient has radiographic evidence of hip osteoarthritis, the patient may also have an inflamed bursa or tensor fascia lata tendinitis that relates pain to the hip.[47] It is imperative that the therapist assess this to treat it appropriately. If the patient's hip abductors are weak, they may be carrying the body's weight differently and irritating the bursas or the tendons around the hip area.[91] A thorough examination of

these areas will help achieve an appropriate targeted treatment plan.

In arthritis of the hip, the patient will complain of an aching sensation, especially with weight bearing by the hip, and there will be corresponding radiographic evidence. The treatment for hip osteoarthritis includes alleviating stress, through the use of a cane, to decrease weight bearing until a person increases his or her strength. This can be followed by strengthening exercises to the areas around the hip, especially for the abductors and extensors, to increase the shock-absorbing system of the hip joint.[62]

Proper range of motion, stretching to the joint capsule, and ergonometric modifications may also be helpful, as can biomechanical alterations. According to Neumann and associates,[91] a patient can decrease the hip force by carrying loads on the same side or with both hands. If a patient is carrying a purse on the uninvolved side, it may actually increase the pain felt by the patient.[91] Strengthening and range-of-motion exercises have also been shown to be very beneficial for patients with osteoarthritis.[53]

Hip Fracture

Hip fracture is the most common acute orthopedic condition of the elderly. Tinetti et al.[92] found that active elderly persons fell less frequently than those were inactive, but when they did fall, it was more serious. Kampa[93] said, "Every 10 minutes someone dies from a hip fracture, and one out of every 20 women over 65 will suffer hip fracture."[93] In the United States, there are 267,000 fractures per year, and 97% of these involve persons 65 years or older, and two-thirds are women.[94]

A study by Cummings and Nevitt[94] raised some interesting points about the relationship of osteoporosis to falls. They found that osteoporosis alone does not explain the exponential increase in the incidence of falls among the elderly. They proposed that four conditions cause elderly people to fall and fracture their hips:

1. The faller is positioned so that impact occurs near the hip.
2. The faller's protective responses fail.
3. Local soft tissue absorbs less shock than necessary to prevent the fracture.
4. The residual energy of the fall exceeds the strength of the femur.

Frequently, a fracture in older people occurs in the neck and intertrochanteric area of the femur where there is less of a blood supply and the bone is of the cancellous rather than the cortical type. Due to the distal arterial supply from the circumflex artery to this area, often these fractures result in nonunion. Subtrochanteric fractures occur with very high-velocity falls and thus are rarely seen in the elderly population. The orthopedic surgeon has a multitude of choices in the types of fixation used, ranging from screws, to pins, to rods and plates. Table 11.4 lists some of these devices and the method of weight-bearing progression that can be used by therapists.[95] It is imperative that the therapist get the older patient to bear weight on the limb as soon as possible so as to enhance normal walking patterns, proprioception, and the integrity of the bone.[96]

Hip fractures are usually treated on a protocol basis.

For a total hip fracture protocol that is commonly used in departments around the United States, see Figure 11A.1 on the CD.

Baker and co-workers[97] showed that treadmill gait retraining following a fracture of the neck of the femur can significantly increase gait strength in patients.[97]

Total Hip Replacement

The third hip pathology of the elderly is total hip replacement. Total hip replacements may be used for hip fractures as well as for patients who have very severe rheumatoid arthritis, osteoarthritis, or carcinomas. Patients receiving total hip replacements tend to do well. They are usually put on a specific protocol procedure.

For an example of this protocol, see CD.

Depending on the approach used by the surgeon, various simultaneous motions need to be avoided by the patient so as not to cause dislocation. Unfortunately, there is no definitive time frame for dislocation, and some orthopedic surgeons may put patients on precaution protocols for anywhere from three months to the rest of their lives.

Some of the best predictors of outcomes for both hip fractures and total hip replacements are the number of visits that the patient makes to physical therapy.[98–100] It is imperative that patients who have had hip replacements or hip fractures receive adequate instruction in both exercise, activities of daily living, and proper precautions and methods of improving their weight-bearing status.

TABLE 11.4   Most Frequently Used Hip Fixation Devices

Device	Characteristics	Weight Bearing Precautions	Comments
Rods Enders	Three rods stablize hip fracture. Rods are inserted into femoral condyle to knee joint.	PWB-PO day 2 FWB—as tolerated	Can cause toe-out posture. Rehab of hip and knee crucial.
Nails Jewett Smith-Peterson	Long stainless steel rods are used to stablize intertrochanteric fracture.	TDWB-PO 2–5 days FWB—when totally healed	Strict weight bearing secondary to fixation possibly piercing femoral head.
Pins Knowles	Sharp stainless stell rod used to reduce non-com minuted intracapsular fracture.	TDWB-PO 2–5 days FWB—6th–7th week	Strict weight bearing secondary to fixation, possibly piercing femoral head.
Screws & Plates Richard's Compression	Most commonly chosen device for intertrochanteric fixation.	PWB-PO day 2 FWB—6th–7th week	The screwing mechanism enhances healing.

PWB = Partial weight bearing; FWB = Full weight bearing; TDWB = Touch down weight bearing; PO = Postoperative.
(Modified and reproduced with permission from Zimmer Product Encyclopedia. *Warsaw IN: Zimmer USA; December 1999.[95])*

See Appendix 11 for evidence-based evaluation and treatment ideas.

THE KNEE

The knee, similar to the hip, has been shown to lose strength with age.[101] According to Borges,[101] older patients showed a significant decrease in torque values likely to be generated at the knee. The knee, however, shows only a very slight decrease in range of motion with age.[89]

Osteoarthritis

Osteoarthritis of the knee is defined as a wearing away of the articular cartilage of the knee.[102] The articular cartilage softens, fissures occur, osteophytes form, and the synovium becomes fibrous. The capsule also thickens.[102] Barrett[103] found that older patients tend to have a slight decrease of proprioception in the knee; however, there was a significant decrease in patients who had osteoarthritis of the knee in this study. This study also found that when patients receive a joint replacement, they have an improvement in proprioception in the knee, but it is still not at the same level as normal.[103]

The important points to consider in osteoarthritis of the knee are the pain and other difficulties encountered by the patient. Frequently, the pain will occur with weight bearing, and the patient will have difficulty with gait activities and simple weight bearing. Therapists, again, need to work on decreasing forces on the knee joint until the patient is strong enough for daily activities.

According to the work of Radin,[104] the major shock-absorbing mechanism of the joint is not the cartilage but is in fact the muscle, which absorbs 80% of the shock. Therefore, a very comprehensive exercise program to improve the strength around the joint will be helpful. According to the work of Fisher and associates[47] and Kreindler and Lewis,[48] strengthening around the joint can improve range of motion and strength. Therefore, a non-weight-bearing strengthening program should be initiated early.

An article by Steinlan and co-workers[105] showed that infrared therapy helps to decrease pain in patients with osteoarthritis of the knee. In this study, patients used home infrared units for twenty minutes every eight hours with significant pain relief.[105]

According to Liang and Fortin,[46] when therapists evaluate osteoarthritis problems of the knee, they must consider other causes for the pain, such as patellar-femoral problems, bursitis, as well as tendonitis and inflammation of the ligament around the knee. If it is a patellar-femoral problem, the patient needs to work on patella-femoral tracking exercises to stimulate the vastus medialis.[106] The simplest exercise to facilitate this is a combination hip abduction with quadricep setting (Figure 11.5).

Prior to starting any strengthening program, however, the therapist must consider decreasing the swelling of the knee joint. This treatment is based on reflex inhibition due to joint extension that may cause difficulty initiating a proper contraction.[5] This can be achieved with ice or electrical modalities. In addition, the patient may complain of stiffness after sitting for long periods of time. This may be caused by an inflammatory response in the knee joint, causing cross-linking of the collagen or synovial thickening. Simply having the person roll the foot back and forth on a soda bottle or something similar can help to increase extensibility of this tissue.

Total Knee Replacement

For intervention protocols for total knee replacement, see figure 11A.2 on the CD.

The next pathology to be discussed here is the total knee replacements, which have been extremely successful in the United States.[107] The intervention protocols for total knee replacements are specific and work with patients on active range-of-motion exercises, various passive exercises, as well as strengthening exercises to improve the range of motion.

For the older patients, it is extremely important to encourage frequent but limited bouts of exercise and to emphasize range of motion. Therapists need to be aware that total knee replacements are very painful operations and are more prone to infection than are total hip replacements.[107] Therefore, the therapist needs not only to work on range of motion and strength but also to check for infection and utilize pain management techniques. Frequently, the use of ice and various weight-bearing protocols has been shown to be effective.[106]

See Appendix 12 for evidence-based evaluation and treatment ideas.

THE FOOT AND ANKLE

The foot requires a special introduction from Arthur Helfand:

> Have you ever imagined the difficulties you might encounter if your feet were in such condition that you could not walk or stand without chronic pain? The foot has received less attention than any other part of the human anatomy, possibly because injuries, disorders of the foot are seldom causes of mortality.[108]

White and Mulley found that 30% of community-dwelling elderly complain of pain in their feet.[109] Common foot disorders and deformities can cause a great deal of pain and severely curtail ambulation activities.[110] Ill-fitting or worn-out shoes can also lead to ulceration and discomfort during weight-bearing activities. Many simple and inexpensive modifications of shoes, and fabrication of

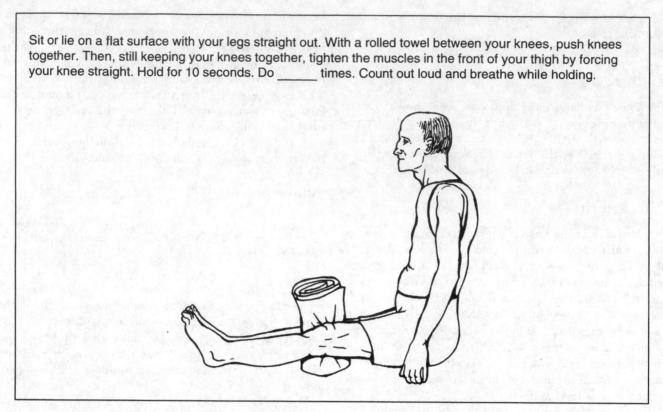

Sit or lie on a flat surface with your legs straight out. With a rolled towel between your knees, push knees together. Then, still keeping your knees together, tighten the muscles in the front of your thigh by forcing your knee straight. Hold for 10 seconds. Do _____ times. Count out loud and breathe while holding.

Figure 11.5   Exercise for facilitating a combination of hip abduction with quadriceps setting.

shock absorbing, total contact orthotics to redistribute weight evenly on the plantar surface, can greatly enhance mobility for an older adult.[111]

When evaluating feet, therapists must first check the skin for dryness and calluses. If they note that they are dry, rough, or callused, the therapist should encourage patients to use creams, unless there are open lesions. The therapist should also check the skin for the integrity of vibratory, temperature, and protective sensations; and hair growth and color to determine diminished circulation or changes consistent with metabolic disorders such as diabetes.[112]

The skin on the feet should be checked for corns and calluses. These are layers of compacted skin that have built up over irritated areas. Calluses are usually found on the soles of the feet or heels. Corns are cone-shaped areas that occur on the toes and are caused by friction and pressure from the skin rubbing against bony areas, such as when the patient wears ill-fitting shoes. The person should be encouraged to wear shoes that fit properly.[111]

The bony alignment of the foot also needs to be checked. The therapist should check for lesser toe deformities such as claw-like hammer toes, mallet toes, dislocated, and/or overlapping toes. These lesser toe deformities are usually the result of weakness in the soft tissue surrounding metatarsal heads, which can lead to tendonitis or capsulitis. Treatment is aimed at relieving pressure. Interventions, such as metatarsal bars or "cookies" (pads) to splay the metatarsal heads, intrinsic exercises to strengthen the foot,

such as toe spreads and stretches, as well as anti-inflammatory medication can be very helpful.[111,113] Hallux valgus, another bone deformity, is an inward deviation of the first metatarsal, coupled with an outward deviation and rotational deformity of the great toe.[110] A person can develop osseous enlargements and joint pain. Treatments include: ultrasound, whirlpool, iontophoresis, joint mobilization, and exercise to the great toe. Orthotics are extremely important for redistributing the forces under the second metatarsal head and for assisting these patients in pressure and pain relief.[111]

Circulation and sensation should be checked in the foot. Patients complaining of cramping and fatigue should receive special attention. For these patients, it is important that they inspect their feet, that they keep them warm and dry, and that they do not wear circular garters that cut off the blood supply to the feet. Patients also need to be careful about any type of medication used on their feet, so as to not cause skin damage. Buerger-Allen exercises may be helpful in improving circulation in the aging foot.

There are strength and joint mobility changes in the foot, Vandervoort and Hayes[114] showed a slowing and a decrease in torque generation applied to foot and ankle flexors in old persons of 71%, when compared with younger persons.[115] This means that older people will be significantly weaker in their plantarflexion strength, which may be a very important factor in balance. (See also Chapter 3.) In addition, ankle and foot range of motion decrease with age, limiting adaptability of the foot to changing walking surfaces.[89]

The approach for foot problems is a thorough evaluation and then treatment of the appropriate problem with modalities and exercises as needed. The importance of properly fitting shoes cannot be stressed enough. Frequently, older persons have been purchasing inappropriately sized shoes for many years, and it will be difficult to convince them they need different-sized shoes. To instruct an older person in the proper shoe fit, the following criteria should be used: When a person stands, a thumb (rule of thumb) should fit between the end of the longest toe to the end of the shoe. When the therapist squeezes the person's shoe (while he or she is standing) at the metatarsal head, a slight give should be felt prior to feeling the metatarsal heads. The metatarsal heads should never be in contact with the lateral borders of the toe box of the shoe.[115] In approximately 99% of cases, patients have poor-fitting shoes. In addition, the shoes should have a strong, supportive sole made of rubber or crepe, so that they do not slip. The sole should have a wide base, and high heels should be strongly discouraged.[1]

See Appendix 13 for evidence-based evaluation and treatments ideas.

Appendix A

STRENGTH

Evaluation Ideas

Strength Testing in Elderly Women Using a Portable Dynamometer; by Karner; *PT Can*; 98[116]

■ Portable dynamometry is reliable.
  • interrater—.860
  • intrarater—716

The Reliability of Upper and Lower-Extremity Strength Testing in a Community Survey of Older Adults; by Ottenbacher; *Arch Phys Med Rehabil*; 10-02[117]

With six intensive hours of training with a physical therapist, laypersons could learn to collect reliable data with dynamometry.

Treatment Ideas

Once-Weekly Resistance Exercise Improves Muscle Strength and Neuromuscular Performance in Older Adults; by Taaffe; *J Am Geriatr Soc*; 10–99[118]

A 1RM program done once or twice a week was as efficacious as a 3x/wk program.

Progressive Resistance Muscle Strength Training of Hospitalized Frail Elderly; by Sullivan; *Am J Phys Med Rehabil*; 7–01[119]

■ A carefully monitored program of PREs is safe and effective for frail elderly recuperating from an acute illness.
  • 10 weeks
  • Weeks 1 and 2 low intensity
  • 3–10 weeks = 80% of 1RM
  • Monitor HR, BP

Effects of Regular and Slow Speed Resistance Training on Muscle Strength; by Westcott; *J Sports Med Phys Fit*; 6–01[120]

■ Super slow training resulted in a 50% greater increase in strength than did regular training.
■ Protocol:
  • 4–6 repetitions per set
  • 14 sec each
  • 10 sec lifting
  • 4 sec lowering
  • at % 80 of 1RM

The Efficacy of Aquatic Exercise in Increasing Strength; by White; *Sports Med Train Rehabil*; 9–99[121]

■ 8 weeks
■ 3×/wk
■ Showed increased strength in the experimental but not the control group
■ Jogging, goose step, striding, straddles
■ 40 minutes

Appendix B

FLEXIBILITY

Evaluation Ideas

The Reliability and Validity of a Chair Sit-and-Reach Test as a Measure of Hamstring Flexibility in Older Adults; by Jones; *Res Quart Ex Sport*; 98[122]

- It is reliable and valid.
- Sit on edge of 17-in folding chair.
- Extend preferred leg; heel to floor and D/F to 90°.
- Other leg's sole of foot flat on floor.
- Hands on top of each other; palms down.
- Try to touch toes.
- Measure from middle finger to end of shoe.

Treatment Ideas

The Effect of Duration of Stretching of the Hamstring Muscle Group for Increasing Range of Motion in People Aged 65 Years or Older; by Feland; *Phys Ther*; 5–01[123]

A 60-second stretch produced greatest rate of gain in range of motion.

- 5 × wk
- 6 weeks
- 4 times each session

Appendix C

OSTEOPOROSIS

Evaluation Ideas

A Questionnaire to Evaluate Disability in Osteoporotic Patients with Vertebral Compression Fracture; by Helmes; *Journal of Gerontology*; 3–95[124]

Conclusions: The OFDQ is a reliable instrument which correlates well with objective measures of osteoporotic spinal damage.

Treatment Ideas

Effects of High-Intensity Strength Training on Multiple Risk Factors for Osteoporotic Fractures; by Nelson; *JAMA*; 12–94[125]

- Conclusions: High-intensity strength training is an effective and feasible means to preserve bone density while improving muscle mass, strength, and balance in postmenopausal women.
- Program:
  - 50–80% 1RM (increasing weight until unable to lift)
  - 3 sets of 8 reps (6–9 seconds on the contraction with 3 seconds rest, 120 seconds rest between sets)
  - 2 days for 50 weeks

Long-term Exercise Using Weighted Vests Prevents Hip Bone Loss in Postmenopausal Women; by Snow; *J Gerontol Med Sci*; 8–2000[126]

- Experimental:
  - 9 months
  - weighted vest and jumping
  - 3×/wk
  - over 5 years continued at 32 weeks for 5 years
- Control:
  - Same as above but only active exercise

Effects of One Year of Resistance Training on the Relation Between Muscular Strength and Bone Density in Elderly Women; by Rhodes; *Brit J Sports Med*; 2000[127]

Significant relations were recorded between dynamic leg strength and BMD of the femoral neck and lumbar spine.

Can Strong Back Extensors Prevent Vertebral Fx in Women with Osteoporosis?; by Sinaki; *Mayo Clin Proc*; 12–96[128]

There is a negative correlation between back extensor strength and both kyphosis and number of vertebral fractures.

Relationship Between Grip Strength and Radial Bone Mineral Density in Young Athletes; by Tsuji; *Arch Phys Med Rehabil*; 3–95[129]

Conclusions: Grip strength is one of the determinant factors of radial BMD in the dominant forearm of young athletes.

Regular Tai Chi Chuan Exercise May Retard Bone Loss in Postmenopausal Women; by Qin; *Arch Phys Med Rehabil*; 10–02[130]

Women aged 50–59 years with over 4 years of regular T'ai Chi exercise had significantly higher BMD than age-matched nonexercising controls.

Effects of Exercise Training Added to Ongoing HRT on BMD in Frail Elderly Women; by Villareal; *J Am Geriatric Soc*; 7–03[131]

- 9-month program sig ^ strength and BMD.
- Program—Low-Intensity Exercise as a Modifier of Physical Frailty in Older Adults; Brown; *Arch Phys Med Rehabil*; 7–2000
  - 3 phases   complete 36 sessions at each phase before progressing to the next; 3×/wk; 90–120 minutes
    - phase 1 — 22 functional exercises.
    - phase 2—Added progressive resistance to the 22 exercises.
    - phase 3—Endurance exercises added to 1 and 2—individually prescribed walking, cycling, rowing, initial goal 15 min to 30; 65–75% peak heart rate

Community-Based Exercise Program Reduces Risk Factors for Falls in 65- to 75-Year-Old Women with OP: RCT; by Carter; *Can Med Assoc J*; 10–02[132]

- Relative to controls, participants experienced ^ in balance and strength.
- 2×/wk for 20 weeks.
- 40 minutes of PRE and stretches.
- www.osteofit.org.

High-Frequency Vibration Training ^ Muscle Power in Postmenopausal Women; by Russo; *Arch Phys Med Rehabil*; 12–03[133]

- Participants stood for three 2-minute sessions; (12hz–28Hz); 1 minute rest.
- 2×/wk for 6 months.
- Muscle strength ^ 5% but no change in BMD.

The Impact of a Senior Dancing Program on Spinal and Peripheral Bone Mass; by Kudlacek; *Am J Phys Med Rehabil*; 12–97[134]

The dance group with OP showed a significant increase in BMD, whereas the dance group without OP remained unchanged.

- The effect of muscle strength on bone mass is more systemic than site specific.
- Spinal BMD is more affected by weight bearing than strength.

Exercise: A Prevention and Treatment for Osteoporosis and Injurious Falls in the Older Adult; by Smith; *J Aging Phys; Act.* 3–95[135]

- Conclusions: If physical activity is within a rather broad normal range for the individual, BMD is not affected.
- Exercise prescription will need to be accompanied by pharmacological and nutritional interventions in order to secure a clinically meaningful increase in BMD.

Osteoporosis Functional Disability Questionnaire

Population:	Patients with osteoporosis and back pain due to vertebral fractures.
Description:	The Osteoporosis Functional Disability Questionnaire (OFDQ) is a specific instrument that was developed to measure disability in 5 domains; quantitative indices of pain, a standard 20-item depression scale, a 26-item functional ability questionnaire, a scale of social activities, and questions regarding the confidence that the patient places in the ability of the prescribed treatment to reverse disability.
Mode of Administration:	The OFDQ is a self-administered paper and pencil questionnaire.

Scoring:

Time to Complete:	Approximately 25 minutes.
Time to Score:	Approximately 10 minutes.
Scoring:	There are certain questions which make up each domain and different ranges to score each of the domains.

Back Pain: The back pain score is made up of four questions: *General health (exclusive of osteoporosis)* is question 1.7 and the range of scores is 1–5. *Visual analogue pain score* is question 1.5 and the possible score is between 0–100. *Pain interference with usual daily activities* is question 1.1 and the score can be 1–7. *Ranked pain score* is question 1.2 and the score can range from 1–5.

Depression Score: The depression score is derived from question 4. There are 20 items about how people sometimes feel. The patient circles the number 0–3, which corresponds to his/her feelings for each item. The score is derived from the total of the items. The range of score is from 0–60. **(Note: The responses for items d, h, l, and p must be reversed. For example, if a patient circles 0 for item d, then the score is actually a 3.**

Activities of Daily Living Score: The patient circles the number 0–4, which best describes his/her ability to do the activities listed. The responses from the 26 items in question 8 are summed to give the ADL score. The score can range from 0–104.

Social Activities Score: This score is derived from the number of activities or clubs the patient checks in question 3.2 $\times$ 0.5. The score can range from 0–10.

Confidence in Program Benefit Score: This is the score from question 2.3 and the range is from 1–5.

Interpretation:	For all the domains, with the exception of the ADL items, an increasing score means increasing disability. In the ADL domain, an increasing score represents decreasing disability. Currently the authors of the OFDQ are working on a way to derive an overall score for osteoporosis functional disability.
Reliability:	Reliability was determined using the test-retest and internal consistency methods. The results showed that the test-retest reliabilities ranged from .76 to .93 with internal consistencies form .57 to .96.
Validity:	Criterion validity was assessed by correlating disability against radiographic evidence of vertebral fractures. Construct validity was demonstrated through comparisons of 81 patients with osteoporosis and fractures to 37 health age-matched controls. The OFDQ was able to clearly distinguish the osteoporotic patients from the healthy controls in 4 of the 5 domains.
Reference:	Reprinted with permission from Anthony, B., Hodsman, M.B., Professor of the Department of Medicine, St Joseph's Health Centre London, Ontario.

Osteoporosis Functional Disability Questionnaire

1. Please answer the following Questions by writing the NUMBER that <u>best</u> fits your feelings in the space provided.

1.1 How often does your back pain interfere with, or limit your usual activity over the past month. Would you say:
   1. never
   2. rarely
   3. not very often
   4. some times
   5. often
   6. very often
   7. all the time

   ANSWER: _____

1.2 How would you rate the severity of your back pain over the last month? Would you say that it is:
   1. not at all severe
   2. not very severe
   3. somewhat severe
   4. severe
   5. very severe

   ANSWER: _____

1.3 Would you tell me how your back pain has changed over the past year. Would you say it is:
   1. a lot better
   2. somewhat better
   3. about the same
   4. somewhat worse
   5. a lot worse

   ANSWER: _____

1.4 During the past two months, how many days did your back pain keep you from work, housework, or other activities at all?

   ANSWER: _____ days

   ANSWER: _____ none

1.5 The line below is a graphic representation of the possible range of pain you have experienced over the past month. Please indicate how severe you consider your pain to be by placing a slash through the line.

least
possible
pain

| 0 | 25 | 50 | 75 | 100 |

worst
possible
pain

I would like to find out how your pain changes during the week. Please circle the number that best indicates the nature of your pain.

Using this scale tell me about your pain.

	None	Mild	Distressing	Horrible	Excruciating
a) Right now	0	1	2	3	4
b) At its worst	0	1	2	3	4
c) At its best	0	1	2	3	4

From time to time people may experience illnesses that vary in both seriousness and duration. Keeping these kinds of illnesses in mind, and excluding your problem with back pain, how would you describe your general health over the past year? Would you say your health has been:

1. excellent
2. good
3. fair
4. poor
5. very poor

   ANSWER: _____

In the last three months have you had any other health condition that has caused you pain? Please check either No or Yes.

No _____

Yes _____   Specify: _____

There appears to be a number of reasons why people decide to participate in the Osteoporosis Program. It is important for us to find out why you did join it. Please read the following list and choose three of the most important reasons for your decision to enter the Osteoporosis Program by assigning number 1 for the most important, 2 for the second most important, and 3 for the third most important reason. Please choose only the three most important reasons.

_____ to reduce or eliminate pain
_____ to lose weight
_____ to improve my health in general
_____ to look better
_____ to get away
_____ to meet and socialize with people
_____ to help myself be able to work
_____ to please the person who recommended this program
_____ other (specify) _____

2.2 Do you really believe this program will:

a) improve your health in general   _____ yes   _____ no
b) reduce or eliminate your pain   _____ yes   _____ no
c) help you lose weight   _____ yes   _____ no
d) help you feel better about yourself   _____ yes   _____ no
e) help you to be able to work   _____ yes   _____ no
f) provide meaningful social life   _____ yes   _____ no
g) improve your physical activities in general _____ yes   _____ no

2.3 To what extent are you confident about the program? Choose one response category that best describes your feeling about this program.

    1. I am absolutely certain it will be helpful.
    2. I am somewhat confident about the program.
    3. I hope it is helpful, but not sure about it.
    4. I am somewhat doubtful about the effect of the program.
    5. I am almost certain that it would not help me to much.

ANSWER: _____

3.1 When you think of your overall financial situation, how difficult would you say it is to meet each of the following commitments? Please circle each commitment according to whether it is: very difficult, somewhat difficult, or not at all difficult.

	very difficult	somewhat difficult	not at all difficult
a) housing	0	1	2
b) food	0	1	2
c) personal expenses	0	1	2
d) transportation	0	1	2
e) medical expenses	0	1	2
f) any other commitment that is difficult to meet (specify) _____	0	1	2

Now I would like to ask you some questions about clubs or organizations you may belong to.

3.2 Do you belong to one or more groups, itemized in the categories listed below (a–f)? Make a check mark for all activities in which you actively participate or attend.

TYPE	ACTIVITY	Check all relevant items
a) CHURCH RELATED GROUP	Board/Standing Committee	_____
	Mens'/Womens' Group	_____
	Voluntary Services	_____
	Choir, Usher	_____
b) JOB RELATED ASSOCIATION	Farmers' Organization	_____
	Business Professional	_____
	Organization	
	Labor Union	_____
c) RECREATIONAL	Bowling League	_____
	Womens' Club	_____
	Card Club, Golf Club	_____
d) FRATERNAL-SERVICE	Mason's or Eastern Star	_____
	Service Club (e.g. Lions, Rotary)	_____
	Hospital Auxiliary	_____
e) CIVIC-POLITICAL	Parent-Teachers Association	_____
	Political Party Club	_____
	Chamber of Commerce	_____
f) OTHER ORGANIZATIONS	Adult leader of a youth group (e.g. Boy Scouts, Brownies)	_____
	Veterans' Organizations	_____
	Board member of a community agency	_____
	Any other group not yet mentioned	_____

4. You are going to read some sentences that say something about how people sometimes feel. Please circle the number that best indicates how often you have felt this way in the past 7 days.

    Have you felt this way:

        0. rarely or none of the time (less than 1 day)
        1. some or a little of the time (1 to 2 days)
        2. occasionally or a moderate amount of the time (3 to 4 days)
        3. most or all of the time (5 to 7 days)

During the past seven days:

a) I was bothered by things that usually don't bother me.	0	1	2	3
b) I did not feel like eating; my appetite was poor.	0	1	2	3
c) I felt that I could not shake off the blues even with the help from my family or friends.	0	1	2	3
d) I felt that I was just as good as other people	0	1	2	3
e) I had trouble keeping my mind on what I was doing.	0	1	2	3
f) I felt depressed.	0	1	2	3
g) I felt that everything I did was an effort.	0	1	2	3
h) I felt hopeful about the future.	0	1	2	3
i) I thought my life had been a failure.	0	1	2	3
j) I felt fearful.	0	1	2	3
k) My sleep was restless.	0	1	2	3
l) I was happy.	0	1	2	3
m) I talked less than usual.	0	1	2	3
n) I felt lonely.	0	1	2	3
o) People were unfriendly.	0	1	2	3
p) I enjoyed life.	0	1	2	3
q) I had crying spells.	0	1	2	3
r) I felt sad.	0	1	2	3
s) I felt that people disliked me.	0	1	2	3
t) I could not get "going."	0	1	2	3

5. I would like some information about your ability to do a number of day to day activities on your own, and without help. Please circle the number that best shows whether you were able to do these things, as follows: 0. absolutely unable to do, 1. very difficult to do, 2. can do with help, 3. able to do without help, but with some discomfort, 4. able to do without effort. There may be activities that do not apply to you. In this case, draw a line through them.

	0	1	2	3	4
a) Get in and out of bed	0	1	2	3	4
b) Use the toilet.	0	1	2	3	4
c) Bath yourself.	0	1	2	3	4
d) Dress and put on your shoes.	0	1	2	3	4
e) Cut your toenails.	0	1	2	3	4
f) Prepare light meals.	0	1	2	3	4
g) Prepare large meals for family or entertainment.	0	1	2	3	4
h) Wash up the dishes.	0	1	2	3	4
i) Do laundry.	0	1	2	3	4
j) Do light housework.	0	1	2	3	4
k) Do vacuuming.	0	1	2	3	4
l) Do heavy housework	0	1	2	3	4
m) Go shopping.	0	1	2	3	4
n) Go on social outings.	0	1	2	3	4
o) Walk around the house.	0	1	2	3	4
p) Climb stairs.	0	1	2	3	4
q) Walk down stairs.	0	1	2	3	4
r) Hold a book to read.	0	1	2	3	4
s) Walk outdoors for over 15 minutes.	0	1	2	3	4
t) Pursue an active interest in your hobby (_____).	0	1	2	3	4
u) Ride a bus.	0	1	2	3	4
v) Drive an automobile.	0	1	2	3	4
w) Do gardening.	0	1	2	3	4
x) Bend down.	0	1	2	3	4
y) Reach overhead.	0	1	2	3	4
z) Difficulty sitting down.	0	1	2	3	4

Reprinted with Permission of Dr. Anthony Hodsman, St. Joseph's Health Center, London, Ontario, based on research by: E. Helmes, PhD; D.A. Lazowski, BScPT; A.B. Hodsman, MB; A. Rhardwei, MD.

Routine for:
Created by:

OSTEOPOROSIS-1 The Body Extender

Extend arms over head or as far as possible. Push entire body down. Count out loud while pushing _____ seconds. Relax _____ seconds.
Repeat _____ times. Do _____ sessions per day.

OSTEOPOROSIS-2 Shoulder Pinch

Pinch shoulder blades together.

Hold _____ seconds while counting out loud.

Repeat _____ times.
Do _____ sessions per day.

OSTEOPOROSIS-3 Axial Extension (Chin Tuck)

Gently pull chin in while lengthening back of neck.

Hold _____ seconds while counting out loud.

Repeat _____ times.
Do _____ sessions per day.

OSTEOPOROSIS-4 Elbow Back

Place hands behind head and pull elbows back as far as possible. Hold _____ seconds while counting out loud.
Repeat _____ times. Do _____ sessions per day.

OSTEOPOROSIS-5 Arm Reach

Bring arms straight up over had and back as far as possible, causing back to arch gently.

Repeat _____ times.
Do _____ sessions per day.

OSTEOPOROSIS-6 Back Archer

Clasp hands at lower back and arch back while pulling hands away from body.

Hold _____ seconds.

Repeat _____ times.
Do _____ sessions per day.

OSTEOPOROSIS-7 Buttocks Squeeze

Sitting, lying or standing, squeeze buttocks together while counting out loud to 10.

Repeat _____ times.
Do _____ sessions per day.

OSTEOPOROSIS-8 Back Wall Slide

With feet _____ inches from wall, lean as much of back against the wall as possible. Gently squat down _____ inches, keeping back against wall.

Hold _____ seconds while counting out loud.

Repeat _____ times.
Do _____ sessions per day.

OSTEOPOROSIS-9 Toe Up

Leaning against wall, go up and down on toes.

Repeat _____ times.
Do _____ sessions per day.

245

WOMAC

Population: Adult population, osteoarthritis of the hip or knee

Description: WOMAC is a self-administered health survey which was designed to measure the disability of patients with osteoarthritis of the hip or knee.

Mode of Administration: WOMAC is a paper and pencil self administered exam.

Completion:

Time to Complete: 10 to 15 minutes

Time to Score: 5 minutes

Scoring: The patient marks their response on a 10 cm Visual Analog Scale. Individual items are scored in relation to the mark the patient made. The final score is computed by adding the individual scores together.

Interpretation: The higher the patients score on the WOMAC the more severe their level of disability.

Reliability: In a study of 57 patients, 28 of which received isoxicam and 29 received piroxicam, the individual subsets were examined both independently and then as a total measure to test for internal consistency using Cronbach's alpha. With the exception of the pain subset the other received a value greater than 0.85 demonstrating strong internal consistency. The pain section had a computed value of 0.73 for the alpha coefficient, which is moderate.

Scores for test-retest reliability were found to be slightly lower than those computed for internal consistency. However, the results of calculating the Kendall tau c statistic indicates that the WOMAC has a moderate level of test-retest reliability.

Validity: Content validity of the WOMAC was established based on the theoretical observations of a literature review of pertinent material and the input from 100 osteoarthritis patients.

Construct validity was established through the comparison of the WOMAC to other indices which cover the same content as the WOMAC. The comparative indices were the Modified Doyle Score, the Lequesne Index, the Bradburn Index and the MHIQ index. Through this comparison the WOMAC was refined until it met acceptable standards.

Reference: Bellamy, N., Buchanon, W., Goldsmith, C.H., Campbell, J., Stitt, L. Validation Study of WOMAC: A Health Status Instrument for Measuring Clinically Important Patient Relevant Outcomes to Antirheumatic Drug Therapy in Patients with Osteoarthritis of the Hip or Knee. *Journal of Rheumatology.* 1988; 15(12):1833–1840.

THE WESTERN ONTARIO AND McMASTER UNIVERSITIES OSTEOARTHRITIS INDEX

WOMAC

Pain

		RATE		0 = None
1	Walking	RATE		0 = None
2	Stair climbing	DIFFICULTY		1 = Slight
3	Nocturnal			2 = Moderate
4	Rest			3 = Very
5	Weight bearing			4 = Extreme

Stiffness

1   Morning stiffness
2   Stiffness occurring later in the day

Physical Function   RATE   Unbearable Pain
1   Descending stairs   PAIN
2   Ascending stairs
3   Rising from sitting
4   Standing
5   Bending to floor
6   Walking on flat
7   Getting in/out of car
8   Going shopping
9   Putting on socks
10 Rising from bed
11 Taking off socks
12 Lying in bed
13 Getting in/out of bath
14 Sitting
15 Getting on/off toilet
16 Heavy domestic duties
17 Light domestic duties

Social Function
1   Leisure activities
2   Community events
3   Church attendance
4   With spouse
5   With family
6   With friends
7   With others   No pain

Emotional Function
1   Anxiety
2   Irritability
3   Frustration
4   Depression
5   Relaxation
6   Insomnia
7   Boredom
8   Loneliness
9   Stress
10 Well-being

Reprinted with permission. Bellamy et al. *Journal of Rheumatology* 1988; 15:1833–1840.

Appendix D

Osteoarthritis

Evaluation Ideas

> WOMAC—The Western Ontario and McMaster Universities Osteoarthritis Index[136]

Treatment Ideas

> **Physical Therapist–Based Group Exercise/Education Program to Improve Functional Health in Older HMO Members with Arthritis; by Gunther; *J Ger Phys Ther*; 03[137]**
>
> - 90 minutes for 9 weeks 26(1)
> - 60 minutes of exercise
> - 15 minutes stretching
> - 15 minutes strengthening
> - 15 minutes endurance
> - 15 minutes balance
> - 30 minutes education
> - Diet, stress, medication, community resources
> - Body mechanics, energy conservation, etc.
> - Group showed functional and psychological improvement.

> **Effects of T'ai Chi Training on Function and Quality of Life Indicators in Older Adults with Osteoarthrits; by Hartman; *J Am Geriatr Soc*; 12–2000[138]**
>
> - RCT of a 2×/wk program for 12 weeks
> - 10–15 minute warm-up
> - 35–45 minutes of T'ai Chi practice
> - 5 minutes cool down
> - 15 min/day practice at home
>
> Improved in both function and quality of life

Appendix E

Rheumatoid Arthritis

Evaluation Ideas

> **Development of an Instrument to Measure Pain in RA; by Anderson; *Arthritis Care Res*; 8–01[139]**
>
> - The RAPS is a reliable and valid instrument for measuring rheumatoid arthritis pain.
> - 0–6 Likert scale for 24 questions.
> - The lower the score, the worse the pain.

Treatment Ideas

> **Persistent Functional and Social Benefit 5 Years After a Multidisciplinary Arthritis Program; by Schloten; *Arch Phys Med Rehabil*; 10–99[140]**
>
> - A 9-day program given by a rheumatologist, orthopedist, PT, and SW led to significant improvement in outcome.
> - Program:
>   - Pathogenesis and drug therapy.
>   - Pt + jt protection, exercise, stress management.
>   - Surgery and coping and efficacy.
>   - Each session has a 10-minute exercise session.

> **A Randomized Controlled Trial to Evaluate the Efficacy of Community Based Physical Therapy in the Treatment of People with Rheumatoid Arthritis; by Bell; *J Rheumatol*; 5–98[141]**
>
> Four hours of community based physical therapy intervention delivered over six weeks significantly improved self-efficacy, disease management knowledge, and morning stiffness.

Rheumatoid Arthritis Pain Scale (RAPS)

DIRECTIONS: The following items relate to pain and arthritis. For each item, choose one number from 0 (never) to 6 (always) to describe how you have felt in the last week.

0	1	2	3	4	5	6
Always						Never

1. I would describe my pain as gnawing. _____
2. I would describe my pain as aching. _____
3. I would use the word exhausting to describe my pain. _____
4. I would describe my pain as annoying. _____
5. I am in constant pain. _____
6. I would describe my pain as rhythmic. _____
7. I have swelling of at least one joint. _____
8. I have morning stiffness of one hour or more. _____
9. I have pain on motion of at least one joint. _____
10. I cannot perform all the everyday tasks I normally would because of pain. _____
11. Pain interferes with my sleep. _____
12. I cannot decrease my pain by using methods other than taking extra medication. _____
13. I would describe my pain as burning. _____
14. I find that I guard my joints to reduce pain. _____
15. I brace myself because of the pain. _____
16. My pain is throbbing in nature. _____
17. I would describe my pain as sharp. _____
18. I would say my pain is severe. _____
19. I feel stiffness in my joints after rest. _____
20. My joints feel hot. _____
21. I feel anxious because of pain. _____
22. I would describe my pain as tingling. _____
23. I feel my pain is uncontrollable. _____
24. I feel helpless to control my pain. _____

When looking at the scale below, overall I would rate my pain as. _____

0	1	2	3	4	5	6	7	8	9	10
NONE										SEVERE

Your doctor will complete your score based on his/her examination of your joints.
Total joint score: _____

Exercise can Reverse Quadriceps Sensorimotor Dysfunction that is Associated with RA without Exacerbating Disease Activity; Similar Rx and results; Bearne; *Rheumatology*; 02[142]

■ A short-term intensive exercise program in active RA is more effective in improving muscle strength than is a conservative exercise program, and it does not have deleterious effects on disease activity.
■ Intensive program:
  • isometric and PRE to UE and LE 5x/wk
  • cycling 3×/wk
  • mean age 60, disease duration 8 years, Rx lasted 30 days

A Randomized and Controlled Trial of Hydrotherapy in RA; by Hall; *Arthitis Care Res*; 6–96[143]

■ Hydrotherapy, land exercise, and progressive relaxation all improved physically and emotionally.
  • 2×/wk
  • 4 weeks
■ Improvements lasted over 3 months.

Appendix F

LUMBAR STENOSIS

Evaluation Ideas

Measurement Properties of a Self-Administered Outcome Measure in Lumbar Spinal Stenosis; by Stucki; *Spine*; 96[144]

■ 3 subscales; total score 17–79 (higher = worse)
■ Symptom severity: 1 = none; 2 = mild; 3 = moderate; 4 = severe; 5 = very severe
■ Balance: 1 = none; sometimes = 3; often = 5
■ Physical function: no = 4; with pain = 3; some pain = 2; comfortably = 1
■ Satisfaction: very = 1; somewhat = 2; somewhat dissatisfied = 3; very dissatisfied = 4

Treatment Ideas

Surgical and Nonsurgical Management of Lumbar Spinal Stenosis; by Atlas; *Spine*; 3–2000[145]

■ Patients had more severe sx at baseline, yet had better outcomes four years later.
■ Nevertheless, 40% of surgical patients and 60% of nonsurgical patients had unsatisfactory outcomes.

A Nonsurgical Treatment approach for Patients with Lumbar Spinal Stenosis; by Fritz; *Phys Ther*; 9–97[146]

■ Patients were treated with flexion exercises and unloading ambulation.
■ Improvements were noted in all outcome measures after 6 weeks of PT and 1 month later.

Appendix G

VERTEBRAL COMPRESSION FRACTURES

Evaluation Ideas

See evaluation ideas for osteoporosis above.

Treatment Ideas

Compression Fractures Due to Osteomalacia, OP or Osteopenia; by Morgan; *Phys Ther Case Rep*; 9–2000[147]

■ Eval = rolling with difficulty, supine to sitting ^ pain, arms longer than trunk, hands hang anterior of body, reduced lung capacity, decreased shoulder flexion, abduction, hip flexion too painful to test
■ Rx = proper positioning, bed rest max 3 days, ice, TENS, rib mobs, diaphragmatic breathing, PRE to Trapezius, Latissimus Dorsi, cervical spine, Thoracic spine horizontal abduction PRE, sitting push-ups

Patient Questionnaire for Lumbar Spinal Stenosis

Population:	Patients with lumbar spinal stenosis.
Description:	The questionnaire is divided into threee scales; seven questions on symptom severity, five questions on physical function, and six questions on patient satisfaction. The measure is intended to complement existing generic measures of spinal-related disability and health status.
Mode of Administration:	Each of the questionnaires are self-administered paper and penell exams.

Scoring:

Time to Complete: 5 minutes for all three scales.

Time to Score: 5 minutes

Scoring: All but one item in the seven symptom severity questions has a Likert response scale with 5 categories scored from 1–5. (none, mild, moderate, severe, very severe). The balance disturbance question has three categories; none, sometimes, and often. The scores for this question are 1, 3, 5, respectively. The score is calcuated as the unweighted mean of all answered items in the questionnaire. If there are more than two answers missing, the the scale score is also considered missing. The overall scale score range is from 1 to 5.

The physical function questions were also set up with Likert scale responses, with the exception of one of the five questions. There are four response options with scores from 1–4 (no could not perform; yes, but always with pain; yes, but sometimes with pain; yes, comfortably). The overall score is the unweighted mean of all answered items as long as there are no more than two items missing. The range is from 1–4.

The satisfaction questions all have Likert response scales with four categories with scores ranging from 1–4 (very satisfied, somewhat satisfied, somewhat dissatisfied, and very dissatisfied). The satisfaction scale score was the unweighted mean of the responses as long as the number of responses exceeded four. The range of the scale is from 1–4, with I being the most satisfied.

Interpretation:	In the symptom severity scale, a higher score is indicative of more severe symptoms. In the physical function scale, a high score reflects less ability to function. In the satisfaction scale, a low score reflects satisfaction, whereas a high score indicates dissatisfaction.
Reliability:	Internal consistency was measured with Cronbach's coefficient alpha on cross-sectional data from 193 patients before surgery. The range was from 0.64 to 0.92. Test-retest reliability was also assessed using a random sample of 23 patients. Spearman's rank correlation coefficient was used and the results ranged from 0.82 to 0.96.
Validity:	In order to assess construct validity, the physical function scale was compared to the SIP (Sickness Impact Profile). This relationship was tested with Spearman rank correlation coefficients. To establish construct validity in the symptom severity scale, the pain domain was compared with pain measured on a visual analogue scale and to the SIP using Spearman correlation coefficients. Finally, the satisfaction scale was compared with the patient's opinion of whether he/she would choose to have surgery again if able to make the decision over again. Results were analyzed using Spearman rank correlation coefficients. The physical function scale was moderately correlated with the global SIP, $r = 0.43$. The symptom severity scale was strongly correlated with pain measured on a visual analogue scale, $r = 0.52$. The satisfaction scale score was highly correlated with whether patients would elect to have surgery if given a chance to choose again, $r = 0.70$.
Reference:	Daltroy, L., Fossel, A.H., Katz, J.N., Liang, M.H., Lipson, S.J., Stucki, G. Measurement properties of a self-administered outcome measure in lumbar spinal stenosis. *Spini.* 1996; 21(7):796–803.

Physical Function Scale (Before Surgery)

In the Last Month, on a Typical Day:
How far have you been able to walk?

Over 2 miles
Over 2 blocks, but less than 2 miles
Over 50 feet, but less than 2 blocks
Less than 50 feet

Have you taken walks outdoors or in malls for pleasure?

Yes, comfortably
Yes, but sometimes with pain
Yes, but always with pain
No

Have you been shopping for groceries or other items?

Yes, comfortably
Yes, but sometimes with pain
Yes, but always with pain
No

Have you walked around the different rooms in your house or apartment?

Yes, comfortably
Yes, but sometimes with pain
Yes, but always with pain
No

Have you walked from your bedroom to the bathroom?

Yes, comfortably
Yes, but sometimes with pain
Yes, but always with pain
No

Satisfaction Scale

How satisfied are you with:
The overall result of back operation?

Very satisfied
Somewhat satisfied
Somewhat dissatisfied
Very dissatisfied

Relief of pain following the operation?

Very satisfied
Somewhat satisfied
Somewhat dissatisfied
Very dissatisfied

Your ability to walk following the operation?

Very satisfied
Somewhat satisfied
Somewhat dissatisfied
Very dissatisfied

Your ability to do housework, yardwork, or job following the operation?

Very satisfied
Somewhat satisfied
Somewhat dissatisfied
Very dissatisfied

Your strength in the thighs, legs, and feet?

Very satisfied
Somewhat satisfied
Somewhat dissatisfied
Very dissatisfied

Your balance, or steadiness on your feet?

Very satisfied
Somewhat satisfied
Somewhat dissatisfied
Very dissatisfied

Outcome Measure in Lumbar Spinal Stenosis

Symptom Severity Scale

In the Last Month, How Would you Describe:
The Pain you have had on average including pain in your back, buttocks and pain that goes down the legs?

None
Mild
Moderate
Severe
Very severe

How often have you had back, buttock, or leg pain?

Less than once a week
At least once a week
Everyday, for at least a few minutes
Everyday, for most of the day
Every minute of the day

The pain in your back or buttocks?

None
Mild
Moderate
Severe
Very severe

The pain in your legs or feet?

None
Mild
Moderate
Severe
Very severe

Numbness or tingling in your legs or feet?

None
Mild
Moderate
Severe
Very severe

Weakness in your legs or feet?

None
Mild
Moderate
Severe
Very severe

Problems with your balance

No, I've had no problems with my balance
Yes, sometimes I feel my balance is off, or that I am not sure footed
Yes, often I feel my balance is off, or that I am not sure-footed

Reprinted with permission from Stucki, G., Daltrey, L., Lisng, M., Lipson, S., Fossel, A., Katz, J. Measurement properties of a self-administered outcome measure in lumbar spinal stenosis. *Spine.* 1996; 21(7):796–803.

Posture Training Support: Preliminary
Report on a Series of Patients with
Diminished Symptomatic Complications
of Osteoporosis; by Kaplan;
Mayo Clin Proc; 12–93[148]

■ Conclusions: The posture training support may
be of considerable symptomatic and prophylactic
value to patients with osteoporosis who cannot
tolerate conventional back supports.

Appendix H

Neck

Evaluation Ideas

Neck Disability Index[149]

Population: Adult population, patients with neck pain

Description: The Neck Disability Index is a revised form of the Oswestry Low Back Pain Index and is designed to measure the activities of daily living in persons with neck pain. It is useful in both clinical practice and in a research setting.

Mode of Administration: The Neck Disability Index is a paper and pencil exam.

Completion:

   Time to Complete: 5 to 10 minutes

   Time to Score: Approximately 5 minutes

   Scoring: Each section is scored on a five point ordinal scale. (See Oswestry scoring instructions for exact scoring mechanism.) The scores of each section are added together to achieve a total score.

Interpretation: A high score indicates that there is an extreme amount of functional disability caused by neck pain.

Reliability: In a study of 48 patients the Neck Disability Index is found to have a strong level of test-retest reliability. The correlation coefficient was computed at 0.89.

   The total index was found to have a high degree of internal consistency, with an alpha coefficient of 0.80. All of the individual subsets had an alpha coefficient larger than 0.76 with the highest items including the sections of, headaches, lifting, recreation, reading and driving.

Validity: Face validity was established based on feedback from a group of peers and patients.

   A moderate level of concurrent validity was established in a study of 48 subjects. The changes in the Neck Disability Index in pre and posttreatment scores were compared with those of an improvement. Visual Analog Scale.

Reference: Vernon, H., Mior, S. The Neck Disability Index: A Study of Reliability and Validity. *Journal of Manipulative and Physiological Therapeutics.* 1991; 14:409–415.

Neck Disability Index

Name _____ Date _____ Therapist _____

This questionnaire has been designed to give your therapist information as to how your neck pain has affected you in your everyday life activities. Please answer each section, marking only ONE box which best describes your status today.

Section 1—Pain Intensity
☐ I have no pain at the moment.
☐ The pain is very mild at the moment.
☐ The pain is moderate at the moment.
☐ The pain is fairly severe at the moment.
☐ The pain is very severe at the moment.
☐ The pain is the worst imaginable at the moment.

Section 2—Personal Care (Washing, dressing, etc.)
☐ I can look after myself normally without causing extra pain.
☐ I can look after myself normally but it causes me extra pain.
☐ It is painful to look after myself and I am slow and careful.
☐ I need some help but manage most of my personal care.
☐ I need help every day in most aspects of self care.
☐ I do not get dressed, Wash with difficulty and stay in bed.

Section 3—Lifting
☐ I can lift heavy weights without extra pain.
☐ I can lift heavy weights but it gives extra pain.
☐ Pain prevents me from lifting heavy weights off the floor, but I can manage if they are conveniently positioned, for example on a table.
☐ Pain prevents me from lifting heavy weights but I can manage light to medium weights if they are conveniently positioned.
☐ I can lift only very light weights.
☐ I cannot lift or carry anything at all.

Section 4—Reading
☐ I can read as much as I want to with no pain in my neck.
☐ I can read as much as I want to with slight pain in my neck.
☐ I can read as much as I want with moderate pain in my neck.
☐ I can't read as much as I want because of moderate pain in my neck.
☐ I can hardly read at all because of severe pain in my neck.
☐ I cannot read at all.

Section 5—Headache
☐ I have no headache at all.
☐ I have slight headaches which come infrequently.
☐ I have moderate headaches which come infrequently.
☐ I have moderate headaches which come frequently.
☐ I have severe headaches which come frequently.
☐ I have headaches almost all the time.

Section 6—Concentration
☐ I can concentrate fully when I want to with no difficulty.
☐ I can concentrate fully when I want to with slight difficulty.
☐ I have a fair degree of difficulty in concentrating when I want to.
☐ I have a lot of difficulty in concentrating when I want to.
☐ I have a great deal of difficulty in concentrating when I want to.
☐ I cannot concentrate at all.

Section 7—Work
☐ I can do as much as I want to.
☐ I can only do my usual work but no more.
☐ I can do most of my usual work, but no more.
☐ I cannot do my usual work.
☐ I can hardly do any work at all.
☐ I can't do any work at all.

Section 8—Driving
☐ I can drive my car without any neck pain.
☐ I can drive my car as long as I want with slight pain in my neck.
☐ I can drive my car as long as I want with moderate pain in my neck.
☐ I can't drive my car as long as I want because of moderate pain in my neck.
☐ I can hardly drive at all because of severe pain in my neck.
☐ I can't drive my car at all.

Section 9—Sleeping
☐ I have no trouble sleeping.
☐ My sleep is slightly disturbed (less than 1 hour sleep loss).
☐ My sleep is mildly disturbed (1–2 hour sleep loss).
☐ My sleep is moderately disturbed (2–3 hours sleep loss).
☐ My sleep is greatly disturbed (3–5 hours sleep loss).
☐ My sleep is completely disturbed (5–7 hours sleep loss).

Section 10—Recreation
☐ I am able to engage in all my recreational activities with no neck pain at all.
☐ I am able to engage in all my recreational activities with some pain in my neck.
☐ I am able to engage in most but not all of my usual recreational activities because of pain in my neck.
☐ I am able to engage in a few of my usual recreational activities because of pain in my neck.
☐ I can hardly do any recreational activities because of pain in my neck.
☐ I can't do any recreational activities at all.

Comments: _____
_____
_____
_____
_____

Adapted from and reprinted with permission. Vernon, H., Mior, S. The Neck Disability Index: A Study of Reliability and Validity. *Journal of Manipulative and Physiological Therapeutics.* 1991; 14(7):409–415.

Treatment Ideas

**Intensive Training, PT, or Manipulation
for Patients with Chronic Neck Pain;
by Jordan; *Spine*; 98[150]**

■ All groups improved (pain, disability, meds use) at 4 and 12 months.
■ IT = 5-minute warm-up and cool down, PRE neck, shoulder, thoracic (1 hr).
■ PT = modal, mob, ex (30 min).
■ Chiro = manipulation and TP (15 min).
■ All had Neck School and HEP.

**A Randomized Trial of Chiropractic
Manipulation and Mobilization for
Patients with Neck Pain; by Hurwitz;
Am J Pub Health; 10–02[151]**

Cervical spine manipulation and mobilization yield comparable clinical outcomes.

Postural and Symptomatic Improvement After PT in Patients with Dizziness of Suspected Cervical Origin; by Karlberg; *Arch Phys Med Rehabil*; 9–96[152]

- PT significantly reduced neck pain and intensity and the frequency of dizziness.
- PT Rx:
  - soft tissue work
  - stabilization exercises
  - mobilization
  - HEP
  - 5–20 weeks
  - 5–23 Rx

Manual Therapy, Physical Therapy, or Continued Care by a GP for Patients with Neck Pain; by Hovig; *Ann Int Med*; 5–02[153]

- 183 patients, RCT, 6 weeks
- Manual therapy (eclectic) 1×/wk
- Physical therapy (exercises: ROM, PRE, relaxation, postural, functional) 2×/wk
- Advice and encouragement from GP every 2 weeks
- At 7 weeks, more favorable outcomes as follows: 68% for MT, 51% for PT, 39% for GP
- Measurement—NDI and pain scale

Efficacy of Home Cervical Traction Therapy; by Swezey; *Am J Phys Med Rehabil*; 99[154]

- 5 minutes, 2×/wk, 3–4 weeks.
- 81% of patients with mild to moderate sx had significant sx relief.
- Authors believe the benefit was derived from pain inhibitor effect of stretching of neurovascular fascia and ligament tissue.

Active Neck Muscle Training in the Treatment of Chronic Neck Pain in Women; by Ylinen; *JAMA*; 5–03[155]

- RCT of 180 chronic neck pain patients (9 sessions): Strength and endurance ^ dramatically versus control; strength even more so.
- Endurance group
- supine neck flexion, 3 sets of 20
- Strength group
  - sitting flexion with T-band 15 times and on diagonals
- Both groups
  - aerobic exercise 3×/wk
  - stretching for 20 minutes
  - dynamic exercises for shoulders and UE
    - dumbbell rows, flys, pullovers, presses, curls, shrugs
    - endurance did 3 sets of 20
    - strength did 80% of 1RM 15 repetitions
- Control group
  - told to do aerobic exercise
  - given instruction in the same stretches

Chronic Neck Pain: A Comparison of Acupuncture Treatment and PT; by David; *Brit J Rheum*; 98[156]

Both acupuncture and PT are effective forms of treatment.

Active Treatment of Chronic Neck Pain: A Prospective Randomized Intervention; by Taimela; *Spine*; 8–00[157]

- The benefit = active > home > control (F-8-C)
- Active group;
  - 2×/wk, 12 weeks for 45 minutes
  - cervicothoracic stabilization
  - relaxation training
  - behavioral support
  - eye fixation exercises
  - seated wobble board
- HEP = 1× lecture and 2× group exercise instruction
- Control = 1× instruction

Randomized Controlled Trial of PT
and Feldenkrais Interventions in Female
Workers with Neck-Shoulder Complaints;
by Lundblad; *J Occ Rehabil*; 99[158]

- 3 groups
  - PT group (ergonomic program): 50 min/2×/ wk/16wks
  - Feld group: Education individual sessions 4×, 12 group sessions (50 min)
  - Control group: nothing
- Feld group had less c/o pain. No change in physical signs or function of any group

Appendix I

SHOULDER

Evaluation Ideas

Measuring Shoulder Function with
the Shoulder Pain and Disability Index;
by Williams; *J Rheumatol*; 3–95[159]

Conclusions: The SPADI is responsive to change and accurately discriminates among patients who are improved or worsened.

Shoulder Pain and Disability Index (SPADI)	
Pain Scale: How severe is your pain? **0 = no pain 10 = worst pain imaginable**	
1. At its worst?	
2. When lying on the involved side?	
3. Reaching for something on a high shelf?	
4. Touching the back of your neck?	
5. Pushing with the involved arm?	
Disability Scale: How much difficulty do you have? **0 = no difficulty 10 = so difficult it required help**	
1. Washing your hair?	
2. Washing your back?	
3. Putting on an undershirt or pullover sweater?	
4. Putting on a shirt that buttons down the front?	
5. Putting on your pants?	
6. Placing an object on a high shelf?	
7. Carrying a heavy object of 10 pounds?	
8. Removing something from your back pocket?	

Williams, J.W.: Measuring Shoulder Function with the Shoulder Pain and Disability Index. *J of Rheumatology* 1995: 22(4):727–732.

Treatment Ideas

Ultrasound Therapy for Calcific Tendinitis of the Shoulder; Ebenbichler; *N Engl J med*; 5–99[160]

- At end of Rx experimental group
  - decreased pain
  - ^ function
- Rx:
  - 15 minutes
  - mechanical US
  - 5×/wk for 3 weeks, then 3×/wk for 3 weeks

The Effect of Medical Exercise Therapy on a Patient with Chronic Supraspinatus Tendonitis: A Case Study; by Torstensen; *JOSPT*; 12–94[161]

Conclusions: This case study is of a 73-year-old patient with a one-year history of shoulder pain who improved completely of symptoms and regenerated the supraspinatus tendon with two months of a specific active exercise regime.

Comparison of Supervised Exercise with and Without Manual Physical Therapy for Patients with Shoulder Impingement Syndrome; by Bang; *JOSPT*; 2000[162]

- Manual therapy applied by experienced PTs combined with supervised exercise is better than exercise alone for increasing strength and function and decreasing pain.
- Both groups—2×/wk for 3 weeks.
- Manual Rx:
  - Enhance caudal glide in flexion or abduction.
  - Direct toward movement limitations.
  - If plateau, change vigor or technique.

A Randomized Controlled Trial Comparing 2 Instructional Approaches to Home Exercise Instruction Following Rotator Cuff Repair; by Roddey; *JOSPT*; 11–02[163]

- Group 1 = video exercise instruction (PT available for questions) and 3 follow-up visits
- Group 2 = 4 one-on-one instruction sessions with PT
- Results: similar outcomes

The Immediate Effects of Soft Tissue Mobilization with PNF on G/H ER and Overhead Reach; by Godges; *JOSPT*; 12–03[164]

- The treatment group improved an average of 16 degrees in one treatment session compared to controls.
- Rx:
  - subscap STM
  - C/R IR and ER
  - PNF patterns

Rehabilitation After Two-Part fractures of the Neck and Humerus; by Hodgson; *J Bone Joint Surg.*; 03[165]

- 16 weeks after fracture.
- The group that received PT within 1 week versus 3 weeks:
  - ^ function
  - ^ ROM
  - less pain
- By 52 weeks the effects were less but still significant.

A Randomized, Controlled Clinical Trial of a Treatment for Shoulder Pain; by Ginn; *Phys Ther*; 8–97[166]

Stretching, strengthening, and work on SHR are effective in improving shoulder function as opposed to spontaneous recovery.

Appendix J

Lower Joints of the Upper Extremity

Evaluation Ideas

> ### Development and Validation of a Rheumatoid Hand Functional Disability Scale That Assesses Functional Handicap; by Duruoz; *J Rheumatol*; 7–96[167]
>
> - 18 items
> - Scored 0–5
> - 0 = no difficulty
> - 5 = impossible
> - 0 = best, 90 = worst score

Rheumatoid Hand Functional Disability Scale

Population:	Patients with rheumatoid arthritis
Description:	The rheumatoid hand functional disability scale is a practical instrument that can be used to assess functional disability due to the rheumatoid hand.
Mode of Administration:	The questionnaire can be administered by the clinician.
Scoring:	
Time to Complete:	The questionnaire takes about 3 ± 1 minutes to answer.
Time to Score:	The total score can be calculated in less than a minute.
Scoring:	The questionnaire is designed on a Likert scale with 6 levels of answers (0-5). 0 = without difficulty and 5 = impossible. The 18 responses are added for an overall score that can range from 0 – 90.
Interpretation:	A lower score reflects less difficulty or less disability whereas a higher score reflects more difficulty and disability.
Reliability:	Intrarater and interrater reliability were assessed. The intrarater reliability was tested on a group of 25 patients. Each patient was interviewed by the same rater twice with a 24 hour interval between interviews. The result was 0.97, using intraclass correlation coefficients. Interrater reliability was also assessed using intraclass correlation coefficients. Two raters interviewed 68 patients at 24 hour intervals. The result was 0.96.
Validity:	Face validity was determined by asking the patients from a sample group if they understood the questions.
	Content validity was determined by dividing the patients daily environment into five subsets (in the kitchen, dressing, hygiene, in the office, and other). Each item on the questionnaire corresponded to a subset and each subset was represented by several questions.
	Criterion referenced validity was determined by comparing the scale scores with the visual analog scale for functional handicap (VAS Hd). The range on the VAS Hd was from 0 – 100. 0 = no handicap and 100 = maximum handicap. The question asked was "During the last month and considering your needs for daily life, what is your handicap level due to hand involvement." The result showed that the scale was well correlated with the VAS Hd. Nonparametric Spearman rank correlation coefficients were used to assess the correlation.
	Construct validity was also determined by assessing convergent and divergent validity and by performing factor analysis. The scale was determined to have good convergent validity with RFI (Revel's Functional Index) and HFI (Hand Functional Index). Yet, the scale only showed a moderate, fair, or no correlation with morning stiffness, disease duration, hand joint swelling age, and pain measures such as VAS-PESN (pain in elbows, shoulders, and neck) and VAS-PH (pain in hands and wrists) and tenderness. Factor analysis was performed using the principal component analysis to extract factors. 3 factors were extracted with eigenvalues > 1, which accounted for 64.1% of total variance.
Reference:	Duroz, M.T., Poiraudeau, S., Fermanian, J., Menkes, C.J., Amor, B., Dougados, M., & Revel, M. (1996). Development and validation of a rheumatoid hand functional disability scale that assesses functional handicap. *The Journal of Rheumatology, 23*(7), 1167–1172.

Rheumatoid Hand Functional Disability Scale that Assesses Functional Handicap

Answers to the questions:
 0 = Yes, without difficulty
 1 = Yes, with a little difficulty
 2 = Yes, with some difficulty
 3 = Yes, with much difficulty
 4 = Nearly impossible to do
 5 = Impossible

Answer the follow questions regarding your ability without the help of any assistive devices:

C1 - In the kitchen
 1. Can you hold a bowl?
 2. Can you seize a full bottle and raise it?
 3. Can you hold a plate full of food?
 4. Can you pour liquid from a bottle into a glass?
 5. Can you unscrew the lid from a jar opened before?
 6. Can you cut meat with a knife?
 7. Can you prick things well with a fork?
 8. Can you peel fruit?

C2 - Dressing
 9. Can you button your shirt?
10. Can you open and close a zipper?

C3 - Hygiene
11. Can you squeeze a new tube of toothpaste?
12. Can you hold a toothbrush efficiently?

C4 - In the Office
13. Can you write a short sentence with a pencil or ordinary pen?
14. Can you write a letter with a pencil or ordinary pen?

C5 - Other
15. Can you turn a round door knob?
16. Can you cut a piece of paper with scissors?
17. Can you pick up coins from a table top?
18. Can you turn a key in a lock?

Reprinted with permission. Duruoz, M.T., Poiraudeau, S., Fermanian, J., Menkes, C., Amor, B., Dougados, M., and Revel, M. Development and Validation of a Rheumatoid Hand Functional Disability Scale That Assesses Functional Handicap. *Journal of Rheumatology* 1996; 23:7.

Treatment Ideas

Physical and Exercise Therapy for Treatment of the Rheumatoid Hand; by Buljina; *Arthritis Care Res*; 8–01[168]

- RCT—3 weeks
  - PT—modalities and exercise
  - Exercise group—exercise
  - Control—nothing
- PT group significant improvement in motion, strength, function, joint tenderness
- Exercise group = maintained
- Control = decline

Joint Protection and Home Hand Exercises Improve Hand Function in Patients with Hand OA: A RCT; by Stamm; *Arthritis Care Res*; 02[169]

- Grip strength, function, and pain improved.
- Program led by OT:
  - Joint protection instruction
  - HEP instruction—fist, PIP/DIP flex, MP flex, touch tip of each finger to thumb, finger abduction, and adduction and opposition
  - 1 time and reevaluate in 3 months

Appendix K

*H*IP

Evaluation Ideas

Harris Hip Score[170,171]

Population: Adult population, hip replacement patient

Description: The Harris Hip Score was designed to assess the level of pain and functional impairment of hip replacement patients. The evaluation consists of 4 sections which encompass the areas of pain, function, deformity and range of motion.

Mode of Administration: The patient is evaluated with the Harris Hip Score sheet by a trained therapist.
Completion:
   Time to Complete: 15 to 30 minutes

   Time to Score: Time to score is included in time to complete.

   Scoring: The Harris Hip Score evaluation has a maximum level of points at 100 points with each category having the following maximum point values:

	pain	44
	function	47
	deformity	4
and	range of motion	5.

Interpretation: The higher the patient's score on the Harris Hip Score the lower the patient's level of disability. The evaluation was designed in four parts so that pain and functional capacity may be the prime consideration. Pain and function are often the primary consideration in deciding whether a patient's treatment should involve surgery. For the purpose of the Harris evaluation they may be considered independently to allow for this decision.

Reliability: not reported

Validity: The Harris Hip Score was validated through a comparison of its results to that of the Larson System and the Shepard System, both previously validated and accepted measures. The results of this comparison indicate that the three tools all reasonably measure the same content, thus validating the Harris Hip Score.

References: Harris, W.E. Traumatic Arthritis of the Hip after Dislocation and Acetabular Fractures: Treatment by Mold Arthroplasty. *Journal of Bone and Joint Surgery* 1969; 51A(4):737–755.

Harris, W.E. Preliminary Report of Results of Harris Total Hip Replacement. *Clinical Orthopaedics and Related Research* 1973; 95:168–173.

Treatment Ideas

Home Exercise to Improve Strength and Walking Velocity After Hip Fx; by Sherrington; *Arch Phys Med Rehabil*; 2–97[172]

- 7 months after hip fracture
- Improved on: quad strength, walking velocity, weight-bearing ability, fall risk
- Intervention: step up on taped phone books (5 cm each, 1–2), 5–50 reps daily, 2 PT visits (initially and in 7 days), 1 month

---

Intensive Physical Training in Geriatric Patients After Severe Falls and Hip Surgery; by Hauer; *Age and Ageing;* 02[173]

- Progressive functional training and PRE sig improved strength, function, and balance.
- Rx:
  - 3 days/wk for 12 weeks.
  - 70–80% 1RM to major muscle groups.
  - Walking, stepping, sitting were taught efficiently and safely and then when mastered they were ^ in complexity and challenge (i.e., ball toss, diagonals, backward, faster, etc.).
  - 45 minutes.

Harris Hip Score—Synopsis of the Evaluation System

I. Pain (44 possible)

  A. None or ignores it   44

  B. Slight, occasional, no compromise in activities   40

  C. Mild pain, no effect on average activities, rarely moderate with pain with unusual activity, may take aspirin   30

  D. Moderate pain, tolerable but makes concession to pain. Some limitation of ordinary activity or work. May require occasional pain medicine stronger than aspirin.   20

  E. Marked pain, serious limitation of activities   10

  F. Totally disabled, crippled, pain in bed, bedridden   0

II. Function (47 possible)

  A. Gait (33 possible)

    1. Distance Walked

      a. Unlimited   11

      b. 4–6 blocks   8

      c. 2–3 blocks   5

      d. indoors only   2

      e. unable to walk   0

    2. Limp

      a. None   11

      b. Slight   8

      c. Moderate   5

      d. Severe   0

    3. Support

      a. None   11

      b. Cane for long walks   7

      c. Cane most of the time   5

      d. One crutch   3

      e. Two canes   2

      f. Two crutches   0

      g. Not able to walk (specify reason)   0

  B. Activities (14 possible)

    1. Stairs

      a. Normally without using a railing   4

      b. Normally using a railing   2

      c. In any manner   1

      d. Unable to do stairs   0

    2. Shoes and Socks

      a. With ease   4

      b. With difficulty   2

      c. Unable   0

    3. Sitting

      a. Comfortably in ordinary chair one hour   5

      b. On a high chair for one-half hour   3

      c. Unable to sit comfortably in any chair   0

    4. Enter public transportation   1

III. Absence of deformity points (4) are given if the patient demonstrates:

  A. Less than 30° fixed flexion contracture

  B. Less than 10° fixed adduction

  C. Less than 10° fixed internal rotation in extension

  D. Limb-length discrepancy less than 3.2 centimeters

IV. Range of motion (index values are determined by multiplying the degrees of motion possible in each are by the appropriate index)

A. Flexion 0–45 degrees $\times$ 1.0
   45–90° $\times$ 0.6
   90–110° $\times$ 0.3
B. Abduction 0–15° $\times$ 0.8
   15–20° $\times$ 0.3
   over 20° $\times$ 0

C. External rotation in ext. 0–15 $\times$ 0.4 over 15° $\times$ 0

D. Internal rotation in extension any $\times$ 0
E. Adduction 0–15° $\times$ 0.2

To determine the overall rating or rating for range of motion, multiply the sum of the index values $\times$ 0.05. Record Trendelburg test as positive, level, or neutral.

Reprinted with permission. Harris, W.H. Traumatic Arthritis of the Hip After Dislocation and Acetabular Fractures: Treatment by Mold Arthroplasty. *Journal of Bone and Joint Surgery* 1969; 51A(4):737–755.

A RCT of Weight-Bearing versus Non-Weight Bearing Exercise for Improving Physical Ability After Usual Care for Hip Fracture; by Sherrington; *Arch Phys Med Rehabil*; 5–04[174]

- RCT compared WB, NWB, and control after usual care—HEP designed by PT
- WB much better
- WB program
  - sit to stand—different heights
  - lateral step-up
  - foot taps while supporting weight on other foot
  - decrease support, ^ reps, ^ height

Effects of External Hip Protectors on Hip Fractures; by Lauretzen; *Lancet*; 1–93[175]

Conclusions: External hip protectors can prevent hip fractures in nursing home residents.

Systematic Home-Based Physical & Functional Therapy for Older Persons After Hip Fx; by Tinetti; *Arch Phys Med Rehabil*; 11–97[176]

- 6-month decreasing frequency program (24 PT visits and 7 OT visits).
- Participants improved in balance, strength, ADL, and gait.
- Program in HO-D-29.
- Cost = $3100 ($100/visit).

Home-Based Multicomponent Rehabilitation Program for Older Persons After Hip Fx: A Randomized Trial; by Tinetti; *Arch Phys Med Rehabil*; 8–99[177]

- Compared usual home care to Tinetti program.
- Usual care received more rehabilitative services and had a higher rate of recovery.

Perioperative Exercise Programs Improve Early Return of Ambulatory Function After THA; by Wang; *Am J Phys Med Rehabil*; 11–02[178]

- Ex group had better gait velocity and distance and ^ stride length at 3 and 24 weeks s/p sx.
- Rx—individualized;
  - strengthening
  - aerobic
  - stretching
  - 1 hour; pain free

Comparison of Two Home Care Protocols for TJR; by Weaver; *J Am Geriatr Soc*; 4–03[179]

- The more "efficient" protocol was as effective as the existing protocol.
- Efficient Rx = 2 nurse and 6 PT visits; 8 total.
- Existing Rx = 11–29 combined visits.
- For TKR:
  - efficient = 11 visits
  - existing = 29–47

Exercise Improves Early Functional Recovery After THA; by Gilbey; *Clin Orth Res*; 3–03[180]

- Compared an 8-weeks pre-op and post sx customized ex program to control who received only in patient rehab.
- Ex group compared to control showed significant improvement throughout the treatment and after.
- Rx = 30 minutes of aerobic and PRE and 30 minutes of mobility and gait training (in pool).

An Analysis of the Relationship Between the Utilization of Physical Therapy Services and Outcomes of Care for Patients After THA; by Freburger; *Phys Ther*; 5–2000[181]

PT intervention was directly related to total cost of care, which was less than expected due to an increased probability of discharge home.

Appendix L

KNEE

Evaluation Ideas

Knee Society Knee Score[112]

Population: Patients with knee infirmities.

Description: The Knee Society developed a stringent evaluation form that provides a knee score that rates only the knee joint itself and a functional score that rates the patient's ability to walk and climb stairs. The knee score is divided into three sections; pain, stability, and range of motion. Flexion contracture, extension lag, and misalignment are dealt with as deductions. The functional score considers only walking distance and stair climbing.

Mode of Administration: The Knee Score is administered by the clinician.

Scoring:

Time to Complete: 20 minutes to one-half hour.

Time to Score: Included in time to complete

Scoring: The maximum knee score is 100 points; 50 points are allotted for pain, 25 for stability, and 25 for range of motion. Points can be found on the test. Once that subtotal is derived, the clinician should deduct for flexion contracture, extension lag, and alignment according to the points on the test in order to arrive at an overall knee score. The maximum function score is also 100 points. Deductions can be taken for one cane, two canes, and crutches or a walker. Again, the deductions should be subtracted from the walking and stairs subtotal for an overall function score.

Interpretation: For the knee score, 100 points can be obtained by a patient with a well-aligned knee with no pain, 125° of motion, and negligible anteroposterior and mediolateral instability. The maximum functional score can be obtained by a patient who can ascend and descend stairs without holding a railing.

Reliability: Reliability was not discussed.

Validity: Validity was not discussed.

Reference: Insall, J.N., Dorr, L.D., Scott, R.D., Scott, W.N. Rationale of the knee society clinical rating system. *Clin Orthop Relat Res.* 1989; 248: 13–14.

Knee Score

Patient Category
  A. Unilateral bilateral (opposite knee successfully replaced)
  B. Unilateral, other knee symptomatic
  C. Multiple arthritis or medical infirmity

Pain	Points	Function	Points
None	50	Walking	50
Mild or occasional	45	Unlimited	40
Stairs only	40	>10 blocks	30
Walking and stairs	30	5–10 blocks	20
Moderate		<5 blocks	10
Occasional	20	Housebound	0
Continual	10	Unable	
Severe	0	Stairs	
		Normal up & down	50
Range of Motion		Normal up; down with rail	40
(5° = 1 point)	25	Up & down with rail	30
		Up with rail; unable down	15
Stability (maximum movement in any position)		Unable	0
Anteroposterior		Subtotal	_____
<5 mm	10		
5–10 mm	5	Deductions (minus)	
10 mm	0	Cane	5
Mediolateral		Two Canes	10
<5°	15	Crutches or Walker	20
6°–9°	10		
10°–14°	5	TOTAL DEDUCTION	_____
15°	0		
Subtotal	_____	FUNCTION SCORE	_____
Deductions (minus)			
Flexion contracture			
5°–10°	2		
10°–15°	5		
16°–20°	10		
>20°	20		
Extension lag			
<10°	5		
10°–20°	10		
>20°	15		
Alignment			
5°–10°	0		
0°–4°	3 pts each degree		
11°–15°	3 pts each degree		
Other	20		

TOTAL DEDUCTION   _____

KNEE SCORE   _____
(If total is a minus number, score is 0)

Reprinted with permission by Insall, J., Dorr, L., Scott, R., Scott, W. The rationale of The Knee Society Rating System *Clinical Orthopedics and Related Research.* 1989; 248:14.

Routine for:
Created by:

TOTAL HIP-1 Heel Slide

Bend knee and pull heel toward buttocks. Hold _____ seconds. Return. Repeat with other knee.

Repeat _____ times. Do _____ sessions per day.

TOTAL HIP-2 Abduction

Slide one leg out to side. Keeep kneecap up. Gently bring leg back to pillow. Repeat with other leg.

Repeat _____ times. Do _____ sessions per day.

TOTAL HIP-3 Internal/External Rotation

With pillow between legs, gently turn legs and feet in and out.

Repeat _____ times. Do _____ sessions per day.

TOTAL HIP (ADVANCED)-4 Abduction

Lift leg up toward ceiling. Return. Use _____ lbs on ankle.
Repeat _____ times each leg. Do _____ sessions per day.

TOTAL HIP (ADVANCED)-5 Extension

Lift leg up in the air and bring it back down.
Use _____ lbs on ankle. Repeat with other leg.

Repeat _____ times. Do _____ sessions per day.

TOTAL HIP (ADVANCED) - 6 Standing Hip Abduction

Lift leg out to side, bring back to midline. Use _____ lbs on ankle.

Repeat with other leg.

Repeat _____ times.
Do _____ sessions per day.

TOTAL HIP (ADVANCED)-7 Standing Hip Extensions

Bring leg back as far as poss ble.
Use _____ lbs on ankle.

Repeat with other leg

Repeat _____ times.
Do _____ sessions per day.

Treatment Ideas

Effects of Electrical Stimulation or Voluntary Contraction for Strengthening the Quadriceps Muscle Strength in an Aged Male Population; by Caggiano; *JOSPT*; 7–94[183]

Conclusions: Electrical stimulation has the same potential as traditional exercise to provide improved strength for aged males. Future research should examine electrical stimulation in older persons with compromised ability to exercise using traditional methods.

A Home-Based Protocol of ES for Quadriceps Muscle Strength in Older Adults with OA of the Knee; by Talbot; *J Rheumatol*; 03[184]

Home-based ES showed significant ^ in strength.

The Effects of 16 Months of Angle-Specific Isometric Strengthening Exercises in Midrange on Torque of the Knee Extensor Muscles in OA of the Knee; by Marks; *JOSPT*; 8–94[185]

Conclusions: Angle-specific strengthening in midrange may be sufficient to strengthen the extensors surrounding an osteoarthritic knee through a wide range of motion, and may therefore prove useful in the rehabilitation of patients with knee OA who are unable to exercise their weakened quadriceps at other angles due to pain or swelling.

A Randomized Trial Comparing Aerobic and Resistance Exercise . . . ; by Ettinger; *JAMA*; 1–97[186]

- Older persons with knee OA improved with either an aerobic or resistance exercise program. Exercise should be prescribed as part of Rx of OA.
- Note: PRE was not 1RM.

The Effects of High-Intensity and Low-Intensity Cycle Ergometry in Older Adults with Knee Osteoarthritis; by Mangione; *J Gerontol*; 4–99[187]

- 3×/wk, 10 weeks, 25 minutes, 40–70% MHR.
- Low intensity and high intensity were as effective in improving function, gait; decreasing pain; and increasing aerobic capacity.

Published Trials of Nonmedicinal and Noninvasive Therapies for Hip and Knee Osteoarthritis; by Puett; *Ann Int Med*; 7–94[188]

Conclusions: Exercise reduces pain and improves function in patients with osteoarthritis of the knee. Topically applied capsaicin and laser treatment may reduce pain associated with osteoarthritis and diabetic polyneuropathy.

The Effects of a Physical Training Program on Patients with OA of the Knees; by Rogind; *Arch Phys Med Rehabil*; 11–98[189]

- PT designed 3 mo/2×/wk (fitness, PRE, stretch, balance, coordination).
- Improvements in function, pain, gait, speed, and crepitus.
- Program had high compliance (100%).
- Good for patients with severe OA.

OA of the Knee: Isokinetic Quadriceps Exercise Versus Educational Intervention; by Maurer; *Arch Phys Med Rehabil*; 10–99[190]

- Both groups improved in outcome measures including strength.
- Isokinetic group = 3×/wk; 90, 120, 150 cps for 8 weeks
- Education group = MD lecture @ OA, video on jt protection, nutrition, coping strategies

Effectiveness of Home Exercise on Pain and Disability from OA of the Knee: A Randomised Controlled Trial; by O'Reilly; *Ann Rheum Dis*; 99[191]

- A simple program of home exercise can significantly improve pain and function
- Program:
  - quad sets (5 sec up to 20 times)
  - midrange quad holds (as above)
  - knee bends (side-lying or prone) (as above)
  - #2 above with Theraband (as above)
  - walking up and down one stair step (as above)
- Exercises done daily
- Nurse taught and monitored at 2, 6, 12 weeks

Effectiveness of Manual Physical Therapy and Exercise in OA of the Knee (RCT); by Deyle; *Ann Int Med*; 2–2000[192]

- Rx group = manual therapy + therex (see HO-E-11)
- Control = subtherapeutic US
- 2×/wk for 4 weeks
- Results = Rx grp had significant improvement in walking distance, WOMAC score, surgery

Appendix M

*F*OOT

Evaluation Ideas

Assessment and Management of Foot Disease in Patients with Diabetes; by Caputo; *N Engl J Med*; 9–94[193]

Conclusions: All patients with diabetes should be assessed with a nylon monofilament (pressed against the skin to the point of buckling) to identify patients who have lost protective sensation.

Ankle Osteoarthritis Scale

- 2 subscales
- 18 questions
- graded on VAS
  Higher score = greater impairment

Treatment Ideas

Effect of Therapeutic Footwear on Foot Reulceration in Patients with Diabetes; by Reiber; *JAMA*; 5–02[195]

- Custom footwear or inserts offered no significant ulcer reduction compared to normal footwear.
- This study suggests that careful attention to foot care by health care professionals may be more important than therapeutic footwear.

Conservative Treatment of Plantar Heel Pain: Long-Term Follow-up; by Wolgin; *Foot Ankle*; 12–94[196]

- Conclusions: 82 of 100 patients recovered completely, most with conservative means.
  - Average time for resolution of symptoms was 5.7 months.
  - Stretching of plantarfascia and achilles, as well as a cushioned inserts, showed the best results.

Routine for:
Created by:

270

TOTAL KNEE-1 Straight Leg Raise

Bend __right__ leg. Keep other leg as straight as possible and tighten muscles on top of thigh. Slowly lit straight leg ____ inches from bed and hold ____ seconds. Lower it, keeping muscles tight ____ seconds. Relax.
Repeat ____ times. Do ____ sessions per day.

TOTAL KNEE-2 Short Arc Quad

Place a large can or rolled towel under __right__ leg. Straighten leg. Hold ____ seconds.
Repeat ____ times. Do ____ sessions per day.

TOTAL KNEE-3 Hamstring Stretch

Sitting with operated leg straight on bed, and foot of other leg on floor, lean forward toward toes of straight leg.
Hold ____ seconds.
Repeat ____ times. Do ____ sessions per day.

TOTAL KNEE-4 Chair Knee Flexion

Keeping feet on floor, slide foot of operated leg back, bending knee.

Hold ____ seconds.

Repeat ____ times.
Do ____ sessions a day.

TOTAL KNEE-5 Partial Knee Bend

Holding on to stable object, slightly bend knees and slowly straighten.

Repeat ____ times.
Do ____ sessions per day.

TOTAL KNEE-6 Wall Slide With

both feet against wall and buttocks ____ inches from wall, slowly "walk" down wall, bending knees as far as possible.

You may give operated leg a gentle push with other leg on top.

Hold ____ seconds.

Repeat ____ times.
Do ____ sessions per day.

TOTAL KNEE-7 Range of Motion

Place __right__ foot on smooth surface. Slowly slide foot back as far as possible. Hold ____ seconds.

Repeat ____ times. Do ____ sessions per day.

Ankle Osteoarthritis Scale

A. Name:_____ Age:_____ Gender:_____ Weight:_____ Occupation:_____

PAIN

The line next to each item represents the amount of pain you typically had in each situation. On the far left is "No pain" and on the far right is "The worst pain imaginable". Place a mark on the line to indicate how bad your ankle pain was in each of the following situations during the past week. If you were not involved in one or more of these situations, mark that item NA.

HOW SEVERE WAS YOUR ANKLE PAIN: NA

1. At its worst?   No pain _____ Worst pain imaginable   _____
2. Before you get up in the morning?   No pain _____ Worst pain imaginable   _____
3. When you walked barefoot?   No pain _____ Worst pain imaginable   _____
4. When you stood barefoot?   No pain _____ Worst pain imaginable   _____
5. When you walked wearing shoes?   No pain _____ Worst pain imaginable   _____
6. When you stood wearing shoes?   No pain _____ Worst pain imaginable   _____
7. When you walked wearing shoe inserts or braces?   No pain _____ Worst pain imaginable   _____
8. When you stood wearing inserts or braces?   No pain _____ Worst pain imaginable   _____
9. At the end of the day?   No pain _____ Worst pain imaginable   _____

B. Name: _____ Date_____/_____/_____

DISABILITY

The line next to each item represents the amount of difficulty you had performing an activity. On the far left is "No difficulty" and on the far right is "So difficult, unable". Place a mark on the line to indicate how much difficulty you had performing each activity because of your ankle during the past week. If you did not perform an activity during the past week, place an "X" in the NA column.

HOW MUCH DIFFICULTY DID YOU HAVE: NA
1. Walking around the house?   No difficulty _____ So difficult unable _____
2. Walking outside on uneven ground?   No difficulty _____ So difficult unable _____
3. Walking for more than four blocks?   No difficulty _____ So difficult unable _____
4. Climbing stairs?   No difficulty _____ So difficult unable _____
5. Descending stairs?   No difficulty _____ So difficult unable _____
6. Standing on tip toes?   No difficulty _____ So difficult unable _____
7. Getting out of a chair?   No difficulty _____ So difficult unable _____
8. Climbing up or down curbs?   No difficulty _____ So difficult unable _____
9. Walking fast or running?   No difficulty _____ So difficult unable _____

_____/_____=_____%

The Ankle Osteoarthritis Scale consists of 18 items. Patients respond by placing a mark along a 100-mm horizontal line to depict their level of pain for the described condition. Each subscale, pain (A) or disability (B), consists of nine items. The sums of the responses for the nine-item subscales are tailed to generate each subscale's total score and overall score. In cases of "NA," the responses are dropped so that normalized total scores are calculated.

Domsic, R.T., Saltzman, C.L., "Ankle Osteoarthritis Scale." Foot and Ankle International. 19(7):466–471;1998.

References

1. Steinberg FU. Principles of geriatric rehabilitation. *Arch Phys Med Rehabil.* 1989; 70(1):67–68.

2. Eva P, Lyyra AL, Viitasalo JT, et al. Determinants of isometric muscle strength in men of different ages. *Eur J Appl Physiol.* 1992; 64(1):84–91.

3. Frontera W, Hughes VA, Lutz KS, et al. A cross-sectional study of muscle strength and mass in 45- to 78-year-old men and women. *J Appl Physiol.* 1992; 72(2):644–650.

4. Hakkinen K, Hakkinen A. Muscle cross-sectional area, force production and relaxation characteristics in women at different ages. *Eur J Appl Physiol.* 1991; 62(4):410–414.

5. De Andrade J, Grant C, Dixon, et al. Joint distension and reflex muscle inhibition in the knee. *J Bone Joint Surg.* 1965; 47A(2):312–322.

6. Healy L. Late-onset rheumatoid arthritis vs. polymyalgia rheumatica in blacks may be an artifact. *J Am Geriatr Soc.* 1990; 38(9):824–826.

7. Thompson LV. Physiological changes associated with aging. In: Guccione AA. *Geriatric Physical Therapy.* 2nd ed. St. Louis: Mosby; 2000: 28–55.

8. Bottomley JM. Extension equals function. *GeriNotes.* September 2000; 7(5):1–4.

9. Lewis CB, Bottomley JM. Musculoskeletal changes with age: Clinical implications. In: Lewis CB, ed. *Aging: Health Care's Challenge.* 2nd ed. Philadelphia: FA Davis; 1990: 135–160.

10. Bottomley JM. Age-related bone health and pathophysiology of osteoporosis. *Ortho Phys Ther Clinics No Amer.* 1998; 7(2):117–132.

11. Geusens P, Dequeker J, Verstraeten A, Nijs J. Age, sex-, and menopause-related changes of vertebral and peripheral bone: Population study using dual- and single-photon absorptiometry and radiogrammetry. *J Nucl Med.* 1986; 27:1540–1549.

12. Riggs BL, Wahner HW, Dann WL. Differential changes in bone mineral density of the appendicular and axial skeleton with aging. *J Clin Invest.* 1981; 67:328–335.

13. Riggs BL, Wahner HW, Melton LJ III. Rates of bone loss in the appendicular and axial skeletons of women. *J Clin Invest.* 1986; 77:1487–1491.

14. Snow-Harter C, Marcus R. Exercise, bone mineral density, and osteoporosis. *Exercise Sport Sci Rev.* 1991; 19:351–388.

15. Dalsky GP. Effect of exercise on bone: Permissive influence of estrogen and calcium. *Med Sci Sports Exer.* 1990; 22(3):281–285.

16. Buchanan JR, Myers C, Lloyd T. Determinants of trabecular bone density in women: The role of androgens, estrogen, and exercise. *J Bone Miner Res.* 1988; 3:673–680.

17. Grove KA, Londeree BR. Bone density in postmenopausal women: High-impact versus low-impact exercise. *Med Sci Sports Exer.* 1992; 24(11):1190–1194.

18. Suominen H. Bone mineral density and long-term exercise. *Sports Med.* 1993; 16(5):316–330.

19. Sanborn CF. Exercise, calcium, and bone density. *Gatorade Sports Sci Exchange.* 1990; 2(24):1–5.

20. Nilsson BE, Westline NE. Bone density in athletes. *Clin Orthop.* 1991; 97:179–182.

21. Dalsky GP, Stocke KS, Ehsani AA. Weight-bearing exercise training and lumbar bone mineral content in postmenopausal women. *Ann Intern Med.* 1988; 108:824–828.

22. Block JE, Friedlander AL, Brooks GA. Determinants of bone density among athletes engaged in weight-bearing and non-weight-bearing activity. *J Appl Physiol.* 1989; 67(3):1100–1105.

23. Aisenbrey JA. Exercise in the prevention and management of osteoporosis. *Phys Ther.* 1987; 67(1):100–104.

24. Lips P, Courpron P, Meunier PJ. Mean wall thickness of trabecular bone: Changes with age. *Calcif Tissue Res.* 1988; 26:13–17.

25. Rudman D, Kutner MH, Rogers CM, Lubin MF, Fleming GA, Bain RP. Impaired growth hormone secretion in the adult population: Relation to age and adiposity. *J Clin Invest.* 1991; 77:1361–1369.

26. Centrella M, Canalis E. Local regulators of skeletal growth: A genetic perspective. *Endocr Rev.* 1985; 6:544–551.

27. Wheeler M. Osteoporosis. *Med Clin North Am.* 1996; 80(6):1213–1224.

28. Greger K, Krystofiak M. Phosphorus intake of Americans. *Food Technol.* 1992; 46:78–84.

29. Frost HM. Structural adaptations to mechanical usage. Redefining Wolff's Law. *Anat Rec.* 1990; 226:403–422.

30. Heinrich Ch, Going RW, Parmenter CD, Perry T, Boyden W, Lohman TG. Bone mineral content of cyclically menstruating female resistance and endurance trained athletes. *Med Sci Sports Exerc.* 1990; 22:558–563.

31. Jacobsoen PC, Beaver W, Grubb SA, Taft TN, Talmadge RV. Bone density in women: College athletes and older athletic women. *J Orthop Res.* 1994; 2:328–332.

32. Pocock N, Eisman JA, Gwinn T. Muscle strength, physical fitness and weight but not age, predict femoral neck bone mass. *J Bone Miner Res.* 1989; 4:441–446.

33. Snow-Harter C, Bouxsein M, Lewis BT, Charette S, Weinstein S, Marcus R. Muscle strength as a

predictor of bone mineral density in women. *J Bone Miner Res.* 1990; 5:589–595.

34. Sinaki M, Mikkelson BA. Postmenopausal spinal osteoporosis. Flexion versus extension exercises. *Arch Phys Med Rehabil.* 1984; 65:593–596.

35. Sinaki M. Musculoskeletal challenges of osteoporosis. *Aging.* 1998; 10(3):249–262.

36. Kanis JA, Melton LF III, Christiansen C, Johnson CC, Khaltev N. The diagnosis of osteoporosis. *J Bone Miner Res.* 1994; 9:1137–1141.

37. Kribbs PJ, Smith DE, Chestnutt CH III. Oral findings in osteoporosis. Part II: Relationship between residual ridge and alveolar bone resorption and generalized skeletal osteopenia. *J Prosthet Dent.* 1983; 50(5):719–724.

38. Shapiro S, Bomberg TJ, Benson BW, et al. Postmenopausal osteoporosis: Dental patients at risk. *Gerodontics.* 1985; 1(5):220–225.

39. Wical EE, Swoope CC. Studies of residual ridge resorption. Part II: The relationship of dietary calcium and phosphorus to residual ridge resorption. *J Prosthet Dent.* 1974; 32(1):13–22.

40. Gunta KE. Alterations in skeletal function: Congenital disorders, metabolic bone disease, and neoplasms. In: Porth C, ed. *Pathophysiology: Concepts of Altered Health States.* 4th ed. Philadelphia: Lippincott; 1994: 1230–1235.

41. Hahn BH. Osteopenic bone diseases. In: McCarty DJ, Koopman WJ, eds. *Arthritis and Allied Conditions.* Vol 2, 12th ed. Philadelphia; Lea & Febiger; 1994: 1935–1938.

42. James J, Steijn-Myagkaya GL. Death of osteocytes. Electron microscopy after in vitro ischemia. *J Bone Joint Surg.* 1986; 68:620–624.

43. Jones JP. Osteonecrosis. In: McCarthy DJ, Koopman WJ, eds. *Arthritis and Allied Conditions.* Vol 1. 12th ed. Philadelphia: Lea & Febiger; 1993: 1677–1696.

44. Schiller AL. Bones and joints. In: Rubin E, Farber JL, eds. *Pathology.* 2nd ed. Philadelphia: Lippincott; 1994: 1273–1347.

45. Pigg JS, Bancroft DA. Alterations in skeletal function: Rheumatic disorders. In: Mattson-Porth C, ed. *Pathophysiology.* 4th ed. Philadelphia: Lippincott; 1994: 1267–1268.

46. Liang MH, Fortin P. Management of osteoarthritis of the hip and knee. *N Eng J Med.* July 11, 1991; 325(2):125–126.

47. Fisher N, Pendergast DR, Calkins EC, et al. Maximal isometric torque of the knee extension as a function of muscle length in subjects of advancing age. *Arch Phys Med Rehabil.* 1990; 71(9):729–734.

48. Kreindler H, Lewis CB. The effects of three exercise protocols on osteoarthritis of the knees. *Top Geriatr Rehabil.* 1989; 4(3):389–409.

49. Felson DT. Weight and osteoarthritis. *Am J Clin Nutr.* 1996; 63(5):430–432.

50. Schumacher RH, ed. *Primer on the Rheumatic Diseases.* 10th ed. Atlanta, GA: Arthritis Foundation; 1993.

51. Gandy S, Payne R. Back pain in the elderly: Updated diagnosis and management. *Geriatrics.* 1986; 41(12):59–72.

52. Hayashi K, Okada K, Hamada M. Etiological factors of mylopathy: A radiographic evaluation of the aging changes in the cervical spine. *Clin Ortho.* 1987; 214(1):200–209.

53. Rider R, Daly J. Effects of flexibility training of enhancing spinal mobility in older women. *J Sports Med Phys Fit.* 1991; 3(2):213–217.

54. Twomey LT, Taylor JR. *Physical Therapy of the Low Back.* New York: Churchill Livingston; 1987.

55. Fast A. Low back disorders conservative management. *Arch Phys Med Rehabil.* 1988; 69(10):880–891.

56. Bottomley JM. The use of T'ai chi as a movement modality in orthopedics. *Ortho Phys Ther Clin No Amer.* 2000; 9(3):361–374.

57. Frost H. Clinical management of the symptomatic osteoporotic patient. *Ortho Clin No Amer.* 1981; 12 (3):671–681.

58. Turner P. Osteoporotic back pain—Its prevention and treatment. *Physiotherapy.* 1991; 77(9):642–646.

59. Sinaki M, McPhee MC, Hodgson SF. Relationship between bone mineral density of spine and strength of back extensors in health postmenopausal women. *Mayo Clin Proc.* 1986; 61(2):116–122.

60. Payne R. Neck pain in the elderly: A management review, part I. *Geriatrics.* 1987; 42(1):59–65.

61. Payne R. Neck pain in the elderly: A management review, part II. *Geriatrics.* 1987; 42(2):71–73.

62. Lewis CB, McNerney T. Neck pain and the elderly. *Phys Ther Practice.* 1992; 1(1):43–53.

63. Furman JM, Whitney SL. Central causes of dizziness. *Phys Ther.* 2000; 80(2):179–187.

64. Cote P, Kreitz BG, Cassidy JD, Thiel H. The validity of the extension-rotation test as a clinical screening procedure before neck manipulation: a secondary analysis. *J Manipulative Physiol Ther.* 1996; 19:159–164.

65. McGregor M, Haldeman S, Kohlbeck FJ. Vertebrobasilar compromise associated with cervical manipulation. *Top Clin Chiro.* 1995; 2:63–73.

66. Terrett AG. *Vertebrobasilar Stroke Following Manipulation.* West Des Moines, IA: Nat Chiro Mutual Co; 1996.

67. Di Fabio RP. Manipulation of the cervical spine: risks and benefits. *Phys Ther.* 1999; 79(1):50–65.

68. Bolton PS, Stick PE, Lord RS. Failure of clinical tests to predict cerebral ischemia before neck manipulation. *J Manipulative Physiol Ther.* 1989; 12: 304–307.

69. Dix M, Hallpike C. The pathology, symptomatology and diagnosis of certain common disorders of the

vestibular system. *Ann Otol Rhinol Laryngol.* 1952; 61:341–354.

70. Whitney SL. Treatment of the older adult with vestibular dysfunction. In: Herdman SJ, ed. *Vestibular Rehabilitation.* 2nd ed. Philadelphia: FA Davis; 1999: 512–543.

71. Borello-France DF, Whitney SL, Herdman SJ. Assessment of vestibular hypofunction. In: Herdman SJ, ed. *Vestibular Rehabilitation.* Philadelphia: FA Davis; 1994: 247–286.

72. Harsh G, Sypert GW, Weinstein PR. Cervical spine stenosis secondary to ossification of the posterior longitudinal ligament. *J Neurosurg.* 1987; 67(3): 349–357.

73. Bassey E, Morgan K, Calloso HM, et al. Flexibility of the shoulder joint measured at range of abduction in a large representative sample of men and women over 65 years of age. *Eur J Appl Physiol.* 1989; 58: 353–360.

74. Faulkner C, Jensen RH, Nosse L. The aging rotator cuff: Internal/external rotation torques for youth vs. senior citizen. *Phys Ther.* June 1991; 71(6): (suppl S75).

75. Sundstrom W. Painful shoulders: Diagnosis and management. *Geriatrics.* March 1983; 38(3):77–96.

76. Warren R, O'Brien S. Shoulder pain in the geriatric patient, part 11: Treatment options. *Ortho Rev.* 1989; 18(2):248–263.

77. Warren R, O'Brien S. Shoulder pain in the geriatric patient, part 1: Evaluation and pathophysiology. *Ortho Rev.* 1989; 18(1):129–135.

78. Simon E, Hill J. Rotator cuff injuries. *Orthop Sport Ther.* April 1989; 10(10):394–399.

79. Harrell L, Massey E. Hand weakness in the elderly. *J Am Geriatr Soc.* 1983; 31(4):223–227.

80. Imrhan S. Trends in finger pinch strength in children, adults and elderly. *Human Factors.* 1989; 31 (6):689–701.

81. Kallman D, Plato CC, Tobin JD, et al. The role of muscle loss in the aging related decline of grip strength cross-sectional and longitudinal perspectives. *J Gerontol.* 1990; 45(3):M82–M88.

82. Denham M, Modkinson MH, Furesh KN, et al. Loss of grip in the elderly. *Gerontol Clin.* 1973; 15: 286–271.

83. Balogun J, Akinloye AH, Adeneola SA, et al. Grip strength as a function of height, body weight and quetelet index. *Physiotherapy Theory and Practice.* 1991; 7:111–119.

84. Sobel JS. Elbow injuries: A rehabilitation perspective. In: Lewis CB, Knortz K, eds. *Orthopedic Asssessment and Treatment of the Geriatric Patient.* St. Louis: Mosby Year Book; 1993: 133–144.

85. Maring J. Effects of mental practice on rate of skill acquisition. *Phys Ther.* March 1990; 70(3):165–172.

86. Villar R, Marsh D, Rushton N, et al. Three years after Colles' fracture. *J Bone Joint Surg.* 1987; 69B (4):635–638.

87. Douvall S. Hand injuries: A rehabilitation perspective. In: Lewis CB, Knortz K, eds. *Geriatriczithopedics: Surgical and Rehabilitative Management.* St. Louis: Mosby Year Book; 1992.

88. Maddali-Bongi S, Giuidi G, Cencett A, et al. Treatment of carpo-metacarpal joint osteoarthritis by means of a personalized splint. *Pain Clinic.* 1991; 4(2):119–123.

89. James B, Parker A. Active and passive mobility of lower limb joints in elderly men and women. *Am J Phys Med Rehabil.* August 1989; 68(4):165.

90. Kramer J, Vaz MD, Vandervoort AA, et al. Reliability of isometric hip abductor torques during examiner and belt-resisted tests. *J Gerontol.* 1991; 46(2): M47–M51.

91. Neumann D, Cook TM, Sholty RL, et al. An electromyographic analysis of hip abductor muscle activity when subjects are carrying loads in one or both hands. *Phys Ther.* March 1992; 72(3): 207–217.

92. Tinetti ME, Williams TF, Mayewski R. Fall risk index for elderly patients based on number of chronic disabilities. *Am J Med.* 1986; 80(3):429–434.

93. Kampa K. Mortality of hip fracture patients within one year of fracture . . . an overview. *Geritopics.* April 1989; 14(1):10–11.

94. Cummings S, Nevitt M. A hypothesis: The causes of hip fractures. *J Gerontol Med Sci.* 1989; 44(4): M107–Mlll.

95. *Zimmer Product Encyclopedia.* Warsaw, IN: Zimmer USA; December 1999.

96. Zuckerman JD, Zetterber C, Kummer FJ, Frankel VH. Weight bearing following hip fractures in geriatric patients. *Top Geriatr Rehabil.* December 1990; 6(2):34–50.

97. Baker P, Evans OM, Lee C, et al. Treadmill gait training following fractured neck-of-femur. *Arch Phys Med Rehabil.* 1991; 72(8):649–652.

98. Bohannon RW, Kloter KS, Cooper JA. Outcome of patients with hip fracture treated by physical therapy in an acute care hospital. *Top Geriatr Rehabil.* 1990; 6(2):51–58.

99. Barnes B, Dunovan K. Functional outcomes after hip fracture. *Phys Ther.* 1987; 67(11):1675–1679.

100. Bonar S, Tinnetti ME, Speechley M, et al. Factors associated with short versus long-term skilled nursing facility placement among community living hip fracture patients. *J Am Geriatr Soc.* 1990; 38(10): 1139–1144.

101. Borges O. Isometric and isokinetic knee extension and flexion torque in men and women aged 20–70. *Scand J Rehab Med.* 1989; 21(1):45–53.

102. Altman R. Development of criteria for the classification and reporting of osteoarthritis of the knee. *Arthritis Rheum.* 1986; 29(8):1039–1049.

103. Barrett D. Joint proprioception in normal osteoarthritis and replaced knees. *J Bone Joint Surg.* 1991; 73B(1):53–56.

104. Radin E. Mechanical aspects of osteoarthritis. *Bull Rheumatic Dis.* 1975–1976; 26(7):862–865.

105. Steinlan J, Gil I, Habot B, et al. Improvement of pain and disability in elderly patients with degenerative osteoarthritis of the knee treated with narrow-band light therapy. *J Am Ger Soc.* 1992; 40(1):23–26.

106. Knortz K. Knee injuries: A rehabilitative perspective. In: Lewis CB, Knortz K, eds. *Orthopedic Assessment and Treatment of the Geriatric Patient.* St. Louis: Mosby Year Book; 1993:301–322.

107. Berry G. Assessment and treatment of knee injuries with particular attention to the hamstring muscles and joint swelling. *Physiotherapy.* 1989; 75(8):690–693.

108. Helfand A. Podiatry in a total geriatric health program: Common foot problems of the aged. *J Am Geriatr Soc.* 1967; 15(6):593–599.

109. White EG, Mulley GP. Foot care for very elderly people: A community survey. *Age and Aging.* 1989; 18(4):275–279.

110. Herman H, Bottomley JM. Anatomical and biomechanical considerations of the elder foot. *Top Geriatr Rehabil.* 1992; 7(3):1–13.

111. Bottomley JM, Herman H. Making simple, inexpensive changes for the management of foot problems in the aged. *Top Geriatr Rehabil.* 1992; 7(3):62–77.

112. Evans S, Nixon BP, Lee I, et al. The prevalence and nature of podiatric problems in elderly diabetic patients. *J Am Geriatr Soc.* 1991; 39(3):241–245.

113. Helfand A. The aging foot. *Focus on Ger Care and Rehab.* April 1989; 2(10).

114. Vandervoort A, Hayes K. Plantarflexor muscle function in young and elderly women. *Eur J Appl Physiol.* 1989; 58(4):389–394.

115. Bottomley JM. Footwear: Foundation for lower extremity orthotics. In: Lusardi MM, Nielson CC. *Orthotics and Prosthetics in Rehabilitation.* Boston: Butterworth-Heinemann; 2000.

116. Karner PM, et al. Strength testing in elderly women using a portable dynamometer. *Physiother Can.* Winter 1998: 35–39.

117. Ottenbacher KJ, Branch LG, Ray L, Gonzales VA, Peek KM, Hinman MR. The reliability of upper and lower extremity strength testing in a community survey of older adults. *Arch Phys Med Rehabil.* 2002; 83:1423–1427.

118. Taaffe DR, Duret C, Wheeler S et al. Once-weekly resistance exercise improves muscle strength and neuromuscular performance in older adults. *J Am Geriatr Soc.* 1999; 47:1208–1214.

119. Sullivan DH, Wall PT, Bariola JR, Frost YM. Progressive resistance muscle strength training of hospitalized frail elderly. *Am J Phys Med Rehabil.* 2001; 80:503–509.

120. Wescott WL, Winett RA, Anderson ES, Wojcik JR, Loud RLR, Cleggett E, Glover S. Effects of regular and slow speed resistance training on muscle strength. *J Sports Med Phys Fit.* 2001; 41:154–158.

121. White T, Smith BS. The efficacy of aquatic exercise in increasing strength. *Sports Med Train Rehabil.* 1999; 9(1):51–59.

122. Jones CJ, Rikli RE, Max J, Noffal G. The reliability and validity of a chair sit-and-reach test as a measure of hamstring flexibility in older adults. *Res Quart Ex Sport.* 1998; 69(4):338–343.

123. Feland JB, Myrer JW, Schulthies SS, Fellingham GW, Meason GW. The effect of duration of stretching of the hamstring muscle group for increasing range of motion in people aged 65 years or older. *Phys Ther.* 2001; 81(5):1100–1117.

124. Helmes E, et al. A questionnaire to evaluate disability in osteoporotic patients with vertebral compression fractures. *J Am Geriatr Soc.* 1995; 50A(2): M91–M98.

125. Nelson ME, et al. Effects of high-intensity strength training on multiple risk factors for osteoporotic fractures. *JAMA.* December 28, 1994; 272(24): 1909–1914.

126. Snow CM, Shaw JM, Winters KM, Witzke KA. Long-term exercise using weighted vests prevents hip bone loss in postmenopausal women. *J Gerontol Med Sci.* 2000; 55A(9):M489–M491.

127. Rhodes EC, Martin AD, Taunton JE et al. Effects of one year of resistance training on the relation between muscular strength and bone density in elderly women. *Brit J Sports Med.* 2000; 34:18–22.

128. Sinaki M, Wollan PC, Scott RW, et al. Can strong back extensors prevent vertebral fractures in women with osteoporosis? *Mayo Clin Proc.* 1996; 71:951–956.

129. Tsuji S, et al. Relationship between grip strength and radial bone mineral density in young athletes. *Arch Phys Med Rehabil.* 1995; 76:234–238.

130. Qin L, et al. Regular Tai Chi Chuan exercise may retard bone loss in postmenopausal women: A case-control study. *Arch Phys Med Rehabil.* 2002; 83: 1355–1359.

131. Villareal DT, Binder EF, Yarasheski KE, Williams DB, Brown M, Sinacore DR, Kohrt WM. Effects of exercise training added to ongoing hormone replacement therapy on bone mineral density in frail elderly women. *J Am Geriatr Soc.* 2003; 51:985–990.

132. Carter ND et al. Community-based exercise program reduces risk factors for falls in 65- to 75-year-old women with osteoporosis: Randomized controlled trial. *Can Med Assoc J.* 2002; 167(9):997–1004.

133. Russo CR, Lauretain F, Bandinelli S, Bartali B, Cavazzini C, Guralnik JM, Ferrucci L. High-frequency vibration training increases muscle power in postmenopausal women. *Arch Phys Med Rehabil.* 2003; 84:1854–1857.

134. Kudlacek, S, Pietschmann F, Bernecker P, Resch H, Willvonseder R. The impact of a senior dancing program on spinal and peripheral bone mass. *Am J Phys Med Rehabil.* 1997; vol 76:477–81.

135. Smith, EJ. Exercise: A prevention and treatment for osteoporosis and injurious falls in the older adult. *J Aging Phys.* 1995; 3:178–192.

136. Bellamy N, Buchanon W, Goldsmith CH, Campbell J, Stitt L. Validation study of WOMAC: A health status instrument for measuring clinically important patient relevant outcomes to antirheumatic drug therapy in patients with osteoarthritis of the hip or knee. *J Rheumatol.* 1988; 15(12):1833–1840.

137. Gunther JS. Physical therapy-based exercise/education program to improve functional health in older individuals with arthritis. *J Geriatr Phys Ther* 2003; 26(1).

138. Hartman CA, Manos TM, Winter C, Hartman DM, Li B, Smith JC. Effects of T'ai Chi training on function and quality of life indicators in older adults with osteoarthritis. *J Am Geriatr Soc.* 2000; 48:1553–1559.

139. Anderson DL. Development of an instrument to measure pain in rheumatoid arthritis: Rheumatoid arthritis pain scales (RAPS). *Arthritis Care Res.* 2001; 45:317–323.

140. Schloten, C, et al. Persistent functional and social benefit 5 years after a multidisciplinary arthritis training program. *Arch Phys Med Rehabil* 1999; 80 (10):1282–1287.

141. Bell MJ, et al. A randomized controlled trial to evaluate the efficacy of community based physical therapy in the treatment of people with rheumatoid arthritis. *J Rheumatol.* 1998; 25(2):231–237.

142. Bearne LM, Scott DL, Hurley MV. Exercise can reverse quadriceps sensorimotor dysfunction that is associated with rheumatoid arthritis without exacerbating disease activity. *Rheumatology.* February 2002; 41(2):157–166.

143. Hall J, Skevington SM, Maddison PJ, Chapman K. A randomized and controlled trial of hydrotherapy in rheumatoid arthritis. *Arthritis Care Res.* June 1996; 9(3).

144. Stucki G, Daltroy L, Liang M, Lipson S, Fossel A, Katz J. Measurement properties of a self-administered outcome measure in lumbar spinal stenosis. *Spine.* 1996; 21(7):796–803.

145. Atlas SJ, Keller RB, Robson D, et al. Surgical and nonsurgical management of lumbar spinal stenosis. *Spine.* 2000; 25(5):556–562.

146. Fritz JM, Erhard RE, Vignovic M. A nonsurgical treatment approach for patients with lumbar spinal stenosis. *Phys Ther.* September 1997; 77(9):962–973.

147. Morgan V, Chevan J, Gilberto M, Koftler M. Compression fractures due to osteomalacia, osteoporosis or osteopenia. *Phys Ther Case Rep.* 2000; 3(4): 181–183.

148. Kaplan RS, et al. Posture training support: Preliminary report on a series of patients with diminished symptomatic complications of osteoporosis. *Mayo Clin Proc.* December 1993; 68.

149. Vernon H, Mior S. The neck disability index: A study of reliability and validity. *J Man Physiol Therap.* 1991; 14:409–415.

150. Jordan A, et al. Intensive training, physiotherapy, or manipulation for patients with chronic neck pain. *Spine.* 1998; 23(3):311–319.

151. Hurwitz EL, Morgenstern H, Harber P, Kominski GF, Yu F, Adams AH. A randomized trial of chiropractic manipulation and mobilization for patients with neck pain: Clinical outcomes from the UCLA neck-pain study. *Am J Pub Health.* 2002; 92(10): 1634–1641.

152. Karlberg M, et al. Postural and symptomatic improvement after physiotherapy in patients with dizziness of suspected cervical origin. *Arch Phys Med Rehabil.* September 1996; 77.

153. Hovig, JL, et al. Manual therapy, physical therapy, or continued care by a general practitioner for patients with neck pain. *Ann Int Med.* 2002; 136(10) 713–722.

154. Swezey RL, Swezey AM, Warner K. Efficacy of home cervical traction therapy. *Am J Phys Med Rehabil.* 1999; 78(1).

155. Ylinen J, et al. Active neck muscle training in the treatment of chronic neck pain in women. *JAMA.* May 21, 2003; 289(19).

156. David J, et al. Chronic neck pain: A comparison of acupuncture treatment and physiotherapy. *Brit J Rheum.* 1998; 37:1118–1122.

157. Taimela S. Active treatment of chronic neck pain: A prospective randomized intervention. *Spine.* 2000; 25(8)1021–1027.

158. Lundblad I, Elert J, Gerdle B. Randomized controlled trial of physiotherapy and Feldenkrais interventions in female workers with neck-shoulder complaints. *J Occ Rehabil.* 1999; 9(3):179–194.

159. Williams JW, Holleman D. Measuring shoulder function with the shoulder pain and disability index. *J Rheumatol.* 1995; 22(4).

160. Ebenbichler GR, et al. Ultrasound therapy for calcific tendinitis of the shoulder. *N Eng J Med.* 1999; 340:1533–1538.

161. Torstensen TA, Meen HD, Stiris M. the effect of medical exercise therapy on a patient with chronic supraspinatus tendinitis. Diagnostic ultrasound–tissue regeneration: A case study. *JOSPT.* December 1994; 20(6).

162. Bang MD, Deyle GD. Comparison of supervised exercise with and without manual physical therapy for

patients with shoulder impingement syndrome. *JOPST.* 2000; 30(3):126–137.

163. Roddey TS, Olson SL, Gartsman GM, Hanten WP, Cook KF. A randomized controlled trial comparing 2 instructional approaches to home exercise instruction following arthroscopic full-thickness rotator cuff repair surgery. *JOSPT.* 2002; 32:548–559.

164. Godges JJ, Mattson-Bell M, Thorpe D, Shah D. The immediate effects of soft tissue mobilization with proprioceptive neuromuscular facilitation on glenohumeral external rotation and overhead reach. *JOSPT.* 2003; 33:713–718.

165. Hodgson SA, Mawson SJ, Stanley D. Rehabilitation after two-part fractures of the neck and humerus. *J Bone Joint Surg.* 2003; 85B:419–422.

166. Ginn K, Herbert RD, Khouw W, Lee R. A randomized, controlled clinical trial of a treatment for shoulder pain. *Phys Ther.* August 1997; 77(8).

167. Duruoz MT, Poraudeau S, Fermanian J, Menkes CJ, et al. Development and validation of a rheumatoid hand functional disability scale that assesses functional handicap. *J Rheumatol.* 1996; 23(7).

168. Buljina AI, Taljanovic MS, Avdic DM, Hunter TB. Physical and exercise therapy for treatment of the rheumatoid hand. *Arthritis Care Res.* 2001; 45: P392–P397.

169. Stamm TA, Machold KP, Smolen JS, Fischer S, Redlich K, Graninger W, Ebner W, Erlacher L. Joint protection and home hand exercises improve hand function in patients with hand osteoarthritis: A randomized controlled trial. *Arthritis Care Res.* 2002; 47:44–49.

170. Harris WE. Traumatic arthritis of the hip after dislocation and acetabular fractures: Treatment by mold arthroplasty. *J Bone Joint Surg.* 1969; 51A(4): 737–755.

171. Harris, WE. Preliminary report of results of Harris total hip replacement. *Clin Orthopaed Rel Res.* 1973; 95:168–173.

172. Sherrington C, Lord SR. Home exercise to improve strength and walking velocity after hip fracture: A randomized controlled trial. *Arch Phys Med Rehabil.* February 1997; 78.

173. Hauer K, Specht N, Schuler M, Bartsch P, Oster P. Intensive physical training in geriatric patients after severe falls and hip surgery. *Age Ageing.* 2002; 31(1):49–57.

174. Sherrington C. A RCT weight-bearing vs. non-weight bearing exercise for improving physical ability after usual care for hip fracture. *Arch Phys Med Rehabil.* 2004; 85(5):710–716.

175. Lauretzen JB, et al. Effects of external hip protectors on hip fractures. *Lancet.* January 2, 1993; 341.

176. Tinetti ME. Systematic home-based physical and functional therapy for older persons after hip fracture. *Arch Phys Med Rehabil.* 1997; vol 78:1331–1337.

177. Tinetti ME, et al. Home-based multicomponent rehabilitation program for older persons after Hip fracture: A randomized trial. *Arch Phys Med Rehabil.* August 1999; 80:916–922.

178. Wang AW, Gilbey HJ, Ackland TR. Perioperative exercise programs improve early return of ambulatory function after total hip arthoplasty. *Am J Phys Med. Rehabil.* 2002; 81:801–806.

179. Weaver FM, Hughes SL, Almagor O, Wixson R, Manheim L, Fulton B, Singer R. Comparison of two home care protocols for total joint replacement. *J Am Geriatr Soc.* 2003; 51:523–528.

180. Gibley HJ et al. Exercise improves early functional recovery after total hip arthroplasty. *Clin Orth Res.* 2003: (408):193–200.

181. Freburger JK. An analysis of the relationship between the utilization of physical therapy services and outcomes of care for patients after total hip arthroplasty. *Phys Ther.* May 2000; 80(5):448–458.

182. Insall, JN, Dorr LD, Scott RD, Scott WN. Rationale of the knee society clinical rating system. *Clin Orthop Relat Res.* 1989: 248:13–14.

183. Caggiano E, et al. Effects of electrical stimulation or voluntary contraction for strengthening the quadriceps femoris muscles in an aged male population. *JOSPT.* July 1994; 20(1).

184. Talbot LA, Gaines JM, Ling SM, Metter EJ. A home-based protocol of electrical muscle stimulation for quadriceps muscle strength in older adults with osteoarthritis of the knee. *J Rheumatol.* 2003; 30:1571–1578.

185. Marks R. The effects of 16 months of angle-specific isometric strengthening exercises in midrange on torque of the knee extensor muscles in osteoarthritis of the knee: A case study. *JOSPT.* August 1994; 20(2).

186. Ettinger WH, Burns R, Messier SP, Applegate W, Rejeski WJ, Morgan T, et al. A randomized trial comparing aerobic exercise and resistance exercise with a health education program in older adults with knee osteoarthritis: The fitness arthritis and seniors trial (FAST). *JAMA.* January 1, 1997; 277(1):25–31.

187. Mangione KK, McCully K, Gloviak A et al. The effects of high-intensity and low-intensity cycle ergometry in older adults with knee osteoarthritis. *J Gerontol.* 1999; 54A(4):M184–M190.

188. Puett DW, Griffin MR. Published trials of nonmedicinal and noninvasive therapies for hip and knee osteoarthritis. *Ann Int Med.* July 15, 1994; 121(2): 133–140.

189. Rogind, H, et al. The effects of a physical training program on patients with osteoarthritis of the knees. *Arch Phys Med Rehabil.* 1998; 79:1421–1427.

190. Maurer B, Stern A, Kinossian B, et. al. Osteoarthritis of the knee: Isokinetic quadriceps exercise versus educational intervention. *Arch Phys Med Rehabil.* October 1999; 80:1293–1299.

191. O'Reilly SC, et al. Quadriceps weakness in knee osteoarthritis: The effect on pain and disability. *Ann Rheum Dis.* 1998; 57:588–594.

192. Deyle GD, Henderson N, Matekel RL et al. Effectiveness of manual physical therapy and exercise in osteoarthritis of the knee. *Ann Int Med.* February 1, 2000; 132(3):173–181.

193. Caputo GM, et al. Assessment and management of foot disease in patients with diabetes. *N Engl J Med.* September 29, 1994; 331(13).

194. Domsic RT, Saltzman CL. Ankle osteoarthritis scale. *Foot and Ankle International.* 1998; 19(7):466–471.

195. Reiber GE, Smith DG, Wallace C, Sullivan K, Hayes S, Vath C, Maciejewski ML, Yu O, Heagerty PJ, LeMaster J. Effect of therapeutic footwear on foot reulceration in patients with diabetes. *JAMA.* May 15, 2002; 287(19):2552–2558.

196. Wolgin M, Cook C, Graham C, Mauldin D. Conservative treatment of plantar heel pain: Long-term follow-up. *Foot Ankle.* 1994; 15:97–102.

PART II

Patient Care Concepts

12

Neurological Considerations

Pearls

- Parkinson's disease is the number-one neurological disease in the elderly, and the most common symptoms of Parkinson's disease are slowness with ADLs, shuffling, tremor, difficulty with speech, and erratic movements.

- When assessing and treating Parkinson patients, it is imperative to thoroughly assess and discriminate between direct, indirect, and composite impairments when designing treatment interventions.

- Parkinson patients may respond to a specific evaluation and treatment progression of exercise and gait programs.

- Numerous methods exist for assessing older patients with strokes. Therapists should choose tools that have the greatest functional emphasis and applicability to geriatric rehabilitation.

- Treatment strategies for patients with stroke are varied and some are modified for the aged.

- Exercise should consist of functionally oriented activities in the Alzheimer's population.

- The maintenance of posture and the ability to move about the environment depend on orientation and balance, and the postural control system receives information from receptors in the proprioceptive, visual, and vestibular systems.

INTRODUCTION

This chapter will build on the discussion of specific biological changes that occur with age or pathology, as developed in Chapters 3 and 5. This section will discuss a model for looking at neurological dysfunction, followed by sections on mobility, balance and coordination, weakness, and tremor. The major pathologies that will be discussed are Parkinson's disease and cerebral vascular accidents (CVA), which will be discussed in terms of prevalence, efficacy of treatment interventions, evaluation, and treatment strategies. This will be followed by a discussion of evaluation and treatment of the common neurological pathology—Alzheimer's disease—which requires special consideration. The last section of this chapter will focus on balance and falls, evaluation of the numerous causes of dizziness and physical changes that increase the risk of falling, and treatment interventions aimed at decreasing the incidence of falls.

The model for neurological dysfunction used is that of Schenkman and Butler.[1] Figure 12.1 illustrates the progression of the stages that result in ultimate disability.

This model is best explained using an example; therefore, a patient with a CVA in which the neuroanatomic pathology is a parietal lobe lesion will be discussed. The impairment's direct effects might include a motor loss from the parietal lesion resulting in hypotonicity of the shoulder. An indirect pathological effect could be a rotator cuff tear, and the resulting impairment would be a subluxed shoulder. The impairment's composite effects would be decreased use of the upper extremity and pain on movement, as well as movement dysfunction in the upper and lower extremities. The resultant functional disability is the patient's inability to dress or walk independently, or sleep without discomfort.

The therapist can then use this model to examine where physical or occupational therapy can benefit the patient. In this example, the therapist may have little effect on the insult or neuroanatomic pathology, but the therapist could positively affect the other areas. Using this information, the therapist can choose the most effective intervention for the problem. This problem-solving model should be kept in mind when reviewing the subsequent dysfunctions.

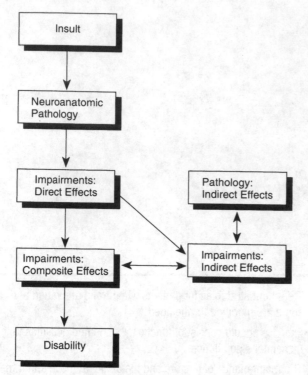

Figure 12.1 Outline of model for evaluating, interpreting, and treating individuals with neurologic dysfunction. (Reprinted with permission from Schenkman, B., Butler, R.B. A model for multisystem evaluation, interpretation and treatment of individuals with neurologic dysfunction. *Physical Therapy.* 1989; 69(7):538–547.)

PARKINSON'S DISEASE

Parkinson's disease is the primary neurological disease of the elderly.[2] It affects 1% of people over 50 years of age, and 50,000 new cases are diagnosed annually.[2] The description of Parkinson's disease and its causes have been covered in detail in Chapter 5. The most common symptoms in Parkinson's disease are:

- Slowness in ambulation and dressing.
- Difficulty in getting out of a chair and in turning in bed.
- Shuffling.
- Stooping when walking or falling to one side when sitting.
- Difficulty with speech.
- Tremor and handwriting changes.
- Difficulty initiating movements.[3]

Medical management of Parkinson's disease revolves mainly around the use of drugs such as L-dopa. It is important to note that the side effects associated with L-dopa's use are less virulent in the elderly and, therefore,

it can be prescribed at the onset.[4] The literature is filled with controversy as to dosage and side effects of anti-Parkinson medications (again see Chapter 7 for the side effects). The most noteworthy and deleterious side effects in the elderly are mental side effects, such as disorientation and confusion.[5]

The medical management of Parkinson's disease depends on the stage of disability. The Hoehn and Yahr[6] stages are as follows:

Stage I: Is characterized by minimal or no functional impairment and unilateral involvement only.

Stage II: Is characterized by bilateral involvement without any type of balance impairment.

Stage III: Is characterized by mild to moderate disability; here, the patient may lose righting reflexes as evidenced by unsteadiness on turns.

Stage IV: Is characterized by moderate to severe disability. The patient can still walk and stand unassisted, but is not stable.

Stage V: Is severe disability and here the patient is confined to bed or a wheelchair.[6]

The medical literature has shown that medication alone is not adequate treatment for this disease and that rehabilitation therapy is an important adjunct to medical treatment.[4–8]

Physical therapy has been shown to be efficacious for these patients.[8] In a study by Banks, Parkinson's patients with all degrees of impairment and duration of the disease improved in walking and other mobility skills after physical therapy.[8]

Evaluation

Schenkman and Butler have developed a model for the evaluation of patients with Parkinson's disease (Figure 12.2).[9]

This model can be used as a guideline for evaluating Parkinson patients. The therapist can begin by assessing the direct effects of the nervous system, such as tremor rigidity, hypokinesis, and autonomic nervous system effects. While it is important to note these, it is also important to recognize that these impairments will respond less dramatically to physical therapy procedures than the indirect effect impairments.[9] The indirect effect impairments are changes in the musculoskeletal system, such as flexibility, strength, and vital capacity. The combined changes of these two areas make up the major impairments listed in composite effects.

Evaluation Form. Figure 12.3 is an evaluation form that highlights and expands on the relevant impairments. This form affords the therapist the ability to differentiate between the various types of impairment.

Under the impairment categories the therapist looks for the following:

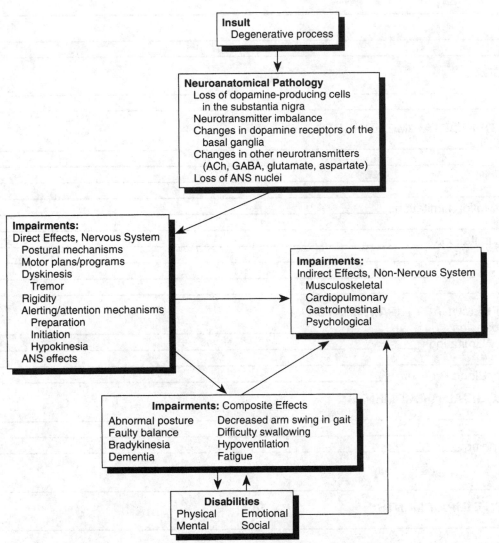

Figure 12.2   Overview of model for evaluation and treatment of patients with Parkinson's disease. ACh, acetylcholine, GABA, gamma-aminobutyric acid; ANS, autonomic nervous system. (Reprinted with permission from Schenkman, M., Butler, R. A model for multisystem evaluation treatment for individuals with Parkinson's disease. *Physical Therapy.* 1989; 69(11):932–943.

1. **Musculoskeletal impairments**

   Trunk mobility—unilateral and then bilateral trunk limitation. Increased kyphosis, decreased lumbar extension.

   Pelvic mobility—decreased rotation, decreased ability to tilt the pelvis.

   a. Range-of-motion limitations: Decreased motion in the plantar flexors, hip flexors, and neck rotators.

   b. Strength limitation: Weak hip extensors, dorsi/plantar flexors, and trunk extensors.

   c. Postural limitations: Forward head, rounded shoulders, kyphosis, increased hip and knee flexion.

2. **Cardiopulmonary impairments:** Decreased chest expansion and increased heart rate and blood pressure.

   a. Slowed movements and difficulty breathing.

   b. Increased fatigue and orthostatic hypotension.

3. **Neurological impairments:** Increased rigidity, resting tremor, slowness of movement, difficulty initiating movement, and increased drooling and flushing.

   a. Balance impairment: Increased loss of balance.

   b. Gait impairment: Shuffling, festination, retropulsion, no arm swing, slow pace.

   c. Swallowing impairments: Increased difficulty swallowing.

Name _____

History _____

FUNCTIONAL

Complaint _____
_____

MUSCULOSKELETAL IMPAIRMENTS

Trunk mobility _____
_____

Pelvic mobility _____
_____

Range of Motion Limitations _____
_____

Strength Limitations _____
_____

Limitations _____
_____

CARDIOPULMONARY IMPAIRMENTS

Chest Expansion _____

Pulmonary Limitations __._____
_____

Heart rate, Blood Pressure _____

NEUROLOGICAL IMPAIRMENTS

Rigidity _____

Tremor _____

Motor Planning _____

ANS

Function _____

COMPOSITE IMPAIRMENTS

Balance _____

Gait _____

Swallowing _____

Bradykinesia _____
_____

Hypoventilation _____
_____

Fatigue _____
_____

Goals _____
_____
_____
_____

Treatment Plan _____
_____
_____
_____
_____
_____
_____

Figure 12.3   Parkinson Evaluation Form. (© Carole B. Lewis)

Even with an extremely comprehensive form such as Figure 12.3, there are still areas that require special mention. Tremor, for example, may be overlooked because it is only present intermittently, minimally, or in one joint. Because tremor may be difficult to assess, the therapist should have the patient sit with arms resting on legs. The patient is then instructed to count backward by 2 from 100. This activity stresses the patient and brings out the resting tremor, which the therapist can then observe. Once the therapist has observed the tremor, placing the hands over the moving part will elicit the four- to seven-second tremor and confirm the resting tremor.[10]

A good test for bradykinesia is to have the patient sit with both hands in his or her lap. The patient then supinates and pronates the forearms as rapidly as possible on one side and then the other. If the symptoms are unilateral the therapist should start with the uninvolved side. The patient must do this activity for at least twenty seconds with the therapist observing for quality of movement. There may be no noticeable impairment at first; however, after three to four seconds, the patient will begin to substitute by shortening the arc, or will fail to flip hands over completely, and movement will generally slow. If this is noted, bradykinesia is confirmed.[10]

Hand posture can be checked by standing above and behind the patient, grasping both wrists, and shaking both hands up and down. The therapist observes for looseness and thumb position. If the patient fails to show general looseness or opposition of the thumb while shaking this may be a sign of early stage involvement. As the disease progresses, the patient will display finger adduction and flexion of the metacarpals, interphalangeal extension, and ulnar deviation. In the very advanced stages, the wrist may be drawn into flexion and pronation.[10]

Rigidity should be assessed in the neck, trunk, and all the extremities. Assessment for rigidity simply involves moving the part through the range of motion, making sure the patient is relaxed and not tensing the muscles. The therapist then notes any resistance or tension. All normal muscle movements should float.[10]

Weinrich and associates[11] noted that limitations in the wrist and head in axial rotation related to the improvement of symptoms of Parkinson's disease. Therefore, this measure may be an important tool in assessment.

Gait Evaluation Gait changes in Parkinson patients deserve special mention. According to the works of Murray and co-authors,[12] there are significant changes in the Parkinson's gait as compared to the normal gait. These changes are:

1. Decreased step length.
2. Wider stride width.
3. Increased knee flexion in the standing position. (Normally, 3° of hyperextension at the knee is observed in standing. Parkinson patients tend to stand in 3°, 6°,

and 12° of flexion for mild, moderate, and severely disabled groups, respectively.
4. Decreased mean total amplitude for flexion-extension used during free walking (degrees respectively in disabled Parkinson patients).[12]
5. Simultaneous thoracic and pelvic rotation in free speed walking.
6. Decreased heel floor angle at heel strike (norms 21° to 16°, 11° to 6° for Parkinson patients).[12]

Functional Assessment. A final area of evaluation of the Parkinson patient is functional assessment. In a study by Henderson and associates,[13] functional or activities of daily living (ADL) assessments were shown to be good for assessing functional deficits. The study did find, however, that if a description of the disease were sought, then an assessment of the actual signs of the disease would be better.[13]

Two ratings scales that incorporate both signs and ADL assessment are found in Table 12.1 and Figure 12.4.[10,14]

Once the therapist has conducted a thorough evaluation then the treatment can be initiated. See Appendix 1 for evidence-based support for the functional evaluation tools.

Treatment Considerations

When designing a treatment program for patients with Parkinson's disease, the model of Schenkman and co-authors[15] can be useful. The therapist must keep in mind which deficits can be corrected and which respond minimally to physical therapy. Rigidity, for example, may be temporarily relaxed in order to facilitate muscle stretching. However, the permanent effects of relaxation training on muscle rigidity will be minimal.[16] Therefore, prior to initiating a program the therapist must prioritize the problems and interpret the goals in terms of what is efficacious. Table 12.2 is an example of this process.[15]

Schenkman's Approach. Schenkman suggests the following treatment progression:

- Relaxation.
- Breathing exercises.
- Passive muscle stretching and positioning.
- Active range of motion and postural alignment.
- Weight shifting.
- Balance responses.
- Gait activities.
- Patient home exercises.[15]

As mentioned previously, relaxation can be used to temporarily decrease rigidity and increase flexibility. Relaxation of the muscles can be induced by slow rhythmic

TABLE 12.1   Parkinson's Disease Rating Scale

Directions: Apply a gross clinical rating to each of the ten listed items, assigning value ratings of 0–3 for each item, where (0) = no involvement and (1), (2), and (3) are equated to early, moderate, and severe disease, respectively. Refer to the discussion in the text for details of the examination and the ratings.

Bradykinesia of Hands—Including Handwriting

(0) No involvement.

(1) Detectable slowing of the supination–pronation rate evidenced by beginning difficulty in handling tools, buttoning clothes, and handwriting.

(2) Moderate slowing of supination–pronation rate, one or both sides, evidenced by moderate impairment of hand function. Handwriting is greatly impaired, microphagia present.

(3) Severe slowing of supination–pronation rate. Unable to write or button clothes. Marked difficulty in handling utensils.

Rigidity

(0) Nondetectable

(1) Detectable rigidity in neck and shoulders. Activation phenomenon is present. One or both arms show mild, negative, resting rigidity.

(2) Moderate rigidity in neck and shoulders. Resting rigidity is positive when patient is not on medication.

(3) Severe rigidity in neck and shoulders. Resting rigidity cannot be reversed by medication.

Posture

(0) Normal posture. Head flexed forward less than 4 inches.

(1) Beginning poker spine. Head flexed forward up to 5 inches.

(2) Beginning arm flexion. Head flexed forward 6 inches. One or both arms raised but still below waist.

(3) Onset of simian posture. Head flexed forward more than 6 inches. One or both hands elevated above waist. Sharp flexion of hand, beginning interphalangeal extension. Beginning flexion of knees.

Upper Extremity Swing

(1) One arm definitely decreased in amount of swing.

(2) One arm fails to swing.

(3) Both arms fail to swing.

Gait

(0) Steps out well with 18–30 inch stride. Turns about effortlessly.

(1) Gait shortened to 12–18 inch stride. Beginning to strike one heel. Turn around time slowing. Requires several steps.

(2) Stride moderately shortened—now 6–12 inches. Both heels beginning to strike floor forcefully.

(3) Onset of shuffling gait, steps less than 3 inches. Occasional stuttering-type or blocking gait. Walks on toes—turns around very slowly.

Tremor

(0) No detectable tremor found.

(1) Less than one inch of peak-to-peak tremor movement observed in limbs or head at rest or in either hand while walking or during finger to nose testing.

(2) Maximum tremor envelope fails to exceed 4 inches. Tremor is severe but not constant and patient retains some control of hands.

(3) Tremor envelope exceeds 4 inches. Tremor is constant and severe. Patient cannot get free of tremor while awake unless it is a pure cerebellar type. Writing and feeding are impossible.

TABLE 12.1   Parkinson's Disease Rating Scale (Continued)

Facies

(1) Detectable immobility. Mouth remains closed. Beginning features of anxiety or depression.

(2) Moderate immobility. Emotion breaks through at markedly increased threshold. Lips parted some of the time. Moderate appearance of anxiety or depression. Drooling may be present.

(3) Frozen facies. Mouth open 1/4 inch or more. Drooling may be severe.

Seborrhea

(0) None.

(1) Increased perspiration, secretion remaining thin.

(2) Obvious oiliness present. Secretion much thicker.

(3) Marked seborrhea, entire face and head covered by thick secretion.

Speech

(0) Clear, loud, resonant, easily understood.

(1) Beginning of hoarseness with loss of inflection and resonance. Good volume and still easily understood.

(2) Moderate hoarseness and weakness. Constant monotone, unvaried pitch. Beginning of dysarthria, hesitancy, stuttering, difficulty to understand.

(3) Marked harshness and weakness. Very difficult to hear and understand.

Self Care

(0) No impairment.

(1) Still provides full self-care but rate of dressing definitely impeded. Able to live alone and often still employable.

(2) Requires help in certain critical areas, such as turning in bed, rising from chairs, etc. Very slow in performing most activities but manages by taking much time.

(3) Continuously disabled. Unable to dress, feed him- or herself, or walk alone.

Reprinted with permission from Webster, D. Critical analysis of the disability in Parkinson's disease. Mod Treat. 1969; 5:257–282.

Parkinson's Disease Quality of Life Questionnaire (PDQL)

Population:	Patient's with Parkinson's disease.
Description:	The Parkinson's Disease Quality of Life Questionnaire (PDQL) is a 37-item instrument used to measure quality of life in patients with Parkinson's disease. There are four subscales that make up the questionnaire; Parkinsonian symptoms, Systemic symptoms, Emotional function, and Social function.
Mode of Administration:	The PDQL is a self-administered paper and pencil questionnaire.
Scoring:	
Time to Complete:	5 to 10 minutes
Time to Score:	5 minutes
Scoring:	The patient fills out the questionnaire using a 5-point Likert scale for response options (All of the time, Most of the time, Some of the time. A little of the time, and Never). The mean scores for each subscale are calculated by dividing the subscale score by the number of items in the subscale. An overall quality of life score can be obtained by adding the mean scores and dividing by the number of items in the questionnaire. The range is from 1–5.
Interpretation:	A lower score indicates higher disease severity and thus, lower quality of life whereas a higher score indicates less disease severity and better quality of life.

Figure 12.4

Reliability:	Reliability was tested by investigating the consistency of the results of the PDQL with Cronbach's alpha coefficient. The results were high for each of the subscales, 0.80–0.87. The overall PDQL score alpha was 0.94.
Validity:	In order to evaluate discriminant validity, three groups of varying severity of disease were compared. ANOVA (analysis of variance) was employed to test for statistical significance. As expected, all subscale and overall scores were lower in patients with higher disease severity. To test convergent validity, the PDQL scores were compared with standard indices of quality of life; the MOS-24 subscales (Medical outcome studies-24), the social support survey, and the CES-D depression scale (Center for Epidemiologic Studies). Product moment correlation coefficients were used to assess linear relationships between the PDQL and the other indices. All correlations were statistically significant, exceeding the 0.40 criterion for conceptually related scales.
Reference:	De Boer, A. de Haes, J., Speelman, J.D., Wijker, W.: Quality of life in patients with Parkinson's disease: development of a questionnaire. J Neurol Neurosurg Psychiatry 61:70–74, 1996.

The Parkinson's Disease Quality of Life Questionnaire (PDQL)

We translated the questionnaire from Dutch into English, following the guidelines for cross cultural adaptation of life measures of Guyatt and Guillemin *et al.*
To obtain semantic, idiomatic, and conceptual equivalence in translation techniques. This involved using native English and Dutch speakers who translated the questionnaire into their mother tongue. A small committee of members compared source and back translation versions and produced a final version as follows:

Response options:

1) All the time 2) Most of the time 3) Some of the time 4) A little of the time 5) Never

How often during the last three months did you have trouble with:

1) stiffness (P)
2) feeling generally unwell (Sys)
3) that you are no longer able to do your hobbies (Soc)
4) being tense (P)
5) feeling insecure of yourself due to your physical limitations (E)
6) shaking of the hand(s) (P)
7) feeling worn out or having no energy (Sys)
8) difficulties in doing sport or leisure activities (Soc)
9) clumsiness (P)
10) feeling embarrassed because of your illness (E)
11) shuffling (P)
12) having to postpone or cancel social activities because of your illness (Soc)
13) a feeling of extreme exhaustion (Sys)
14) difficulties turning around while walking (P)
15) being afraid of possible progressing of the illness (E)
16) difficulties writing (P)
17) being less able to go on holiday than before your illness (Soc)
18) feeling insecure of yourself around others (E)
19) difficulties getting a good night's rest (Sys)
20) "on/off" periods (P)
21) difficulty with accepting your illness (E)
22) difficulties talking (P)
23) difficulties signing your name in public (Soc)
24) difficulties walking (Sys)
25) drooling (P)
26) feeling depressed or discouraged (E)
27) difficulty with sitting still (for long periods) (P)
28) often needing to urinate and/or wetting yourself (Sys)
29) difficulties with transport (Soc)
30) sudden extreme movements (P)

Figure 12.4   (Continued)

31) difficulties concentrating (E)
32) difficulties getting up from a chair (P)
33) constipation (Sys)
34) difficulties with your memory (E)
35) difficulties turning around in bed (P)
36) that your illness inhibits your sex life (Soc)
37) feeling worried about (the possible consequences of) an operation in connection with your illness (E)

(P): Parkinson symptoms (Sys): Systemic symptoms (Soc): Social functioning (E): Emotional functioning

Parkinson Activity Scale

I. Chair Transfers

1. Getting up *(From arm chair; first trial without using arms; then second trial with using arms)*
—normal, without apparent difficulties ☐ 4
—without arms, mild difficulties (toes dorsiflex to maintain balance) ☐ 3
—without arms, impossible or several attempts needed, with arms normal ☐ 2
—with arms, difficult (several attempts, hesitation) ☐ 1
—dependent on physical assistance ☐ 0

2. Sitting down *(First trial without hands, second trial with hands when necessary)*
—normal, without apparent difficulties ☐ 4
—without arms, mild difficulties (uncontrolled landing) ☐ 3
—without arms, abrupt landing or ending in an uncomfortable position, with arms normal ☐ 2
—with arms, abrupt landing or ending in an uncomfortable position ☐ 1
—dependent on physical assistance ☐ 0

II. Gait Akinesia

3. Gait initiation *(Tested after rising from a chair)*
—normal, without apparent difficulties ☐ 4
—hesitation or short festination ☐ 3
—unwanted arrest of movement with or without festination lasting 5 s or less ☐ 2
—unwanted arrest of movement with or without festination lasting more than 5 s ☐ 1
—dependent on physical assistance to start walking ☐ 0

4. Turning 360° *(Testing in a situation provoking difficulties in daily life)*
—normal, without apparent difficulties ☐ 4
—hesitation or short festination ☐ 3
—unwanted arrest of movement with or without festination lasting 5 s or less ☐ 2
—unwanted arrest of movement with or without festination lasting more than 5 s ☐ 1
—dependent on physical assistance to start walking ☐ 0

III. Bed Mobility

5. Lying down *(The patient is asked to lie down on his or her back)*
—normal, without apparent difficulties ☐ 4
—1 difficulty, with lifting legs, moving trunk, or reaching adequate end position ☐ 3
—2 difficulties, with lifting legs, moving trunk, or reaching adequate end position ☐ 2
—3 difficulties, with lifting legs, moving trunk, and reaching adequate end position ☐ 1
—dependent on physical assistance ☐ 0

6. Rolling onto the side *(The patient is asked to roll over to the side)*
—normal, without apparent difficulties ☐ 4
—1 difficulty, with turning, shifting trunk, or reaching adequate end position ☐ 3
—2 difficulties, with turning, or shifting trunk, or reaching adequate end position ☐ 2
—3 difficulties, with turning, shifting trunk, and reaching adequate end position ☐ 1
—dependent on physical assistance ☐ 0

7. Rising *(The patient is asked to get up and sit on the edge of the bed)*
—normal, without apparent difficulties ☐ 4
—1 difficulty, with moving legs or trunk or reaching adequate end position ☐ 3
—2 difficulties, with moving legs or trunk or reaching adequate end position ☐ 2
—3 difficulties, with moving legs and trunk and reaching adequate end position ☐ 1
—dependent on physical assistance ☐ 0

IV. Bed Mobility with Cover

8. Lying down with cover *(The patient is asked to lie down on his or her back under the covers)*
—normal, without apparent difficulties ☐ 4
—1 difficulty, with either moving body, adjusting cover, or reaching adequate end position ☐ 3
—2 difficulties, with moving body, adjusting cover, or reaching adequate end position ☐ 2
—3 difficulties, with moving body, adjusting cover, and reaching adequate end position ☐ 1
—dependent on physical assistance ☐ 0

Figure 12.4   (Continued)

9. Rolling onto the side with cover *(The patient is asked to roll onto his or her side under he covers)*	—normal, without apparent difficulties	☐ 4
	—1 difficulty, with turning body, adjusting cover, or reaching adequate end position	☐ 3
	—2 difficulties, with turning body, adjusting cover, or reaching adequate end position	☐ 2
	3 difficulties, with turning body, adjusting cover, and reaching adequate end position	☐ 1
	—dependent on physical assistance	☐ 0
10. Rising with cover *(The patient is asked to get up and sit on the edge of the bed)*	—normal, without apparent difficulties	☐ 4
	—1 difficulty, with moving body, adjusting cover, or reaching adequate end position	☐ 3
	—2 difficulties, with moving body, adjusting cover, or reaching adequate end position	☐ 2
	—3 difficulties, with moving body, adjusting cover, and reaching adequate end position	☐ 1
	—dependent on physical assistance	☐ 0

Figure 12.4 (Continued)

(Reprinted with permission from De Boer, A., Wijker, W., Speelman, J., de Haes, J. Quality of life in patients with Parkinson's disease: Development of a questionnaire. *Journal of Neurol Neurosurg Psychiatry. 1996; 61: 70–74.*)

TABLE 12.2 Examples of Problems, Interpretations, and Goals for Patients With Parkinson's Disease

Problem[a]	Quantitative	Descriptive	Interpretation	Goal
Gait	Ambulates 25 ft[b] in 18 sec (18 steps)	Small steps; decreased left heel-strike; decreased trunk rotation; left knee in flexion from weight acceptance to push-off; no left arm swing	Problems attributable to limitations in left knee and ankle range of motion and decreased available trunk rotation combined with trunk and limb rigidity with motor programming and planning deficits	Ambulate 25 ft in 10 sec (12 steps); improved heel-strike, pushoff, trunk rotation, and arm swing
Bed mobility (supine to sitting)	7 sec to complete task	Lacks trunk rotation and dissociation of pelvic complex from shoulder complex; appears fearful of losing balance	Problems attributable to combination of limited available trunk ROM, rigidity, and impaired balance	2 sec to complete task; improved trunk rotation with dissociation of shoulder complex from pelvic complex
Transfers (sitting to standing from low treatment table)	Sitting to standing from mat takes 10 sec	Lack of anterior pelvic tilt and of scooting forward on mat; excessive use of arms for push-off from mat	Problems attributable to lack of lumbopelvic mobility, rigidity, and difficulty motor planning and programming	Patient will accomplish task in 5 sec, use anterior tilt, scoot forward, and decrease need for use of arms
Decreased hip ROM	Straight leg raise (left leg: 0°–50°; right leg: 0°–45°; internal rotation (left leg: 0°–25°; right leg: 0°–30°)		Problems result from rigidity and improper posturing	Hip ROM within normal limits
Rigidity[c]		Moderate[d]	Attributable to primary impairments of disease	Patient will self-relax rigidity for increasing ROM

[a]*Patient problems may relate to disabilities or impairments.*
[b]*1 ft = 0.3048 m.*
[c]*Rigidity is listed as a problem because of its causal role in most impairments of Parkinson's disease; however, objective measures of rigidity do not exist, and physical therapy does not appear to affect long-term changes.*
[d]*Feldman, R., Lannon, M. Parkinson's disease and related disturbances. In: Feldman, R., ed.* Neurology: The Physician's Guide. *New York: Thieme Medical Publishers; 1984: 147–162.*
Reprinted with permission from Schenkman, M., et al. Management of individuals with Parkinson's disease: Rationale and case studies. Phys Ther. *November 1989; 69(11)944–955.*

rotating movements beginning with very small motions and progressing to larger ones. Other techniques, such as biofeedback, contract-relax stretch, and deep breathing, can be helpful. The relaxation will be more effective if the approach begins supine and progresses to sitting and standing; and the more supported the individual is, the better will be the ability to relax. In addition, relaxation is better if it is begun passively and is progressed to active. Finally, the relaxation is more effective if the patient is taught to relax individual functional segments (for example, the head on the thorax, the shoulder on the thorax, and the lower extremity on the pelvis).

Breathing or breathing control should be encouraged throughout the various stages of treatment. The patient is taught to take deep relaxed breaths while doing the relaxation exercises. Once the patient has achieved some degree of relaxation in the thoracic area, then deeper breathing combined with trunk stretching can help to increase chest expansion.

Passive muscle stretching is another commonly used modality for physical therapy. What is different for the patient with Parkinson's disease is the mode and area of application. As with relaxation, the most effective stretch will be with the body in the most supported position due to the patient's decreased protective responses; therefore, begin with stretching in the supine or side-lying position. Areas requiring special stretching are:

- Lumbopelvic extensions are important for balance.
- Rotation and lateral flexion of the pelvis.
- Hamstring and plantar flexion.
- Cervical and thoracic extension rotation, and lateral flexion.
- Hip extension, external rotation, and abduction.
- Elbow extension and supination.
- Finger flexion and extension.

To achieve passive stretching, contract-relax stretching and passive stretching using Gustaffson's principle of fifteen- to thirty-second stretches gives the best results.[17] Stretching is followed by active range of motion and postural alignment.

The key to achieving the best results in active range of motion and postural alignment is repetition. According to Nelson,[18] for a movement to become assimilated by the nervous system it needs millions of repetitions, which equates to hundreds to thousands of repetitions a day. Therefore, the patient should do the activity for five to ten minutes instead of five to ten times. Some of the most useful active motion activities for these areas are (1) pelvic clocks to enhance pelvic and lumbar motion, (2) isolated lateral and anterior pelvic tilts, and (3) clocks around any joint in the body. If the patient has limitation in the lumbar spine, the patient may substitute for lumbopelvic motion with pelvic-femoral motion. Therefore, evaluate and treat any loss of mobility in the lumbar spine.

Once the patient is able to actively move the various body parts in a supine and then a standing position following stretching, then weight shifting in a standing position with the pelvis in a balanced position is practiced. Weight shifting, like the previous sequences, can be practiced from the supine to the standing positions.

Finally, balance activities and responses must be stressed. Here the patient's balance can be challenged intrinsically and extrinsically. Methods of challenging the patient's intrinsic balance include having the patient reach overhead, from side to side, and backward in a rotational direction when sitting and standing. For extrinsic balance challenges, the therapist can apply an outside stress, such as a gentle shove, to disturb the patient's balance. Both are needed for everyday activity and should be practiced when sitting and standing.

Function is the final area of treatment and must always be kept in mind when designing the exercise program, because exercises are most effective if they relate to function. For example, trunk rotation should be followed by rolling in bed as an active functional activity that the patient can do on his or her own at home. Anterior pelvic tilting when standing is another useful home exercise employing a needed functional activity. When designing a home exercise program, be sure to stress the functional carry-over. This way when the patient does daily activities, he or she is constantly doing the exercise program.

Flewitt-Handford Exercises. Another well-known program for Parkinson patients are the Flewitt-Handford exercises. These exercises were developed to help improve the gait of Parkinson patients. The developers of the exercises believe that the gait seen is a result of adaption to gain control of forward progression and balance. Parkinson patients have plenty of propulsion, but they lack a braking mechanism. Flewitt-Handford exercises are directed to reteach heel strike, improve weight transference, increase motion of the hip and knee, and prevent stiffness of the lower extremity (Table 12.3).[19]

Patient education is an important component for the treatment of the Parkinson patient. The Parkinson's Disease Foundation is an excellent resource for information and assistance for the patient and the families. It has developed an exercise videotape for Parkinson patients called "Get-up and Go," which is a useful tool for helping patients maintain the benefits of a rehabilitation program in a fun and interesting way.

Group Rehabilitation. Another treatment consideration is group rehabilitation.[20] Table 12.4 is a sample group evaluation and exercise progression.

See appendix 1 for evidence-based treatment ideas.

TABLE 12.3 The Flewitt-Handford Exercises

1. **Long sitting.** Alternate flexion/extension of toes, feet, and knees.

2. **Crook lying.** Rolling knees from side to side.

3. **Lying.** Alternate hip and knee flexion/extension, lift each foot off the plinth.

4. **Stand** facing and holding onto either parallel bars in a gym, or a heavy chair, table, or mantelpiece at home.

   a. High stepping.

   b. With straight knees and not leaning backward alternate feet dorsiflexion.

   c. Cross the left leg in front of the right and vice versa each time trying to touch the floor heel first.

   d. If in the gym, the patient should practice weight transference by walking sideways up and down the parallel bars. Then the same again, but crossing the legs over each other.

5. **Standing** at right angles to the parallel bars or chair, practice taking strides from toe off to heel-strike of first one leg, then the other. Pay attention to hip extension and proper heel-strike.

   When walking, patients must learn to put their heels down first with every step. Many patients become "stuck" while walking. They can easily unstick themselves by rocking backwards so their weight is going through their heels. Though taking a step backwards or sideways, they will find themselves able to move forwards again.

Reprinted with permission from Handford, F. *The Flewitt-Handford exercises for Parkinson's Gait. Physiotherapy.* August 1986; 72(8): 382.

STROKE

Even though stroke is not the major neurological problem of old age, it is significant because it is such a functionally devastating disease. In the United States alone between 250,000 and 300,000 persons have CVAs a year.[21,22] Most strokes occur late in life; forty-three percent of stroke patients are over the age of 74.[22,23]

In absolute numbers, women and men over age 75 are almost equally afflicted with CVAs; however, because the ratio of women to men is so much greater (3:2), statistically men have a greater likelihood of developing stroke.[24] Blacks and Japanese Americans are more likely to have strokes than whites, and the geographic area with the highest percentage of strokes is the southern United States.[22,25]

Besides causing tremendous morbidity (it is estimated that 20% to 40% of stroke patients die within 30 days),[26] nearly 40% of people with this disease report limitations in their activities. Cerebral vascular disease results in an average of 36 days of restricted activity for stroke victims.[27]

There are three major types of strokes. The cerebral thrombosis occurs when an artery that supplies blood to the brain becomes narrowed by plaque and deposits. The blood may coagulate and form a clot that does not allow sufficient blood through to the area. A cerebral emboli is caused by a blockage of some foreign object in the bloodstream, such as a clot, that can become wedged where it obstructs blood flow to the brain. The final type of stroke is a cerebral hemorrhage, where the artery is not blocked but bursts and blood seeps into the surrounding brain tissue. Depending on the extent of the damage, a cerebral hemorrhage is usually the most severe type of stroke, followed by thrombosis, then emboli. The severity of the stroke also depends on what area of the brain is affected and the extent and duration of the blockage of blood. Table 12.5 shows the clinical symptoms of vascular lesions and neurovascular disease.[28]

TABLE 12.4 Parkinsonism Evaluation

Occupational Therapy	
Upper Extremity Function	*Activities of Daily Living*

1. Drawing concentric circles
   a. number in 30 sec
   b. size of circles
   c. line quality
2. Alternating finger flexion/extension: number of complete repetitions in 10 sec
3. Grasp strength
	1. Dressing (in seconds)
	   a. put on shirt
	   b. fasten three buttons
	   c. put one shoe
	   d. tie one shoelace
	2. Transfers (in seconds)
	   a. standing to supine

TABLE 12.4   Parkinsonism Evaluation (Continued)

4. Signature: time, legibility	b. supine to standing
	c. standing to sitting
	d. sitting to standing
	3. Mobility (in seconds)
	  a. rolling supine to prone
	  b. standing 360° turn
	  c. opening/entering doors
	  d. ascending/descending stairs

Physical Therapy

Muscle Tightness	*Balance*
1. Pectorals—active range 2. Hamstrings—passive range 3. Hip flexors—passive range 4. Hip adductors—passive range	1. Quadruped-balance on opposite arm and leg, 5 sec 2. Standing on one foot, 5 sec 3. Propulsion (push patient forward) 4. Retropulsion (push patient backward)

Reciprocation (repetitions in 30 sec)
1. Supine
2. Gait
3. Stop start walk: sec/15 m
	Posture
	1. Standing
	  a. anterior–posterior
	  b. lateral
	2. Walking
	3. Supine

Phase I:
  Warm-up exercises for range of motion, reciprocality, and mobility.
  Mat exercises: bridging, trunk rotation, side leg raises, and reciprocal movements
  Parallel bars: knee bends, side leg raises, balancing.
  Bicycle/pulleys.

Phase II:
  Activities for mobility and equilibrium.
  Range of motion exercises for all major joints.
  Facial exercises.
  Static and dynamic balance: *Hokey Pokey, Alley Cat*

Phase III:
  Activities for coordination and socialization:

Week 1: Special exercises for breathing
    Alley Cat
    Shuffleboard
    Frisbee
	Special exercises for face, lips
	Marching
	Hot potato
	Instrument playing
	Tic-Tac-Toe

Week 2: *Hokey Pokey*
  Ball: reciprocal bouncing, tossing, kicking,
    pass and reverse, beach ball
	Subgroup *a: Alley Cat*
	cotton ball blow
	hand-clapping patterns
	Subgroup *b*: individual tasks: perceptual
	    tasks, dexterity boards, tracing

Week 3: Beanbag toss Sitting relay: overhead, sideways	Horseshoes Hot potato
Week 4: *Hokey Pokey* Bowling	Special exercises for arms, hands Wang passing Basketball

Reprinted with permission from Davis, J. Team management of Parkinson's disease. Am J Occup Ther. *May–June 1977;*
31(5)300–308.

TABLE 12.5   Clinical Symptoms of Cerebral Vascular Lesions and Neurovascular Disease

Vessel	Clinical Symptoms	Structures Involved
Cerebral Vascular Lesions		
Middle cerebral artery	Contralateral paralysis and sensory deficit	Somatic motor area
	Motor speech impairment	Broca's area (dominant hemisphere)
	"Central" asphasia, anomia, jargon speech	Parietoccipital cortex (dominant hemisphere)
	Unilateral neglect, apraxia, impaired ability to judge distance	Parietal lobe (nondominant hemisphere)
	Homonymous hemianopsia	Optic radiation deep to second temporal convolution
	Loss of conjugate gaze to opposite side	Frontal controversive field
	Avoidance reaction of opposite limbs	Parietal lobe
	Pure motor hemiplegia	Upper protion of posterior limb of internal
	Limb-kinetic apraxia capsule	Premotor or parietal cortex
Anterior cerebral artery	Paralysis—lower extremity	Motor area—leg
	Paresis in opposite arm	Arm area of cortex
	Cortical sensory loss	Sensory area
	Urinary incontinence	Posteromedial aspect of superior frontal gyrus
	Contralateral grasp reflex, sucking reflex	Medial surface of posterior frontal lobe
	Lack of spontaneity motor inaction, echolalia	Uncertain
	Perseveration and amnesia	Uncertain
Posterior cerebral	Homonymous hemianopsia	Calcarine cortex or optic radiation
	Bilateral homonymous hemianopsia, cortical blindness, inability to perceive objects not centrally located, ocular apraxia	Bilateral occipital lobe
		Inferomedial portions of temporal lobe
	Memory defect	Nondominant calcarine and lingual gyri
	Topographic disorientation	
Central area	Thalamic syndrome	Posteroventral nucleus ophthalmus
	Weber's syndrome	Cranial nerve III and cerebral peduncle
	Contralateral hemiplegia	Cerebral peduncle
	Paresis of vertical eye movements, sluggish pupillary response to light	Supranuclear fibers to cranial nerve III
Internal carotid artery	Contralateral ataxia or postural tremor	Uncertain
	Variable signs according to degree and site of occlusion—middle cerebral, anterior cerebral, posterior cerebral territory	

TABLE 12.5   Clinical Symptoms of Cerebral Vascular Lesions and Neurovascular Disease (Continued)

Vessel	Clinical Symptoms	Structures Involved
Basilar artery		Middle and superior cerebellar peduncles
Superior cerebellar	Ataxia	Vestibular nucleus
	Dizziness, nausea, vomiting, horizontal nystagmus	Decending sympathetic fibers
		Spinal thalamic tract
	Horner's syndrome on opposite side, decreased pain and thermal sensation	Medial lemniscus
	Decreased touch, vibration, position sense of lower extremity greater than upper extremity	Vestibular nerve
Anterior inferior cerebellar artery	Nystagmus, vertigo, nausea, vomiting	Cranial nerve VII
	Facial paralysis on same side	Auditory nerve, lower coclear nucleus
	Tinnitus	Middle cerebral peduncle
	Ataxis	Fifth cranial nerve nucleus
	Impaired facial sensation on same side	Spinal thalamic tract
	Decreased pain and thermal sensation on opposite side	
Hemorrhage		CT scan can detect hemorrhages greater than 1.5 cm in cerebral and cerebellar hemispheres; they are diagnostically superior to arteriography; they are especially helpful in diagnosing small hemorrhages that do not spill blood into cerebrospinal fluid; with massive hemorrhage and increased pressure, cerebrospinal fluid is grossly bloody; lumbar puncture in necessary when CT scan is not available; radiographs occasionally show midline shift (this is not true with infarction); EEG shows no typical pattern, but high volt to age and slow waves are most common with hemorrhage; urinary changes may reflect renal disease
Hypertensive hemorrhage	Severe headache	
	Vomiting at onset	
	Blood pressure > 170/90; usually "essential" hypertension but can be from other types	
	Abrupt onset, usually during day, not in sleep	
	Gradually evolves over hours or days according to speed of bleeding	
	No recurrence of bleeding	
	Frequency of blacks with hypertensive hemmorage is greater than frequency of whites	
	Hemorrhaged blood absorbs slowly—rapid improvement of symptoms is not usual	
	If massive hemorrhage occurs, client survive a few hours or days, secondary brain stem compression	

(continued)

TABLE 12.5   Clinical Symptoms of Cerebral Vascular Lesions and Neurovascular Disease (Continued)

Vessel	Clinical Symptoms	Structures Involved
Ruptured saccular aneurysm	Asymptomatic before rupture	CT scan detects localized blood in hydrocephalus if present; cerebrospinal fluid is extremely bloody; radiographs are usually negative; carotid and vertebral arteriography are performed only if certain of diagnosis
	With rupture, blood spills under high pressure into sub-arachnoid space:	
	Excruciating headache with loss of consciousness	
	Sudden loss of consciousness	
	Decerebrate rigidity with coma	
	If severe—persistent deep coma with respiratory arrest, circulatory collapse leading to death; death can occur within 5 minutes	
	If mild—consciousness regained within hours then confusion, amnesia, headache, stiff neck, drowsiness	
	Hemiplegia, paresis, homonymous hemianopsia, or aphasis usually absent	
Basilar artery Complete basilar syndrome	Bilateral long tract signs with cerebellar and cranial nerve abnormalities	_____
	Coma	_____
	Quadriplegia	_____
	Pseudobulbar palsy	_____
	Cranial nerve abnormalities	
Vertebral artery	Decreased pain and temperature on opposite side	Spinal thalamic tract
	Sensory loss from a tactile and proprioceptive	Medial lemniscus
	Hemiparesis of arm and leg	Pyramidal tract
	Facial pain and numbness on same side	Descending tract and fifth cranial nucleus
	Horner's syndrome, ptosis, decreased sweating	Descending sympathetic tract
	Ataxia	Cranial nerve XII
	Spinal cerebellar tract	Cranial nerves IX and X
	Paralysis of tongue	Uncertain
	Weakness of vocal cord, decreased gag	
	Hiccups	
Neurovascular Disease		
Thrombosis	*Extremely variable*	
	Preceded by a prodromal episode	Cerebrospinal fluid pressure is normal
	Uneven progression	

TABLE 12.5   Clinical Symptoms of Cerebral Vascular Lesions and Neurovascular Disease (Continued)

Vessel	Clinical Symptoms	Structures Involved
TIAs	Onset develops within minutes, hours, or over days ("thrombus in evolution") 60% occur during sleep—awaken unaware of problem, rise, and fall to floor Usually no headache but may occur in mild form Hypertension, diabetes, or vascular disease elsewhere in body Linked to atherosclerotic thrombosis Proceeded or accompanied by stroke Occur by themselves Last 2–30 minutes Experience a few attacks or hundreds Normal neurological examination between attacks If transient symptoms are present on awakening, may indicate future stroke	Cerebrospinnal fluid is clear EEG: limited differential diagnostic value Skull radiographs are not helpful Arteriography is the diffinitive procedure, it demonstrates site of collateral flow CT scanning is helpful in chronic state when cavitation has occurred Usually none
Embolism	*Extremely variable*	
Cardiac	Occurs extremely rapidly— seconds or minutes	Generally same as thrombosis except for following:
Noncardiac Atherosclerosis	There are no warnings	If embolism causes a large hemorrhagic infarct, cerebrospinal fluid will be bloody
Pulmonary thrombosis Fat, tumor, air	Branches of middle cerebral artery are involved most frequently, large embolus will block internal carotid artery or stem of middle cerebral artery If in basilar system, deep coma and total paralysis may result Often a manifestation of heart disease, including atrial fibrillation and myocardial infarction As embolis passes through artery, client may have neurological deficits that resolve as embolis breaks and passes into small artery supplying small or silent brain area	30% of embolic strokes produced small hemorrhagic infarct without bloody cerebrospinal fluid

Reprinted with permission and adapted from Ryerson, S. Hemiplegia resulting from vascular insult or disease. In: Umphred, D., ed. Neurological Rehabilitation. *St. Louis: Mosby: 2001: 476.*

Risk factors associated with stroke are similar for young and old. Spriggs and co-workers[29] noted such factors as previous cerebral vascular disease, taking certain prescribed medicines, and regular cigarette smoking as high-risk factors. Family history was also a factor but was not found to be significant in the older population.[22,29]

Perceptual deficits occur in varying degrees with a stroke. Table 12.6 is a chart of these deficits.

A central problem in tone occurs in approximately 10% of stroke patients. This condition, which severely affects gait and balance in the hemiplegic, has been termed the Pusher syndrome.[30] This problem is one of postural imbalance due to ipsilateral pushing or lateropulsion. The patient pushes strongly away from the unaffected side toward the hemiplegic side. Ipsilateral pushing varies in severity from mild to severe and may be transient or pronounced and prolonged.[31] If severe, pushing occurs in all positions, supine, sitting, and standing, and during remission or resolution pushing typically disappears first in the supine position, then in the sitting position, and finally in the standing position. Pushing increases in intensity with the difficulty of the postural challenge.[32] The most apparent problem of this syndrome is that is represents a threat to safety during standing and transfers, as the hemi side cannot effectively support body weight.

It has been suggested that the damage from the stroke lesion occurs in the subcortical sensory pathways.[31,32] Pusher syndrome affects sensory feedback in relationship to posture and gravity leading to a misperception of the individual's position in space. In other words, the patient reflexively compensates for a false feeling of leaning toward the unaffected side by leaning in the opposite direction.[30]

Before a therapist can begin evaluating and treating a stroke patient, a thorough understanding of the various stages of recovery of limb tone is essential. In the majority of cases, the predominant abnormality on admission in both upper and lower extremity is flaccidity.[33] The recovery of tone goes through stages of progression occurring mainly in the first seven to fourteen days. By day 28, a total of 20% of the patients had normal upper limb tone and 28% of the patients had normal lower limb tone.[34]

Table 12.7 shows the recovery of limb tone at 28 days.[33]

Many of the following evaluative techniques are for assessing tone. It is imperative to realize that the greatest recovery occurs within the first seven days, and many patients do regain spontaneous motor recovery within that time. Studies as of yet have not shown a difference in this early recovery stage between young and old.[33]

The efficacy of rehabilitation techniques for stroke patients has been questioned by legislative as well as administrative personnel. Nevertheless, there are several references that point to the efficacy of physical therapy.[34–36] Lehman, in the *Archives of Physical Medicine Rehabilitation*, showed that there are excellent improvements

TABLE 12.6   Perceptual Deficits in CNS Dysfunction

LEFT HEMIPARESIS: right hemisphere—general spatial-global deficits

Visual-perceptual deficits
  Hand-eye coordination
  Figure-ground discrimination
  Spatial relationships
  Position in space
  Form constancy

Behavioral and intellectual deficits
  Poor judgment, unrealistic behavior
  Denial of disability
  Inability to abstract
  Rigidity of thought
  Disturbances in body image and body scheme
  Impairment of ability to self-correct
  Difficulty retaining information
  Distortion of time concepts
  Tendency to see the whole and not individual steps
  Affect lability
  Feelings of persecution
  Irritability, confusion
  Distraction by verbalization
  Short attention span
  Appearance of lethargy
  Fluctuation in performance
  Disturbances in relative size and distance of objects

RIGHT HEMIPARESIS: left hemisphere—general language and temporal ordering deficits

Apraxia
  Motor
  Ideational

Behavioral and intellectual deficits
  Difficulty initiating tasks
  Sequencing deficits
  Processing delays
  Directionality deficits
  Low frustration levels
  Verbal and manual perseveration
  Rapid performance of movement or activity
  Compulsive behavior
  Extreme distractibility

Reprinted with permission from Ryerson, S. Hemiplegia resulting from vascular insult or disease. In: Umphred, D., ed. Neurological Rehabilitation. St. Louis: Mosby; 2001, 476.

TABLE 12.7   Recovery of Limb Tone at 28 Days

Admission limb tone	Limb tone at 28 days					
	No.	*Normal*	*Flexor*	*Extensor*	*Flaccid*	*Dead*
Upper limb						
Normal	19	16	0	0	0	3
Flexor	43	10	14	1	4	14
Extensor	8	4	1	1	0	2
Flaccid	87	17	20	3	17	30
Lower limb						
Normal	47	38	0	2	0	7
Flexor	11	4	1	0	1	5
Extensor	45	15	5	9	3	13
Flaccid	54	15	4	4	7	24

Reprinted with permission from Gray, C., French, J., Bates, D. Motor recovery following acute stroke. Age Ageing. *1900; 19:179–184.*

for stroke patients over the age of 80 who are discharged to the home for up to 2 years.[37] Longitudinal studies are needed to determine the long-term effects of rehabilitation. Older patients can improve on a stroke rehabilitation program if it is properly applied. Evaluation and treatment techniques for the older patient will be described next.

Evaluation

Several models for evaluating stroke patients can be used. As mentioned in the Parkinson's disease section, Schenkman focuses on impairments and direct and indirect effects of the disease as well as on functional disability.[38] This model stresses that there are certain areas where physical therapy will be more beneficial.

Other authors have developed extensive forms and methods of evaluating stroke patients, and one interesting model developed by Tripp divides assessment into the following areas:[39]

1. Motor neuron response: Evaluates tone in terms of spasticity and ability to activate and relax muscle, with associated reactions.
2. Fractionated movement: Evaluates the ability of the patient to move individual limb segments.
3. Movement consistency: Evaluates whether or not the patient's ability to perform gross motor activities is consistent with his or her ability to form isolated movements.
4. Mental status: Looks at ability to follow commands and ability to learn safety and judgment.

5. Functional assessment: Includes mobility and gross upper extremity function.[39]

Two excellent functional assesment tools for older pateints that have suffered a stroke are the Frenchay Activities Index and the Rivermead ADL Scale.[40,41] The Rivermead was specifically designed for older patients. See Figure 12.5 for the explanation of the Frenchay Activities Index (FAI) and Figure 12.6 for the Frenchay tool. See Figure 12.7 for the Rivermead ADL Scale explanation and Figure 12.8 for the Rivermead tool.

Carr and Shepherd Evaluation. Carr and Shepherd,[42] physical therapists from Australia, have a different way of analyzing patients who have sustained strokes. These therapists have developed an entire strategy based on motor relearning. Their strategy is to eliminate unnecessary movements and to better organize the movement patterns. It is important to understand this principle when looking at their evaluation strategies. In evaluating upper limb function, for instance, instead of grading the function in terms of synergies or range-of-motion deficits, this approach outlines common problems and compensatory strategies. For example, in the arm, common problems are (1) poor scapular movement and persistent depression of the shoulder girdle; (2) poor muscular control of the glenohumeral joint caused by a lack of abduction, flexion, and inability to sustain position; and (3) excessive and unnecessary elbow flexion, internal rotation, shoulder, and forearm supination.

In looking at the hand, this approach would consider the following dysfunctional movement patterns:

The Frenchay Activities Index (FAI)

Population: Stroke patients.

Description: The Frenchay Activities Index (FAI) was developed to measure the disability and handicap in stroke patients. The FAI includes 15 items, regarding an activity that requires the patient to make decisions and organize both inside and outside of the home. The FAI measures activities that reflect both independence and social survival.

Mode of Administration: The FAI can be completed either by the clinician through an interview or it can be filled out by the patient.

Scoring:

Time to Complete: 5 minutes.

Time to Score: 5 minutes.

Scoring: Each individual section of the index includes a scoring code. The sum of the scores for all 15 items is the total score for the FAI. The scores can range from 15 to 60. Three subscale scores can also be derived for domestic, leisure/work, and outdoors.

Interpretation: Higher scores on the FAI reflect more independence by the patient.

Reliability: Internal consistency was measured by Cronbach's alpha indicating homogeneity in the FAI. Reliability coefficients met the standards for sufficient correlation for both the total FAI and its three subscales. Reliability improved when items 14 and 15 were deleted from the index and when two subscale scores were created; domestic and outdoor activities.

Validity: Construct validity was established by measuring correlations between the FAI, Sickness Impact Profile, and the Barthel Index. There was a substantial convergent relationship between the FAI total scores, the Barthel Index disability scores, and the subscales of household activities and physical functioning in the Sickness Impact Profile.

Discriminant validity was established by the low correlations between the subscales of emotional behavior and alertness and the FAI.

Figure 12.5

(Reprinted with permission from Schuling, J., de Haan, R., Limburg, M., Groenier, K.H. The Frenchay Activities Index: 2. Assessment of functional status in stroke patients. *Stroke.* 1993; 24(8):1173–1177.)

1. Difficulty in grasping;
2. Difficulty in extending and flexing metacarpal phalangeal joints;
3. Difficulty with abduction and rotation of the thumb;
4. Difficulty cupping the hand;
5. Inability to hold different objects while moving the arm;
6. Tendency to pronate the forearm;
7. Excessive extension of the fingers and thumbs;
8. Inability to release objects;
9. Difficulty with abduction and rotation with the thumb in order to grasp.

During assessment the therapist would look at these deficits, identify them, and treat them.

Carr and Shepherd's method[42] of assessing lower extremity and trunk deficits is to describe them in terms of functional tasks, such as walking, balance, standing, standing from sitting, and sitting over the edge of the bed. In an analysis of sitting over the side of the bed, Carr and Shepherd identified two common problems: (1) flexion of the hip and knee on the affected side; and (2) flexion of the shoulder and protraction of the shoulder girdle, which results in the patient's inability to use the appropriate body mechanics to get out of bed.

This analysis can then be easily transferred to the appropriate treatment strategies for working with these patients. More specific evaluative and treatment information is available in Carr and Shepherd's *A Motor Re-Learning Programme for Stroke.*[42] In a subsequent section of this chapter, a specific form developed by Carr and Shepherd will be examined that goes over some of these points.[42]

In evaluating strength deficits, several studies have made a comparison between extension and torque in the knees, as well as various other joints of the body, and it can be a reliable and valid measure in stroke patients. Therefore, therapists can use manual muscle tests or dynamometry readings to assess strength in their elderly patients with a stroke.[43–45]

Olney and Colbourne's Gait Assessment. Another consideration that is extremely important in the area of stroke is

The Frenchay Activities Index

Item	Code
In the last 3 months:	
1. Preparing main meals	1 = Never
	2 = < 1 time per week
2. Washing up	3 = 1–2 times per week
	4 = most days
3. Washing clothes	1 = Never
	2 = 1–2 times in 3 months
4. Light housework	3 = 3–12 times in 3 months
	4 = ≥ 1 time per week
5. Heavy housework	
6. Local shopping	
7. Social outings	
8. Walking outside > 5 minutes	
9. Actively pursuing hobby	
10. Driving car/bus travel	
In the last 6 months:	
11. Outings/car rides	1 = Never
	2 = 1–2 times in 6 months
	3 = 3–12 times in 6 months
	4 = ≥ 1 time per week
12. Gardening	1 = Never
	2 = Light
13. Household/car maintenance	3 = Moderate
	4 = All necessary
14. Reading books	1 = None
	2 = 1 in 6 months
	3 = <1 in 2 weeks
	4 = >1 in 2 weeks
15. Gainful work	1 = None
	2 = <10 hours/week
	3 = 10–30 hours/week
	4 = >30 hours/week

Figure 12.6
(Reprinted with Permission. Schuling, J., de Haan, R., Limburg, M., Groenier, K. The Frenchay Activities Index: Assessment of functional status in stroke patients. *Stroke.* Vol. 24, No. 8. August 1993. © American Heart Association.)

the analysis of gait. In a particularly valuable journal article, Olney and Colbourn describe some of the deficits in gait and discuss methods of treating the gait problem. They also divide the gait pattern into phases. The first phase, "late swing to foot flat," identifies three problems for stroke patients: (1) inability to attain full hip flexion during swing, (2) inability to extend the knee fully, and (3) inability to activate ankle dorsiflexor muscles. In addition, stroke patients may hyperextend the knee to avoid the problem of instability.

The next phase of gait that presents problems is "foot flat to heel off." Problems noted here are the decreased use of hip extensor muscles, limited hip extension motion, and that ankle plantar flexors contract inappropriately.

The next phase, "push off, pull off in early swing," causes residual weakness of ankle plantar flexors and hip flexors. It also results in the stance phase of the affected side being longer than normal, and the body's weight being transferred to the lower limb through push off.[46]

An excellent clinical tool for assessing gait in older patients with stroke is the Wisconsin Gait Scale. See Figure 12.9 for the instructions and the tool.[47]

Rivermead ADL Scale (Revised)

Population: Adult stroke patients, elderly

Description: The Rivermead ADL scale was designed to assess the activities of daily living for stroke
                           patients. One advantage of this scale is that the total score reflects not only the level of dis-
                           ability but also the problem areas. The revised ADL may be used either for inpatient ther-
                           apy or after discharge.

Mode of Administration: This is a task performance exam.

Completion:

   Time to Complete: 30 to 60 minutes

   Time to Score: Scoring is completed while test is administered.

   Scoring: Independent item scores are assigned as follows:
                           1 independent
                           0v patient requires verbal assistance
                           0 dependent.
                           The scores for each section are then added to achieve a total score.

Interpretation: The higher the total score the more independent the patient is.

Reliability: not reported

Validity: Validity of the Rivermead ADL Scale was established through Guttman scaling. In a study
                           of 150 stroke patients, of which 103 were over the age of 65, the self care section was
                           proven to be valid. Problems arose in the test on the Household section primarily because
                           of where the patients resided.

Figure 12.7
(Reprinted with permission from Lincoln, N.B., Edmans, J.A. A re-validation of the Rivermead ADL Scale for Elderly Patients
with Stroke. *Age and Ageing.* 1990; 19:19–24.)

Pusher Syndrome Assessment. Common findings of sensory deficits on the hemi side of a patient with Pusher syndrome are hemianopsia, problems with proprioception, and somatosensory deficits which contribute to postural inattention and difficulties with postural adjustments.[48] Perceptual dysfunction includes unilateral neglect and agnosia. Cognitive function is usually decreased with significant memory impairments, impulsivity with decreased attention (typical of left hemiplegia), lack of insight or understanding of problems, and apraxia.

Motor function in Pusher syndrome includes overuse of extension on the sound side with ipsilateral pushing and predominance of a flexion synergy pattern in the affected lower extremity.[30,31,48] Posturally, the head and trunk are held toward the hemi side with increased weight bearing on the involved side and shifting of the trunk away from the sound side. The patient's balance is severely disturbed with an inability to find a midline orientation. In fact, the patient resists all attempts to assist in centering of the center of motion within the base of support. The patient pushes back strongly when weight transfer is attempted.

Typically, the individual shows no concern or fear of falling and does not automatically compensate for loss of balance with adjustments to support body weight. During the stance phase of gait, the patient demonstrates inadequate extension of the involved leg. During stepping, the patient is unable to transfer the weight efficiently onto the sound limb, and the hemi leg typically adducts strongly during swing (scissors).[30–32,48] Functional assessment reveals profound difficulties with sit to stand and transfers. The patient is often unable to stand without assistance.

Motor Assessment Scale. Specific compacted tests for the assessment of stroke patients are somewhat difficult to find, but they do exist. Carr and Shepherd have developed the Motor Assessment Scale in Figure 12.10A. All items on the form are constructed so that a score of 6 indicates optimal motor behavior. The criteria for scoring are listed in Figure 12.10B. These particular criteria are self-explanatory and give the examiner a 6-point scale from which to assess the patient and show improvement in a very simple form.[49]

When evaluating a stroke patient, it is important to choose the tools that will appropriately reflect the patient's status and the methods to be used in the evaluation treatment progression. Several different types of tools have been provided and will be considered next.

ADL Assessment: Instructions
All aids supplied or recommended to be stated on the form. Decide where to start. If patient can do that item, go back three to make sure patient can do these as well, and forward three until three consecutive failures—then stop. This applies to each section. Instructions should be strictly followed.

Self care
Drinking. A full cup of hot liquid, not spilling more than one eighth of the contents.
Comb hair. To be presentable on completion.
Wash face and hands. At basin (not with bowl), including putting in plug and managing taps and patient drying self (all materials to hand).
Make up or shave. Shaving to be done by patient's preferred method.
Clean teeth. Unscrewing toothpaste–putting toothpaste on brush. Managing tap.
Eating. A slice of cheese on toast eaten with knife and fork (this was chosen as being reasonably tough to cut and an easy snack to prepare).
Undress. Dressing gown, pajamas, socks and shoes to be taken off.
Bed to chair. From lying covered, to chair with arms within reach.
Lavatory. Mobility to WC (less than 10 metres). To include managing pants and trousers, cleaning self and transferring.
Indoor mobility. Moving from one room to another—turns must be to left. Distance of 10 metres.
Dressing. Does not involve fetching clothes. Clothes to be within reach in a pile but not in any specific order. All essential fastenings to be done up by patient.
Wash in bath. Showing movements, i.e. ability to wash all over. Ability to manage taps and plugs.
Overall wash. Not in bath—at basin (not with bowl). Patient must be able to wash good arm, stand up, and touch toes from sitting, in order to be able to wash overall.
Outdoor mobility. To cover a distance of 50 metres and to include going up a ramp and through a door.
Floor and chair. From lying, to upholstered chair without arms, seat 15 in high.
In and out of bath. A dry bath.

Household
Cope with money. Match coins to packet of sugar, cornflakes and margarine. Ask for change of 34p from 50p (16p); 72.5p from £ 1 (27.5p); £ 3.21 from £ 5 (£ 1.79p).
Preparation of hot drink. Fill electric kettle, everything to be ready on working surface.
Washing. Handwash smalls at sink.
Get in and out of car. Front seat of any car except sports model.
Preparation of snack. Making a sandwich—materials to be easily reached. Washing and clearing work surface to be done afterwards.
Light cleaning. Cleaning and tidying surfaces—height 13–37 in.
Preparation of a meal. Peel a potato, fry sausage. Frozen vegetable from fridge. Open tin.
Bedmaking. Putting on sheet and blanket, straightening and tucking in. Bed 21 inches high.
Ironing. Not with steam iron. Organize ironing surface (board or table).
Carry shopping. 1/2 lb butter, 14 oz tin and money.
Hang out washing. On rail indoors, away from sink, no pegs.
Crossing roads. Cross at traffic lights with kerbs—no pedestrian crossing.
Transport self to shop and back—distance of 1/2 mile.
Public transport. Travel on bus (not Park and Ride). Distance at least 1 mile with minimum three stops before destination.
Heavy cleaning. Vacuum, sweep and dustpan/brush in 11 ft square room, moving dining-room chairs only.

Scoring   1 Independent, with or without aid. All aids should be listed on each page of form.
          0v Verbal assistance only.
          0 Dependent (if not assessable, if patient medically unfit, if not safe to try, or too soon to try, if time taken is beyond practical bounds).

Figure 12.8
(Reprinted with permission from Lincoln, N.B., Edmans, J.A. A Re-validation of the Rivermead ADL Scale for elderly patients with stroke. *Age and Ageing.* 1990; 19:19–24.)

Wisconsin Gait Scale (WGS)

Population:	Patients with chronic hemiplegia.
Description:	The Wisconsin Gait Scale (WGS) consists of 14 observable variables measuring clinically relevant components of gait.
Mode of Administration:	The clinician observes the subject walking toward and away from the clinician and from side to side.

Scoring:

Time to Complete:	5 minutes
Time to Score:	Included in time to complete.
Scoring:	Scores for each item are included on the test. Individual items are totaled for an overall score. Items 1 and 4 are weighted by 3/5 and 3/4, respectively, before adding them to the overall score.
Interpretation:	A lower score indicates better gait than a higher score.
Reliability:	Total score ratings were found to be highly consistent. Among the subjects tested for rater consistency, the largest deviation from the mean of 4 gait ratings, was 26% of that subject's mean total score. Total scores for each of the raters did not differ significantly from each other before or after gait training.
Validity:	The average WGS score improved significantly after gait training. Statistically significant differences were found between pretraining and posttraining mean scores $p < .05$ for stance time, step length, hip extension, stance width, and weight shift. In addition, pretraining WGS scores were significantly associated with the ratings on the Physical Functioning Scale of the Health Status Questionnaire (HSQ). Thus, lending validity to the WGS in that WGS ratings were significantly associated with the subject's own appraisal of the physical limitation of the stroke more than 1 year later.

Gait Assessment Scale Documentation

Observe subject walking toward and away from observer, and from the side.

Stance Phase Affected Leg

1.) Use of a hand held gait aid
   1 = No gait aid
   2 = Minimal gait aid used — Gait aid used optionally with minimal weight transferred on to it, narrow base of support.
   3 = Minimal gait aid, wide base — Gait aid used minimally, may rock the legs of a quad cane as weight transfers forward. Distance between unaffected foot to cane is greater than distance between affected and unaffected foot (wide support base).
   4 = Marked use — Weight through the aid, narrow base of support.
   5 = Marked use, wide base — Transfers weight through the aid, wide support base.

2.) Stance time on impaired side
   1 = Equal — An equal amount of time is spent on the affected leg compared to the unaffected leg during the single leg stance.
   2 = Unequal — The subject remains on the affected leg for a shorter period of time compared to the unaffected leg during single leg stance.
   3 = Very brief — The subject spends the least amount of time on the affected leg necessary to accomplish advancing the unaffected leg.

3.) Step length of unaffected side
   1 = Step through — The heel of the unaffected foot clearly advances beyond the toe of the affected foot.
   2 = Foot does not clear — The heel of the unaffected foot does not advance beyond the toe of the affected foot.
   3 = Step to — The unaffected foot is placed behind or up to, but not beyond the affected foot.

Figure 12.9

4.) Weight shift to the affected side, with or without a gait aid.

1 = Full shift	The subject's head and trunk shift laterally over the affected foot during single stance.
2 = Decreased shift	The subject's head and trunk crosses midline, but not over the affected foot.
3 = Very limited shift	The subject's head and trunk does not cross midline, minimal weight shift in the direction of the affected side.

5.) Stance width (measure distance between feet prior to toe off of affected foot)

1 = Normal	Up to one shoe width between feet.
2 = Moderate	Up to two shoe widths between feet.
3 = Wide	Greater than two shoe widths between feet.

Toe Off Affected Leg

6.) Guardedness (pause prior to advancing affected foot)

1 = None	Good forward momentum with no hesitancy noted.
2 = Slight	Slight pause prior to toe off.
3 = Marked hesitation	Subject pauses prior to toe off

7.) Hip extension of affected side (observe gluteal crease from behind subject)

1 = Equal extension	Hips equally extend during push off. Maintains erect posture during toe off.
2 = Slight flexion	Hips extend at least to neutral, but less than unaffected side.
3 = Marked flexion	Forward trunk and hip flexion at toe off.

Swing Phase Affected Leg

8.) External rotation during initial swing

1 = Same as unimpaired leg	
2 = Increased rotation	Externally rotates the leg <45°, but more than the uninvolved side.
3 = Marked	Externally rotates the leg >45°.

9.) Circumduction at mid swing (observe path of affected heel)

1 = None	Affected foot adducts no more than unaffected foot during swing.
2 = Moderate	Affected foot adducts up to one shoe width during swing.
3 = Marked	Affected foot circumducts more than one shoe width during swing.

10.) Hip hiking at mid swing

1 = None	Pelvis slightly dips during swing.
2 = Elevation	Pelvis is elevated during swing phase.
3 = Vaults	Little true hip flexion, subject contracts lateral trunk muscles and elevates hip during swing.

11.) Knee flexion from toe off to mid swing

1 = Normal	Affected knee flexes equally to unaffected side.
2 = Some	Affected knee flexes, but less than unaffected knee flexion.
3 = Minimal	Minimal flexion noted in affected knee (flexion barely seen).
4 = None	Knee remains in extension throughout swing.

12.) Toe Clearance

1 = Normal	Toe clears the floor throughout swing.
2 = Slight drag	Toe drags slightly during beginning of swing phase.
3 = Marked	Toe drags during the majority of the swing.

13.) Pelvic rotation at terminal swing

1 = Forward	The pelvis is rotated forward to prepare for heel strike.
2 = Neutral	Posture is erect with pelvis in neutral position.
3 = Retracted	Pelvis has marked lag behind the unaffected pelvis.

Heel Strike Affected Leg

14.) Initial foot contact

1 = Heel strike	Heel makes initial contact with the floor.
2 = Foot flat	Foot lands with weight distributed over entire foot.
3 = No contact of heel	Foot lands on lateral border of the foot or toes.

Figure 12.9   (Continued)

*Items 1 and 4 are weighted by 3/5 and 3/4, respectively, before adding individual items for a total score.

Reprinted with permission from Rodriquez, A., Black, P., Kile, K., Sherman, J., Stellberg, B., McCormick, J., Roszkowski, J., Swiggum, E. Gait training efficacy using a home-based practice model in chronic hemiplegia. *Arch Phys Med Rehabil.* August 1996; 77.

MOTOR ASSESSMENT SCALE

NAME _____

MOVEMENT SCORING SHEET

DATE	0	1	2	3	4	5	6
1. SUPINE TO SIDE LYING							
2. SUPINE TO SITTING OVER SIDE OF BED							
3. BALANCED SITTING							
4. SITTING TO STANDING							
5. WALKING							
6. UPPER-ARM FUNCTION							
7. HAND MOVEMENTS							
8. ADVANCED HAND ACTIVITIES							
9. GENERAL TONUS							

COMMENTS (IF APPLICABLE)

Figure 12.10A
Reprinted with Permission Carr, J., Shepherd, R., et al. "Investigation of a New Motor Assessment Scale for Stroke Patients." *Physical Therapy*, Vol. 65, #2, Feb. 1985.

Criteria for Scoring

1. Supine to Side Lying onto Intact Side

1. Pulls himself into side lying. (Starting position must be supine lying, not knees flexed. Patient pulls himself into side lying with intact arm, moves affected leg with intact leg.)
2. Moves leg across actively and the lower half of the body follows. (Starting position as above. Arm is left behind.)
3. Arm is lifted across body with other arm. Leg is moved actively and body follows in a block. (Starting position as above.)
4. Moves arm across body actively and the rest of the body follows in a block. (Starting position as above.)
5. Moves arm and leg and rolls to side but overbalances. (Starting position as above. Shoulder protracts and arm flexes forward.)
6. Rolls to side in 3 seconds. (Starting position as above. Must not use hands.)

2. Supine to Sitting over Side of Bed

1. Side lying, lifts head sideways but cannot sit up. (Patient assisted to side lying.)
2. Side lying, to sitting over side of bed. (Therapist assists patient with movement. Patient controls head position throughout.)
3. Side lying to sitting over side of bed. (Therapist gives stand-by help [see Appendix 2] by assisting legs over side of bed.)
4. Side lying to sitting over side of bed. (With no stand-by help.)
5. Supine to sitting over side of bed. (With no stand-by help.)
6. Supine to sitting over side of bed within 10 seconds. (With no stand-by help.)

3. Balanced Sitting

1. Sits only with support. (Therapist should assist patient into sitting.)
2. Sits unsupported for 10 seconds. (Without holding on, knees and feet together, feet can be supported on floor.)
3. Sits unsupported with weight well forward and evenly distributed. (Weight should be well forward at the hips, head and thoracic spine extended, weight evenly distributed on both sides.)
4. Sits unsupported, turns head and trunk to look behind. (Feet supported and together on floor. Do not allow legs to abduct or feet to move. Have hands resting on thighs, do not allow hands to move onto plinth.)
5. Sits unsupported, reaches forward to touch floor, and returns to starting position. (Feet supported on floor. Do not allow patient to hold on. Do not allow legs and feet to move, support affected arm if necessary. Hand must touch floor at least 10 cm [4 in] in front of feet.)
6. Sits on stool unsupported, reaches sideways to touch floor, and returns to starting position. (Feet supported on floor. Do not allow patient to hold on. Do not allow legs and feet to move, support affected arm if necessary. Patient must reach sideways not forward.)

4. Sitting to Standing

1. Getting to standing with help form therapist. (Any method.)
2. Gets to standing with stand-by help. (Weight unevenly distributed, uses hands for support.)
3. Gets to standing. (Do not allow uneven weight distribution or help form hands.)
4. Gets to standing and stands for 5 seconds with hips and knees extended. (Do not allow uneven weight distribution.)
5. Sitting to standing to sitting with no stand-by help. (Do not allow uneven weight distribution. Full extension of hips and knees.)
6. Sitting to standing to sitting with no stand-by help three times in 10 seconds. (Do not allow uneven weight distribution.)

5. Walking

1. Stands on affected leg and steps forward with other leg. (Weight-bearing hip must be extended. Therapist may give stand-by help.)
2. Walks with stand-by help from one person.
3. Walks 3 m (10 ft) alone or uses any aid but no stand-by help.
4. Walks 5 m (16 ft) with no aid in 15 seconds.
5. Walks 10 m (33 ft) with no aid, turns around, picks up a small sandbag from floor, and walks back in 25 seconds. (May use either hand.)

6. Walks up and down four steps with or without an aid but without holding on to the rail three times in 35 seconds.

6. Upper-Arm Function

1. Lying, protract shoulder girdle with arm in elevation. (Therapist places arm in position and supports it with elbow in extension.)
2. Lying, hold extended arm in elevation for 2 seconds. (Physical therapist should place arm in position and patient must maintain position with some external rotation. Elbow must be held within 20° of full extension.)
3. Flexion and extension of elbow to take palm to forehead with arm as in 2. (Therapist may assist supination of forearm.)
4. Sitting, hold extended arm in forward flexion at 90 degrees to body for 2 seconds. (Therapist should place arm in position and patient must maintain position with some external rotation and elbow extension. Do not allow excess shoulder elevation.)
5. Sitting, patient lifts arm to above position, holds it there for 10 seconds, and then lowers it. (Patient must maintain position with some external rotation. Do not allow pronation.)
6. Standing, hand against wall. Maintain arm position while turning body toward wall. (Have arm abducted to 90° with palm flat against the wall.)

7. Hand Movements

1. Sitting, extension of wrist. (Therapist should have patient sitting at a table with forearm resting on table. Therapist places cylindrical object in palm of patient's hand. Patient is asked to lift object off the table by extending the wrist. Do not allow elbow flexion.)
2. Sitting, radial deviation of wrist. (Therapist should place forearm in midpronation-supination. ie, resting on ulnar side, thumb in line with forearm and wrist in extension, fingers around a cylindrical object. Patient is asked to lift hand off table. Do not allow elbow flexion or pronation.)
3. Sitting, elbow into side, pronation and supination. (Elbow unsupported and at a right angle. Three-quarter range is acceptable.)
4. Reach forward, pick up large ball of 14-cm (5-in) diameter with both hands and put it down. (Ball should be on table so far in front of patient that he has to extend arms fully to reach it. Shoulders must be protracted, elbows extended, wrist neutral or extended. Palms should be kept in contact with the ball.)
5. Pick up a polystyrene cup from table and put it on table across other side of body. (Do not allow alteration in shape of cup.)
6. Continuous opposition of thumb and each finger more than 14 times in 10 seconds. (Each finger in turn taps the thumb, starting with index finger. Do not allow thumb to slide from one finger to the other, or to go backwards.)

8. Advanced Hand Activities

1. Picking up the top of a pen and putting it down again. (Patient stretches arm forward, picks up pen top, releases it on table close to body.)
2. Picking up one jelly bean from a cup and placing it in another cup. (Teacup contains eight jellybeans. Both cups must be at arms' length. Left hand takes jellybean from cup on right and releases it in cup on left.)
3. Drawing horizontal lines to stop at a vertical line 10 times in 20 seconds. (At least five lines must touch and stop at the vertical line.)
4. Holding a pencil, making rapid consecutive dots on a sheet of paper. (Patient must do at least 2 dots a second for 5 seconds. Patient picks pencil up and positions it without assistance. Patient must hold pen as for writing. Patient must make a dot not a stroke.)
5. Taking a dessert spoon of liquid to the mouth. (Do not allow head to lower towards spoon. Do not allow liquid to spill.)
6. Holding a comb and combing hair at back of head.

9. General Tonus

1. Flaccid, limp, no resistance when body parts are handled.
2. Some response felt as body parts are moved.
3. Variable, sometimes flaccid, sometimes good tone, sometimes hypertonic.
4. Consistently normal response.
5. Hypertonic 50 percent of the time.
6. Hypertonic at all times.

Figure 12.10B
Reprinted with Permission Carr, J., Shepherd, R., et al. "Investigation of a New Motor Assessment Scale for Stroke Patients." *Physical Therapy*, Vol. 65, #2, Feb. 1985.

Treatment Interventions

There are a number of treatment techniques commonly used by physical therapists ranging from the classic therapeutic exercise to the proprioceptive neuromuscular facilitation (PNF) to the Bobath and Brunnstrom techniques. A brief discussion of Carr and Shepherd's work will follow in the next section. Treatment considerations for gait will also be discussed, as will research on various types of ancillary modalities that can be used for the treatment of stroke deficits.

Carr and Shepherd's Approach. Their treatment revolves around five principles:[49]

1. Elimination of unnecessary muscle activity.
2. Any human activity becomes better organized and more effective when it is practiced.
3. A muscle response depends on the condition of the muscle at the moment with the following perimeters: length, velocity, temperature, and joint ankle.
4. The body must have the ability to adjust to gravity and change segmental alignment for all motor activities. Therefore, the person must be trained to preserve balance.
5. A learned task is not just doing the task in front of a therapist. A learned task is when a person can do it in a situation without actually thinking.

In their treatment approach, Carr and Shepherd go through four steps: (1) analyze the task, (2) practice the missing component, (3) practice the task as a whole, and (4) transference of training.

An example of this would be a patient who has difficulty standing. First, analyze the difficulty (e.g., hip position). Second, practice the missing component. For instance, the difficulty in standing comes from the patient's hip position (i.e., work with the hip). Third, practice this task (i.e., standing with proper hip position). Fourth, transfer to another activity with the same problem (i.e., standing in the proper position with a slight bend on a stool or a wedge under the foot).[49]

During treatment, motor tasks are practiced in their entirety. There is no "technique"; the person is just instructed and manually guided through various deficits. The patient may first be passively placed in the proper position, and then the patient takes over active control. As the patient develops more control, the therapist does less.

The most important component of Carr and Shepherd's approach is the patient's contribution to the effort. Patients are encouraged to do the exercises as often as possible and to keep a notebook of their efforts and responses. In the notebook, the patients are encouraged to write down their actual program progression.[49]

Shoulder Problems in Hemiplegia. Shoulder pain in hemiplegia has always been a concern and several clini-

cians have suggested that excessive distraction on the shoulder may lead to pain.[28,40,49]

In an article by Kumar and associates,[50] the use of overhead pulleys is described as the highest risk of developing shoulder pain for patients with hemiplegia, and it was suggested that this should be strongly discouraged with these patients.[50] In training upper extremity problems, it is preferred to provide increased weight training through the upper extremity, as well as facilitating proper positioning.[40,49]

Bohannon and associates[51] found that it is not necessarily the position that explained the "synergistic" increased force of the elbow strength, but possibly the length of the muscle in various positions. Therefore, in working with the upper extremity, it is important to look not only at the neurological factors, such as tone, but also at the length-to-tension relationship of the muscles. Therapists should facilitate range of motion and proper posture, as well as encourage weight bearing through the upper extremity in the proper position.

Gait Treatment Suggestions. The upright control evaluation mentioned earlier differentiated different gait variations. In addition, in the same study from Rancho Los Amigos, the authors outlined a specific program for lower extremity problems.[47] Their treatment techniques revolve around the use of ankle-foot orthotics with various types of dorsiflexion stops, as well as electrical stimulation to the weak areas. For example, if a therapist notices stance deviation of inadequate hip and knee extension, he or she can suggest ankle-foot orthotics with dorsiflexion stops and electrical stimulation to the quadriceps or gluteus maximus for strengthening and facilitation. Inhibitive casting is used for excessive plantarflexion or with increased tone. Prolonged icing is suggested to inhibit tone. The treatment approach is to divide the various phases of gait and treat each separately according to deficit.

Treatment of gait disturbances in the patient with Pusher syndrome requires intact cognition and active patient participation. The focus needs to be on early resumption of upright postures (sitting and standing), transitional movements (supine to sit and sit to stand), and a concentration on active movements (guided or assisted). The goal is basically to "recalibrate" the patient's perception of upright posture by providing him or her with feedback about movement outcomes and positional correctness. Maximizing tactile and proprioceptive inputs facilitates correct muscle contraction. Emphasizing stability during early standing with biofeedback for regaining a symmetrical and stable midline position can be accomplished through physical and verbal cues.[52]

In the area of gait, it appears that weight shifting is one of the biggest problems. Patients must be taught the concept of proper weight shifting, which can be done using bicycle ergonometry or EMG for proper muscle use.[51,53]

Despite the various techniques suggested for stroke intervention (ranging from therapeutic exercise to biofeedback), the therapist must be careful to check the efficacy of the various treatment programs.[54] For example, Sackley[55] showed that symmetry and weight shifting strongly correlated with motor function. These components appear to be very important and should be treated vigorously with weight-shifting exercises. In contrast, Trueblood and coworkers[56] showed that pelvic positioning exercises were helpful while the patient did the exercise. However, after the exercise session, stroke patients did not carry the pelvic position into daily activities.[56]

Finally, Logigian and associates[57] showed that both facilitation and traditional exercise improved functional and motor performances and that there was no difference between the two exercises.[57] This study provides food for thought, especially for those working with the geriatric patient. Finding the most appropriate program, working within the patient's tolerance, and reviewing the results that accompany the treatment progression are extremely important for achieving the optimal outcomes.

See Appendix 2 for evidence-based treatment ideas.

ALZHEIMER'S DISEASE

A concise discussion of the incidence and etiology of Alzheimer's disease (AD) is provided in Chapter 5. This discussion focuses on evaluation, staging, and intervention in patients with AD. The challenge for the geriatric rehabilitation therapist working with AD patients is to apply creative solutions to the problem of finding activities that maintain physical health. Keeping these individuals active enough to generate fitness benefits should be the primary goal of intervention in this population. Avoiding restraints is crucial. While this patient population may appear physically healthy, they are susceptible to falls and other accidents resulting in orthopaedic and other types of injuries. The clinical features of patients with AD are a gradual but relentless onset of symptoms including impairment of recent memory, disorientation, confabulations, and retrogressive loss of remote memories.[58] Over time, reasoning ability, concentration, speech, and handwriting degenerate. In the early phases of the disease motor function is well maintained; however, as the disease progresses neurological involvement often renders the AD patient bedridden. In late stages, patients can deteriorate to a nonfunctional, vegetative state.

Alzheimer's disease is generally staged based on the progression of the disease. Various staging strategies are used, employing as few as three stages and as many as twelve stages, depending on the setting.[59] This therapist uses a four-stage progression scale, which is provided in Table 12.8. This staging breaks the disease into early, middle, late, and terminal stages based on symptomatology. Staging allows the health care team to quantify changes in functional and cognitive abilities over time, which helps in establishing a patient's treatment plan. It must be noted, however, that from an outcomes viewpoint, it is unclear whether AD patients do in fact pass through a specific sequence of deterioration. It is unlikely that the "staging" of

a patient has any prognostic implications in terms of speed of decline. Staging basically captures a moment in time; that is, the point at which the initial and subsequent evaluations occurred. Nevertheless, there is considerable practical utility in developing some formulation of the patient's current functional status since this directly influences decisions for management.

Six different, although overlapping, functional spheres are affected and need to be evaluated in the AD patient. (1) Cognitive or intellectual disturbance is the clinical hallmark of Alzheimer's dementia. This includes symptoms of

TABLE 12.8 Stages of Alzheimer's Disease

Stages	Signs and Symptoms
Early Stage (I)	Forgetfulness
	Mild memory deficit
	Difficulty with novel or complex tasks
	Apathy and social withdrawal
Middle Stage (II)	Moderate to severe objective memory deficit
	Disorientation to time and place
	Language disturbance
	Visuoconstructive difficulty
	Apraxia
	Personality and behavioral changes
	Requires supervision
Late Stage (III)	Intellectual functions virtually untestable
	Verbal communication severely limited
	Incapable of self-care
	Incontinence of bladder and bowel
Terminal Stage (IV)	Unaware of environment
	Mute
	Bedridden
	Joint contractures
	Pathological reflexes
	Myoclonus
Associated Coexisting Neurological Disorders	Increased tone
	Seizures
	Movement disorders
	Gait disorders

memory impairment, language disorder, apraxia, visuoconstructive difficulty, and problems with abstract thinking. Common symptoms such as getting lost, failure to recognize familiar faces, and certain types of hallucinations are also manifestations of cognitive disturbance. Tools for testing cognition are presented in Chapter 10. (2) Another important functional domain to assess is the noncognitive function. Changes in affect, personality, and behavior are extremely common, though this aspect of the syndrome is rarely evaluated in any formal manner. There are scales, such as the Blessed Performance of Everyday Activities[60] and the Alzheimer's Disease Assessment Scale,[61] which do measure features such as irritability, apathy, hyperactivity, and bothersomeness. Depression, anxiety, and delusions may be apparent on psychiatric assessment; however, noncognitive symptoms occur sporadically and do not necessarily coincide with the time of the examination. (3) Neurologic function is usually preserved through the early and middle stages of AD, although seizures, gait disorders, and tremors may occur at any time. In the later stages of the disease, neurologic signs include hyperactive reflexes, increasing primitive tone (gegenhalten), flexion contractures, and primitive reflexes. These are tested just as they are tested in neurologically impaired pediatric patients. (4) Activities of daily living (ADL) are affected by cognitive, noncognitive, and elementary neurologic changes. This is another important functional domain to explore in assessing the status of the patient with AD. Tools for assessing function are discussed in Chapter 10. (5) As patients gradually lose the ability to perform many ADL, there is a corresponding increase in their need for assistance. In addition to determining the availability of family members to assist with personal care, one must also probe caregivers' understanding of their patient's deficits and their physical and emotional capability to cope satisfactorily with them. (See Chapter 8.) (6) Finally, all diseases occur in a psychosocial context, and this aspect assumes special importance in Alzheimer's disease (see Chapter 4). Psychosocial evaluation provides objective data on the patient's social circumstances, as well as an impression of the patient's family and its structure, sociocultural beliefs, attitudes to health and disease, myths, patterns of communication, and degree of psychopathology, if any. Through assessment one can identify the situation and psychosocial stressors that impact on the patient and family, and define the coping strategies that they use to meet them, including their ability to seek out appropriate community resources.[62]

> For additional information on release signs and reflexes related to AD, see CD.

Treatment Interventions

Treatment in the AD patient is focused on maintaining the highest level of function. Although physical and occupational therapists don't treat the disease itself, when caring for an elderly patient who has Alzheimer's, caregivers can call on their knowledge, compassion, and understanding to help patients achieve rehabilitation goals, despite the challenges associated with this difficult disease. It is rarely indicated in the literature that physical therapy has a direct impact on the course of Alzheimer's; however, therapists can play a primary role in mitigating the disease's impact as a complicating factor throughout the rehabilitation process.

In the early stages of the disease, maintaining physical fitness and providing as much neurosensory stimulus as possible assists in improving functional capabilities and enhancing overall well-being. In addition to exercise, focus should be placed on good nutrition and minimizing the use of drugs, both prescribed and over-the-counter medications. Providing a structured, protected environment with warmth and emotional support is crucial. Maintenance of a familiar environment is helpful. For instance, if AD patients are admitted to a nursing home, having their own furniture moved into the facility often helps to improve patient responsiveness and connectedness with their surroundings (see Chapter 4).

Exercise should consist of functionally oriented activities. Walking, performing ADL, dancing, gardening, and the like can be activities that translate into physical fitness. This therapist has found that the use of T'ai Chi, which is similar to dance, is a wonderful means of stimulating a cardiovascular response and has the added benefits of promoting calm and relaxation. Though the use of calisthenic exercises may be employed, the exercise sessions need to be set in a calm environment (paying attention to noise and color—see Chapter 8) and instructions should be kept simple and accompanied by demonstration. Music (classical or new age) is often helpful in the background as it has a calming effect.

The use of a rocking chair also facilitates muscle contraction through reflexive activity. Sundowning, which is a phenomenon unique to the AD patient, is a syndrome characterized by restlessness, excitement, increased confusion, hallucinations, and agitation seen in the late afternoon or early evening in patients in the middle and late stages of Alzheimer's disease.[62]

A primary emphasis in treating the AD patient must be the prevention of falls. As with any aging patient, falls in people with AD are often precipitated by a number of intrinsic risk factors. Additionally, AD is associated with specific cognitive and systemic effects that place individuals at increased fall risk. Any significant loss of cognitive function can result in:

- Lack of understanding and awareness of their potential for falls;
- Need for assistance;
- Judgmental errors, inability to recognize dangers, and misperception of environmental hazards;
- Overestimation of capacity for safe mobility resulting in attempts to do things without assistance;

- Failing to remember limitations in ADL;
- Insistence on performing activities, such as getting out of bed or going to the bathroom without assistance because of forgetfulness or failure to understand the intervention (such as the use of bed rails);
- Inability to ask for assistance with mobility because of communication problems, such as word finding or aphasia;
- Refusing or forgetting to use assistive devices (canes, walkers, grab rails) when indicated;
- Inability to understand the correct use of assistive devices (Note: the authors of this book avoid using assistive devices whenever possible due to the inherent dangers);
- Behavioral manifestation such as wandering, pacing, agitation, restlessness, disorientation, hallucinations, delusions, irritability, and anxiety, which can result in attention deficits and worsening cognition;
- Sundowning—disruptive behaviors that appear during the late afternoon or evening (associated with dusk and darkness).

With respect to visual performance, AD is associated with an excess of dysfunction that is beyond what would be expected on the basis of age or underlying disease as discussed above. Significant visual problems that may lead to falls in the AD patient include:

- Restriction of visual fields (loss of peripheral vision; homonymous hemianopia);
- Decrease in visuospatial function (ability to match and integrate the position of self and objects in the environment);
- Decline in depth perception (ability to judge distances and relationship among objects in the visual field);
- Loss of contrast sensitivity (ability to perceive colors and dark from light);
- Agnosia (decreased recognition of familiar objects and places).

Last, numerous gait and balance abnormalities are associated with AD and include:

- Apraxia (inability to perform routine motor tasks);
- Loss of proprioception (awareness of posture, movement, and changes in equilibrium)—
  - Decreased stride length;
  - Decreased step height, shuffling;
  - Decreased speed of walking with bradykinesia and latent balance reactions;
- Cautious gait. Alzheimer's patients have a classic gait pattern generally characterized by a wide base of support, flexed posture, and short, shuffling steps that are especially prominent when turning. They can be uncertain of their step or foot placement, and may hold arms tightly to their sides or crossed in front of them without arm swing (appears in early stages of AD).
- Frontal lobe gait disorder characterized by a wide base of support, slightly flexed posture, and small, shuffling, hesitant steps (appears in late stages of AD);
- Gait initiation failure characterized by a delay during the first few steps of walking; as a result, the body sometimes moves forward before the feet start to move, placing individuals at risk for balance loss;
- Motor impersistence in which normally automatic motions (e.g., left foot–right foot alternating foot pattern) are frozen or abruptly stopped;
- Motor incoordination in which normally automatic motions such as alternating foot pattern are disrupted, so that patient takes two or three steps with the right foot without moving the left (may be completely thrown off center of gravity);
- Disequilibrium failure—characterized by an inability to maintain stability during postural challenges, such as standing on one foot or stepping over obstacles in the path.

While these factors by themselves increase fall susceptibility, their relationship to the likelihood of falling is more accurately reflected by their effects on mobility—the ability of the AD person to ambulate and transfer independently and safely in the living environment.

The risk of fall-related injury in AD is dependent on several intrinsic and extrinsic factors operating simultaneously. For example, the risk of sustaining a hip fracture is enhanced by the presence of poor vision, neuromuscular diseases resulting in a loss of protective reflexes, difficulty rising from a chair, osteoporosis, decreased adipose tissue surrounding the hip, the height from which the fall occurs (e.g., elevated beds, climbing over side rails, falling down stairs), and falls against harder surfaces (e.g., nonabsorptive linoleum, concrete, or wooden floors).

The management approach advocated for all older persons who fall, or are at risk, is appropriate for AD patients. These strategies are discussed in the subsequent section of this chapter.

The accumulated effects of medical diseases, altered cognition, medications, and resulting functional abilities, combined with extrinsic factors, predispose many AD patients to falls and subsequently cause them. However, the degree of individual fall risk and the etiology, or causes, of falls among persons with AD varies considerably. Because of interindividual variability, both assessment and intervention should be customized to meet each AD patient's needs.

Patients with chronic neuromuscular disorders affecting gait and balance may respond to a number of rehabilitative strategies. These include exercise, proper footwear, hip-protective pads (this therapist uses ice hockey shorts), and limited use of ambulation devices to assist with mobility when warranted.

In AD patients, a daily program of walking can offset altered gait and balance problems that usually result from inactivity (e.g., strength, coordination, postural control). Also, habitual exercise may improve cognitive functioning and reduce falls that result from poor judgment. Low-intensity strengthening, stretching, and range-of-motion exercises can improve muscle strength and joint flexibility; help to maintain or restore cardiovascular conditioning and endurance; and improve functional capabilities (e.g., ambulation, transfers) and safety.

BALANCE AND FALLS

In the elderly, falls often precipitate a series of events with catastrophic potential. The fear of falling is a major concern for many elderly persons. This fear is restrictive and constraining and often results in functional losses and substantially increases the risk of falls. It results in withdrawal, a progressive decrease in activity, and a steady decline in the quality of life and mental well-being.[63]

The maintenance of posture and the ability to move about the environment depend on orientation and balance.[64] Orientation, the awareness of the relationship of the body and body parts to each other and to the environment in a dynamic and reciprocal interaction, is a complex function that relies on multiple sensory input and central nervous system integrity. Likewise, balance is the process by which individuals maintain and move their bodies in relationship to the environment, and requires an automatic and unconscious process to resist the destabilizing effect of gravity. Balance is essential for purposeful movement and effective function. Many central nervous system disorders affect both.

The complexity of the integrated neurosensory system, as the following discussion reveals, translates to balance problems in the elderly. Dysfunction in any one of the components of balance will affect motor control. An older person may have postural changes affecting her or his center of gravity; mobility of the neck, thoracic, and lumbar spines may be limited. Elders frequently have poor neck rotation and extension capabilities. Muscles may be weak and inflexible. Joints may be restricted or contracted. Vision may be diminished. The vestibular system may not be working correctly due to dehydration, either due to self-restriction of fluids (to prevent incontinence), medical restriction of fluids (often related to the use of diuretic drugs), or drugs that cause dehydration. Gait patterns may be slow, with poor foot clearance or inaccurate foot placement. The older adult may be confused and misinterpret neurosensory and neuromuscular cues. Numerous pathologies can lead to a higher likelihood of falling.

To achieve balance, the body's center of gravity (COG) must be perpendicular to the center of support. This is accomplished through the integration by the central nervous system of information received from sensory organs and through the execution of coordinated and synchronized movements.[65] A loss of balance occurs when the sensory information about the position of the COG is inaccurate, when the execution of automatic right movements is inadequate, or when both are present. The postural control system receives information from receptors in the proprioceptive, visual, and vestibular systems. All of these systems, in addition to appropriate motor function, need to be intact for ultimate balance control.

Somatosensory inputs provide information about the position of the body and body parts relative to each other and to the support surface. The somatosensory input the brain receives from muscles and joints stems from sensory receptors called proprioceptors. These proprioceptors are sensitive to pressure and the stretching motion in the tissues that surround them. For instance, the impulses that come from the mechanoreceptor in the neck, which indicate head position and movement, and impulses that come from the ankles and the bottom of the feet, which indicate the movement of the body over the base of support, are important in maintaining balance. Somatosensory inputs are the dominant sensory information for balance when the body is standing still on a fixed, firm surface, or moving through the environment. Conditions that alter sensory input, such as cerebral vascular accidents, peripheral neuropathies, or nutritional deficits (see Chapter 6), may affect input and subsequent interpretation of somatosensory information.[48]

Vision informs the individual about the physical environment and the relation of the body relative to the surroundings. Visual input is the primary backup when the somatosensory system is deficient.[66] It is not uncommon for an older adult to have visual changes or pathologies (see Chapters 3 and 5), which can play a major role in balance loss when the support system is precarious. Balance also involves the ability to stabilize gaze.

The vestibular system originates in the inner ear from five balance receptor sites. These sites are located in three semicircular canals (anterior, horizontal, and posterior) and two sacs (the saccule and the utricle). Each semicircular canal lies roughly perpendicular to the other two. When a person rotates her or his head in the plane of a particular canal, the endolymphatic fluid within the canal lags behind the movement of the canal. The fluid pushes against sensory receptors (hair cells) in the canal and temporarily bends them. This bending of the hair cells in the inner ear sends impulses to the brain via the nervous system. This mechanism varies slightly when people change their head position or move their head in a straight line. Calcium carbonate crystals produced naturally by the body make the hair cells of the saccule and utricle react to the pull of gravity or to translational movement of the head. The hair cells in the saccule and utricle send messages to the CNS. When both inner ears are functioning properly, the vestibular system sends symmetrical messages to the brain.

The vestibular system has both a sensory and a motor function, and measures the head's angular velocity and linear acceleration and detects head position relative to the gravitational axis. This is a sensory function. Head angular velocity is measured by the cristae of semicircular canals, while the maculae of the statolabyrinth (utricle and saccule) register linear acceleration and changes in gravitational force. Because the vestibular system senses head motion, it is less sensitive to body sway than is the visual or the somatosensory system.[67] When somatosensory and visual information are adequate, the vestibular system plays a minor role in the control of the COG position. Its role is dominant when there is a conflict between visual and somatosensory information and during ambulation.[64,68]

The component of motor function controlled by the vestibular system input is muscular activity. During erect posture, it initiates transitory muscular contractions and controls muscle tone. In addition, it assists in stabilizing gaze during head and body movements by generating conjugate, smooth eye movements opposite in direction and approximately of equal velocity to head movements.[69] The vestibulo-ocular reflex stabilizes gaze during target fixation and unsuspected perturbation of head and body position. Gaze stabilization is essential for clear vision; it results from the combined effect of the vestibulo-ocular reflex on the nuclei of the extraocular muscles, neck proprioception, and the position of images on the retina.[64]

The vestibulospinal reflex initiates the compensatory body movements necessary to maintain posture and to stablize the head over the trunk.[65] There are positional, acceleratory, and righting vestibulospinal reflexes.[69] The positional reflexes are initiated by a change in the support surface. The acceleratory reflexes, attributed to the semicircular canals, assist in tilt detection and sway displacement. Righting reflexes tend to keep the head in an upright position and facilitate contraction of the neck receptors and the axial musculature.[70]

The central neurological component, termed the vestibular-nuclear complex, is located in the pons and consists of four major nuclei and seven minor ones. It processes information from the peripheral vestibular system and the visual, proprioceptive, tactile, and auditory system. The vestibular nuclei are extensively connected to the cerebellum, to the nuclei of the extraocular muscles, and to the reticular formation in the brain stem.[70]

The cerebellum plays a prominent role in regulating the output of the vestibulospinal system through extensive reciprocal connections with the vestibular nuclei. Cerebellar lesions can result in severe postural disturbance.[71]

Located beneath the skin, pressure sensors measure the intensity of contact made by the different parts of the body with the environment. These sensors play a dominant role in the maintenance of balance as they relay information about the base of support.[67]

The inertial-gravitational reference provided by the vestibular system is critical to the resolution of sensory conflicts between visual and vestibular inputs and between spinal and vestibular inputs. The vestibular inputs are critical to the selection of appropriate postural movement strategies. The cerebellum and basal ganglia help to mediate visual, vestibular, and proprioceptive interactions and coordinate the proprioceptive reflexes subserving balance.[69] Information from proprioceptive, visual, vestibular, auditory, tactile, and stretch receptors in various organs is integrated to create a picture of the position and movements of the body parts relative to each other and to the environment. This picture is stored and constantly upgraded. It is the essence for all body movement and the determinant for sudden and rapid corrective motor activity.

Impaired balance, often seen in older patients, is the result of inaccurate information about the position of the COG, inadequately executed movements to bring the COG to a balanced position, or a combination of both. Vestibular information for body orientation is particularly important for an elderly individual who lacks good somatosensory or visual cues for orientation. Equilibrium is maintained through a flexible postural synergy.[72] When deterioration in the function of one or more systems subserving the balance function is progressive, as frequently seen in aging, balance remains unaffected as long as the central nervous system is able to adapt and to compensate for these functional changes. Disequilibrium is the consequence of inadequate balance function.[73] Imbalance will not manifest as long as compensation is adequate for the tasks at hand. Whenever the demands on the system exceed the function capabilities, however, instability becomes evident. As functional competence continues to deteriorate, imbalance becomes more prevalent. Chronic instability occurs when the compensating strategies can no longer offset the functional decline.

Falls occur whenever the righting reflexes are either insufficient or too slow to counter the force of attraction exerted by the earth's gravity on an individual. In the elderly, falls are usually the result of the accumulation of multiple chronic disabilities. Falling is a clinical entity in its own right in the practice of geriatrics. Falls are potentially preventable if the causative factors can be recog-nized and addressed.[74] Diminished alertness, poor concentration, general fatigue, drug-induced sedation or dizziness, and impaired situational judgment increase the likelihood of falls.

Age-related morphologic changes occur in all body systems, including those essential for the maintenance of posture. As discussed in Chapter 3, aging has been shown to be associated with a significant loss of hair cells in the vestibular sensors, a decrease of primary vestibular neurons, a diminution in the neuronal cell density of the cerebral cortex, and a decrease in the number of Purkinje's cells in the cerebellum. In addition, there are degenerative changes in the sensory and motor systems, in the tendon receptors of the lower extremities, and in the musculoskeletal system.

The vestibulo-ocular reflex gain and dominant time constant decrease with age.[75] This is probably the result of a combination of age-related changes in the hair cells at the center of the cristae,[76] a relatively selective loss of large-diameter primary vestibular afferents, and neuronal loss in the superior vestibular nuclei.[76,77] The superior vestibular nucleus is a major relay for the canal-ocular reflex.

Changes in the vestibulospinal reflex are difficult to assess because of functional overlap with sensory and motor functions. Distinction among vestibulospinal, visual, and somatosensory dysfunction is difficult in the elderly.[78] The increased body sway seen after the age of 60 is the consequence of cumulative degenerative changes in the vestibular, proprioceptive, sensory, and musculoskeletal systems.[79] Increased body sway shrinks the limits of stability. As the COG moves rapidly, the momentum of the body acts as an additional destabilizing force.

The visual system is of most importance in the control of balance, especially in the aged.[77] Degenerative ocular changes, such as macular degeneration and cataracts, decrease the visual acuity and contribute to instability. Because vision operates slowly, when an older person loses balance, the visually guided postural reflexes do not react quickly enough to prevent a fall.

The elderly have a tendency to walk flexed forward, with the head fixed to the trunk or flexed at the neck and the eyes fixating on the ground in front of them. Such a stance places the COG in a forward position—that is, close to the anterior periphery of the limits of stability. In addition, this impairs orientation by limiting the visual field. The forward position of the head also alters the position of the statolabyrinth relative to the gravitational axis.

Instability manifests as an exaggeration of the COG sway and is the expression of the difficulty encountered in resisting the destabilizing effects of gravity. It is the consequence of the interaction between normally functioning and abnormally functioning components that results in functionally inappropriate and/or ineffective balance response.[69] As the destabilizing forces increase or the corrective measures become inadequate, or both, sway oscillations increase.

The amplitude of the COG sway, therefore, is representative of an individual's difficulty in achieving balance, and the amplitude and velocity of the sway are proportional to the difficulty experienced counteracting gravity.

The COG sway can be measured by computer analysis of information received from a force plate on which the individual stands, or can be assessed using the Romberg's test or the Functional Reach Test.[80–84]

The evaluation of an elderly patient with a vestibular disorder can be a most challenging task. The great overlap that exists between the different systems that subserve the balance function renders the interpretation of measurements of the vestibulo-ocular and the vestibulospinal reflexes difficult. Because of the effects of adaptation and habituation, these measurements do not reflect an organic loss but rather a functional loss that remains uncompensated for at the time the measurements are made.

In the evaluation of vestibular disorders in the elderly, there is no gold standard; rather, experienced clinicians make use of the history, physical examination, assessment of drug regimes and diet, and a medley of laboratory tests, as well as their own best judgment regarding a particular individual. For instance, clinical experience has taught that subtle differences in testing outcomes occur. When testing for vestibular involvement, head movements are used to elicit nystagmus of the eyes, a positive finding. Vertebral artery impingement testing, as well as central nervous system involvement, also results in nystagmus of the eyes as a positive indicator of involvement. How do you differentiate? When the nystagmic movements are jerky, it is usually vestibular involvement. When the nystagmic movements are smooth and rhythmical, the patient generally has central nervous system or circulatory involvement. It is important to thoroughly question the older adult relative to the circumstances that cause dizziness. Table 12.9 provides a summary of some of the complaints older persons may relay to their therapist regarding episodes of dizziness; determining what those symptoms "feel like" may assist the clinician in pinpointing the causes of dizziness.

In the elderly, the causes of unsteadiness and falls are multifactoral and overlapping. The approach to the management of an elderly individual with unsteadiness encompasses more than the diagnosis of the disease entity or entities that are causing the problem. Often, there is no consistent relationship between anatomic abnormalities and physical signs, nor between physical signs and resulting function. The presence of fear of falling can greatly confound any evaluative tests. Nonetheless, comprehensive assessment and evaluation of an elderly patient with balance problems should include:

- Measurement of the functional competence of the vestibular, visual, proprioceptive, sensory, auditory, and musculoskeletal systems;
- Evaluation of gait and movement patterns;[85]
- Evaluation of cognitive function and psychological characteristics;
- Determination of the impact of the functional loss (physiologic, functional, social, and societal) on the particular individual.

See Appendix 3 for evidence-based evaluation tools.

Treatment Interventions

The goal of a treatment program in rehabilitation is to prevent impairments by optimizing function. The authors strongly believe that many of the balance and fall problems seen in an older adult population are related to inactivity. In other words, patients fall when they are attempting to perform activities that they have not practiced in a long while. Therefore, balance reorganization strategies are the cornerstone of the management of balance disorders, especially in the elderly. Intervention should promote orientation, gaze stabilization, postural realignment, muscle strength, and joint mobility. Practicing activities, such as standing on one foot or varying the walking surfaces, enhance the integration of the input or affect the way the brain responds to a deficit in one or more of the three

TABLE 12.9   Elder's Description of Dizziness: Pinpointing the Cause

Patient Complaint	Possible Cause
Dizziness "Feels Like" Vertigo	
❑ Certain head positions trigger it.	Benign paroxysmal positional vertigo (BPPV), in which small calcium stones in the inner ear's otolith (gravity detectors) become dislodged and start floating.
❑ Ringing in the ears or hearing loss.	Ménière's syndrome, a result of fluid buildup in the inner ear (with pain, pressure, or fullness). In rare cases, could be a slow-growing tumor pressing on the auditory nerve.
❑ Dizziness provoked by loud noises.	The result of head trauma or, in rare cases, thinning of the bony cover of the inner ear, which can lead to a fistula, or abnormal opening through which fluids can pass.
❑ Difficulty swallowing or speaking, or feel weakness or numbness in face or limbs.	Stroke or a tumor.
❑ Recent cold or flu.	A viral infection in the inner ear (labyrinthitis).
❑ Taking medications.	Drug side effects. Long-term use or high doses of many drugs (sleeping pills, alcohol, tranquilizers, antidepressants, blood pressure medications) can cause dizziness, and sometimes vertigo.
Dizziness "Feels Like" Physical Loss of Balance	
❑ Neurological or neuroendocrine disease.	Neuropathy.
❑ Age-related changes.	Multisensory deficit, a blunting of neurosensory input, such as vision, hearing, proprioception, kinesthetic sense. Decrease in muscle strength, endurance, flexibility. Poor posture. Cardiovascular changes.
Dizziness "Feels Like" Lightheadedness or Near Fainting	
❑ Sweating, racing heart, fast breathing.	Anxiety, which can cause dizziness as blood pressure drops, hyperventilation, tachycardia.
❑ High blood pressure, heart or vascular disease.	Insufficient blood to brain due to poor circulation.
❑ Dizzy when standing.	Orthostatic hypotension, hypothyroidism, anemia, B12 deficiency, or diabetes.
❑ Sweating, trembling, feel shaky and hungry.	Low blood sugar from poor food ingestion or diabetes.
❑ Taking medications.	Side effects of drugs. Polypharmacy—drug interactions.

sensory systems (e.g., somatosensory, visual, vestibular). The improvement to be expected depends on accurate assessment of the multisystem causes of the imbalance, functional conceptualization of the exercises, severity of the impairments, the general physical and mental health of the patient, patient motivation, and family support.

Patients should be encouraged to incorporate exercises that challenge their COG into their daily routines and to use new strategies in their everyday activities. The home environment should be made safe, as discussed in Chapter 8. Despite all efforts, when the COG can no longer be maintained over the base of support provided by the two feet, the base of support may need to be extended with the use of a cane, walker, or other assistive devices.

Too many elderly individuals with imbalance and dizziness receive inappropriate and ineffectual care, simply because of the bias that they are falling because they are old. Falls are not an inevitable consequence of aging changes, although age-related changes may predispose an older individual to falls. In many cases, falls can be prevented. Table 12.10 provides a list of age-related changes that increase the risk of falls. Strengthening, flexibility, postural, and balance-challenging activities can actually decrease the risk of falling. Home modifications with a focus on safety can be made, especially for activities such as walking to the bathroom at night (providing night lighting, a clear path), going up or down stairs (providing railings and sufficient lighting on nonskid stairs), cooking activities (placing most commonly used utensils in an easily accessible location, improving kitchen lighting, providing a stool for counter activities). Counseling and balance reorganization strategies have proven successful in the management of balance dysfunction in the elderly.

Intervention does not necessarily need to be a formal exercise program. Simply increasing daily activities may be the trick to practicing movement. Many times elderly people fall because they are so inactive. Because inactivity reduces muscle function, flexibility, and strength, as exercise program which focuses on the involved muscle groups can greatly help an elderly person. A study by Tinetti and associates[86] confirmed the importance of activity. This study found that community-dwelling people at least 75 years old with low mobility test scores were nearly twice as likely to fall as those who had high mobility scores. Staying in shape can prevent the "trip and fall" syndrome commonly caused by the deteriorating sensory system associated with inactivity. Exercise/activity prevents this deterioration and keeps the fine motor sensory system finely tuned and increases overall muscle strength and endurance.

TABLE 12.10   Age-Related Changes that Increase the Risk of Falls

Gait Changes	**Hearing Reduced**
❑ Decreased step height, poor foot clearance	❑ Reduced ability to hear high frequency sounds
❑ Narrow-based waddling gait pattern	❑ Reduced tendency to notice approaching car, bicycle on sidewalk, bus, siren, etc.
❑ Shorter step, wider base	❑ Startles easily
❑ Slower movement (stop/start gait pattern)	**Sense of Touch Diminished**
❑ Shuffling (no heel-strike or push-off)	❑ Somatosensory loss
❑ Decreased ankle dorsiflexion	❑ Unable to detect change in support surface
Postural Instability	**Cognitive Changes**
❑ Increase in body sway, both lateral and anterior-posterior	❑ Confused by environment
❑ Decreased responsiveness of sensory receptors that alert muscle to contract when movement is away from the center of gravity	❑ Inattentive
	❑ Decreased level of alertness
❑ Co-contraction of antagonists and agonists upon balance perturbation	❑ Poor judgement
	Orthostatic Hypotension
❑ Weakening of muscles (anterior tibialis, knee extensors and flexors, hip extensors and abductors, trunk and neck extensors)	❑ Drop of 20 mm Hg in systolic blood pressure when assuming upright position
❑ Forward flexed posture shifting center of gravity beyond toes	❑ Decrease blood supply to brain with lightheadness upon standing
Vision Diminished	❑ Decreased efficiency of baroreceptors
❑ Decrease light entering eye secondary to opacities	**Nocturia**
❑ Cataracts	❑ Decreased bladder capacity
❑ Presbyopia (far sightedness)—increased time required for near/far adaptation	❑ Delay in signal to void
	❑ Post mictoration syncope
❑ Increase in interocular pressure (black "floaters" in field of vision) secondary to dehydration or hypertension	❑ Urgency to reach bathroom
	❑ Frequency during the night—half asleep or with poor lighting
❑ Diminished color perception, especially blue-green perception (cataracts—can't see red, orange)	
❑ Increased time required for light/dark adaptation	
❑ Increased glare (especially with macular degeneration)	

Intervention should be directed toward sensory and motor, peripheral, and central impairments specific to the individual. It is important to identify those impairments which can be rehabilitated and those which will require compensation strategies. Cognition as well as perceptual problems may affect the ability to relearn skills or acquire new ones. Optimal learning for motor control, skilled movements, and balance requires:

- Patient's knowledge of abilities and limitations;
- Patient's knowledge of the environmental risks and advantages;
- Knowledge of the critical components of the task to be performed;
- Problem-solving abilities, using the knowledge sets listed above;
- The ability to modify and adapt movements as the task and environment changes.

With older individuals, using practice and feedback to teach motor skills requires repetition of the activity, as well as modifying lighting, surfaces, background distractions, and other environmental conditions that challenge their concentration as well as their balance. Treatment should be multi-impairment oriented with tasks and environments selected to stimulate involved systems.

The less sensory information available, the more difficult the task of balancing. Initially, treatment might start by providing adequate sensory inputs (somatosensory, visual, vestibular) with augmented feedback if sensory channels are deficient. Progression of the treatment would then add the challenge of manipulating visual, somatosensory, or vestibular inputs so that equilibrium is taxed in varying conditions.

To stimulate the somatosensory system, a stable surface for standing can be provided and the other senses modified (eyes open, eyes closed, practicing in low lighting). Eyes closed with weight shifting during standing can further challenge the somatosensory system.

To stimulate the use of visual inputs, treatments that disrupt the somatosensory system (destabilize) are helpful. For instance, the use of rocker boards, BAPS boards, Fitters™, and foam pads will provide differing stimuli to the somatosensory system and encourage the visual system to assume a dominant role in determining where the individual is in relation to the environment. Varying the surface for walking with different levels of light can also challenge this system.

The vestibular system can be stimulated by practicing activity on unstable or compliant surfaces with vision either absent (eyes closed), destabilized (eye movements or head movements), or confused (background movements, activity). Adding head movements to any activity will place the vestibular organ at different angles in relationship to gravity. Gaze stabilization (keeping a stationary object in focus) while moving the head or body is also a helpful approach in the elderly. Starting slow and gradu-

ally increasing the rate of head or body movement is a excellent stimulus to the vestibular system. Gaze stabilization with head movement while standing or walking on uneven surfaces increases the challenge. Head movements should be practiced in whatever direction provokes dizziness. Though it is beyond the scope of this chapter to discuss all the possible exercise protocols for treating vestibular disorders, in general, quick movements of the head, head tilts, or forward/backward and side to side will progressively challenge and improve the vestibular response to movement.[87] It is also important to keep in mind the importance of proper hydration.

Challenging the center of gravity should be done in sitting, sit to stand and stand to sit, standing balance, strategy training (e.g., stimulating the ankle, hip, and stepping responses with sternal nudges or decentralizing activities), and during gait (e.g., obstacle courses).

Another treatment consideration should be footwear. An older person should be fitted with supportive, flat-soled, nonslip and nonstick soles, with a good heel counter and adequate room in the shoe for the foot. Elderly individuals often fall because of poor foot gear.

Many balance exercises can be incorporated into home activities. The older persons should be instructed to do things, such as standing tasks, in a corner or near a counter to initially enhance their stability. The community setting is a natural challenge for gaining postural control. Grocery or library aisles, public transport systems, elevators, escalators, lawns, beaches, ramps, trails, hills, and varied environmental conditions can provide a challenge to the balance with significant functional relevance.

See Appendix 3 for evidence-based balance and fall treatment strategies.

Appendix A

*P*ARKINSON'S DISEASE

Evidence-Based Evaluation Support

Quality of Life in Patients with Parkinson's Disease; by DeBoer; *J Neurol Neurosurg Psychiatry* 96[88]

Parkinson's Disease Quality of Life Questionnaire (PDQL)

- Score range 37–185.
- Higher scores indicate less disease severity and better QOL.

The Effect of a Home Physiotherapy Program for Persons with Parkinson's Disease: by Nieuwboer; *J Rehabil Med*; 11–2001[89]
Parkinson Activity Scale

- 10 items rated 0–4
- The higher the score, the better the function
- Can be used to evaluate "on-off" phases

Evidence-Based Treatment Ideas

The Effect of Temperature on Hand Function in Patients with Tremor; by Cooper; *J Hand Ther*; 12–00[90]

- Use of cooling temporarily decreases tremor.
- 5 minutes in 59° water.

The Effects of Balance Training and High-Intensity Resistance Training on Persons with PD; Hirsch; *Arch Phys Med Rehabil*; 8–03[91]

- RCT compared balance and PRE and balance training: 3×/wk for 10 weeks.
- Combined program ^ more in both strength and balance.
- PRE = 60–80% 1RM all muscle groups.
- Balance = standing on foam and nonfoam, eyes open and closed, head, body turns, weight shifts, swaying to limits of stability all directions.

Treadmill Training with Body-Weight Support: Its Effect on PD; by Miyai; *Arch Phys Med Rehabil*; 7–2000[92]

- Training with body weight support produces greater improvement in ADL, motor performance, and gait than PT.
- Rx = 20%, 10%, 0% —12 minutes each.
- PT = general conditioning, ROM, ADL and gait.

Long-Term Effect of Body-Weight-Supported Treadmill Training in PD; by Miyai; *Arch Phys Med Rehabil*; 10–02[93]

Showed treadmill effective for lasting effects on short-step gait.

Immediate Effects of Speed-Dependent Treadmill Training on Gait Parameters in Early PD; Pohl, *Arch Phys Med Rehabil*; 12–03[94]

- Speed and stride length can be improved through a single intervention on a treadmill for 30 minutes.
- No ^ noted with conventional PT.

Resistance Training and Gait Function in Patients with Parkinson's Disease; by Scandalis; *Am J Phys Med Rehabil*; 01–01[95]

- Patients with mild to moderate Parkinson's
- 2×/wk for 8 weeks
- Exercises:
  - leg press (60% 1RM)
  - toe raise
  - leg curl/extension
  - crunches
- ^ Strength, posture, and gait

Tertiary Prevention in Parkinson's Disease; by Blackinton; *Neuro Report*; 9–02[96]

6-week balance, flexibility, and "strengthening" program showed no benefit over a social meeting program.

Effect of Exercise on Perceived Quality of Life of Individuals with PD; by Baatile; *J Rehabil Res Dev*; 9–2000[97]

8-week polestriding exercise program showed increases in function and QOL.

- 3 ×/wk for 37 minutes
- Exerstrider (like Nordic Track)

Trunk Muscle Performance in Early Parkinson's Disease; by Bridgewater; *Phys Ther*; 6–98[98]

- People with PD exhibit less axial range of motion and isometric torque.
- This study suggests the importance of initiating a strengthening program early to delay the decline in function.

<table>
<tr><td>

Short-Term Effects of Behavioral Treatment on Movement Initiation and Postural Control in Parkinson's Disease; by Muller; *Movement Dis*; 9–97[99]

- Behavioral Rx in PD may improve motor disability in moderately advanced PD.
- Behavioral Rx = (20 sessions):.
  - relaxation training (Jacobson PMR).
  - specific training of motor performance tailored to problems reported by the patient (patient videotaped and analyzed).
  - role playing for difficult social interactions.
  - lots of positive reinforcement.

</td><td>

The Role of Sensory Cues in the Rehabilitation of Parkinsonian Patients: A Comparison of Two Physical Therapy Protocols; Marchese; *Movement Dis*; 5–00[100]

- Two groups received PT.
- One group received additional sensory cues.
- Both groups improved; however, the cued kept the benefit after Rx termination.
- The incorporation of sensory cues can extend the short-term benefit of rehabalitation.

</td></tr>
</table>

Main Items of the Rehabilitation Program

Items	Protocol A ("non-cued")	Protocol B ("cued").
1. Segmental exercises of active or assisted mobilization (flexo-extension, pronosupination) to increase strength, motility, and coordination of four limbs	With open eyes, patients were requested to exert an active and attentional control of movement	Patients were requested to perform the same exercise as in protocol A but with closed eyes, recognizing perceptively the limb position requested
2. Exercises to improve equilibrium (in quadrupedic position)	Patients were requested to extend together upper limb + contralateral lower limb (alternating the side) while supporting themselves on the other two limbs	Patients were requested to perform the same exercise as in protocol A with the help of visual feedback (minor) or rhythmic acoustic feedback (metronome)
3. Exercise to improve control of posture in different positions (sitting, standing)	Patients were requested to maintain balance during unexpected pushes on a basculating plane, with advance knowledge of perturbation direction	Patients were requested to trace with the index finger visual tracks while maintaining balance during postural perturbations on a basculating plane
4. Training exercises for alternate and pendular movements of the upper limbs	In quadrupedic and standing position without any feedback	In quadrupedic position with visual (mirror) control and in standing position with rhythmic acoustic feedback (metronome).
5. Training exercises for walking on level ground or between parallel bars	Patients were requested to walk with wide base and long strides and to exert voluntary control for limb raising	Patients were requested to walk with the aid of lines drawn along the floor and to pass burdles with rhythmic acoustic feedback (metronome)

Effects of Physical Training on Straightening-up Processes in Patients with Parkinson's Disease; by Vlliani; *Disabil Rehabil*; 99[101]

- Motor program
- 2×/week
- 5 weeks
- Significant improvement in:
  - supine to sit
  - sit to supine
  - supine rolling
  - sit to stand
- Exercises to relieve functional disability related to rigidity and bradykinesia:
- Exercise to arise from a chair:

  Slide forward on the seat, leaning from the hips so that the body is at a 45° angle. Position one foot under the edge of the chair seat and the other foot one-half step forward. Next, position hands at the side of the seat near the front legs of the chair, and push with the arms while stepping forward, all in one continuous motion.
- Exercise to sit down in a chair:

  Reverse the process described for rising from the chair. Turn one's back to the chair, place one foot behind the other, bend the torso to a 45° angle, then sit slowly but smoothly while grasping the sides of the chair with the hands.
- Exercise for stooped posture:

  Stand with one's back to the wall, with the head; shoulders, buttocks, and heels all touching the wall. After holding the position for 30 seconds, walk away from the wall and then return, assuming the same position.

These exercises should be repeated 5 to 10 times every morning and evening to improve functional ability.

Active Music Therapy in Parkinson's Disease: An Integrative Method for Motor and Emotional Rehab; by Pachetti; *Psychosom Med*; 2000[102]

- Happiness and emotional measures improved for up to 2 months after Rx in MT group.
- PT improved rigidity only.
- MT group seen 2 hrs/week—**listening, singing, breathing, rhythmic movements, and body expression to music.**
- PT group seen 1½ hrs/wk— **stretching, joint mobilization, balance training, posture work, motor tasks for hypokinesis.**

The Effect of Trager Therapy on the Level of Evoked Stretch Response in Patients with PD; by Duval; *JMPT*; 9–02[103]

- The level of ESR was reduced 36% immediately after RS and remained 32% lower than pretest values 11 minutes after Rx.
- 20-minute sessions to whole body.

Gentle rhythmic rocking 1–4 cm in amplitude confined to 1–2 articulation.

RCT of the Alexander Technique for PD; by Stallibrass; *Clin Rehab*; 02[104]

- 24 lessons in Alexander Technique lead to sustained benefit in PD.
- Using skilled hand contact, a teacher observes and assesses changes in muscle activity, balance, and coordination resulting from mental activity, and provides immediate feedback. Participants learn to recognize and adopt better thinking strategies for control of movement.

Exercise to Improve Spinal Flexibility and Function for People with PD: A Randomized Control Trial; by Schenkman; *J Am Geriatr Soc*; 10–98[105]

- A 10-week exercise program for early and mid-stage PD improves:
  - functional reach
  - axial rotation
- No difference was noted in supine to sit time.

Axial Mobility Exercise Program

Week 1
Stage I: Relaxation While Increasing Range of Motion—Supine
                   Deep Breathing
                   Knee Rocks (Full)
                   Hip abduction (1 leg at a time)
                   Bell Ringer
                   Neck Rotation in axial extension

Week 2
Stage II: Segmental Motion of the Spine and Upper Quadrant with Emphasis on the Thorax
                   Combination Knee Rock-Bell Ringer
                   Sidelying Thoracic Rotation
                   Sidelying Forward and Backward Arm Reaches
                   Sidelying Thoracic Rotation with Forward and Backward Arm Reaches

Week 3
Stage III: Segmented Motion of the Spine and Isolated Motion of the of the Lower Extremity on a Stable Pelvis
                   Prone Wiggle
                   Prone Props
                   Prone Hip Internal Rotation

Weeks 4–5
Stage IV: Segmental Motion of the Spine and Pelvis: Quadruped
                   Cat and Camel
                   All Fours Isolated Lumbar Extension
                   All Fours Backward Rocking in Sagittal Plane
                   All Fours Backward Rocking Diagonal Plane

Weeks 6–7
Stage V: Segmental Motion of the Spine and Pelvis Sitting
                   Sitting Anterior and Posterior Tilt
                   Siting Forward Trunk Flexion Over Stable Base
                   Sitting Diagonal Trunk Flexion over a Stable Base
                   Sitting Lateral Tilt of Trunk and Pelvis
                   Sitting Pelvic Clock
                   Sitting Chin Tucks

Week 8
Stage VI: Coordinated Trunk and Upper Extremity Movement in an Unsupported Position
                   Sitting Trunk Rotation
                   Sitting Trunk Flexion and Extension with Bell Ringer
                   Sitting Trunk Flexion and Extension with Arms in the Diagonal Plane

Weeks 9–12
Stage VII: Axial Mobility in Standing
                   Standing Lateral Trunk Flexion
                   Standing Trunk Rotation with Arm Swing
                   Standing Isolated Lower Trunk Rotation
                   Standing Isolated Upper Trunk Rotation
                   Standing Pelvic Tilt
                   Standing Forward and Backward Weight Shifts
                   Standing Ball Throw
                   Standing Golf Swing
                   Standing Ball Kick

Stretches: Hamstring and Gastrocnemius Stretch

Schenkman, M., Keysor, J., Chandler, J., Laub, K.C., MacAller, H. *Axial Mobility Exercise Program. An Exercise Program to Improve Functional Ability.* Claude Pepper Older American's Independence Center, Durham, NC, 1994.

Routine for: _____
Created by: _____

PARKINSON-1 Axial Extension (Chin Tuck)

Gently pull chin in while lengthening back of neck.

Hold _____ seconds while counting out loud.

Repeat _____ times.
Do _____ sessions per day.

PARKINSON-2 Knee Rock

With knees bent and feet flat, roll knees form side to side about _____ inches.

Repeat _____ times.
Do _____ sessions per day.

PARKINSON-3 Standing Rock

Using support, with one foot in front of other, rock back and forth shifting weight from foot to foot _____ times.

Reverse foot position and repeat.

Repeat _____ times.
Do _____ sessions per day.

PARKINSON-4 Trunk Twist

Place hands on shoulders and gently twist head, neck and trunk to one side as far as possible.

Hold _____ seconds while counting out loud.

Repeat to other side.

Repeat _____ times.
Do _____ sessions per day.

PARKINSON-5 Getting Up/Sitting Down-Chair

Holding chair, scoot to front of seat. Lean forward from hips. Slide one foot under the edge of chair, other foot one-half step forward. Push with arms and stand in one continuous motion.

Reverse process to sit.

Repeat _____ times.
Do _____ sessions per day.

Appendix B

Stroke

Evidence-Based Treatment Ideas

Evaluation of a Home-Based Exercise and Training Programme to Improve Sit to Stand in Patients with Chronic Stroke; by Monger; *Clin Rehab*; 02[106]

- Stroke patients who were at least 1 year status/post stroke and 6 months out of rehab.
- 3×/wk, for 3 weeks
- 20-minute program supervised by a PT.
- Patients were asked to do exercises 20 minutes every day.
- HEP = Sit-stand-sit (10).
- Step-ups (8 cm × 30×), calf stretch (2 min × 10).

High-Intensity Strength Training Improves Strength and Functional Performance After Stroke; Suzuki; *Am J Phys Med Rehab*; 8–2000[107]

- Rx:
- 12 weeks
- 2×/wk
- 70% 1RM
  - 1 year after stroke
  - 68% ^ in strength
  - Improved chair stands, balance, and motor performance

A Yoga-Based Exercise Program for People with Chronic Poststroke Hemiparesis; by Bastille; *Phys Ther*; 04[108]

Subjects showed ^ in movement, QOL, and balance.

- 8-week intervention.
- ^ 9 months s/p stroke
- 1½ hrs/2×/week

Yoga Therapy Session Format

Activity	Description
Education (5–10 min)	Subjects were given a brief description of basic anatomical structures (musculoskeletal, nervous, and circulatory structures) and explanations of yoga concepts related to the week's theme. The goal was to facilitate a greater understanding of one's physical body and thought processes.
Body awareness (10–15 min)	The instructor verbally led the subject through bringing conscious awareness to various parts of the body and to notice one's thoughts. The goal was to promote awareness of body sensation, position, and awareness of the activity of the mind.
Pranayama (breathing) (5 min)	Voluntary breathing activities were taught and practiced such as diaphragmatic breathing, 3-part complete breath, *ujjayi* (breathing with the throat partially closed to create a snoring sound), and *nadhi shodhana* (alternate nostril breathing). The goals were to promote awareness of the sensations of the breath in the body and awareness of how the breath can facilitate movement of body segments and to promote concentration.
Asana (physical poses) (30–40 min)	The subjects were instructed and assisted as necessary in performing a variety of modified yoga poses related to the week's theme. The goal was to improve in flexibility, muscle force, endurance, balance, and coordination of body segments.

(continued)

Yoga Therapy Session Format (Continued)

Activity	Description
Guided imagery/relaxation (10–15 min)	The subjects were read a guided imagery script incorporating visualization and then allowed to rest in silence. The goal was to elicit a relaxation response.
Seated silent meditation (5 min)	The subjects were asked to return to a seated position on the floor, in a chair, or at bedside and to remain in this position in silence, focusing on the sound of the breath. The goal was to promote mental clarity (clear one's mind of extraneous thoughts).
Expression/sharing (5 min)	The subjects were invited to express their experiences of each session verbally or through drawing. The goal was to integrate the experiences of the session and facilitate awareness of any physical, mental, or emotional changes that may have occurred.

Weekly Themes	Focus
Week 1 Establishing a solid foundation	Ankle flexibility
Week 2 Activating the power of the legs	Strengthening the thighs
Week 3 Opening the hips	Hip flexibility
Week 4 Aligning the spine	Postural alignment and spinal flexibility
Week 5 The flow of life	Circulatory system and emotions
Week 6 Integrating the senses	Energy pathways/*prana-vayus* (yoga philosophy of main pathways of energy flow through the body)
Week 7 Creating better balance	Postural stability/mind-body connection
Week 8 Creating peace of mind	Relaxation and peace

Task-Related Circuit Training Improves Performance of Locomotor Tasks in Chronic Stroke: A Randomized Controlled Pilot Trial; Dean; *Arch Phys Med Rehabil*; 2000[109]

- Chronic (at least 3 months status post by stroke).
- 3×/wk for 4 weeks.
- Exp—strengthening and functional task for LE.
- Control—UE tasks.
- Exp had sig and retained (2 months) improvement in walking speed, endurance, strength, sit to stand.

Strength Programs for Patients with Cerebrovascular Disease

Research Based Practices

Resistance Bands and Cuff Weight Program

Mode of Resistance	◆ 8 levels of resistance bands
	◆ Cuff weights
Exercises	◆ Hip flexion
	◆ Knee flexion
	◆ Knee extension
	◆ Ankle dorsiflexion
	◆ Ankle plantarflexion
Intensity	◆ 50% 1 RM × 1 week
	◆ 80% 1 RM 9 weeks
Repetitions	◆ 10
Sets	◆ 3
Frequency	◆ Three times a week
Duration	◆ 10 weeks
Criteria for Advancing	◆ Every two weeks
Strength Gains	◆ 42.3% average
Other Program Components	◆ Warm Up (5 minutes): calisthenics, mild stretching, and ROM
	◆ Aerobic Exercise: graded walking, plus steps or cycle at 70% max HR
Time Required	◆ 60 minutes

Teixeira-Salmela, L.F., et al. Muscle strengthening and physical conditioning to reduce impairment and disability in chronic stroke survivors. *Arch Phys Med Rehabil.* 1999; 80:1211–1218.

Isokinetic Program

Mode of Resistance	◆ Orthotron at speeds of 30, 60, and 120°/sec
Exercises	◆ Knee flexion
	◆ Knee extension
Intensity	◆ Maximal reciprocal contractions
Repetitions	◆ 6–8
Sets	◆ 3
Frequency	◆ Three times a week
Duration	◆ 6 weeks
Criteria for Advancing	◆ Not applicable
Strength Gains	◆ 15–20% average
Other Program Components	◆ Warm Up (5 minutes): bike, 15 second stretches
	◆ Cool down: same stretches as warm up
Time Required	◆ 40 minutes

Sharp, S.A., Brouwer, B.J. Isokinetic strength training of the hemiparetic knee: effects on function and spasticity. *Arch Phys Med Rehabil.* 1997; 78:1231–1236.

Randomized Clinical Trial of Therapeutic Exercise in Subacute Stroke

Pamela Duncan, PhD, FAPTA; Stephanie Studenski, MD, MPH; Lorie Richards, PhD;

Conclusions—This structured, progressive program of therapeutic exercise in persons who had completed acute rehabilitation services produced gains in endurance, balance, and mobility beyond those attributable to spontaneous recovery and usual care. (*Stroke*, 2003; 34:2173–2180.)

Components of the Intervention Program

Range of Motion and Flexibility	Range of motion and stretching to the shoulder, elbow, wrist, fingers, hip, ankle, and trunk
Strengthening	Active motion in PNF unilateral patterns with manual resistance progressing to Theraband repetitions (2 sets of 10) in anatomical planes. Targeted movements for Theraband exercises were shoulder flexion/external rotation, elbow flexion/extension, wrist extension, hip abduction, knee flexion/extension, and ankle dorsiflexion. Once exercise was completed with little difficulty, the resistance of the band used was increased.
Balance	Step-ups: repeated stepping anteriorly and laterally onto a step: up with affected LE and down with unaffected LE, progressing to higher step and decreasing upper extremity support.
	Chair rises: repeated rising from a seated position, progressing from using arms to not using arms and from high surface to lower.
	Wall exercise: repetitions of standing from a wall and falling backwards with the trunk straight to contact the wall with the upper back and bouncing upright again, progressing to greater distances from the wall.
	Marching: repeated marching in place, progressing from UE support to no support.
	Toe rises: repeated rising up on toes, progressing from UE support to no support and from bilateral rises to unilateral rises on affected LE only.
	Other: kicking a ball with either foot, simulated batting/golfing, abrupt stops and turns while walking.
UE Functional Use	Practicing the use of the UE in real-life tasks with an emphasis on increasing coordination requirements, eg. washing countertops, opening drawers, putting away dishes, folding towels, closing blinds, counting change, writing.
Endurance	Riding a stationary bike, progressing in time up to 30 min with increasing speed and resistance.
	Exercise duration was initially increased in 2- to 5-min-increments until 20 to 30 min of continuous cycling at 40 rpm was achieved. Interval training was then instituted and used periods of increased speed to achieve a higher heart rate. Intervals were completed in blocks of 5 minutes (ie, 1-min interval at 50 rpm and 4-min interval at 40 rpm; 1½ min at 50 rpm and 3½ min at 40 rpm; 2 min at 50 rpm and 3 min at 40 rpm). Resistance was increased once the subject could complete 4 2-min intervals. Next phase of endurance training began with continuous cycling at 40 rpm for 25 to 30 min at next level of resistance. Progression continued with interval training as previously described.

PNF indicates proprioceptive neuromuscular facilitation: LE = lower extramity and UE = upper extremity

Constraint-Induced Movement Therapy for Motor Recovery in Chronic Stroke Patients; by Kunkel; *Arch Phys Med Rehabil*; 6–99[110]

- CI therapy is effacious (**taubtraining@uabmc.edu**).
- CI Rx = restraint of unaffected UE in a sling for 14 days combined with 6 hours of training a day (shaping part-task practice done 10× with encouragement and concentration and not excessive effort).
- To be included must be able to extend at least 20° at the wrist and 10° at the MP and IP joints.

Longer versus Shorter Daily Constraint-Induced Movement Therapy of Chronic Hemiparesis: An Exploratory Study; by Sterr; *Arch Phys Med Rehabil*; 10–02[111]

- 3-hour CIMT significantly improved motor function, but it was less effective than the 6-hour training schedule.

Modified Constraint-Induced Therapy in Chronic Stroke; by Sisto; *Am J Phys Med Rehab*;[112]

- 1/2 hour of PT and OT 3×/wk for 10 weeks (case study but did show improvements)

Effect of Trunk Restraint on the Recovery of Reaching Movements in Hemiparetic Patients; by Michaelsen; *Stroke*; 8–01[113]

- During trunk restraint, ranges of elbow and shoulder motion, as well as interjoint coordination, increased.
- A harness was secured to the back of a chair that minimized trunk movement and shoulder girdle movement.

The Effect of Shoe Wedges and Lifts on Symmetry of Stance and Weight Bearing in Hemiparetic Individuals; by Rodriquez; *Arch Phys Med Rehabil*; 4–02[114]

- A shoe wedge or shoe lift applied to unaffected limb can help overcome the learned disuse of the affected limb.

Obstacle Training Programme for Individuals Post Stroke; Bassile; *Clin Rehab*; 03[115]

- 2×/wk; substantial ^ in gait and disability level after obstacle training
- 10 m increasing to 750 m walking over obstacles, 1/3 of path

Effects of Perceptual Learning Exercises on Standing Balance Using a Hardness Discrimination Task in Hemiplegic Patients Following Stroke: A RCT; by Morioka; *Clin Rehab*; 03[116]

- Balance ^ in exp group
- Rx—rehab +
  - blindfolded and explained the ascending hardness of sponges 5—15 mm, then descending
  - 3 trials to guess the hardness with immediate feedback
  - 30 seconds later; 10 trials in random order
  - done for 10 days in 2 weeks
- Control—rehab only

A New Approach to Retrain Gait in Stroke Patients Through Body Weight Support and Treadmill Stimulation; by Visintin; *Stroke*; 1998; 29:1122–1128[117]

- Retraining gait in patients with stroke while a percentage of their body weight was supported resulted in better walking abilities than gait training while the patients were bearing full weight.
- Hesse; *Arch Phys Med Rehabil*; 4–99; Barbeau; *Arch Phys Med Rehabil*; 10–03: similar findings[118]

STROKE-1 Sitting Extension

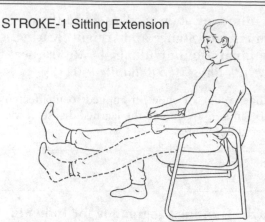

Straighten knee as far as possible. Slowly bend it slightly, and then bring it back up to full extension. Repeat with other leg.
Repeat _____ times. Do _____ sessions per day.

STROKE-2 Hip Adduction

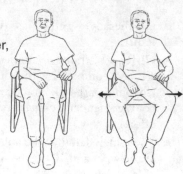

Squeeze knees together, spread them apart and bring them back together. Work within the controllable range, even if only a few inches.

Repeat _____ times.
Do _____ sessions per day.

STROKE-3 Walk To the Side

Step to the side with stronger leg and follow with involved leg. Then return.

Hold chair if necessary.

Repeat _____ times.
Do _____ sessions per day.

STROKE-4 Upper Extremity Reach

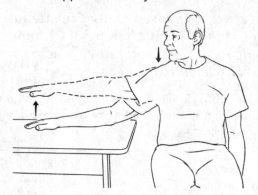

Rest involved arm on table. Attempt to lift arm off table without lifting shoulder.

Repeat _____ times. Do _____ sessions per day.

STROKE-5 Weight Bearing Hand Sit

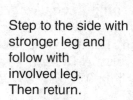
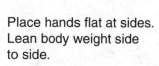

Place hands flat at sides. Lean body weight side to side.

Hold _____ seconds each side.

Repeat _____ times.
Do _____ sessions per day.

STROKE-6 Wall Weight Bearing (Advanced)

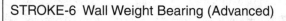
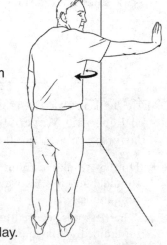

Keep hand of involved arm flat against wall and turn body from side to side.

Repeat _____ times.
Do _____ sessions per day.

Routine for:
Created by:

STROKE-7 Supported Arm Movements

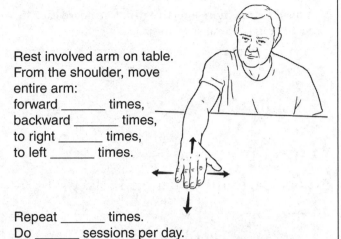

Rest involved arm on table. From the shoulder, move entire arm:
forward _____ times,
backward _____ times,
to right _____ times,
to left _____ times.

Repeat _____ times.
Do _____ sessions per day.

STROKE-8 Sitting Balance (Very Advanced)

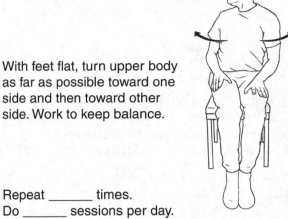

With feet flat, turn upper body as far as possible toward one side and then toward other side. Work to keep balance.

Repeat _____ times.
Do _____ sessions per day.

STROKE-9 Forward Upper Body Weight Shift

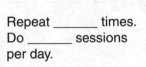

Place both hands on a chair or stool in front. Lean body forward, then return to upright. Try to shift more weight onto involved arm.

Repeat _____ times.
Do _____ sessions per day.

STROKE-10 Beach Ball Kick

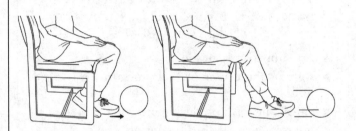

Hook strong leg behind weak leg. Push with strong leg to weak leg kicks ball.

Repeat _____ times. Do _____ sessions per day.

Conventional PT and Treadmill Re-training for Higher-Level Gait Disorders in CVA; by Liston; *Age & Ageing*; 2000; 29:311–318[119]

No difference between conventional PT and treadmill retraining.

Step Training with Body Weight Support Combined with Treadmill Training in Stroke Subjects; by Sullivan; *Arch Phys Med Rehabil*; 5–02[120]

Best to train at normal walking velocities.

Hemiplegic Gait of Stroke Patients: The Effects of Using a Cane; by Kuan; *Arch Phys Med Rehabil*; 1999; 80(7): 777–84[121]

A cane improves gait by:
- shifting the center of body mass toward sound limb
- enhancing push-off during preswing
- improving circumduction during swing

Effect of an Arm Sling on Gait Pattern in Patients with Hemiplegia; by Yavuzer; *Arch Phys Med Rehabil.* 2002; 83(7): 960–963[122]

An arm sling improved gait (walking speed, stance period double support, excursion of the center of gravity, weight bearing on the paretic side).

The Effect of Walking Aids on Balance and Weight-Bearing Patterns of Patients with Hemiparesis in Various Stance Positions; Laufer; *Phys Ther*; 2003; 83(2):112–122[123]

A quad cane is more effective than a standard cane in decreasing postural sway in stance.[123]

Appendix C

*B*ALANCE AND FALLS

Evidence-Based Evaluation Tools

Timed Up and Go

- Fallers—21.5 seconds.
- Nonfallers—11.3 seconds.
- On the modified version—subject arises from a chair without armrests, walks 3 meters, turns and sits in a second chair with armrests, rises from the second chair, and walks back to the first chair, turns around and sits down.
- No reliability measures (O'Brien; *J Gerontol Biolog Sci*; 97[124])
- Community-dwelling elderly between 65 and 85 years old = TUG 12 sec or less (Bischoff: *Age Aging*; 03[125]).

One-Leg Balance Is an Important Predictor of Injurious Falls in Older Persons; by Vellas; *J Am Geriatr Soc*; 6–97[126]

If the person is unable to balance 5 seconds, he or she is at risk for INJURIOUS falls.

Dizziness Handicap Inventory

Instructions: The purpose of this scale is to identify difficulties that you may be experiencing because of your dizziness or unsteadiness. Please answer "yes," "no," or "sometimes" to each question. *Answer each question as it pertains to your dizziness or unsteadiness problem only.*

Item		Response
P1.	Does looking up increase your problem?	_____
E2.	Because of your problem, do you feel frustrated?	_____
F3.	Because of your problem, do you restrict your travel for business or recreation?	_____
P4.	Does walking down the aisle of a supermarket increase your problem?	_____
F5.	Because of your problem, do you have difficulty getting into or out of bed?	_____
F6.	Does your problem significantly restrict your participation in social activities such as going out to dinner, going to movies, dancing or to parties?	_____
F7.	Because of your problem, do you have difficulty reading?	_____
P8.	Does performing more ambitious activities like sports, dancing, household chores such as sweeping or putting dishes away increase your problem?	_____
E9.	Because of your problem, are you afraid to leave your home without having someone accompany you?	_____
E10.	Because of your problem, have you been embarrassed in front of others?	_____
P11.	Do quick movements of your head increase your problem?	_____
F12.	Because of your problem, is it difficult for you to do strenuous housework or yardwork?	_____
P13.	Does turning over in bed increase your problem?	_____
F14.	Because of your problem, is it difficult for you to do strenuous housework or yardwork?	_____
E15.	Because of your problem, are you afraid people may think you are intoxicated?	_____
F16.	Because of your problem, is it difficult for you to go for a walk by yourself?	_____
P17.	Does walking down a sidewalk increase your problem?	_____
E18.	Because of your problem, is it difficult for you to concentrate?	_____
F19.	Because of your problem, is it difficult for you to walk around your house in the dark?	_____
E20.	Because of your problem, are you afraid to stay home alone?	_____
E21.	Because of your problem, do you feel handicapped?	_____
E22.	Has your problem placed stress on your relationships with members of your family or friends?	_____
E23.	Because of your problem, are you depressed?	_____
F24.	Does your problem interfere with your job or household responsibilities?	_____
P25.	Does bending over increase your problem?	_____

Reprinted with permission. Jacobson, G.P., Newman, C.W. The Development of the Dizziness Handicap Inventory. *Arch Otolaryngol Head Neck Surg* 1990; 116:424–427.

Scoring: A "yes" response is scored 4 points
A "sometimes" is scored 2 points
A "no" response is scored 0 points

Reprinted with permission

Total possible points = 100. The higher the score, the worse the disability.

Evidence-Based Treatment Ideas

Occupation and Visual/Vestibular Interaction in Vestibular Rehabilitation; Cohen; *Otolaryngol Head Neck Surge*; 95[127]

- Both the vestibular and the *Purposeful Activity* improved outcomes.
- PA =
- playing Frisbee and catch
- reading signs

Sample Treatment Activities

Therapist can grade any task by changing speed and/or duration of the task, subject's position, or range of motion required.

1. Completeing pegboard designs. Board and pattern can be situated on one side, with pegs on other side, so that subject must rotate the head to find pegs and then rotate the head to the other side to place them in board.
2. Playing catch, with the subject seated on bench or large ball or standing.
3. Simulating housework.
4. Playing Frisbee.
5. Walking and reading signs on walls, ceiling, and floor. Subject can walk at different speeds, with or without volitional head movements, forward, or sideways.
6. Stimulating other movement problems of interest to subject, such as sports or leisure activities.

Effects of Mental Practice on Balance in Elderly Women; Fansler; *Phys Ther*; 9–85[128]

- 3-day intervention.
- Relaxation and ideokinetic facilitation (idealized visual and kinesthetic mental images).
- OSLT × 3, tape, OSLT × 3

Balance Transcript

"Now think about balancing. Remember what it was like to play balancing games as a child. Remember how long you could balance playing hopscotch. Remember how easy and fun it was to walk along a thin wall."

"Think about balance now. Realize that the balance you had as a child is still yours. You can balance; you just need to practice and remind yourself how easy it can be."

"As you stand on one leg, see yourself as a tall oak tree. Feel the support of the roots beneath you. Feel your arms like branches, reaching out to the sky, helping to support you in the air. Enjoy the feeling of standing calm and still in the wind."

"See a large brightly colored bird. Imagine you are that bird. You have long, strong legs. You lift up on one leg and begin to balance. Feel how securely you stand on one leg with other tucked comfortably up beneath you."

Reprinted from *Physical Therapy*, Fransier, et al. September 1985.

Can the Control of Bodily Orientation Be Significantly Improved in a Group of Older Adults with a History of Falls? Rose; *J Am Geriatr Soc*; 2000[129]

- Rehab focused on manipulating individual, task, and environmental constraints sig improve control of body orientation of older adults with history of falls.
- Rehab—stand on narrow surfaces while reaching, reestablish BOS, step forward and backward, inclines, stepping from center, weight shifts, ball catching, head movements, steps, foam.

Yale Ficsit: Risk Factor Abatement Strategy for Fall Prevention; by Tinetti, *J Am Geriatr Soc*; 3–93[130]

- Targeted Risk Factors and Interventions (see next below).

Tinetti Protocol

*4 levels of progressively destabilizing manuevers
with decreasing support*

KAT
1. Wide Circles
2. Small Circles   Decreasing PSI   Decrease BOS
3. Cross
4. Figure 8

BAPTS
1. Forward &
   Backward
2. Side to Side   Foam 1"   Decrease BOS
3. Circle   Foam 1/2"
4. Figure 8   No Foam

FOAM
1. Look Side to Side
2. Turn Side to Side   No Foam   Decrease BOS
3. Squat   Foam 1/2"   (1 leg)
4. Reach   Foam 1"

Progressive Resistive Exercise

*2×/day 15–20 minute sessions when patient is able
to complete 10 repetitions through full range
of motion, increase resistance*

HIP
  Flexion
  Abduction
  Extention

ANKLE
  Pro-stretch

KNEE
  Extention
  Flexion

SHOULDER
  Flexion
  Extention
  Abduction
  Scapular Depression

HAND
  Putty

ELBOW
  Flexion
  Extention

**progress beige, yellow, red, green,
blue, black, grey, gold**

"A Multifactorial Intervention to Reduce the Risk of Falling Among Elderly People Living in the Community". *The New England Journal of Medicine*, Sept. 29, 1994. Vol. 331, No. 13. pp. 822–3.

Balance Exercises

Exercises

Level I	Level II	Level III	Level IV
Sink Toe Stand with both hands	Sink Toe Stand with one hand	Sink Toe Stand with no hands	Standing Arm/Leg March
One Leg Sink Stand with both hands	One Leg Sink Stand with one hand	One Leg Sink Stand with no hands	Cross Over Walk
Sink Hip Circle	Bed Walk with arms	Bed Walk with arms folded	Tandem Walk
Sitting Arms Circles	Sink Side Step with both hands	Sink Side Step with one hand	Heel Toe Walk
Sitting Knee Lifts; Arms to Side	Sitting March	Sink Leg Cross	One Leg Sink Toe Stand
	Sitting Knee Lifts; Arms Across Chest	Sink Leg Swing	
		Sink Leg Lift Heel Stand	

Indications: Less than normal performance during baseline PT assessment in sitting, standing, or reaching balance; transferring lie to sit, sit to stand, or stand to sit; or during gait assessment.

Frequency: Twice per day. Each exercise performed 5 or 10 times per session.

Progression of exercises: All subjects begin at Level I and progress to higher levels when all exercises at lower level are performed correctly, and without significant effort as defined by criteria listed in the procedure manual.

Randomised Factorial Trial of Falls Prevention Among Older People Living in Their Own Homes; by Day; *Brit Med J* 2002; 325:128; 7–02[131]

- 3 interventions were used.
  - group-based exercise (1 hr/wk for 15 weeks, PT designed, of flex, strength, and balance)
  - home hazard management
  - vision improvement
- Outcome—followed for falls for 18 months.
- Group exercise was the most potent single intervention. Adding the others further reduced falls.

The Effect of Land and Aquatic Exercise on Balance Scores in Older Adults; by Douris; *J Geriatr Phys Ther*; 2003; 26[132]

- Regardless of medium, signif ∧ were evidenced on Berg Balance Score
- 2×/wk, 6 weeks, 30 minutes
- Rx:
  - walk forward, back, side, tandem
  - march, squats, Sit to Stand
  - hip flexion, extension, abduction, adduction
  - toe/heel raises

Reducing Frailty and Falls in Older Persons: An Investigation of Tai Chi; by Wolf; *J Am Geriatr Soc*; 1996; 44(5):489–97[133]

T'ai Chi was found to reduce the risk of multiple falls by 47.5%.

The Effects of a 12-week PRE Program on LE Strength and TUG Measures in Community-Dwelling Elderly; by Schiller; *Gerinotes*; 01[136]

- A 12-week, once/week program ^ LE strength, gait velocity, and TUG scores
- Program:
  - Theraband to LE
  - 8 reps, 3 sets
  - Increasing resistance when full ROM and no tiredness or slight tiredness noted

Exercise Training for Rehabilitation and Secondary Prevention of Falls in Geriatric Patients with a History of Injurious Falls; by Hauer; *J Am Geriatr Soc* 2001; 49(1): 10–20[134]

- PRE and prog func training are safe and effective methods for improving impairments and function.
- 10-min warm-up, PRE 3×/wk to LE (hip abd and ext, knee ext, plantarflexion 80% 1RM).
- Stepping, forward, backward, challenges, ball throw, T'ai Chi, chair sits, one legged stand test.
- *Arch Phys Med Rehabil*; 03 found 2 years later all declined.

Effects of Physical Training on the Physical Capacity of Frail, Demented Patients with a History of Falling: A RCT; Toulotte; 03[137]

- 2×/wk for 16 weeks.
- Walking (gait speed), flexibility (sit and reach), balance (OLST and Get-up and Go) were ^ in training group.
- Rx—done by physicians:
  - Theraband PRE
  - sit to stands
  - LAQ
  - OLS
  - stepping over obstacles
  - long sit stretch with leg over big ball or foot on skate
  - avoid ball swung from ceiling

Effects of Balance Training in Elderly Evaluated by Clinical Tests; by Ledin; *J Vestib Res*; 2–91[135]

- Conclusion: The training group significantly improved in balance.
- The training program:
  - walking—forward, backward, toes, heels, sideways
  - walking with sudden turns
  - rising from sitting, one leg standing
  - vis fix with neck motions
  - jumping, ball throwing, bouncing, and catching

Routine for:
Created by:

BALANCE-1 Standing Side Lean

Using support, lean body weight from side to side.

Repeat _____ times.
Do _____ sessions per day.

BALANCE-2 Toe Up

Using support, gently rise up on toes and rock back on heels.

Repeat _____ times. Do _____ sessions per day.

BALANCE-3 Heel Cord Stretch

Place one leg forward, bent other leg behind and straight. Lean forward keeping back heel flat.

Hold _____ seconds while counting out loud.

Repeat with other leg.

Repeat _____ times.
Do _____ sessions per day.

BALANCE-4 One-Legged Stand

Standing on one leg, try to maintain balance _____ seconds or as long as possible without support.

Repeat on other leg.

Repeat _____ times.
Do _____ sessions per day.

BALANCE-5 Eye Motion

Stand with hands out in front of head. Move eyes from one hand to the other as quickly as possible. Stop if you become dizzy or nauseous.

Repeat _____ times. Do _____ sessions per day.

BALANCE-6 Grapevine

Using support, cross one foot over the other. Then bring back boot up beside front foot.

Repeat, going the other direction.

Repeat _____ times.
Do _____ sessions per day.

BALANCE-7 Walking Figure Eight

Practice walking in figure eight. Start with large figures. Make it more difficult by walking in a smaller figure eight.

Repeat _____ times. Do _____ sessions per day.

BALANCE-8 Semi Tandem Standing

Heel on one foot against arch of other: 1. Look right _____ times. 2. Look left _____ times. 3. Look up _____ times. 4. With right arm, reach left, forward and back.

Repeat _____ times. Do _____ sessions per day.

SPECIAL CARD - 1
TARGET HEART RATE (THR)

Exercise for several minutes, stop, and immediately take pulse for 10 seconds at wrist. See beats table to get beats per minute and check against what your current THR should be. Check pulse periodically to maintain THR for the entire workout.

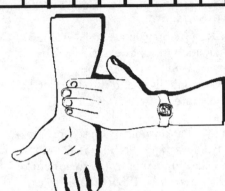

Beats/ 10 Sec.	=	Beats/ Min.
10		60
11		66
12		72
13		78
14		84
15		90
16		96
17		102
18		108
19		114
20		120
21		126
22		132
23		138
24		144
25		150

Your Current Target Heart Rate Should Be Between:

_____ - _____

References

1. Schenkman M, Butler R. A model for multisystem evaluation, interpretation and treatment of individuals with neurologic dysfunction. *Phys Ther.* 1989; 69 (7):538–547.
2. Topp B. Towards a better understanding of Parkinson's disease. *Geriatr Nurs.* July–August 1987; 180–182.
3. Mutch W, Strudwick A, Sisare R, et al. Parkinson's disease: Disability, review and management. *Brit Med J.* 1986; 293(9):675–677.
4. Wilson J, Smith R. The prevalence and aeitology of long-term L dopa side effects in elderly Parkinson's patients. *Age Ageing.* 1989; 18:11–16.
5. Amenoff MJ. Parkinson's disease in the elderly: Current management strategies. *Geriatrics.* 1987; 42(7): 31–37.
6. Hoehn M, Yahr M. Parkinsonism: Onset, progression and mortality. *Neurology.* 1967; 17(5):427–442.
7. Greer M. Recent developments in the treatment of Parkinson's disease. *Geriatrics.* 1985; 40(2):34–41.
8. Banks M. Physiotherapy benefits patients with Parkinson's disease. *Clin Rehab.* 1989; 3:11–16.
9. Schenkman M, Butler R. A model for multisystem evaluation treatment for individuals with Parkinson's disease. *Phys Ther.* 1989; 69(11):932–943.
10. Webster D. Critical analysis of the disability in Parkinson's disease. *Mod Treat.* 1968; 5:257–282.
11. Weinrich M, Koch K, Garcia F, et al. Axial versus distal motor impairment in Parkinson's disease. *Neurology.* 1988; 38(4):540–545.
12. Murray MP, Sepic S, Gardner G, et al. Walking patterns of men with parkinsonism. *Am J Phys Med.* 1978; 57(6):278–294.
13. Henderson C, Kennard C, Crawford S, et al. Scales for rating motor impairment in Parkinson's disease: Studies of reliability and convergent validity. *J Neur Psych.* 1991; 54(1):18–24.
14. Alba A, Trainor F, Ritter W, et al. A clinical disability rating for Parkinson's disease. *J Chron Dis.* 1968; 21:507–522.
15. Schenkman M, Donovan J, Tsubota J. Management of individuals with Parkinson's disease: Rationale and case studies. *Phys Ther.* 1989; 69(11):944–955.
16. Hallet M. Physiology and pathophysiology of voluntary movement. In: Tyler K, Dawson D, eds. *Current Neurology.* Boston: Houghton-Mifflin; 1979: 351–376.
17. Saal JS, ed. *Flexibility Training and Rehabilitation of Sports Training.* Philadelphia: Hardey & Belfus; 1987.
18. Nelson A. *Lecture Notes.* New York: Hospital for Special Surgery; September 1988.
19. Handford F. The Flewitt-Handford exercises for Parkinson's gait. *Physiotherapy.* 1986; 72(8):382.
20. Davis J. Team management of Parkinson's disease. *Am J Occup Ther.* 1977; 31(5):300–308.
21. Rusin M. Stroke rehabilitation: A geropsychological perspective. *Arch Phys Med Rehabil.* October 1990; 71:914–920.
22. Centers for Disease Control and Prevention. *Unrealized Prevention Opportunities: Reducing the Health and Economic Burden of Chronic Disease.* Atlanta, GA: Centers for Disease Control and Prevention, National Center for Chronic Disease Prevention and Health Promotion; 1997.
23. Robins M, Baum H. Incidents. *Stroke.* 1981; 12 (suppl 1):45–57.
24. Kelley R. Cerebral vascular disease. In: Weiner W, Goetz C, eds. *Neurology for the Nonneurologists.* 2nd ed. Philadelphia: Lippincott; 1989: 52–66.
25. Gillum R. Stroke in blacks. *Stroke.* 1988; 19:1–9.
26. Baxter D. Clinical syndromes associated with stroke. In: Brandstater M, Basmajian JV, eds. *Stroke Rehabilitation.* Baltimore: Williams and Wilkins; 1987: 36–54.
27. Dawson D Adams P. Current estimates from the National Health Interview Survey. United States 1986 National Center for Health Statistics. *Vital Health Statistics.* 1987; 10:164.
28. Ryerson S. Hemiplegia resulting from vascular insult or disease. In Umphred D, ed. *Neurological Rehabilitation.* 4th ed. St. Louis: Mosby; 2001.
29. Spriggs D, French J, Murdy J, et al. Historical risk factors for stroke—A case controlled study. *Age Ageing.* 1990; 19:280–287.
30. Ashburn D, Ward C. Asymmetrical trunk posture, unilateral neglect and motor performance following stroke. *Clin Rehab.* 1994; 8(1):48–53.
31. Bohannon R. Correction of recalcitrant lateropulsion through motor relearning. *Phys Ther Case Reports.* 1998; 1:157–159.
32. Gottlieb D, Levine D. Unilateral neglect influences the postural adjustments after stroke. *J Neurol Rehabil.* 1992; 6(1):25–41.
33. Gray C, French J, Bates D. Motor recovery following acute stroke. *Age Ageing.* 1990; 19:179–194.
34. Feigenson JS. Stroke rehabilitation: Effectiveness, benefits, and costs. Some practical considerations. *Stroke.* January–February 1979; 10(l):1–4.
35. Anderson TP, McClure WJ, Athelstan G, et al. Stroke rehabilitation: Evaluation of its quality by assessing patient outcomes. *Arch Phys Med Rehabil.* 1978; 79(4):170–175.
36. Anderson TP, Baldridge M, Ettinger MG. Quality of care for completed stroke without rehabilitation: Evaluation by assessing patient outcomes. *Arch Phys Med Rehab.* 1979; 60(3):103–107.

37. Lehman JF, Delateur BJ, Fowler RS, et al. Stroke: Does rehabilitation affect outcome? *Arch Phys Med Rehabil.* 1975; 56(9):375–382.

38. Schenkman M, Butler RB. A model for multisystem evaluation interpretation and treatment of individuals with neurologic dysfunction. *Phys Ther.* 1989; 69: 538–547.

39. Tripp N, Boudoures K, Dalum A, et al. Initiation of a systemic evaluation to categorize the hemiplegic patient. *Phys Ther.* 1991; 71(Suppl 6):57.

40. Schuling J, deHaan R, Lindberg M, and Groenier KH. The Frenchay Activities Index: 2. Assessment of functional status in stroke patients. *Stroke.* 1993; 8:1173–1177.

41. Lincoln NB, Erdman JA. A revalidation of the Rivermead ADL Scale for Elderly Patients with Stroke. *Age Ageing;* 1990; 19:19–24.

42. Carr J, Shepherd R. *A Motor Re-Learning Programme for Stroke.* Rockville, MD: Aspen Publishers; 1986.

43. Bohannon R. Knee extension torque in stroke patients: Comparison of measurements obtained with a hand-held and a Cybex Dynamometer. *Physiother Can.* November–December 1990; 42(6).

44. Bohannon R. Consistency of muscle strength measurements in patient with stroke: examination from a different perspective. *J Phys Ther Sci.* 1990; 2:1–7.

45. Bohannon R. Is the measurement of muscle strength appropriate in patients with brain lesions? A special communication. *Phys Ther.* March 1989; 69(3): 189–191.

46. Olney S, Colbourne GR. Assessment and treatment of gait dysfunction in the geriatric stroke patient. *Top Geriatr Rehabil.* 1991; 7(1):70–78.

47. Black PO, Kile KA, McCormick J, Rodrguez AA, Roszkowski J, Sherman J, Swiggum E, Stellberg B. Gait training efficacy using a home-based practice model in chronic hemiplegia. *Arch Phys Med Rehabil.* 1996; 77:801–805.

48. Shumway-Cook A, Horak F. Assessing the influence of sensory interaction on balance: Suggestions from the field. *Phys Ther.* 1986; 66(10):1548–1550.

49. Carr J, Shepherd R, Nordholm L, Lynne D. Investigation of a new motor assessment scale for stroke patients. *Phys Ther.* 1985; 65(2).

50. Kumar R, Metter EJ, Mehta AJ, et al. Shoulder pain in hemiplegia. *Am J Phys Med.* August 1990; 69 (4):205 208.

51. Bohannon R, Warren M, Cogman K. Influence of shoulder position on maximum voluntary elbow flexion force in stroke patients. *Occup Ther J Res.* March–April 1991; 11(2):73–79.

52. Davies P. *Steps to Follow.* 2nd ed. New York: Springer Verlag; 2000: 403–428.

53. Brown DA, DeBacher GA. Bicycle ergometer and electromyographic feedback for treatment of muscle imbalance in patients with spastic hemiparesis. *Phys Ther.* 1987; 67(11):1715–1719.

54. Wissel J, Ebersbach G, Gutjahr PDL, et al. Treating chronic hemiparesis with modified biofeedback. *Arch Phys Med Rehabil.* August 1989; 70:612–617.

55. Sackley CM. The relationship between weight-bearing asymmetry after stroke, motor function and activities of daily living. *Physiother Theor Prac.* 1990; 6:179–185.

56. Trueblood PR, Walker JM, Perry J, et al. Pelvic exercise and gait in herniplegia. *Phys Ther.* 1989; 69(l):18–26.

57. Logigian MK, Samuels MA, Falconer J. Clinical exercise trial for stroke patients. *Arch Phys Med Rehabil.* August 1983; 64:364–367.

58. Glenner GG. Alzheimer's disease (senile dementia): A research update and critique with recommendations. *J Am Geriatr Soc.* 1982; 30(1):59–62.

59. Forsyth E, Ritzline PD. An overview of the etiology, diagnosis, and treatment of Alzheimer's disease. *Phys Ther.* 1998; 78(12):1325–1331.

60. Blessed G, Tomlinson BE, Roth M. The association between quantitative measures of dementia and of senile changes in the cerebral grey matter of elderly patients. *Brit J Psychiatry.* 1968; 114:797–911.

61. Rosen WB, Mohs RC, Davis KL. A new rating scale for Alzheimer's disease. *Am J Psychiatry.* 1984; 141: 1256–1364.

62. Boller F, Huff FJ, Querriera R, Kelsey S, Beyer J. Recording neurological symptoms and signs in Alzheimer's disease. *Am J Alzheimer's Care Res.* May–June 1987; 19–29.

63. Bhala RP, O'Connell J, Thoppil E. Ptophobia: Phobic fear of falling and its clinical management. *Phys Ther.* 1982; 62(2):187–190.

64. Hobeika CP. Equilibrium and balance in the elderly. *Ear, Nose, Throat J.* 1999; 78(8):558–566.

65. Horak FB. Clinical measurement of postural control in adults. *Phys Ther.* 1987; 67(12):1881–1885.

66. Dornan J, Fernie GR, Holliday PJ. Visual input: Its importance in the control of postural sway. *Arch Phys Med Rehabil.* 1978; 59(5):586–591.

67. Keshner E, Peterson B. Frequency and velocity characteristics of head, neck, and trunk during normal locomotion. *Soc Neurosci Abst.* 1999; 15(12): 1200–1204.

68. Begbie GH. Some problems of postural sway. In: de Reuck AVS, Knight J, eds. *Myotatic, Kinesthetic, and Vestibular Mechanisms.* Boston: Little, Brown; 1967: 80–92.

69. Horak FB, Shupert CL. Role of the vestibular system in postural control. In: Herdman SJ, ed. *Vestibular Rehabilitation.* 2nd ed. Philadelphia: FA Davis; 2000: 22–46.

70. Hain CH. *Vestibular Rehabilitation.* Philadelphia: FA Davis, 1994.

71. Shimazu H, Smith CM. Cerebellar and labyrinthine influences on singular vestibular neurons identified by natural stimuli. *J Neurophysiol.* 1971; 34(5): 493–508.

72. Mergner T, Becker W. Perception of horizontal self-rotation: Multisensory and cognitive aspects. In: Warren R, Wertheim AH, eds. *Perception and Control of Self-motion.* Mahwah, NJ: Lawrence Erlbaum; 1990: 219–224.

73. Weber PC, Cass SP. Clinical assessment of postural instability. *Am J Otol.* 1993; 14(5):566–569.

74. Tinetti ME, Williams CS. Falls, injuries due to falls, and the risk of admission to a nursing home. *N Engl J Med.* 1997; 337:1279–1284.

75. Wall C, Black FO, Hunt AE. Effects of age, sex and stimulus parameters upon vestibulo-ocular responses to sinusoidal rotation. *Acta Otolaryngol.* 1984; 98:270–278.

76. Rosenhall U. Degenerative patterns in the aging human vestibular neuro-epithelia. *Acta Otolaryngol.* 1973; 76:208–220.

77. Paige GD. Senescence of human visual-vestibular interactions: Smooth pursuit, optokinetic, and vestibular control of eye movements with aging. *Exp Brain Res.* 1994; 98(3):355–372.

78. Keshner EA, Allum JH. Plasticity in pitch sway stabilization: Normal habituation and compensation for peripheral vestibular deficits. In: Bles W, Brandt T, eds. *Disorders of Posture and Gait.* Amsterdam: Elsevier; 1986: 289–298.

79. Allum JH, Keshner EA, Honegger F, Pfaltz CR. Indicators of the influence a peripheral vestibular deficit has on vestibulo-spinal reflex responses controlling postural stability. *Acta Otolaryngol.* 1988; 106:252–263.

80. Black FO, Wall C, O'Leary DP. Computerized screening of the human vestibulospinal system. *Ann Otol Rhinol Laryngol.* 1978; 87:853–860.

81. Romberg MH. *Manual of Nervous Diseases of Man.* London: Sydenham Society; 1853: 395–401.

82. Duncan P. Functional reach: A new clinical measure of balance. *J Gerontol.* 85(5):529–531.

83. Furman JM. Role of posturography in the management of vestibular patients. *Ortolaryngol Head Neck Surg.* 1995; 112(1):8–15.

84. Miller K, Hobeika CP, Sick S. Platform posturography as a predictor or falls. Proceedings of the Association for Research in Otolaryngology. St. Petersburg, FL; 1997.

85. Bottomley JM. Gait in later life. *Ortho Phys Ther Clin North Am.* 2001; 10(1):131–149.

86. Tinetti ME, Speechly M, Ginter SF. Risk factors for falls among elderly persons living in the community. *N Engl J Med.* 1988; 319(26):1701–1707.

87. Furman JM, Cass SP. Benign paroxysmal positional vertigo. *N Engl J Med.* 1999; 341:1590–1596.

88. De Boer AGEM, Wijker W, Speelman JD, de Haes JCJM. Quality of life in patients with Parkinson's disease: Development of a questionnaire. *J Neurol Neurosurg Psychiatry.* 1996; 61:70–74.

89. Nieuwboer A, De Weerdt W, Dom R, Truyen M, Janssens L, Kamsma Y. The effect of a home physiotherapy program for persons with Parkinson's disease. *J Rehabil Med.* 2001; 33:266–272.

90. Cooper C, Evidente VG, Hentz JG, Adler CH, Caviness JN, Gwinn-Hardy K. The effect of temperature on hand function in patients with tremor. *J Hand Ther.* 2000; 13:276–288.

91. Hirsch MA, Toole T, Maitland CG, Rider RA. The effects of balance training in high-intensity resistance training on persons with idiopathic parkinson's disease. *Arch Phys Med Rehabil.* 2003; 84:1109–1117.

92. Miyai I, Fujimoto Y, Ueda Y, Yamamoto H, Nozaki S, Saito T, Kang J. Treadmill training with body-weight support: Its effect on parkinson's disease. *Arch Phys Med Rehabil.* 2000; 81:849–852.

93. Miyai I, Fujimoto Y, Yamamoto H, Ueda Y, Saito T, Nozaki S, Kang J. Long-term effect of body-weight-supported treadmill training in parkinson's disease: A randomized controlled trial. *Arch Phys Med Rehabil.* 2002; 83:1370–1373.

94. Pohl M, Rockstroh G, Ruckriem S, Mrass G, Mehrholz J. Immediate effects of speed-dependent treadmill training on gait parameters in early parkinson's disease. *Arch Phys Med Rehabil.* December 2003; 84.

95. Scandalis TA, Bosak A, Berliner JC, Helman LL, Wells MR. Resistance training and gait function in patients with Parkinson's disease. *Am J Phys Med Rehabil.* 2001; 80:38–43.

96. Blackinton MT, Summerall L, Waguespack K. Tertiary prevention in parkinson's disease: Results from a preliminary study. *Neurol Rep.* 2002; 26:160–165.

97. Baatile J, Langbein WE, Weaver F, Maloney C, Jost MS. Effect of exercise on perceived quality of life of individuals with Parkinson's disease. *Rehabil Res Dev.* 2000; 37(5):529–534.

98. Bridgewater KJ, Sharpe MH. Trunk muscle training and early parkinson's disease. *Physiother Theory Practice.* 1997; 13:139–153.

99. Muller V, et al. Short-term effects of behavioral treatment on movement initiation and postural control in parkinson's disease: A controlled clinical study. *Movement Dis.* 1997; 12(3):306–314.

100. Marchese R, Diverio M, Zucchi F, Lentino C, Abbruzzese G. The role of sensory cues in the rehabilitation of parkinsonian patients: a comparison of two physical therapy protocols. *Movement Dis.* 2000; 15(5):879–883.

101. Viliani T, Pasquetti P, Magnolfi S, Lunardelli M, Giorgi C, Serra P, Taiti P. Effects of physical training on straightening-up process in patients with

parkinson's disease. *Disabil Rehabil.* 1999; 21(2): 68–73.

102. Pacchetti C, Mancini F, Aglieri R, Fundaro C, Martignoni E. Active music therapy in Parkinson's disease: An integrative method for motor and emotional rehabilitation. *Psychosom Med.* 2000; 62: 386–393.

103. Duval C, Lafontaine D, Hebert J, Leroux A, Panisset M, Boucher JP. The effect of trager therapy on the level of evoked stretch response in patients with parkinson's disease and rigidity. *JMPT.* 2002; 25: 455–464.

104. Stalibrass C, Sissons P, Chalmers C. Randomized controlled trial of the Alexander technique for idiopathic parkinson's disease. *Clin Rehab.* 2002; 16: 695–708.

105. Schenkman, Margaret, et al. Exercise to improve spinal flexibility and function for people with parkinson's disease: A randomized controlled study. *J Am Geriatr Soc.* 1998; 46:1207–1216.

106. Monger C, Carr JH, Fowler V. Evaluation of a home-based exercise and training programme to improve sit to stand in patients with chronic stroke. *Clin Rehab.* 2002; 26:361–367.

107. Suzuki T. High intensity strength training improves strength and functional performance after stroke. *Am J Phys Med Rehabil.* 2000; 79(4): 369–376.

108. Bastille JV, Gill-Body KM. A yoga-based exercise program for people with chronic poststroke hemiparesis. *Phys Ther.* 2004; 84:33–48.

109. Dean CM, Richards CL, Moalouin F. Task-related circuit training improves performance of locomotor tasks in chronic stroke: A randomized, controlled pilot Trial. *Arch Phys Med Rehabil.* April 2000; 81:409–417.

110. Kunkle A, et al. Constraint-induced movement therapy for motor recovery in chronic stroke patients. *Arch Phys Med Rehabil.* June 1999; 80:624–628.

111. Sterr A, Elbert A, Berthold I, Kobel S, et al. Longer versus shorter daily constraint-induced movement therapy of chronic hemiparesis: An exploratory study. *Arch Phys Med Rehabil.* 2002; 83:1374–1377.

112. Schenkman M, Keysor J, Chandler J, Laub KD, MacAller H. *Axial Mobility Exercise Program: An Exercise Program to Improve Functional Ability.* Claude Pepper Older American's Independence Center, Durham, NC, 1994.

113. Michaelsen SM, Luta A, Roby-Brami A, Levin MF. Effect of trunk restraint on the recovery of reaching movements in hemiparetic patients. *Stroke.* 2001; 32:1875–1883.

114. Rodriquez GM, Aruin A. The effect of shoe wedges and lifts on symmetry of stance and weight bearing in hemiparetic individuals. *Arch Phys Med Rehabil.* April 2002; 83:478–482.

115. Bassile, CC, Dean C, Boden-Albala B, Sacco R. Obstacle training programme for individuals post stroke: Feasibility study. *Clin Rehab.* 2003; 17: 130–136.

116. Morioka S, Yagi F. Effects of perceptual learning exercises on standing balance using a hardness discrimination task in hemiplegic patients following stroke: A randomized controlled pilot trial. *Clin Rehab.* 2003; 17:600–607.

117. A New Approach to Retrain Gait in Stroke Patients Through Body Weight Support and Treadmill Stimulation, Martha Visintin, Hugues Barbeau, Nicol Korner-Bitensky, and Nancy E. Mayo. Stroke 1998 29: 1122–1128.

118. Barbeau H, Visintin M. Optimal outcomes obtained with body weight support combined with treadmill training in stroke subjects. *Arch Phys Med Rehabil.* 2003; 84:1485–1465.

119. Liston R, Mickelborough J, Harris B, Wynn Hann A, Tallis RC. Conventional physiotherapy and treadmill re-training for higher-level gait disorders in cerebrovascular disease. *Age Ageing.* 2000; 29: 311–318.

120. Sullivan KJ, Knowlton BJ, Dobkin BH. Step training with body weight support: Effect of treadmill speed and practice paradigms and poststroke locomotor recovery. *Arch Phys Med Rehabil.* 2002; 83: 683–691.

121. Kuan, Ta-Shen et al. Hemiplegic gait of stroke patients: The effects of using a cane. *Arch Phys Med Rehabil.* July 1999; 80:777–784.

122. Yavuser G, Ergin S. Effect of an arm sling on gait pattern in patients with hemiplegia. *Arch Phys Med Rehabil.* July 2002; 83:960–963.

123. Laufer Y. The effect of walking aids on balance and weight-bearing patterns of patients with hemiparesis in various stance positions. *Phys Ther,* February 2003; 83:112–122.

124. O'Brien K, Culham E, Pickles B. Balance and skeletal alignment in a group of elderly female fallers and non-fallers. *J Gerontol Biolog Sci.* 1997; 52A(4): B221–B226.

125. Bischoff HA, et al. Identifying a cut-off point for normal mobility: A comparison of the timed "up and go" test in community-dwelling and institutionalised elderly women. *Age Aging.* 2003: B2(3)315–320

126. Vellas BJ, Wayne SJ, Romero L, Baumgartner RN, Rubenstein LZ, Garry PJ. One-leg balance is an important predictor of injurious falls in older persons. *J Am Geriatr Soc.* 1997; 45:735–738.

127. Cohen H, Kane-Wineland M, Miller LV, Hatfiled CL. Occupation and visual/vestibular interaction in vestibular rehabilitation. *Otolaryngol Head Neck Surg.* 1995; 112:526–532.

128. Fansler CL, et al. Effects of mental practice on balance in elderly women. *Phys Ther.* September 1985; 65(9):1332–1338.

129. Rose, D, Clark S. Can the control of bodily orientation be significantly improved in a group of older adults with a history of falls?" *J Am Geriatr Soc.* 2000; 48:275–282.

130. "A Multifactorial Intervention to Reduce the risk of Falling Among Elderly People Living in the

Community". *The New England Journal of Medicine.* Sept. 29, 1994. Vol. 331, No. 13. pp. 822–3.

131. Day L, Fildes B, Gordon I, Fitzharris M, Flamer H, Lord S. Randomised factorial trial of falls prevention among older people living in their own homes. *Brit Med J.* July 20, 2002; 325.

132. Douris P, Southard V, Varga C, Schauss W, Gennaro C, Reiss A. The effect of land and aquatic exercise on balance scores in older adults. *J Geriatr Phys Ther.* 2003; 26(1):043.

133. Wolf SL, et al. Reducing frailty and falls in older persons: An investigation of Tai Chi and computerized balance training. *J Am Geriatr Soc.* May 1996; 44(5).

134. Hauer K, Rost B, Rutschle K, Opitz H, Specht N, Bartsch P, Oster P, Schlierf G. Exercise training for rehabilitation and secondary prevention of falls in geriatric patients with a history of injurious falls. *J Am Geriatric Soc.* 2001; 49:10–20.

135. Ledin T, et al. Effects of balance training in elderly evaluated by clinical tests and dynamic posturography. *J Vestib Res.* 1991; 1(2).

136. Schiller J, Schubert S, Lowe S. The effects of a 12-week progressive resistance program on lower extremity strength and timed up & go measures in community-dwelling elderly: A pilot study. *GeriNotes.* 2001; 8(6):12–20.

137. Toulotte C, Fabre C, Dangremont B, Lensel G, Thevon A. Effects of physical training on the physical capacity of frail, demented patients with a history of falling: A randomised controlled trial. *Age Ageing.* 2003; 32:67–73.

13

Cardiopulmonary and Cardiovascular Considerations

Pearls

- Cardiovascular disease is the major cause of death after age 65, accounting for over 40% of deaths in this population.

- Prolonged inactivity and bed rest quickly and markedly impair cardiovascular functional capacity.

- Cardiopulmonary and cardiovascular changes related to aging include decreases in aerobic capacity, vital capacity, minute volume, maximum cardiac output, maximal obtainable heart rate, stroke volume, maximal oxygen consumption, and an increase in blood pressure.

- The outcomes of aging on the pulmonary system are an increased mechanical workload for breathing, a decrease in the efficiency of gas exchange, and a compromise in the ability to efficiently supply oxygen to peripheral tissues.

- Submaximal stress testing can be done safely for older persons. The various types of tests (step test, modified chair-step test, walking test, treadmill testing, and cycle ergometer testing) are all useful for evaluating cardiovascular status in the elderly.

- Intensity, duration, and frequency—the three major components of exercise prescription—are different for the elderly. Intensity is safe at 60%; duration, which is usually twenty minutes, may need to be cut to four to five minutes initially; frequency should be daily.

- When prescribing exercise for an older person, special considerations and modifications should be made for obese, diabetic, osteoporotic patients; those with pacemakers or on cardiopulmonary medications; and patients with CHF.

INTRODUCTION

Cardiopulmonary considerations are particularly important in treating the elderly population in geriatric rehabilitation settings. Diseases of the heart, lungs, and blood vessels are by far the most prominent causes of morbidity and mortality among elderly individuals, rising logarithmically with age.[1-2] As the number of older individuals at risk for cardiovascular disease continues to rise, and as successful medical treatments for ischemic and hypertensive diseases in the middle-aged population drive up the number of people with known diseases surviving into older age, health care providers will be managing increasing numbers of elderly individuals with cardiopulmonary and cardiovascular disease. Eventually, the process of aging and inactivity takes its toll on the cardiovascular and cardiopulmonary systems and compromises each individual's ability to meet the oxygen demands of activity beyond the resting state.[3]

This chapter covers the cardiopulmonary and cardiovascular changes associated with aging and the physiological aspects of exercise associated with improving cardiopulmonary and cardiovascular health. Evaluation techniques specific to a frailer elderly population are covered, and special considerations when prescribing exercises for people with diseases, including obesity, medications, diabetes mellitus, and osteoporosis are presented.

INCIDENCE OF CARDIOPULMONARY AND CARDIOVASCULAR DISEASE

The projected shift in the age distribution of the population, as described in Chapter 1 of this text, indicates that older individuals comprise an increasing proportion until the middle of the next century, when they will constitute about one-fifth of the total. Currently there are over 33.9 million people in the United States who are 65 years of age and older.[4] Of these, 50% of them have some form of cardiopulmonary or cardiovascular disorders. Indeed, cardiovascular disease is the major cause of death after the age of 65, accounting for over 40% of deaths in this age group.[1] Figure 13.1 demonstrates the rates for leading causes of death among persons aged 65 or older. In 1997, though showing a slight decline in heart disease since 1980, the leading cause of death among persons age 65 or older continues to be heart disease (1832 deaths per 100,000 persons).[2] Elderly people, who contribute 68% of all deaths in the United States annually, account for 78% of deaths attributed to cardiovascular disease.[5] In the most rapidly growing segment of the US population, those 85 years of age and older, cardiovascular and cardiopulmonary diseases account for over 76% of all deaths.[5–6] Morbidity is similarly prevalent in the population over the age of 65. Twenty-eight percent reported significant health impairments related to heart, lung, and vascular conditions, including angina, congestive heart failure, rhythm disturbances, chronic obstructive and restrictive lung diseases, and peripheral vascular disease.[1–2]

The majority of US residents receiving cardiovascular services are believed to be Medicare beneficiaries, and the age-associated increase in prevalence and incidence is true for all forms of cardiovascular and cardiopulmonary disease (except congenital). Although women are often thought to be at lower risk for cardiovascular disease, this relative immunity represents only a 7- to 10-year delay in onset. In fact, as age increases, prevalence rates become more equal with those of men, and ultimately cardiovascular mortality rates in women and men are equivalent.[7] More people in the US population, as a whole, die of cardiovascular disease than the combined total of other leading causes of death (Figure 13.2). As Figure 13.2 depicts, cardiovascular disease tops the list of the ten leading causes of death in the United States and annually kills more Americans than all the other diseases combined, including cancer, diabetes, AIDS, and suicide. One in four Americans, nearly 59 million, suffers from cardiovascular disease. The American Heart Association estimates that the cost per year in health care and lost productivity is approximately $138 billion, which represents about one-seventh of the total health bill. As cardiovascular disease doesn't start in old age (i.e., after the age of 65), preventive measures must be addressed throughout the life cycle.

Implications

The most frequently occurring problem is atherosclerotic heart disease. It is common to find hypertension coexisting with atherosclerotic heart disease. Congestive heart failure, arrhythmias, and electrocardiographic abnormalities have an increased incidence with aging.[8] Cardiac disease in the elderly is complicated by the fact that it rarely occurs in isolation. Pulmonary problems, such as chronic obstructive pulmonary disease (COPD) and emphysema, usually result in death from the cardiac complications they impose, and vascular diseases generally accompany cardiac disease or predispose an individual to the development of cardiovascular and cardiopulmonary pathologies (see Chapter 5). Chronic inactivity, resulting from musculoskeletal or neuromuscular causes, or systemic diseases, further exacerbates the effects of aging on the cardiovascular system. Deaths from cardiovascular disease are only part of the story. The debilitating effects on individuals who survive a stroke or a heart attack lead to a loss in

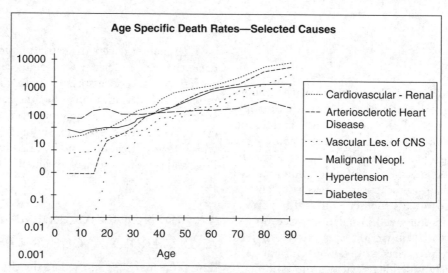

Figure 13.1 Age-specific death rates indicate that cardiovascular causes of death occur most frequently with advancing age. (Source: National Center for Health Statistics. *Health, United States, 1999 with Health and Aging Chartbook.* Hyattsville, MD: National Center for Health Statistics; 1999.)

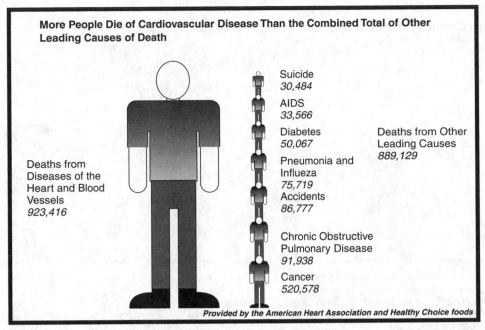

Figure 13.2   Comparison of deaths from cardiovascular disease to other leading causes of death. (Source: American Heart Association and Healthy Choice Foods; 1998.)

functional capabilities and severely impact the individual's ability to maintain independence as depicted in Figure 13.3.

Cardiac rehabilitation is a means of improving the cardiopulmonary response to increased oxygen demands during increased activity through endurance and conditioning exercises. The progression of the aging process eventually evolves into diseases in the cardiovascular and cardiopulmonary systems. Any of the pathologies mentioned above will lead to an inhibition of the cardiopulmonary responses to increased oxygen demands. Functional level of activity decreases as a result of a vicious cycle of inactivity and deconditioning, imposed by a variety of medical problems in the musculoskeletal, neuromuscular, and sensory systems, that can cause cardiovascular disability or may exacerbate underlying cardiac disease.

Prolonged inactivity and bed rest quickly and markedly impair cardiovascular functional capacity.[9-11] All too often, deconditioning of the cardiopulmonary system is potentiated by excessive bed rest and overmedication for the elderly cardiac patient. Even prior to illness, many elderly patients decrease their activity level due to a varied combination of musculoskeletal and neuromuscular problems. Additionally, because of the decreased aerobic capacity with aging, any submaximal task is perceived as requiring increased work because of its increased relative energy cost and resulting fatigue. Relative inactivity thus potentiates the decreased physical work capacity in the elderly, often threatening the possibility of an independent lifestyle. This can be avoided and, indeed, functional capacity can be improved with conditioning and endur-

ance exercises, and the reinstitution of the older person's participation in functional activities of daily living (ADL).

There has been increased interest in research about the effects of exercise on the aged cardiac patient.[9-11] Perhaps this is a result of the growing numbers of the elderly and changing demographic and sociologic patterns.[6] Individuals are living relatively healthy lives well beyond the socially imposed demarcation line that defines old age.[12-13] The expectations of acceptable levels of function for the elderly segment of the population have changed. Research studies have demonstrated that not only is exercise beneficial for maintaining functional baseline condition in the unimpaired elderly individual, but it is also therapeutic for reversing the effects of impairment and improving baselines in individuals who have become deconditioned as a result of symptom limitations (e.g., angina and dyspnea).[11,14]

American society's increased focus on exercise and a corresponding broadening of the expectations among the elderly for an active lifestyle, have increased their participation in physical activity programs. As a result, it is important that physical therapists be involved with the development of clinical procedures that are safe and effective in exercise assessment and prescription for the elderly. Therapeutic evaluation and program planning have now reached the point where the elderly individual, who was once confined to bed because of angina and dyspnea resulting from cardiopulmonary disease, can be evaluated and treated with a total rehabilitation program. This should include an individualized exercise prescription that

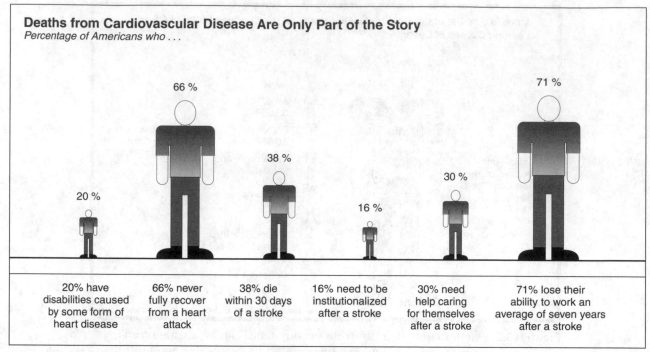

Deaths from Cardiovascular Disease Are Only Part of the Story
Percentage of Americans who . . .

20 %	66 %	38 %	16 %	30 %	71 %
20% have disabilities caused by some form of heart disease	66% never fully recover from a heart attack	38% die within 30 days of a stroke	16% need to be institutionalized after a stroke	30% need help caring for themselves after a stroke	71% lose their ability to work an average of seven years after a stroke

Figure 13.3   Debilitating effects of cardiovascular disease. (Source: American Heart Association and Healthy Choice Foods; 1998.)

considers the severity of disease, attempts symptom reversal, and has functional improvement as its primary goal. Cardiopulmonary considerations are important in the geriatric population for the prescription of any activity, as cardiopulmonary pathological manifestations are most likely to accompany increasing age in close to 100% of the elderly population we see in the clinic.

PHYSIOLOGICAL ASPECTS OF EXERCISE

Human performance is a remarkable integration of all of the systems of the body. Practically no tissue or organ escapes involvement in increasing activity levels. While the muscles perform the work, the heart and peripheral vascular systems deliver the nutrients and, with the assistance of the pulmonary system, provide O_2 to and remove CO_2 from the working tissues. The nervous and endocrine systems integrate all of this activity into meaningful performance. At the cellular level, the mitochondria and numerous enzymes are activated and energy is generated to enable the muscle to contract. Skin acts as the heating and cooling system as activity is prolonged, and the kidneys assist in maintaining a homeostatic fluid balance. It is apparent that any pathological manifestation involving any of the body systems will negatively influence the physiologic response to exercise.[9]

The heart is an amazing organ. Despite its decreased power and ability to contract, slower rate of recovery, diminished cardiac reserve, and the other changes of aging

and disease, the human heart continues to function well as long as it is not overwhelmed by disease. By the time a person is eighty to ninety years of age, the heart has long outperformed the best mechanical pumps devised by man. By the age of one hundred, the human heart has beat more than 3.6 billion times and pumped more than 288 billion cubic centimeters of blood. The ability of the cardiovascular and cardiopulmonary systems to respond to stress admittedly decreases with advancing age, but many elderly people, even with heart disease, can continue their normal routine activities well into older age.

During the normal life span, the cardiovascular and cardiopulmonary systems are subject to a variety of normal physiologic stimuli and processes that may create pathological consequences. In addition, the biologic changes of aging, beginning after the process of growth and development, the evolution of maturity and adulthood, and proceeding into the phases of senescence and old age, modify the anatomic, physiologic, and functional capabilities of the heart, lungs, and vascular systems.

CARDIOPULMONARY CHANGES WITH AGING AND DISEASE

The changes in the cardiopulmonary system related to aging and disease have been discussed in Chapters 3 and 5, respectively, and will only be summarized in this chapter as a foundation for cardiopulmonary treatment considerations in the elderly.

There is some controversy over the degree of physiologic change that is expressly age related as opposed to disease related. Most investigators agree, however, that certain changes in muscle strength and in cardiac and pulmonary function are so common that they may be thought of as universal. Because rehabilitation exercise programs increase the level of activity above resting states, these changes are likely to affect the older person. Aerobic capacity (VO$_2$ max) decreases with advancing age,[14] and declines in aerobic capacity are probably greater in the patient who has become deconditioned during a recent hospital stay or who had poor exercise habits prior to developing a disability. Exercise capacity may be further affected by decreases in vital capacity and minute volume.[15] Additional cardiopulmonary changes related to aging include increased blood pressure and decreased maximum cardiac output.[11,14] Maximal obtainable heart rate and stroke volume decline in relation to the decrease in maximal oxygen consumption (VO$_2$ max).[15] With age, lean muscle mass decreases as does muscle strength[16] and will be discussed in this chapter as it relates to the cardiopulmonary system's need to meet working muscles' energy demands. Orthostatic hypotension is frequently seen, particularly in those recently bedridden. Peripheral vascular resistance rises with age, increasing the risk of developing hypertensive episodes with exercise programs.

The heart demonstrates little change in the size of its chambers, but the left ventricular wall thickens and becomes less compliant.[17] There is a thickening of or a development of nodular ridges along the attachments of the aortic cusps.[18] The conduction system displays relatively little change in the atrioventricular (AV) node or the bundle of His, though the number of proximal bundle fascicles connecting the left to the main bundle may be reduced.[19]

Coronary artery or ischemic heart disease is the most prevalent disease in individuals over the age of 60.[13] In 90% to 95% of the cases, the reduction of blood flow to the heart is the result of atherosclerotic narrowing of the coronary lumen.[17] This reduction in flow creates the manifestations of angina, myocardial infarction, and sudden death. Angina and infarction impair function by decreasing the maximum cardiac output and maximum oxygen consumption. Infarction or necrosis of the heart muscle limits the distensibility of the heart and reduces the stroke volume. Collectively, these pathologic changes produce a self-limiting impediment to cardiac function. Increased systemic demands for oxygen necessitate an increase in cardiac output or myocardial work. Increased work requires an increased supply of O$_2$ to the myocardial muscle. The restricted coronary blood flow results in ischemia, which increases the left end-diastolic pressure, prolongs systole as the heart is unable to relax, and stiffens the ventricle wall. A destructive cycle is instituted as these physiological changes reduce perfusion of the myocardium and increase the degree of ischemia further damaging cardiac tissue.[14] The result of this vicious circle is progressive deconditioning of the heart as angina and dyspnea self-limit and impair functional activity and exercise capacity.

Lung changes are characterized by an increase in residual volume accompanied by a decrease in vital capacity. Declines are seen in maximal voluntary ventilation, the surface area for gas exchange, the rate of diffusion, and the arteriovenous oxygen differential.[20] Both the lung tissue and chest wall lose elasticity. Cardiopulmonary demands usually can be met, but when disease or deconditioning is present, the demands may exceed the available reserve. All of these changes result in reduced tolerance for physical activity and are important to consider with regard to rate and intensity of activities for the older person. Due to the wide variety in lifestyles, the rate and magnitude of changes cannot be predicted and may not be apparent until they impact on ADL.

The anatomic and functional changes seen in COPD mimic those seen in aging. Both are characterized by microtraumas that occur over time, which do not interfere with resting or low-level ventilatory function.[21–22] The pathological tissue changes seen with emphysema and chronic bronchitis are also similar to the tissue changes of advancing age. The degree of impairment is the distinguishing factor between what is considered "normal" aging and the degree of impairment and compromise that is considered pathological. In emphysema there is an abnormal enlargement of the terminal airspaces as a result of a loss in tissue elasticity of the lung. This results is expiratory collapse of the larger airways. Expiration is difficult for the patient with emphysema. Chronic bronchitis is accompanied by a persistant productive cough on a daily basis. The result of these respiratory conditions is an increase in the work of breathing and an inability to meet the energy demands required for functional activities of living, exercise, or both.

Maximal Oxygen Consumption (VO$_2$ max)

The major function of the cardiovascular and cardiopulmonary systems during exercise is to deliver blood to the active tissues, supplying O$_2$ and nutrients, and removing metabolic waste products. If exercise is prolonged, the cardiovascular system also assists in maintaining body temperature.

The cardiac and pulmonary systems integrate a number of component functions in order to adequately acquire and distribute O$_2$ to the working muscles. The muscles of the thorax contract to initiate an increase in thoracic volume and to lower the intrathoracic pressure. A decrease in the intrathoracic pressure creates gas flow from the higher-pressured atmosphere into the conducting tubules where the gas is warmed, filtered, humidified, and mixed with existing gases to produce an alveolar oxygen tension of 90–100 mm Hg.[9] Alveolar oxygen is diffused across the 70-square-meter blood gas interface into pulmonary capillaries via an approximate 40 mm Hg pressure gradient where it combines with hemoglobin and then enters the left atrium.

The heart, through rhythmic contraction, delivers the oxygenated blood to the myocardial muscle first and then to the peripheral tissues. The pressure created by the contraction of the heart (systolic) overcomes systemic pressure and generates blood flow through the arterial vascular system.

Maximal oxygen consumption (VO_2 max) is the best measure of cardiopulmonary fitness. It can be derived by a simple equation: $VO_2 = Q \times (aO_2 - vO_2)$. VO_2 is the amount of oxygen the system absorbs and is equal to cardiac output (Q) multiplied by the arterial oxygen content (aO_2) minus the central venous oxygen content (vO_2). Each link of this multistaged process needs to be adequately functioning in order for the system to efficiently acquire, transport, and deliver O_2. An impairment at any phase as a result of disease, age, or deconditioning limits the amount of O_2 uptake and competent delivery to the working tissues.

Heart Rate

The resting heart rate is influenced by age, body position, the level of cardiopulmonary fitness, and various environmental factors (e.g., temperature, humidity, altitude). Resting heart rate remains relatively constant with age though in advanced age it may show a decline. Better cardiopulmonary fitness results in a decrease in resting heart rate, whereas the resting heart rate will increase in higher environmental temperatures or at an increase in altitude.[23]

Before exercise the heart rate may be increased by an anticipatory response, a reflection of a sympathetic neurohumoral effect. As exercise begins, the heart rate increases, but during low levels of exercise at a constant workload, the heart rate will attain a plateau or steady state. As workload increases, the heart rate increases in a roughly linear manner. At higher workloads, the heart rate takes longer to plateau. For the same workload, the more fit individual will have a lower steady-state value.

The older individual shows a lower response given the same workload, but at progressively higher workloads, will eventually reach a level that is totally exhausting. Prior to this, however, the heart rate will have reached a plateau at its maximum.

The maximum heart rate declines with age. Each individual has a definable maximum heart rate. The equation for maximum achievable heart rate is 220 minus the person's age. Figure 13.4 provides a worksheet for calculating aerobic and anaerobic training ranges. This provides an approximation of the mean maximal heart rate for any one age category with a standard deviation of 10, so this equation should be used cautiously. The decline in maximum heart rate with age has been attributed mainly to changes in the myocardial oxygen supply, but additional factors include pathological impairment of blood flow to the sinus node, producing a lower heart rate during maximal exercise (the "sick sinus" syndrome), and greater stiffness (reduced compliance) of the heart wall, which increases the time required for filling of the ventricles and interferes

with the "feedback" of information on venous filling to the cardioregulatory center.[23]

Heart rate responses will vary at rest and submaximal exercise levels according to the degree of cardiovascular impairment, whereas the maximum achievable heart rate shows a progressive decline with age.[9,23] Heart rate responses to physiologic stimuli such as postural change and cough have also been shown to decrease with age.[18] In an older, frailer population, it is not necessary to reach aerobic heart rate levels to gain improvements in cardiovascular health. Any activity above rest works! The importance of activity beyond the resting level cannot be emphasized enough in an elderly population.

Stroke Volume

The difference between the end-diastolic and end-systolic blood volumes is the stroke volume. The stroke volume response is highly dependent on hydrostatic pressure effects. When sitting or standing, without exercise, the stroke volume is reduced relative to the supine position due to blood pooling in the extremities. The maximum stroke volume attained during exercise in supine or sitting position is only slightly higher. The increase is sufficient to overcome the effect of venous pooling. Stroke volume at rest in the erect position varies between 50 mL and 80 mL. In a highly trained athlete, this volume can be as high as 200 mL. The stroke volume increases linearly with the workload until it reaches its maximum at approximately 50% of the individual's capacity for exercise.[9]

There is some controversy as to whether there is a change in stroke volume with age or if the changes are a result of a decline in VO_2 max, a slower maximum heart rate response, and an increased peripheral resistance that diminishes the ejection fraction.[24] Understanding the significance of stroke volume changes has been hampered to some extent by the inability to accurately measure absolute left ventricular dimensions (i.e., end-diastolic and end-systolic volumes).[25] Studies have suggested that there is no age-related change in stroke volume at rest[26] and that the ejection fraction remains unchanged with age at rest.[27] During exercise, end-diastolic volume and end-systolic volume showed marked age-related increases as higher levels of exercise were achieved according to a study by Rodeheffer and associates.[28] Elderly subjects showed an increase in end-diastolic volume at low levels of exercise and continued to show progressive increases with increasing exercise intensity. End-systolic volume in elderly subjects also increased with exercise, though less dramatically. Younger subjects at high levels of exercise showed no change in the end-diastolic volume from resting levels while end-systolic volume decreased significantly. The implication of these volume changes is that the young population maintains cardiac output by achieving a high heart rate and that healthy older individuals maintain cardiac output by dilating the ventricle and

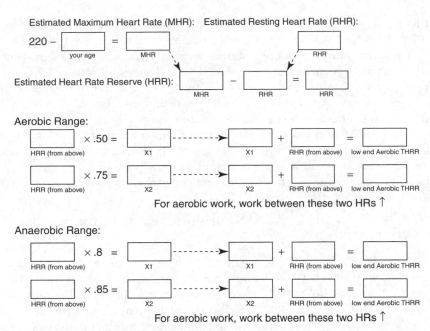

Figure 13.4   Worksheet for calculating aerobic and anaerobic training heart rate ranges. *Aerobic Example: Using 70 years of age with a resting heart rate (RHR) of 80. Maximum Heart Rate (MHR) = 220 − 80 = 140. Subtracting RHR from MHR you get 140 − 80 = 60 for Heart Rate Reserve (HRR). Aerobic training heart rate range (THRR) will lie between 50% and 75% of the HRR added to the RHR: 50% of 60 = 30; 75% of 60 = 45. Adding these figures to the RHR gives: 80 + 30 = 110 and 80 + 45 = 125. Thus the THRR would be 110 to 125 beats per minute. Anaerobic Example: To calculate anaerobic heart rate range take 80% of 60 = 48 and 85% of 60 = 51. Adding these figures to RHR gives: 80 + 48 = 128 and 80 + 51 = 131. Thus the anaerobic threshold THRR is 128 to 131 beats per minute.*

utilizing the Frank-Starling mechanism to increase stroke volume.[28]

Cardiac Output

The cardiac output (CO) at rest is 4 to 6 liters per minute (L/min). It increases linearly with workload. At exercise levels of 40% to 60%, the increase in CO is accomplished through an increase in both the heart rate and the stroke volume. At higher levels of exercise, the increase in CO results solely from the continued increase in heart rate. Maximal values of cardiac output during exercise are dependent on many factors. Body size and the degree of physical fitness appear to have the most prominent influence on CO. For instance, in a small, deconditioned individual the maximum CO during exercise could be as little as 20 L/min, whereas in a large, well-conditioned individual the CO can reach 40 L/min.[14,23]

Physiologic changes in the cardiovascular system primarily involve the determinants of CO. Cardiac output is affected by preload and afterload conditions, which are altered by aging. Early diastolic filling is decreased as a result of mitral valve thickening and/or the decrease in the compliance of the left ventricle.[19] There is an increase in afterload with aging as well. This is possibly produced by an increase in the rigidity of the ascending aorta and a general decrease in the diameter of the peripheral vascular system. This combination of factors increases the overall load on the myocardium and is responsible for the age-associated decrease in cardiac output.

Blood Pressure

The normal response of the blood pressure is a linear increase in systolic pressure with increasing work (200 Hg or higher). Blood pressure changes in aged individuals are dependent on many factors, including extracellular fluid volume, vascular tone and reactivity, the autonomic nervous system, and the arterial baroreceptor reflexes. Each component factor can affect responsiveness in the aged individual somewhat differently. Resting systolic and diastolic blood pressures tend to rise with age; however, the range is quite variable.[19,23] Diastolic blood pressure changes little in healthy elderly individuals. An increase in systemic blood pressure with age is related to the loss of elasticity in the walls of the larger arteries, which raises systolic and depresses diastolic pressures. There is also the increased liability of vasopressor control, which tends to raise both systolic and diastolic pressures. As a result, the systolic arterial blood pressure rises progressively up to the age of 75 years, and the diastolic pressure rises slightly to the age of 60 and then gradually declines.[29]

Arteriovenous Oxygen Differential

The arteriovenous oxygen difference is the difference between the O_2 in the arteries compared to the O_2 content in the veins. It reflects the amount of O_2 that the peripheral tissues extract. The maximum arteriovenous oxygen difference tends to decrease with age.[30] Shepard[14] suggests that factors contributing to this decline with age include: lower levels of physical fitness; a reduction of arterial oxygen saturation; a decreased hemoglobin level; poor peripheral blood distribution; a loss of activity in tissue enzyme systems; and a greater relative blood flow to the skin.

The arteriovenous oxygen difference tends to be larger in the elderly compared to young adults both at rest and at submaximal exercise levels, indicating that there is a decrease in the amount of O_2 extracted in older subjects.[31] Some increase in the stroke volume in combination with a decrease in mechanical efficiency of the cardiopulmonary and cardiovascular systems could explain this. Horvath and Borgia[32] report that there is no reduction in the amount of O_2 saturation/transport capacity of arterial blood. The metabolic potential of skeletal muscle does not decline;[33] however, there is a decrease in the capillary/fiber ratio in the aged muscle[34] and a reduction in the amount of blood that flows to the periphery.[35]

Peripheral Vascular Resistance

Blood flow from the heart varies with tissue needs. During exercise, blood is shunted from areas of little or no metabolic activity (e.g., the gut) to those tissues that are involved in the exercise. Blood to the heart increases proportionally to the increase in metabolic activity.[9] Blood to the skin and muscles is increased, and blood to the stomach and intestines is decreased. The effective blood volume decreases from maximal levels with prolonged work and in a hot and humid environment, because of the increased blood flow to the periphery that promotes both metabolic and environmental heat loss.[14]

Vascular changes of age affect each tissue layer differently. The cells of the intima become irregularly aligned instead of orienting themselves along the longitudinal axis of the vessel.[19] The subendothelial layer becomes thickened due to lipid deposition, calcification, and increased cross-linking of the connective tissue. The media demonstrates increased calcification and fraying of the elastic fibers. These changes all lead to regional differences in vessel diameter and increase in the resistance to blood flow.

The peripheral vascular resistance may be increased by atheromatous plaques in the lumina and, with a loss in vessel elasticity, and a failure to vasodilate in response to increasing activity. Regular exercise can reduce the resting systemic pressure by about 5 mm Hg, but it has little influence on the peripheral pressure during maximum effort.[36]

Neurohumoral Factors

There is a decline in the neurohumoral controls with aging, which reduces the ability to adjust to external and internal stresses.[14] The body hormones contribute to the regulation of circulating fluid volumes and cardiovascular performance. They also mobilize blood glucose, liberate fat, and break down protein to provide energy for increasing activity levels. Neurohumoral factors are important in tissue repair because they are involved with the synthesis of new protein (anabolism), which is important in the healing process at the cellular level.

Fluid loss in prolonged exercise results in a decrease in plasma volume, hemoconcentration of red blood cells (RBCs) and plasma proteins. This hemoconcentration results in an increase in RBCs by 20% to 25%, and there is a shift of fluid from the plasma to the interstitial fluid.[14]

The blood pH shows little change up to approximately 50% intensity of exercise. Past 50%, the pH decreases and the blood becomes more acidic. This decrease in pH is primarily the result of an increase in anaerobic muscle metabolism and corresponds to an increase in blood lactate.

Neurohumoral regulatory changes affect the physiologic response of the elderly individual. Catecholamines function to maintain the systemic pressure, mobilize muscle glycogen to sustain plasma glucose, liberate fatty acids, stimulate gluconeogenesis in the liver, stimulate glucagon secretion, and inhibit insulin secretion.[14] Although there may be an increase in the plasma-catecholamine levels with advancing age,[37] there is a decrease in the end-organ responsiveness to β-adrenergic stimulation.[19] This variation in circulating catecholamines or decrease in neuroresponsiveness may partially account for the decreased heart rate and blood pressure response to activities such as a cough or Valsalva maneuver. This attenuated responsiveness is also partly attributed to decreased baroreceptor sensitivity.[37]

PULMONARY RESPONSE TO EXERCISE

Pulmonary ventilation or minute volume increases from approximately 6 L/min at rest to above 100 L/min during maximal exercise, and in a well-conditioned individual, this can exceed 200 L/min. This is accomplished by an increase in both tidal volume and respiratory frequency. Tidal volume at rest is about 0.5 L/min and can increase to 2.5 to 3.0 L/min during maximal exercise efforts. Resting respiratory frequency ranges from 12 to 16 breaths/minute and increases to 40 to 50 breaths/minute during maximal exercise.[9]

The respiratory system is responsible for ventilation through the coordinated contraction of the diaphragm and associated ventilatory muscles, the displacement of the rib cage, and the expansion of the lungs by the negative pressure created by the contraction of these muscles. The resting length and strength of the ventilatory muscles, the thoracic cage compliance, and the compliance of the lungs are important factors in generating adequate gas flow. Aging produces a progressive decrease in the thoracic wall and bronchiolar compliance.[38] Because of structural changes in bone, cartilage, and elastic structures with age, the chest wall becomes stiff. There is an increase in cross-linking of collagen fibers, a decrease in the resiliency of elastic and cartilaginous tissue, and a decrease in collagen and the annulus fibrosis.[14,36] The elastic fibers within the lung change so that there is an increase in compliance of the lung, but a decrease in its elastic recoil.[39] Superimposed on a decreased compliance of the thoracic wall, this results in a decrease in total lung compliance with age. There is an increase in the size and number of alveolar fenestrae[40] that, in combination with the change in elastic features at the alveolar levels and the loss of tissue from the alveolar walls and septa, results in a decrease in the surface area available for gas exchange. The conducting tubules become more rigid, decreasing their radius and increasing resistance to gas flow.[36] The result is an increased mechanical workload for breathing and a decrease in the efficiency of gas exchange.

The pulmonary systemic changes produced by pathological lung changes as those seen in COPD, emphysema, and chronic bronchitis increase the work of breathing and decrease the energy supply available to working muscles. There is a reduction in vital capacity due to an increased residual volume, a decreased forced expiratory volume, and a reduced arterial oxygen tension with an increase in the carbon dioxide tension.[3,14] In combination with a decrease in thoracic compliance and progressive narrowing of the airways, the force required for the ventilatory muscles to create airflow severely stresses the cardiopulmonary system and compromises the ability to efficiently supply O_2 to peripheral tissues.[41]

BENEFITS OF EXERCISE TRAINING IN THE ELDERLY

Cardiac, vascular, and pulmonary diseases need not be a barrier to better fitness. Too many health care professionals working with the elderly have set their sights low by accepting as normal the reduced ability of aging people who are inactive, sedentary, or incapacitated by subclinical or clinical disease. For instance, a decline in cardiac output is considered a normal process in aging; however, according to noninvasive studies with radioactive thallium nuclear and echocardiographic studies, the decline in cardiac output is absent in physically fit older people without occult coronary artery disease.[28] Most studies dealing with changes in cardiopulmonary response to exercise are done on more sedentary and less physically fit elderly individuals who may very likely have subclinical cardiopulmonary or cardiovascular disease.

There are limited studies on the role of exercise in the prevention of coronary and pulmonary problems in the elderly population. However, epidemiological studies suggest the clear role that increased activities (exercise, occupational, recreational, and leisure) play in decreasing the risk of developing cardiovascular and cardiopulmonary diseases.[9–10,23,42–43] Lack of exercise progressively becomes a more important risk factor in the development of cardiopulmonary and cardiovascular pathologies.[10–11,42–44] The relative body weight has less influence on the chances of developing a fatal heart attack.[45] Shepard[14] suggests that this may reflect the confounding influence of an increasing loss of lean tissue.

For more information on the benefits of exercise training in the elderly, see CD.

BENEFITS OF EXERCISE FOR PERIPHERAL VASCULAR CIRCULATION

Peripheral vascular disease results in increased peripheral vascular resistance due to narrowing and loss of elasticity in the vessel walls. Peripheral arterial insufficiency is present in most elderly individuals in varying degrees.

Indications of poor circulation in the feet include the absence of the dorsal pedal and posterior tibialis pulses, muscle fatigue, cramps in the foot and leg, intermittent claudication, pain, burning, coldness, pallor, paresthesias, atrophy of soft tissues, nail bed alterations, and trophic dermal changes such as dryness and loss of hair on the lower extremities. Prime significance should not be placed on the absence or presence of pedal pulses as the pulses may not be palpable at pressures between 70 and 100 mm Hg and are usually absent below 70 mm Hg. The ankle/brachial index may be lower in some patients with palpable pulses due to hypertension compared to normotensive patients with lower ankle pressures and nonpalpable pulses.

Decreased vascularization increases the likelihood of injury due to fragility of the tissues. Delayed and inadequate healing results because there is a decrease in oxygen supply to the peripheral tissues. Assessment of the two separate vascular beds in the lower extremity should include the major arterial system as well as the small arteries, arterioles, capillaries, and venules which nourish the skin. In most cases the small vessels are dependent on the flow of the major vessels. However, in chronic occlusive vascular disease in which partial or complete occlusion of the major vessels occurs, the blood supply to the tissues may be adequate due to extensive collateral arterial circulation developed by the body as a defense to the slowly progressing ischemia.

The physiological basis for the use of Buerger-Allen exercises is hypothetical and the authors of this book present this theoretical explanation based on clinical experience. The importance of treating individuals with arterial insufficiency is threefold: to enhance peripheral circulation, to prevent limb loss, and to permit healing of wounds. The aim of Buerger-Allen exercises in the treatment of occlusive arterial disease is to improve circulation in a noninvasive therapeutic way.

Buerger-Allen exercises are postural exercises that hypothetically increase local collateral circulation and stimulate circulatory flow through postural changes thereby enhancing tissue nourishment and blood supply.[46] The addition of active muscle contraction during each positional change also appears to improve circulation by stimulating blood flow to the working muscles to increase oxygenation and by the "milking" of the contracting muscles around the vascular structures. Buerger-Allen exercises are based on the theory that the alternating emptying and filling of blood vessels increases the efficiency of transporting blood by stimulating the peripheral vascular system.[47] Research currently underway clearly indicates that there are physiological improvements observed that enhance circulation, facilitate wound healing, and decrease hypersensitivity and pain in the lower extremities of elderly patients with peripheral vascular involvement.[48] Additionally, preliminary results indicate that Buerger-Allen exercises employed in the diabetic population are effective in enhancing circulation in the lower extremities and diminishing, if not eliminating, paresthetic pain in diabetics, in addition to improving muscle function through active foot and ankle pumping.[48]

Buerger-Allen exercises are performed according to the protocol displayed in Figures 13.5 through 13.7. The starting position is with the legs horizontal in supine, as depicted in Figure 13.5. The individual elevates the lower extremities at an angle of 45° until blanching occurs or for a maximum time of three minutes (Figure 13.6). Active pumping and circling of the feet and isometric quadriceps and gluteal contractions are performed for one minute or more (not necessarily a consecutive minute) in the elevated position. Once the blanching has occurred in the elevated position, the subject returns to the horizontal position for three minutes, pumping and circling the feet for one minute of that time. The feet should go from a blanched color to a warm, rosy pink color. The subject then sits up and hangs the legs over the edge of the bed (Figure 13.7). While in this position, again the individual is encouraged to actively plantarflex, dorsiflex, and circle the feet. This position is maintained for a minimum of three minutes or until rubor has occurred. Last, the individual returns to the horizontal position with the lower extremities flat for another three minutes (Figure 13.5). Again, active muscle contraction of the leg muscles is performed for at least one minute in this position. One note of caution: in the elderly, Bottomley recommends assuming the flat/supine position between the elevation and dependent phases to prevent the consequences of orthostatic hypotension. Buerger's original protocol goes from the elevated position directly to the dependent position. The entire sequence is repeated three times in each exercise session (for a total of thirty-six minutes of exercise). Buerger-Allen exercises should be performed once each day for maximum benefit. If the patient is not able to actively contract the muscles in the lower extremities (e.g., peripheral neuropathy is present and active muscle contraction is not possible, patient has a flaccid lower extremity due to hemiplegia), the clinician can passively plantarflex and dorsiflex the foot in each of the respective positions to increase blood flow and facilitate the pumping action of the surrounding musculature. The authors of this book have successfully employed high-frequency electrical stimulation to elicit threshold muscle contractions in the lower extremities of the elderly patient with peripheral neuropathy as well.

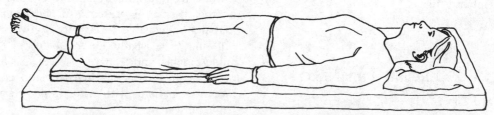

Figure 13.5   Buerger-Allen Protocol—Horizontal Position. Lying flat on back in rest position, pump and circle feet to facilitate circulation. Position maintained for at least three minutes. (Bottomley, J.M. [artist].)

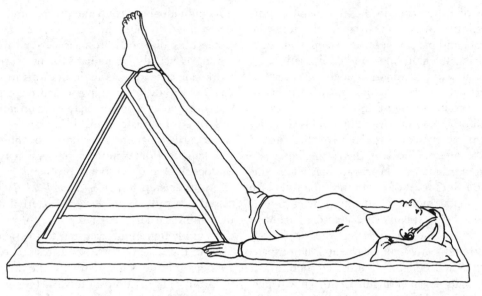

Figure 13.6   Buerger-Allen Protocol—Legs Elevated. Lie on back with legs elevated at least twelve inches higher than the chest and ideally at 45 degrees. Pump and circle feet to enhance circulation. Maintain this position for three minutes.

If the individual is in congestive heart failure (CHF), the Buerger-Allen protocol is modified by omitting the elevated position or having the patient seated upright (in cases of extreme CHF) and moving the lower extremities from a horizontal to a dependent position only. An absolute contraindication in the use of Buerger-Allen exercises is cellulitis.

EXAMINATION, EVALUATION, AND MODIFIED EXERCISE TESTING

In an elderly person's routine cardiopulmonary and vascular physical evaluation, particular attention must be paid to the neuromuscular, musculoskeletal, and sensory examination, because results of these tests will yield valuable information on residual abilities and potential for improvement. Goals of the examination include observation of deviations from normal structure or function, evidence of secondary complications from cardiopulmonary and cardiovascular diseases, and assessment of residual strengths.

Skin should be closely inspected, particularly over bony prominences, for evidence of excessive pressure, friction, or maceration that may lead to breakdown. With the high prevalence of diabetic and arteriosclerotic peripheral vascular disease in the elderly, it is also prudent to inspect the skin of the feet, particularly between the toes.

A musculoskeletal exam should include an evaluation for posture, joint range of motion, flexibility, and tenderness, and muscle strength with an emphasis on existing imbalances or asymmetry. An assessment for any complaints of pain should also be incorporated. Ambulatory status and gait pattern assessment are crucial in developing a reconditioning program.

In a neurological examination, mental status should be routinely evaluated. A routine check on appearance, affect, orientation, and communication is helpful in determining an elderly individual's level of functioning and

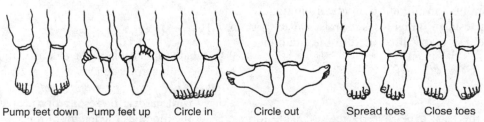

Pump feet down   Pump feet up   Circle in   Circle out   Spread toes   Close toes

Figure 13.7   Buerger-Allen Protocol—Legs Dependent. Sit with legs hanging over side of bed. In this position pump and circle feet, spread toes, then pinch toes together. Maintain the dependent position for three minutes.

safety. Other areas of importance in the neurologic examination include testing of sensation (particularly vibration, protective sensation, and proprioception), deep tendon reflexes, balance (sitting and standing), and coordination.

In the cardiopulmonary examination, a check for orthostatic hypotension may prove valuable, particularly in an older person who is complaining of lightheadedness, dizziness, or episodes of blacking out with falling. This is particularly important in patients on hypertensive medications with orthostatic side effects. Checking the resting heart rate with comparison to a postactivity heart rate may yield valuable clues as to a person's level of endurance and tolerance of exercise. Identifying arrhythmias, murmurs, rales, or evidence of COPD may help explain exercise intolerance with easy fatiguability or dyspnea. Evaluating the respiratory pattern, posture, strength of cough, segmental lung expansion, and diaphragmatic excursion should be a routine part of evaluation, especially in an individual with known pulmonary disease. Cardiopulmonary patients often present with chronic musculoskeletal problems or peripheral adaptations such as clubbing of the fingers and toes, discoloration of the nail beds, or edema in the feet and ankles.

Checking extremity pulses is important, especially if the patient presents with complaints of claudication or peripheral sensory changes. The amount of activity needed to induce claudicant pain should be determined. As objective measures, local blood pressures and the time it takes for claudication to occur are helpful measures for establishing a baseline with which treatment effects can be compared. For instance, in a normal individual, treadmill or walking exercise tends to increase the systolic pressure at the ankle, but in the claudicant individual, the ankle pressure falls to a very low level and is slow to recover.[49]

Stress testing to determine an elderly individual's cardiopulmonary response to exercise is a crucial component of evaluation. There are several means of acquiring a baseline exercise level, which will be discussed in the subsequent section of this chapter. The appropriate stress test protocol and method for exercise testing employed will be determined by the older person's ambulatory and functional status, level of physical fitness, medical status, motivation, mentation, and safety of the test chosen. Many elderly individuals will not tolerate maximal test levels, and submaximal testing should be utilized to determine the level that is safe for prescribing and starting endurance training protocols. The importance of stress testing cannot be overstated.

Another important consideration in determining the protocol that best tests an individual's exercise capacity is the method of exercise that will be used in the endurance training.

Step Tests

Steps are among the least expensive devices available for the administration of an exercise stress test. The most commonly employed step test is the *Master's 2-step exercise*. It requires a platform of two steps each nine inches high.

The individual walks up and down the steps at a given rate determined by age and sex using a metronome to keep pace. This diagnostic test lasts only three minutes. Step testing is usually inadequate for measurement of aerobic work capacity and has its limitations in the elderly, especially with advanced aging. Quadriceps strength and endurance may not be adequate to maintain stepping for the full three-minute period. The test is too strenuous for some cardiac patients, yet does not induce enough stress to adequately determine exercise capacity in elderly without occult cardiopulmonary problems.

Another step test uses a *single platform*, which can be raised vertically to increase the external workload, used to determine cardiovascular reponse to progressive exercise. This graduated multilevel step test parallels the principles used in the design of treadmill tests.[50] A stepping rate of 24 steps/minute is maintained while the platform is raised vertically at periodic intervals (generally 2 cm each minute). The second phase of the step test increases the cadence to 30 steps/minute, again gradually increasing the height of the platform at the same time.

Modified Chair-Step Test for the Elderly

A particularly helpful modification of the step test is employed more commonly in the nursing home setting or with the frail elderly who cannot maintain their balance during step, bicycle, or treadmill testing.[51] This test is done sitting using a bar or a platform of adjustable height placed in front of the seated individual. The feet are alternately lifted and placed on the bar or platform as in stepping at a cadence of 24 to 30 steps/minute. The height of the bar or platform is gradually increased, dependent on physical capabilities of the elder, in three- to six-inch increments every one to three minutes up to the height of eighteen inches. In frail elderly, this author often modifies the increases of the platform height to increments of one to two inches to a maximum of twelve inches and decreases the stepping pace to 18 to 24 steps/minute. If the person is able to reach the twelve- or eighteen-inch height, he or she can continue with the final phase of the testing protocol, which employs upper extremity reaching over the head each time a foot is raised. This has been found to be an effective means of evaluating cardiovascular and cardiopulmonary response to gradually increasing levels of work in the deconditioned elderly.

Walking Tests

A test that is applicable to the elderly without balance problems or ambulatory deficits is the walking test. A *twelve-minute walk*[52] or a *six-minute walk*[53] is employed in the elderly with cardiac or respiratory problems. Once again, this author modifies the length of this test based on the individual's capabilities. For instance, if the elder can ambulate for only three minutes, the length of the walk is decreased accordingly. The walk is accomplished on a level surface at a pace as brisk as the individual can manage and the distance recorded at the end of the timed period. This test is particularly useful in establishing a baseline walking level for those elderly who cannot accomplish either treadmill walking or bicycle riding because of angina or dyspnea.

For the more physically fit elderly, the use of a one-mile walk is a good measure of cardiopulmonary capabilities. The *one-mile walk test*[54] is on a level surface. A brisk pace is established by the individual, and the amount of time it takes the individual to cover the last quarter mile is recorded. The VO_2 max is determined by a formula that incorporates the heart rate during the last quarter mile; the distance covered in the last quarter mile; and the age, sex, and weight of the individual exercise regressed against a constant (see Kline and associates[54] for details).

A *low-level functional walking test* employs a ECG chest strap (e.g., Polaris™) to monitor cardiopulmonary responses during functional activities. The individual is evaluated during activities of daily living. For instance, ambulating from bedroom to bathroom, toileting activities, or dressing activities are monitored for cardiovascular response to those tasks that the elderly individual are required to perform for self-maintenance on a daily basis. Often this assessment can be coordinated with the cardiologist when a *Holter monitor* is utilized to evaluate cardiac response to daily activities over a 24-hour period.[55]

Treadmill Tests

The most commonly used treadmill test for the determination of maximal oxygen intake is the *Bruce* or *modified Bruce protocol*.[56] The modified test, which incorporates a much more gradual increase in the speed and incline of the treadmill, is most frequently employed for elderly individuals. Initially the speed is set at 1.7 mph at a grade of 10% (though in some protocols, the initial grade is set at 5% and increased to 10% during the first three minutes of the test for the more impaired elderly). Every three minutes the speed and the percent of incline is increased in a specified manner until a speed of 5 mph at a grade of 18% is reached. This stress test protocol can be used with relatively fit elderly individuals to accurately measure the cardiopulmonary response to exercise.

The *modified Balke test* is an alternative to treadmill stress testing. The rationale of the test is the same, but the speed of the treadmill is held constant (as determined by the individual's perceived capabilities) and every two minutes the grade is increased from 0% by 3.5% increments.[55]

In both of these protocols, assessment parameters include: expired air analysis, ECG, heart rate, blood pressure, and respiratory rate monitoring. The test is terminated using the following criteria: a decrease in blood pressure, ischemic drop of the ST segment or arrhythmias on the ECG, tachycardia, bradycardia, severe shortness of breath, angina, dizziness, or leg pain. Often the elderly individual's perceived limit of exertion will be the ending point of the stress test.

A *low-level functional treadmill walking test* is an intermittent walking test used with patients with moderate to severe cardiac or respiratory involvement. It is divided into three stages and monitors ECG, blood pressure, respiratory rate, heart rate, O_2 saturation, and pulmonary function tests. Stage I is a six-minute walk on a level surface at a pace of approximately 1.5 to 2.0 mph. The objective of this phase of the assessment is to determine the cardiopulmonary response at this intensity of walking. At the end of six minutes, the patient is allowed to return to baseline heart rate, respiratory rate, and O_2 saturation.

Stage II is a functional ambulation assessment. The treadmill is set at a speed and incline equal to the functional work capacity based on the individual's physiologic and symptomatic response during stage I. This phase is also six minutes long and the patient is allowed to return to baseline before proceeding to stage III.

Stage III is the maximum exercise tolerance component of the test, and it is also six minutes. The treadmill is set to produce a heart rate of 70% to 85% max or a preestablished ventilatory maximum. Termination of the test is based on the following criteria: (1) reaching 85% of the predicted heart rate maximum; (2) O_2 saturation of 85% or below; (3) reaching the predicted ventilatory maximum; (4) development of significant cardiac arrhythmias; or (5) development of significant symptoms. This modified stress test elicits a safe exercise response that produces an actual exercise limit and enables accurate measurement of maximal levels in elderly individuals with severe pulmonary or coronary (or both) impairment. It also allows flexibility in establishing the workload to be accomplished by modification according to the person's physiological and symptomatic response, and establishes an accurate baseline for exercise prescription.

Cycle Ergometer Test

The bicycle ergometer provides another alternative to exercise testing. The advantage is that individuals are supported by the bike and can maintain their balance using the handlebars. The use of a tractor seat in place of a regular bike seat to further facilitate the patient's stability and comfort while on the bike is helpful. For screening an older person for exercise prescription, a continuous test of six to nine minutes of cycling with gradual incremental increases in intensity and speed is employed.[51] The individual should work up to 70% to 85% of his or her predicted maximum heart rate. The same parameters are monitored during the bike stress test as in the treadmill tests.

Buerger-Allen Test for Peripheral Circulation

An objective means of measuring peripheral circulation is to time the emptying and filling times of the lower extremities. This is best accomplished using the *Buerger-Allen Testing*

Protocol for peripheral circulation. In this test, the initial position is in supine with the legs resting in a horizontal plane (see Figure 13.5). Allow the individual to rest in this position for at least three minutes. Note the color of the feet (particularly the color of the nail beds). Ideally, the nail beds will be a healthy pink color. In the presence of peripheral vascular disease, however, the nail beds and skin color of the feet will be progressively deeper shades of pink to red based on the severity of the disease. One objective means of documenting skin color is through the use of photography, using Instamatic film and taking care to keep the light source and distance of the camera from the lower extremities constant, so that subsequent photo documentation will be consistent. Other measures—such as skin temperature, circumference measures, and grading of pitting edema if present, palpate for resting pulse rate and grade the pulse intensity (e.g., 0, 1+, 2+, 3+), sensory testing for protective sensation, and vibratory sensation— are valuable baseline measures to obtain during initial and subsequent examination.

> For an evaluation form and flow sheet for managing the Buerger-Allen exercise protocol, see CD.

Other Evaluations of Circulatory Status

Vascular evaluation should include the palpation and grading of the femoral, popliteal, dorsalis pedis, and posterior tibial pulses, as previously mentioned, and the observation of other clinical signs and symptoms indicating vascular compromise to the lower extremities. These include intermittent claudication, foot temperature (e.g., cold feet), nocturnal pain, rest pain, nocturnal and rest pain relieved by dependency, blanching on elevation, atrophic skin, absence of hair growth, and presence of wounds or gangrene. Any lesions, areas of hyperkeratosis, or discoloration should be observed and documented.[57]

Palpating for the pedal pulses can yield a qualitative measure of the dorsalis pedis or posterior tibial circulation, but the examiner must realize that there can be a substantial decrease in flow to the extremity even though arterial ankle pulses are good. To differentiate an organic disorder, such as blockage of the lumen of the vessel, from a vasospastic condition, temporary dilation of the vessel in question is a useful vascular test. This approach is accomplished by using an arterial tourniquet for one minute and then releasing it. The perfusion distal to the tourniquet should increase if the condition is due to vasospasm.

The evaluation of skin temperatures and circumferential measures are other means of assessing circulatory insufficiency and determining the presence of infection.

Skin temperature measurements are useful if the circulatory problem is asymmetrical though test results may be variable because of ambient temperature. In an individual with peripheral vascular disease, the extremities are often cool to touch and in the presence of infection, there may be "hot spots." The use of a skin temperature monitoring device to obtain precise temperature measures is helpful; however, the therapist can also objectively evaluate skin temperature by touch and grading cold, cool, warm, and hot accordingly.

Circumferential measurements of the lower leg and foot also aid in the assessment of the individual with peripheral vascular involvement. Edema is often present when the peripheral vascular system is involved due to an inability of the involved vessels to efficiently remove waste materials from the interstitial tissues. This edema will increase in the dependent position owing to gravity. Measurement of circumference can be accomplished using Jobst measurement tapes (which are free from your local vendor). Measure around the metatarsal heads, midfoot, figure-8 around the ankle, and incrementally every three inches up the lower leg from the malleolar level to the subpatellar level. Another means of determining the level of edema is volume displacement using a bucket of water with a ruler taped to the inside and measuring the amount of water that is displaced upward when the lower extremity is submerged (in inches or centimeters). This method will give an objective and reproducible means for assessing edema in the lower extremity.

Vibratory and temperature sense are diminished very early in the peripheral vascular disease process compromising proprioception, kinesthesia, and awareness of temperature gradients.

Protective sensation defined by Nawoczenski and Birke[58] is 5.07 grams of pressure using the Semmes-Weinstein monofilaments. Specific evaluation of the entire plantar surface of the foot will determine areas of sensory loss vulnerable to breakdown.[59–60]

The Semmes-Weinstein monofilaments have been found to be a reproducible and accurate mode for testing sensation, and reliable in predicting those individuals at risk for ulceration due to loss of protective sensation.[59–60] The Carville group[59] measured protective sensation using the Semmes-Weinstein monofilaments and found that those individuals who could not feel the 5.07 monofilament were at greater risk for skin breakdown than those who could feel this level of stimulation. They demonstrated that 5.07 grams was the protective sensation threshold. Standardizing of sensory testing is crucial in the evaluation, so that adequate protective measures can be taken to prevent feet at risk from developing ulcers.

EXERCISE PRESCRIPTION

Intensity, duration, and frequency are the three major components of exercise prescription. These three elements are used in formulating an appropriate exercise level based on the results of exercise stress testing. Evidence suggests that the best prescription to improve cardiovascular training effects should incorporate an intensity of 60% or greater of the maximum heart rate and be done for a duration of twenty minutes or more with a frequency of three or more times per week.[10,15,61] In the absence of cardiopulmonary impairment, the elderly can achieve a cardiovascular training effect with aerobic exercise. As a result of the decline in maximum heart rate with age, a training effect occurs at lower relative heart rate increases compared with younger subjects.[14]

Elderly individuals with cardiopulmonary impairment may be restricted in the amount of aerobic activity they can do because of dyspnea or angina. Individuals with comorbidities, such as chronic obstructive lung disease, superimposed on cardiac pathology, may not experience the same training effects as a person with cardiac disease alone. As Irwin and Zadai[21] so aptly put it:

> At the present time, the question remains of whether patients with COPD ever achieve the hallmark "anaerobic threshold" even at the higher heart rates they demonstrate with lower levels of exercise. The improvements seen in COPD patients after exercise training are not consistent with the changes demonstrated by exercising normals (central cardiovascular training effect).

Intensity of exercise is a significant factor in determining the success of improving aerobic capacity with exercise.[15,62] In healthy elderly, usually the heart rate is utilized as a reliable indicator of exercise intensity. Heart rate can be a useful indicator for those people who can palpate their own pulse (or have access to a wrist monitoring device). In prescribing exercise for the elderly, it is important to establish a target heart rate that is 60% plus that achieved during exercise testing in order to obtain the desirable VO_2 max. Once an exercise prescription has been determined that provides the time and the distance necessary to improve endurance at a safe heart rate (usually between 60% to 70% max initially), patients are instructed to maintain that heart rate level throughout their exercise session.

In the elderly individual with cardiopulmonary disease, however, heart rate may be an inadequate reflection of oxygen consumption as the oxygen cost of an ineffective breathing pattern and inefficient cardiac pump can shift the amount of O_2 supply away from the working peripheral muscles. In addition, heart rates are often modified by the medications prescribed for cardiac conditions. It is important to instruct the individual in heart rate monitoring, as the heart rate is correlated with the oxygen demand that produced significant symptoms during the patient's stress test. The elderly individual is instructed, therefore, not to exceed that heart rate during an exercise session. Given the unreliability of the heart rate as an indicator of O_2 consumption during exercise, rather than having these individuals rely on heart rate as an indicator of exercise intensity, the intensity is prescribed by recommending a certain amount of work be accomplished over a given period of time. For instance, a person who was able to walk 0.5

mile in the twelve-minute walking test can continue to walk for endurance with the goal of one mile in thirty minutes. Gradually the distance can be extended as determined by the patient's cardiopulmonary tolerance, self-perceived endurance, and motivation. In endurance terms, the intensity of the exercise is determined by the distance covered in a specific amount of time.

If exercise stress tests are not available, establishing the intensity of exercise in an older adult may be accomplished by using the "communication rule." In this measure, if an individual who is exercising is able to carry on a conversation without shortness of breath, that person is exercising at a level well within his or her physiological capabilities. An individual who is exercising at a submaximal level (40% to 60%) can carry on a conversation, but has apparent shortness of breath and is talking between periods of breaths. When aerobic levels of exercise are reached (60% to 80%), the individual can communicate but would prefer not to. Anaerobic levels of exercise result in the inability to communicate at all. Below is a chart for taking target heart rate.

The primary goal of endurance training is to increase the elderly individual's functional activity level by improving the exercise capacity. In order to improve endurance, the duration of exercise should also to be a part of the prescription. If an elderly individual is able to accomplish only stage I (six minutes) of the low-level functional test, intermittent exercise periods would be a way to incorporate the principle of duration. The initial prescription has a duration time (e.g., twenty minutes) that equals the eventual goal; however, the exercise is performed in four- to five-minute segments with two- to three-minute rest periods in between. As the exercise progresses, the rest periods are gradually decreased until the individual is able to walk the entire twenty-minute period continuously. In the nursing home environment, it is not uncommon to exercise an elderly patient two to three short sessions a day at first, before progressing to one long session. The same principle is applicable for those elderly exercising in the community on their own. Gradually the time of the exercise session can be increased as endurance improves.

Frequency is another consideration in exercise prescription. Initially, especially with the intermittent exercise program, it is recommended that the exercise session be done daily unless the individual is limited by symptoms or the weather. Once the person is able to exercise for twenty to thirty consecutive minutes, four to five times per week is beneficial in maintaining and improving the training effects of exercise.

As previously discussed, recovery times are frequently longer in the elderly due to the increased O_2 demands. Warm-up and cool-down sessions are essential as part of the exercise prescription. Individualized warm-up and cool-down sessions can address muscle imbalances, postural problems, flexibility, and overall strength. Stretching and flexibility exercises can also incorporate breathing exercises to facilitate the mobilization of the thorax and improve ventilation. Balance and coordination are often facilitated with rhythmic aerobic exercises as well.[63]

The importance of *activity* cannot be overemphasized. Daily activities are also beneficial in maintaining and improving cardiac and pulmonary function. Though reaching target heart rates established during stress tests is the most effective means of improving aerobic fitness, the truth of the matter is that *Anything Above Rest Works!* The heart responds to activity like any other muscle. Moderate amounts of regular work can help strengthen the heart and improve circulation. Aerobic activities include raking, gardening, pushing a lawn mower, dancing, walking, and many other activities that are done on a daily routine.

> (See CD for) the metabolic equivalence of various activities of daily living.

Figure 13.8 provides a pictorial representation (just like the food triangle) of activities and exercises based on a

weekly recommendation for increasing fitness and improving health.

SPECIAL CONSIDERATIONS IN PRESCRIBING EXERCISE

Pacemakers and Intracardiac Defibrillators

Pacemakers and intracardiac defibrillators (ICDs) are frequently used in an elderly population to treat abnormally slow heart rhythms and the resulting symptoms of lightheadedness and fatigue. Pacemakers and ICDs are also used in patients with heart failure and those with atrial fibrillation.

Exercise testing can act as a diagnostic and a therapeutic tool in the adjustment of rate-responsive pacemakers. Once a permanent pacemaker with rate-responsive pacing capacity has been implanted, exercise testing is useful in the evaluation of pacemaker behavior, as well as

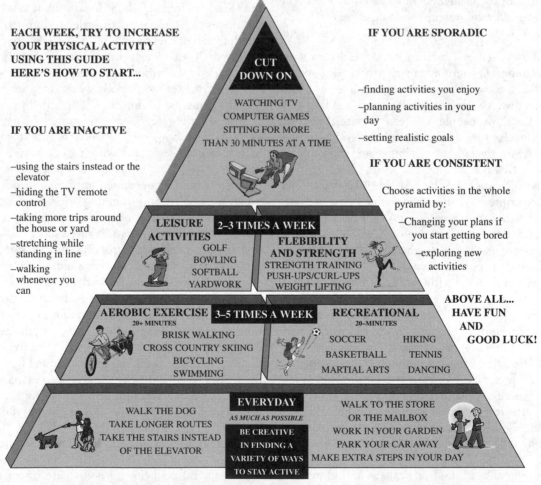

Figure 13.8   Activity Triangle: Recommended Weekly Allowance for Activity and Exercise. (Distributed by: Park Nicollet Health Source (1-800-372-7776). *Copyright © 1996 Institute for Research and Education Health-System, Minnesota.*)

optimizing the pacemaker response. Since most patients with pacemakers are the elderly, the exercise protocol should use gradual increments in workload, such as modified Bruce, Balke, or Naughton protocol. It is important to remember that in patients with pacemaker dependence, ST segment changes do not reflect ischemic changes, and thus other diagnostic tests are required (e.g., thallium scan).[64]

Recent technologic advances have dramatically improved pacemaker function to the point at which they can nearly mimic normal cardiac function at rest and during exercise. Nevertheless, it is important that the exercise training upper heart rate limit be set below the patient's ischemic threshold.

When developing an exercise program for pacemaker patients, basic information about the pacemaker must be understood. Atrial, ventricular, and dual-chamber devices can produce varying exercise responses and impact the exercise prescription. The type of rate-adaptive sensor the pacemaker has will affect the nature of heart response and therefore must be taken into account when prescribing exercise.[65]

Patients with ICDs are at risk of receiving inappropriate shocks during exercise. This can occur if the sinus heart rate exceeds the programmed threshold rate or if the patient develops exercise-induced supraventricular tachycardia. For this reason, patients with ICDs should be closely monitored during exercise to ensure that their heart rate does not approach the activation rate for the device. At least a 10% safety margin between exercise heart rate and rate cutoff for the device is advised.[65]

The elderly patient with an ICD or a pacemaker can benefit from exercise training. In addition to improvements in functional capacity, exercise training can also reduce cardiac risk factors (e.g., cholesterol, high blood pressure) and improve psychosocial outcomes.

> Obesity and Diabetes are related to increased risk for cardiovascular disease in the elderly. For more information, SEE CD.

> For the effects of medications and osteoporosis, see CD.

Congestive Heart Failure/Cardiomyopathy

There was a time in the not-too-distant past when exercise was contraindicated in an individual with cardiomyopathy and congestive heart failure. However, as the research (to follow) indicates, although precautions need to be taken in relation to the pathophysiological cardiovascular dynamics in these patients, exercise, starting just above rest and gradually progressing to the submaximal ranges, is beneficial for those elders with cardiac failure.

Exercise performance in chronic heart failure is severely impaired, due in part to a peripherally mediated limitation.[65] In addition to impaired maximal exercise capacity, the O_2 uptake (VO_2) response during submaximal exercise may be affected, with a greater reliance on anaerobiosis leading to early fatigue. Therefore, exercise periods need to be shorter and at lower intensities in the initial phases of reconditioning. Hepple and associates[66] studied the relationship between oxygen utilization and peripheral response to exercise in a group of elderly patients with chronic heart failure compared to healthy sedentary elderly individuals at submaximal exercise levels. Heart failure subjects displayed a significantly prolonged VO_2 kinetics response at similar absolute workloads compared to healthy controls. In addition, heart failure subjects demonstrated a lower maximal calf blood flow compared to the controls. These results indicate that patients with heart failure have a prolonged VO_2 kinetics on-response compared with healthy subjects at a similar absolute work rate, but not at a similar relative work rate. Thus, despite a reduced maximal calf blood flow response associated with heart failure, it does not appear that this contributes to an impairment of the submaximal exercise response beyond that explained by a reduced maximal exercise capacity [VO_{2max}].[66]

Peripheral microvascular function plays an important role in congestive heart failure (CHF). Decreased exercise blood flow and microvascular dysfunction have been described in the condition and influence exercise capacity in the CHF patient. Sorensen and associates[67] demonstrated that these factors are related to or can be characterized by clinical severity of CHF. Patients with CHF have reduced exercise skeletal muscle blood flow, which is a limiting factor for the reduced maximal exercise capacity. Moreover, microvascular distensibility in skeletal muscle is reduced and correlates to maximal exercise skeletal muscle blood flow.[67] It was determined that skeletal muscle blood flow correlates to exercise time. This implies that increased skeletal muscle microvascular stiffness may contribute to reduced blood flow during exercise, and skeletal muscle blood flow may partly limit length of exercise performance in CHF patients diagnosed with idiopathic dilated cardiomyopathy.[67]

In normal subjects during exercise, there is vasoconstriction of nonexercise resistance vessels and an increase in blood pressure. It has been found that impairment in the reflex venoconstriction in patients with hypertrophic cardiomyopathy is related to syncope or exercise hypotension.[68] Thomson[69] investigated patients with vasovagal syncope with structurally normal hearts and patients with hypertrophic cardiomyopathy compared with normal controls and found a failure of vasoconstriction in both compared groups with normal subjects. This was evidenced by exercise hypotension. There is an association between exercise hypotension and sudden death. The author of this study speculates that in patients with vasovagal syncope and structurally and electrically normal hearts, exercise hypotension is well tolerated. However, in patients with structurally abnormal hearts, exercise hypotension can have catastrophic consequences.[69]

Another concern in cardiomyopic patients is the low ejection fraction and its relationship to potential arrhythmias. The results of a study by Mager and colleagues,[70] however, suggest that patients with a diminished ejection fraction as low as 16% can safely perform an exercise program. A significant improvement in peak VO_2 and maximal work rate was achieved in this study. Moreover, this study suggests that exercise training might diminish the severity of asymptomatic ventricular arrhythmia.[70]

Peripheral adaptations and ventricular abnormalities influence physical performance in chronic heart failure. However, the role of the heart in determining exercise capacity has not been completely elucidated. To define cardiac determinants of exercise capacity in patients with dilated cardiomyopathy, Pepi and associates[71] measured peak exercise oxygen consumption, left ventricular ejection fraction, left and right atrial and ventricular cavity dimensions, and mitral and tricuspid valvular flows.[71] These researchers concluded that in patients with dilated cardiomyopathy, peak VO_2 is related to left and right ventricular dimensions, left and right ventricular filling patterns, and ejection fraction. It was determined that both systolic and diastolic dysfunction influence functional capacity in chronic heart failure patients.[71] Other researchers assessed the ventricular-arterial coupling at peak exercise in patients with dilated cardiomyopathy coupled with respiratory gas analysis and concluded that ventricular arterial coupling is further altered at peak exercise in these patients because of a lack of increase in contractility and is not due to altered effective arterial elastance response.[72]

The utility of metabolic gas exchange measurements in evaluating the severity and determinants of exercise limitation was studied during upright symptom-limited cardiopulmonary exercise with hypertrophic cardiomyopathy and healthy age- and gender-matched subjects.[73] It was concluded that the peak VO_2 is significantly related to the functional class as defined by the New York Heart Association in patients with hypertrophic cardiomyopathy and that peak VO_2 was a superior measure of cardiovascular performance. The data from this study indicate that mechanical obstruction has an adverse pathophysiologic effect on functional capacity and that VO_2 provides an indicator to support treatments aimed at gradient reduction. Low peak VO_2 characteristics suggest that measurement of VO_2 may aid in differential diagnosis between a cardiomyopic and a healthy heart.[73] In chronic heart failure, oxygen delivery during exercise is impaired mainly because of failure of cardiac output to increase normally.[74] Compensatory mechanisms are that hemoglobin concentration increases and there is a rightward shift in the oxyhemoglobin dissociation curve. In addition, as previously mentioned, blood flow redistribution from the nonexercising

organs and muscles to the exercising muscles occurs.[74] Changing the exercising muscle group alters the ventilatory response to exercise in chronic heart failure. The recognized muscle abnormalities previously described in CHF may contribute to the ventilatory abnormalities of this condition during increasing levels of activity.[75]

Constant workload exercise at submaximal levels of exercise intensity is frequently used in physical training programs. Faggiano and associates[76] studied the hemodynamic changes induced at a steady workload in CHF patients and found a marked increase in right heart pressure. Cardiac output and heart rate were significantly higher during submaximal exercise at higher workloads, though the systolic pulmonary artery pressure was not statistically different at increasing levels of exercise. Additionally, the hemodynamic profile during submaximal exercise at the anaerobic threshold was similar to that observed during symptom-limited exercise. It was concluded that in patients with heart failure, submaximal exercise performed at a constant workload, even at low exercise intensity, may determine relevant pressure changes in pulmonary circulation thereby influencing the availability of oxygen and affecting endurance.[76]

Mancini and co-researchers[77] investigated the impact of alteration of glycogen stores and metabolism on exercise performance in patients with heart failure. In normal subjects, muscle glycogen depletion results in increased exertional fatigue and reduced endurance. Skeletal muscle biopsies have revealed reduced glycogen content in patients with congestive heart failure (CHF).[77] Whether glycogen depletion contributes to reduced endurance and abnormal ventilation in CHF patient is not entirely known. The Mancini study indicated that glycogen depletion minimally affects maximal exercise performance, endurance, or ventilation in CHF patients, whereas slowed glycogen utilization markedly enhances exercise endurance. This demonstrates that low-level therapeutic interventions that speed up or slow down use of glycogen stores may have great clinical significance in the individual with cardiomyopic heart failure.[77]

Webb-Peploe and colleagues[78] examined the benefits and complications of a home-based exercise program in patients with ischemic versus idiopathic dilated cardiomyopathy. Training in both groups resulted in a higher peak oxygen consumption, a higher peak heart rate, and an improved sense of well-being. Patients with idiopathic dilated cardiomyopathy showed a significant increase in exercise time and peak oxygen consumption as well as a decrease in left ventricular end-diastolic and end-systolic measures in contrast to those with coronary artery disease, who developed a reduction in septal excursion and shortening following training.[78] Complications of training were more common in those patients with ischemic cardiomyopathy and these individuals experienced greater left ventricular workloads and poorer exercise tolerance with fluid retention and exercise-induced ventricular tachycardia. Conversely, those elders with idiopathic dilated cardiomyopathy, despite poorly functioning left ventricle status, exercised without complications. It was concluded that home-based exercise programs, particularly in those patients with idiopathic origin of the pathology, can proceed safely, with close monitoring for the development of complications.[78]

For Complementary Therapies and Cardiovascular Disease, see CD.

References

1. National Center for Health Statistics. *Health, United States, 1999 with Health and Aging Chartbook.* Hyattsville, MD: National Center for Health Statistics; 1999: 34–35.
2. National Center for Health Statistics. *Health, United States, 1999 with Health and Aging Chartbook.* Hyattsville, MD: National Center for Health Statistics; 1999: 36–37.
3. Shepard RJ. The cardiovascular benefits of exercise in the elderly. *Top Geriatr Rehabil.* 1985; 1(1):1–10.
4. US Bureau of the Census. *Statistical Abstract of the United States: 1997.* 117th ed. Washington, DC. US Bureau of the Census; 1997.
5. Centers for Disease Control and Prevention. *Unrealized Prevention Opportunities: Reducing the Health and Economic Burden of Chronic Disease.* Atlanta, GA: Centers for Disease Control and Prevention, National Center for Chronic Disease Prevention and Health Promotion; 1997.
6. Verbrugge L. Recent, present, and future health of American adults. In: Breslow L, Fielding JE, and Lave LB, eds. *Annual Review of Public Health.* Palo Alto, CA: Annual Reviews Inc.; Vol. 20. 1999.
7. Cheitlin MD, Gerstenblith G. Management of patients over age 75 with cardiovascular disease. Presented at the American Heart Association 72nd Scientific Sessions, Atlanta, GA; November 7–10, 1999. Plenary Session XIII, November 10, 1999.
8. Palmore EB. Trends in the health of the aged. *Gerontologist.* 1986; 26:298–302.
9. Astrand PO. Exercise physiology and its role in disease prevention and in rehabilitation. *Arch Phys Med Rehabil.* 1987; 68:305–311.
10. Lee IM, Paffenbarger RS, Hennekens CH. Physical activity, physical fitness and longevity. *Aging.* 1997; 9(1–2):2–11.
11. Blair SN, Kohl HW III, Barlow CE, et al. Changes in physical fitness and all-cause mortality. A prospective study of healthy and unhealthy men. *JAMA.* 1995; 273(14):1093–1098.
12. Rowe JW, Besdine RW. *Health and Disease in Old Age.* Boston: Little, Brown; 1982.
13. Crimmins EM, Saito Y, Ingegneri D. Changes in life expectancy and disability-free life expectancy in the United States. *Population and Development Review.* 1989; 15(2):235–267.
14. Shepard RJ. *Physical Activity and Aging.* 2nd ed. Gaithersburg, MD: Aspen Publishers; 1987.
15. Bruce RA. Functional aerobic capacity, exercise and aging. In: Andres R, Bierman EL, Hazzard WR, eds. *Principles of Geriatric Medicine.* New York: McGraw-Hill; 1985: 87–103.
16. Cress ME, Schultz E. Aging muscle: Functional, morphologic, biochemical, and regenerative capacity. *Top Geriatric Rehabil.* 1985; 1(1):11–19.
17. Gerstenblith G, Weisfeldt ML, Lakatta, EG. Disorders of the heart. In: Andres R, Bierman EL, Hazzard WR, eds. *Principles of Geriatric Medicine.* New York: McGraw-Hill; 1985: 515–526.
18. Wei JY. Heart disease in the elderly. *Cardiovasc Med.* 1984; 9:971–998.
19. Wei JY. Cardiovascular anatomic and physiologic changes with age. *Top Geriatr Rehabil.* 1986; 2(1): 10–16.
20. Redden WG. Respiratory system and aging. In: Smith EL, Serfass RC, eds. *Exercise and Aging: The Scientific Basis.* Hillside, NJ: Enslow Publishers; 1981: 89–108.
21. Irwin SC, Zadai CC. Cardiopulmonary rehabilitation of the geriatric patient. In: Lewis CB, ed. *Aging: The Health Care Challenge.* 2nd ed. Philadelphia: FA Davis; 1990: 181–211.
22. Zadai CC. Cardiopulmonary issues in the geriatric population: Implications for rehabilitation. *Top Geriatr Rehabil.* 1986; 2:1:1–9.
23. Hurst W. *The Heart, Arteries and Veins.* 9th ed. New York: McGraw-Hill; 1998.
24. Mann DL, Deneberg BS, Gash AK, et al. Effects of age on ventricular performance during graded supine exercise. *Am Heart J.* 1986; 111:108–115.
25. Rodeheffer RJ, Gerstenblith G. Effect of age on cardiovascular function. In: Johnson HA, ed. *Relations Between Normal Aging and Disease.* New York: Raven Press. Aging Series. 1985; 28:85–99.

26. Gerstenblith G, Lakatta EG, Weisfeldt ML. Age changes in myocardial function and exercise response. *Progr Cardiovasc Dis.* 1976; 19:1–21.

27. Port S, Cobb FR, Coleman RE, et al. Cardiac ejection fraction in aging. *N Engl J Med.* 1980; 303:1133–1137.

28. Rodeheffer RJ, Gerstenblith G, Becker LC, et al. Exercise cardiac output is maintained with advancing age in healthy human subjects: Cardiac dilatation and increased stroke volume compensate for a diminished heart rate. *Circulation.* 1984; 69:203–213.

29. Harris R. *Clinical Geriatric Cardiology: Management of the Elderly Patient.* Philadelphia: Lippincott; 1986:29–42.

30. Weisfeldt ML, Gerstenblith ML, and Lakatta EG. Alterations in circulatory function. In: Andres R, Bierman EL, Hazzard WR, eds. *Principles of Geriatric Medicine.* New York: McGraw-Hill; 1985:248–279.

31. Niinimaa V, Shepard RJ. Training and oxygen conductance in the elderly. *J Gerontol.* 1978; 33:354–367.

32. Horvath SM, Borgia JF. Cardiopulmonary gas transport and aging. *Am Rev Respir Dis.* 1984; 129 (suppl):569–571.

33. Aniansson A, Hedberg M, Henning GB, et al. Muscle morphology, enzymatic activity, and muscle strength in elderly men: A follow-up study. *Muscle Nerve.* 1986; 9:585–591.

34. Coggan AR, Spina RJ, King DS, et al. Skeletal muscle adaptations to endurance training in 60–69 year old men and women. *J Appl Physiol.* 1992; 72:1780–1786.

35. Martin WH III, Kohrt WM, Malley MT, et al. Exercise training enhances leg vasodilatory capacity of 65-year-old men and women. *J Appl Physiol.* 1990; 69:1804–1809.

36. Smith EL, Serfass RC, eds. *Exercise and Aging: The Scientific Basis.* Hillside, NJ: Enslow Publishers; 1981.

37. Shimada K, Kitazumi T, Sadakne N, et al. Age-related changes of baroreflex function, plasma, norepinephrine, and blood pressure. *Hypertension.* 1985; 7:113–118.

38. Irwin SC. Cardiac rehabilitation for the geriatric patient. *Top Geriatr Rehabil.* 1986; 2:44–54.

39. Turner JM, Mead J, Wohl ME. Elasticity of human lungs in relation to age. *J Appl Physiol.* 1968; 25(6):664–683.

40. Pump KK. Fenestrae in the alveolar membrane of the human lung. *Chest.* 1965; 65:799–802.

41. Loke J, Mahler DA, Paul-Man SF, et al. Exercise impairment in chronic obstructive pulmonary disease. In: *Symposium on Exercise: Physiology and Clinical Applications. Clin Chest Med.* 1984; 5(1):121–129.

42. Paffenbarger RS, Wing AL, Hyde RT, Jung DL. Physical activity and incidence of hypertension in college alumni. *Am J Epidemiol.* 1983; 117:245–256.

43. Paffenbarger RS, Hyde RT, Wing AL, Hsieh CC. Physical activity, all-cause mortality and longevity of college alumni. *N Engl J Med.* 1986; 314:605–613.

44. Baker PB, Arn AR, Unverferth DV. Hypertrophic and degenerative changes in human hearts with aging. *J Coll Cardiol.* 1985; 5:536A.

45. Krotkiewski M, Lonroth P, Mandroukas K, et al. The effects of physical training on glucose metabolism in obesity and type II (noninsulin-dependent) diabetes mellitus. *Diabetologia.* 1985; 28:881–890.

46. Ebel A, Kim D. Exercise in peripheral vascular disease. In: Basmajian JV, Wolf S, eds. *Therapeutic Exercise.* 4th ed. Baltimore: Williams and Wilkins; 1990:371–386.

47. Wisham MB, Lawrence H, Abramson MD, Arthur S, Ebel A. Value of exercise in peripheral arterial diseases. *JAMA.* 1953; 153:10–12.

48. Bottomley JM. A comparison of the effects of Buerger-Allen exercises, walking, and high galvanic electrical stimulation on lower extremity blood flow in elderly patients. (Submitted to circulation—unpublished)

49. Thiele BL, Strandness DE. Disorders of the vascular system: Peripheral vascular disease. In: Andres R, Bierman EL, Hazzard WR, eds. *Principles in Geriatric Medicine.* New York: McGraw-Hill; 1985:527–535.

50. Nagle FJ, Balke B, Naughton JP. Gradual step tests for assessing work capacity. *J Appl Physiol.* 1965; 20:745–752.

51. Smith EL, Gilligan C. Physical activity prescription for the elderly. *Phys Sports Med.* 1983; 11:91–101.

52. McGavin CR, Cupta SP, McHardy GJR. Twelve-minute walking test for assessing disability in chronic bronchitis. *Brit Med J.* 1976; 1:822–826.

53. Enright PL, Sherrill DL. References equations for the six-minute walk in healthy adults. *Am J Respir and Critical Care Med.* 1998; 158:1384–1387.

54. Kline G, Parcari JP, Hintermeister R, et al. Estimated VO_2 max from a one-mile track walk, gender, age, and body weight. *Med Sci Sports Exerc.* 1987; 19:253–259.

55. Ellestad NH. *Stress Testing: Principles and Practice.* Philadelphia: FA Davis; 1979.

56. Bruce RA. Exercise, functional aerobic capacity, and aging—Another viewpoint. *Med Sci Sports Exerc.* 1984; 16:8–15.

57. Rowbotham JL, Gibbons GW, Kozak GP. Guidelines in examination of the diabetic leg and foot. In: Kozak GP, Hoar CS, Rowbotham JL, et al., eds. *Management of Diabetic Foot Problems.* Philadelphia: WB Saunders; 1984: 9–16.

58. Nawoczenski D, Birke J, Graham S, et al. The neuropathic foot—A management scheme. *Phys Ther.* 1989; 69(4):287–291.

59. Birke JA, Sims DS. Plantar sensory threshold in the ulcerative foot. *Leprosy Rev.* 1986; 57:261–267.

60. Dorairaj A, Reddy R, Jesudasan K. An evaluation of the Semmes-Weinstein 6.10 monofilament as compared with 6 nylon in leprosy patients. *Indian J Leprosy.* 1988; 60(3):413–417.

61. Frontera WR, Evans WJ. Exercise performance and endurance training in the elderly. *Top Geriatr Rehabil.* 1986; 2(1):17–32.

62. Verg JE, Seals DR, Hagberg JM, et al. Effects of endurance exercise training on ventilatory function in older individuals. *J Appl Physiol.* 1985; 58:791–794.

63. Pollock DL. Breaking the risk of falls: An exercise benefit for the older patients. *Phys and Sportsmed.* 1992; 20(11):146–156.

64. Greco EM, Guardini S, Citelli L. Cardiac rehabilitation in patients with rate responsive pacemakers. *Pacing Clin Electrophysiol.* 1998; 21(3):568–575.

65. Sharp CT, Busse EF, Burgess JJ, Haennel RG. Exercise prescription for patients with pacemakers. *J Cardiopulm Rehabil.* 1998; 18(6):421–431.

66. Hepple RT, Liu PP, Plyley MJ, Goodman JM. Oxygen uptake kinetics during exercise in chronic heart failure: Influence of peripheral vascular reserve. *Clin Sci.* 1999; 97(5):569–577.

67. Sorensen VB, Wroblewski H, Galatius S, Haunso S, Kastrup J. Exercise skeletal muscle blood flow is related to peripheral microvascular stiffness in idiopathic dilated cardiomyopathy. *Microvasc Res.* 1999; 58(3):268–280.

68. Thomson HL, Morris-Thurgood J, Atherton J, McKenna WJ, Frenneaux MP. Reflex responses of venous capacitance vessels in patients with hypertrophic cardiomyopathy. *Clin Sci.* 1998; 94(4):339–346.

69. Thomson HL. Exercise vascular responses in health and disease. *Aust NZ J Med.* 1997; 27(4):459–461.

70. Mager G, Reinhardt C, Kleine M, Rost R, Hopp HW. Patients with dilated cardiomyopathy and less than 20% ejection fraction increase exercise capacity and have less severe arrhythmia after controlled exercise training. *J Cardiopulm Rehabil.* 2000; 20(3):196–198.

71. Pepi M, Agostoni P, Marenzi G, et al. The influence of diastolic and systolic function on exercise performance in heart failure due to dilated cardiomyopathy or ischemic heart disease. *Eur J Heart Fail.* 1999; 1(2):161–167.

72. Cohen-Solal A, Faraggi M, Czitrom D, Le Guludec D, Delahaye N, Gourgon R. Left ventricular arterial system coupling at peak exercise in dilated nonischemic cardiomyopathy. *Chest.* 1998; 113(4):870–877.

73. Sharma S, Elliot P, Whyte G, et al. Utility of cardiopulmonary exercise in assessment of clinical determinants of functional capacity in hypertrophic cardiomyopathy. *Am J Cardiol.* 2000; 86(2):162–168.

74. Agostoni P, Wasserman K, Perego GB, et al. Oxygen transport to muscle during exercise in chronic congestive heart failure secondary to idiopathic dilated cardiomyopathy. *Am J Cardiol.* 1997; 79(8):1120–1124.

75. Harrington D, Clark AL, Chua TP, Anker SD, Poole-Wilson PA, Coats AJ. Effect of reduced muscle bulk on the ventilatory response to exercise in chronic congestive heart failure secondary to idiopathic dilated and ischemic cardiomyopathy. *Am J Cardiol.* 1997; 80(1):90–93.

76. Faggiano P, D'Aloia A, Gualeni A, Giordano A. Hemodynamic profile of submaximal constant workload exercise in patients with heart failure secondary to ischemic or idiopathic dilated cardiomyopathy. *Am J Cardiol.* 1998; 81(4):437–442.

77. Mancini D, Benaminovitz A, Cordisco ME, Karmally W, Weinberg A. Slowed glycogen utilization enhances exercise endurance in patients with heart failure. *J Am Coll Cardiol.* 1999; 34(6):1807–1812.

78. Webb-Peploe KM, Chua TP, Harrington DL, Henein MY, Gibson DB, Coats AJ. Different response of patients with idiopathic and ischaemic dilated cardiomyopathy to exercise training. *Int J Cardiol.* 2000; 74(2–3):215–224.

14

Integumentary Considerations

Pearls

- The healing process can easily be remembered by the 3 **R**s of wound healing: **R**eaction (inflammation), **R**egeneration (proliferation and epithelialization), and **R**emodeling.
- The effects of aging and age-associated diseases slow the wound-healing process.
- Thinning and flattening of the epidermis results in an increased vulnerability to trauma from shear and frictional forces in the older adult.
- Inadequate blood supply can result in poor oxidative and nutritive status in the tissues and lead to an arterial ulcer; and ve-

nous ulcerations are caused by venous hypertension, valvular incompetence, and generally accompanied by a history of deep vein thrombosis.

- All pressure ulcers are preventable if attention is directed to insensate areas, malnutrition, skin fragility, and the physical or cognitive inability to accomplish pressure relief without guidance or assistance.
- Treatment approaches for wound healing in the elderly population include physical modalities, debridement, incontinence care, topical dressings, and nutritional interventions.

INTRODUCTION

Older adults are often predisposed to wounds because of poor hydration and nutrition, poor circulation, and inactivity. Skin breakdown can be prevented through proper seating and positioning. Given the right circumstances, older individuals with wounds also heal well, despite age-related problems and nutritional deficiencies.

This chapter will focus on skin and wound care in the elderly patient. From a geriatric rehabilitation perspective, positioning, seating devices and mattresses, and a focus on the prevention of skin breakdown are important components of therapy. Often, in an older population, we encounter wounds that are chronic and slow to heal. The aging of the skin, nutritional status, and hydration, in addition to immobility, will impact the integrity of the external integumentary system. Integumentary conditions that therapists treat will be discussed followed by an appraisal of how a wound repairs itself and what complicating factors in the healing process exist in an aged individual. Evaluation, staging of a wound, and documentation will be discussed. The importance of nutrition and hydration in maintaining skin health and the importance of its role in healing will be presented. The types of ulcers, venous,

arterial, and diabetic, will be reviewed as they impact treatment approaches. Other types of wounds seen in the elderly, such as extravasation sites, abrasions and skin tears, dehisced surgical wounds, fistulas, and radiation burns, will be discussed. Finally, a review of treatment modalities for wound management, surgical indications, and wound care products will be presented.

There are natural delays in the healing of wounds of older individuals.[1] Open wounds contract more slowly and incised wounds gain strength more slowly. Experimental studies indicate that cellular proliferation, wound metabolism, and collagen remodeling occur at a delayed rate in older people.[1,2]

DEFINING INTEGUMENTARY CONDITIONS

Integumentary problems involve any covering or lining of the body. Therefore, the topic of integumentary system conditions could potentially cover skin and wound care to gastrointestinal conditions such as diverticulosis, constipation, or gastric ulceration, and respiratory conditions such as tuberculosis. Though the status of these systems will impact the functional status of our elderly patients and may be affected by exercise, positioning, nutrition, and hydration, physical or occupational therapists primarily treat integumentary problems affecting the external covering of the body (e.g., the skin). Despite this, it is important that the therapist not ignore the other integumentary conditions in assessing, evaluating, and treating the whole patient. It is vital that a therapist is cognizant of integumentary conditions that affect the gastrointestinal or respiratory systems and the influence these conditions might have on mobility and functional capabilities. These pathologies, when they exist, should be cared for as a part of an interdisciplinary team approach to patient care.

THE SKIN AND THE AGING PROCESS

It is well recognized that the skin of the elderly differs in many ways from that of a younger person.[2] While great variance exists among individuals' physiologic responses to aging, certain characteristics are inherent to the aging process. In order to understand gerontodermatological changes and the effects they have on delayed wound healing, it is important to review what is normal so that the changes that take place can be put into perspective.

On average there is approximately 20 square feet of skin (if laid out flat) and the skin is often called "the body's biggest organ." It is the only organ that is exposed to the external environment. It is an all-purpose covering in that it is water-proof (it keeps the water out and in), and it assists in regulating body temperature.

The skin has three distinct layers: the epidermis, dermis, and subcutaneous layers. Figure 14.1 provides a pictorial representation of the layers of normal skin. The epidermis is the uppermost layer of skin. This is divided into the stratum corneum (top layer), stratum spinosum (middle layer), and stratum germinativum (innermost layer). The stratum corneum, or the horny layer, is somewhat acidic and referred to as the acid mantle. It is the major barrier to the environment and effectively prevents the penetration of most environmental substances. The middle layer, or stratum spinosum, is called the prickle-

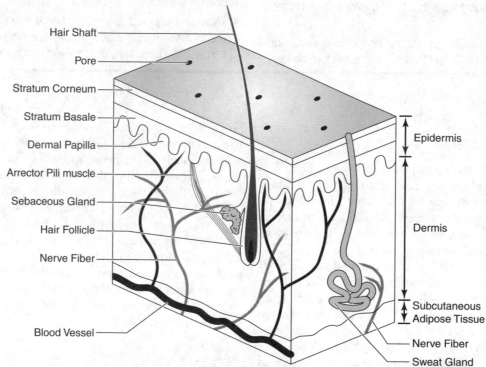

Figure 14.1   Structure of skin, including accessory structures. Hair with the follicles located deep in the dermis are shown with the associated arrector pili muscles that cause the hairs to become erect and form "gooseflesh" in the cold. Sweat glands with their coiled portion deep in the dermis and openings onto the surface of the skin are also depicted. Sebaceous glands are associated with hair follicles and secrete their oily sebum onto the skin to help retain moisture. Also note the relative thickness of the dermis, which is about 10 times thicker than the epidermis, the presence of sensory receptors in the dermis, and blood vessels in the dermis.

cell layer. This is the thickest of the epidermal layers. The cells in the stratum spinosum are squamous cells, which essentially are basal cells that have matured and migrated upward. The basal layer, the stratum germinativum, continuously reproduces new cells. This layer contains basal cells and elanocytes, in addition to melanocytes, the cells which produce melanin (providing the skin color).[3]

The dermis is the second layer. It contains collagen and elastic fibers, which are complex proteins responsible for the support and elasticity of skin. This layer enables the skin to regain its shape after being stretched or deformed. The circulatory supply is contained in the dermis, as well as the nerve endings, and the oil and sweat glands. Skin nutrition and oxygenation are supplied by numerous arteries, veins, and capillaries coursing upward through the dermis. Incredibly, each square inch of the dermis houses numerous small, nutrient-providing blood vessels. Their constriction and dilation, in response to ambient temperature changes, are responsible for keeping the body temperature constant. These small vessels also keep the skin healthy and viable by providing nutrients and remove metabolic waste materials. (See Figure 14.1.)

The subcutis or subcutaneous is the fatty layer, which gives the skin its smooth appearance. It is loosely connected to itself but adheres to the dermis and the underlying fascia. This allows skin to dissipate both pressure and shear forces. In areas where bony prominences such as the greater trochanter or heel are immediately adjacent to the subcutaneous fat layer without any muscle or other soft tissue protection, the ability of the skin to dissipate pressure is compromised. The disproportionate pressure placed on these areas can occlude blood flow, causing tissue breakdown and leading to tissue death. As well as mechanical protection, the subcutaneous layer also provides thermal insulation. Fat also acts as an energy store. By volume, fat stores approximately 20 times as much energy as the storage form of carbohydrate called glycogen.

As the skin ages, there are certain changes which occur that will ultimately impact the healing process in the event of an injury or wound. These changes are summarized in Table 14.1.

Wound Repair

The body's response to injury of the skin, the repair sequence, is the same regardless of the origin of the wound—whether it is a traumatic injury, a pressure sore, a venous stasis ulcer, or a diabetic ulcer. Wound repair starts the moment the tissue is injured. The healing process involves several predictable stages, which are summarized in Figure 14.2. Wound healing consists of four basic phases: inflammation, proliferation, epithelialization, and remodeling.[4,5] This healing process can easily be remembered by the 3 **R**s of wound healing: **R**eaction (inflammation),

Regeneration (proliferation and epithelialization), and **R**emodeling.

The inflammatory response is decreased with age,[6,7] and undoubtedly this bears on some of the alterations in healing that will subsequently be discussed. The proliferative phase traditionally includes cell migration, proliferation, and maturation, all of which are changed with age. Remodeling encompasses the tertiary binding of collagen molecules, whish is also altered with age.[7] Although all of these stages of wound healing differ with age, the changes are qualitative. Events begin later, proceed more slowly, and often do not reach the same level. However, there are neither new events nor an absence of expected events in the healing of wounds in the elderly.

Uninterrupted Wound Repair

After the injury, inflammation allows the destruction of foreign material and microbes. Neutrophils are usually the first cells to the site of injury, and they function to destroy microbes. Macrophages come later, and aid in wound healing by removing debris and attracting and promoting proliferation of fibroblasts. Fibroblasts secrete the molecules that form the ground substance and fibers of the scar tissue that fills the tissue loss. The tissue that is generated forms in small piles, resembling the pebbled surface of a basketball, and because of the formation of leaky, new blood vessels, it is beefy red and shiny. This tissue is called granulation tissue, and from this, fibers are generated in random directions, but provide little of the tensile strength of normal skin (this is scar tissue). During the proliferation phase, myofibroblasts in the wound pull the wound edges toward the middle, producing wound contraction. Concurrent with and continuing after the wound has completed granulation, is the process of epithelialization. As granulation tissue fills in from the sides of the wound, new epithelial cells are regenerated to cover the scar tissue below. Although mature scar tissue has many of the same components of dermis, it lack the accessory structures (sweat glands, sebaceous glands, hair follicles, nails) and blood vessels of natural dermis. The remodeling phase consists of reinforcement of collagen in the direction of stress and removal of collagen bundles that are unstressed so that a mature scar has approximately 80% of the strength of normal skin.[4,5] In fact, during the first two weeks of healing, an acute wound regains one-third to one-half of the skin's original strength. It takes approximately three months for a wound to regain nearly 80% of the tensile strength of the original skin. The maturation or remodeling phase of healing continues for a year or more; thus care must be taken in the older person to protect healed areas from reinjury, particularly in the first three-month period.

An acute wound, such as a surgical incision, may be expected to complete this process in a more rapid and orderly manner than a wound dehiscence or a pressure ulcer

TABLE 14.1   Aging-Related Changes in the Skin that Affect the Healing Process

Aging Change	Result
Thinning and flattening of epidermis	• Increased vulnerability to trauma • Increased susceptibility to shearing stress leading to blisters and skin tears • Decreased tissue barrier properties • Impairment of barrier functions causing problems by allowing certain drugs and irritants to be more easily absorbed
Decreased epidermal proliferation	• The production of new skin cells slows down and the epidermis cannot replace itself as rapidly • Decreased wound contraction • Delayed cellular migration and proliferation
Cells in horny layer become less elastic	• The skin is unable to return to original position when stretched (i.e., like a worn rubber band)
Atrophy of the dermis	• Underlying tissues are more vulnerable to injury • Increased rate of wound dehiscence • Decreased wound contraction
Decreased vascularity of the dermis	• Easy bruising and susceptibility to injury • Poor temperature regulation (usually making skin cool) • Increased vulnerability to trauma • Decreased wound capillary growth • Increased rate of wound dehiscence
Changes and loss in collagen and elastin fibers	• Underlying tissue more vulnerable to injury • Decreased tensile strength • Delayed collagen remodeling
Decrease in number of oil and sweat glands	• The skin is not as moist or as well lubricated
Vascular response is compromised	• Cutaneous immune and inflammatory response are impaired • Reduced ability to clear foreign materials and fluids • Decreased wound capillary growth • Altered metabolic response
Nerve endings become abnormal	• Altered or reduced sensation
Fragility of the subcuteous layer	• Easy bruising and tearing of the skin • Loss of cushion effect of subcutaneous layer • Skin no longer feels as thick

in an elderly malnourished individual. The stages of chronic wound repair may not follow the sequence of an acute wound.

Certain conditions need to be in place in order for a wound to heal in a timely manner. Appropriate cells need to be present, including macrophages, granulocytes, fibroblasts, platelets, and both red and white blood cells. Circulation needs to be adequate in order to provide oxygen and nutrients essential for wound healing. A proper electrolyte and fluid balance creates the ideal healing environment. Sufficient amounts of calories to fuel the very

high-energy expenditure needed for healing should be present, as well as appropriate amounts of vitamins, minerals, and proteins. Finally, in order to heal 100%, wounds need to be free from infection.

The Effects of Aging on Wound Healing

There is a potential for problems in wound healing related to the aging process itself, as well as age-associated disease and slower healing as described in Table 14.1. Elderly individuals may have a decrease in sensory input or neuro-

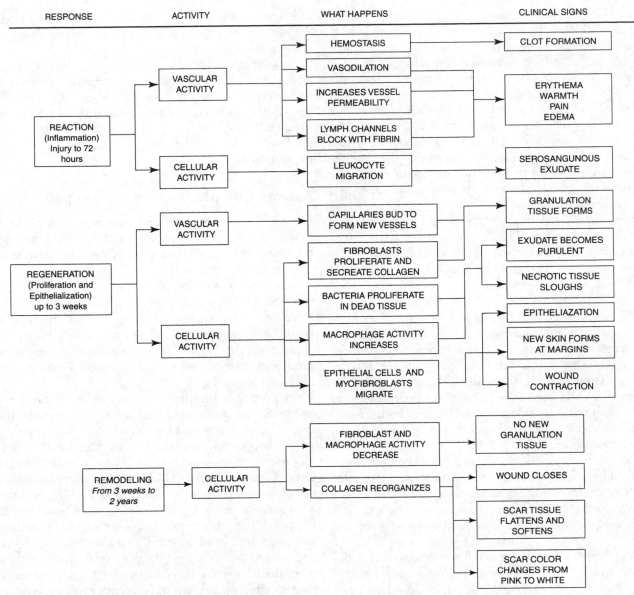

RESPONSE	ACTIVITY	WHAT HAPPENS	CLINICAL SIGNS

REACTION (Inflammation) Injury to 72 hours

VASCULAR ACTIVITY → HEMOSTASIS → CLOT FORMATION

VASODILATION
INCREASES VESSEL PERMEABILITY → ERYTHEMA / WARMTH / PAIN / EDEMA
LYMPH CHANNELS BLOCK WITH FIBRIN

CELLULAR ACTIVITY → LEUKOCYTE MIGRATION → SEROSANGUNOUS EXUDATE

REGENERATION (Proliferation and Epithelialization) up to 3 weeks

VASCULAR ACTIVITY → CAPILLARIES BUD TO FORM NEW VESSELS → GRANULATION TISSUE FORMS

FIBROBLASTS PROLIFERATE AND SECREATE COLLAGEN → EXUDATE BECOMES PURULENT

BACTERIA PROLIFERATE IN DEAD TISSUE → NECROTIC TISSUE SLOUGHS

CELLULAR ACTIVITY → MACROPHAGE ACTIVITY INCREASES → EPITHELIAZATION / NEW SKIN FORMS AT MARGINS

EPITHELIAL CELLS AND MYOFIBROBLASTS MIGRATE → WOUND CONTRACTION

REMODELING From 3 weeks to 2 years

CELLULAR ACTIVITY → FIBROBLAST AND MACROPHAGE ACTIVITY DECREASE → NO NEW GRANULATION TISSUE

COLLAGEN REORGANIZES → WOUND CLOSES / SCAR TISSUE FLATTENS AND SOFTENS / SCAR COLOR CHANGES FROM PINK TO WHITE

Figure 14.2   Reaction • Regeneration • Remodeling • *Wound healing process—The 3Rs.*

logical involvement such as paralysis and peripheral neuropathies that may negatively impact their ability to detect potentially destructive pressures. Older patients may experience decreased cognitive ability, fluctuating mental states, weakness and debilitation, and chronic illnesses that lead to immobility, which may predispose them to skin breakdown.[6,7]

These factors are not the only ones that will affect wound healing in an older population. Tissue and vascular changes related to decreased activity levels will diminish the nutritional health of tissue and increase their vulnerability to injury.

In an older individual with an impaired inflammatory response, blastema cells may appear within days of injury. This is indicative that the tissue repair process is not starting.[8,9] The inflammatory response may also be prolonged in an older patient, lasting from seven to fourteen days following the initial injury (generally lasts around two to four days). The proliferation period is also extended. Typically this phase of healing lasts for about three weeks. In the elderly, it is more commonly five to six weeks in duration.[10] A delay in wound contraction and cellular migration and proliferation may occur in older patients, and the remodeling phase varies, ranging anywhere from two years to five years (sometimes even more).[11] In an older adult, it is also important to keep in mind that the scar tissue is generally weaker and less elastic than that seen in a younger population.

The aging changes affecting tissue repair as depicted in Table 14.1 influence the rate of healing in older adults. Thinning and flattening of the epidermis results in an increased vulnerability to trauma from shear and frictional forces. The skin is more likely to blister or tear, resulting in a partial thickness injury. Additionally, changes in sensation and perfusion allow the skin to become macerated or overhydrated, which can lead to breakdown. Once the epidermis has been damaged, it takes longer for the older adult to replace these tissue layers.[6,7]

Healing also takes longer in the older adult because the epidermal proliferation or turnover time is slowed. The production of new skin cells decreases and the surface layer simply does not replace itself as readily. The end result is delayed wound contraction and decreased cellular migration and proliferation resulting in an inefficient and slower rate of healing.[7]

Atrophy of the dermis results in less elasticity and a thinning of the tissues. This leaves the underlying tissues more exposed and more vulnerable to breakdown. This circumstance also increases the likelihood of dehiscence and delayed wound contraction.[12]

An older individual's skin also shows a decrease in vascularity, not only compromising sensation because of nutrient deficiency but also altering the ability to regulate body temperature. Capillary growth decreases resulting in a reduction in the amount of blood being delivered to the tissues.[6,7] Consequently, the tissues become more susceptible to injury and breakdown. Due to the poor vascularity and nutrient status, the skin is more likely to bruise. Small insults can result in hemorrhages that are disproportional to the actual injury.

The quality of the tissue is also compromised in the elderly. The loss of collagen and elastic fibers and a delay in collagen remodeling leave the underlying tissue more vulnerable to trauma. The scar tissue of a healed wound is less flexible and much more fragile than the original skin tissue.[6,7]

The number of sebaceous and sweat glands also decreases making the skin less moist, lubricated, and resilient. The skin becomes drier, more easily cracked, and is susceptible to infection and fungal development. Because of the loss of hair follicles and touch/pressure receptors, coupled with dehydration, the sensory system is compromised, increasing the chance of injury.

A diminishment in the responsiveness of the vascular system impairs cutaneous immune and inflammatory responses.[6,7] It also results in delayed wound closure. There is a reduction in the ability to clear foreign materials or fluids, a decrease in wound capillary growth, and an alteration of metabolic responses.

With age, the ability to discriminate touch, temperature, and vibration declines. The skin is more prone to trauma and burns, often without perception.

Last, the subcutaneous tissue, which is a natural padding system, is reduced. This leaves bony prominences directly exposed to external forces without a protective layer for shock absorption. Because of the abundant circulatory network in the subcutaneous layer, the loss of this layer of tissue also impacts the ability to regulate systemic temperature through vasodilation and vasocontriction. The elderly are much less efficient at coping with ambient temperature changes.

In addition to alterations in skin condition related to aging, many disease processes will affect the status of the skin. Peripheral vascular disease, for instance, leads to a poor nutritional state and an increased risk for ulceration. Wounds related to the peripheral neuropathy seen in diabetes mellitus are extremely common in the older population.

Factors Complicating Wound Repair

Elimination of exogenous and endogenous impediments to wound repair and meticulous local care are required for humane and cost-effective patient care and satisfactory treatment outcomes.

This section of the chapter provides an overview of factors which might impair healing in an elderly population. Infection, nutrition, and the aging process are the major factors in overall success of wound healing in an older population. Additionally, the patient's complex medical status and potential medical complications may compromise wound healing.

The presence of infection increases the metabolic demands for wound healing and normal cellular functioning.[6] The most common complication of wound repair is wound infection. Due to the changing homeostatic mechanism of core body temperature (see Chapter 3) and decreased responsiveness of blood cell production, the body temperature may not be elevated and white blood cell production may not appear to be increased based on laboratory findings. As a result, the presence of infection may go undetected. It is important, therefore, for the clinician to look for indicators of infection, such as wound color, odor, drainage, pain, and edema, or changes in cognition such as lethargy, confusion, or restlessness. Patients with infection may also report dizziness or lightheadedness. In fact, sometimes a fall is the first indicator of an infection. The therapist must be alert to these signs and symptoms, especially when a wound is present.

Many drugs that an older patient may be on compromise wound repair.[12] These include:

- Steroids
- Nonsteroidal anti-inflammatory drugs (NSAIDs)
- Narcotics and sedatives
- Immunosuppressive agents
- Antineoplastic drugs
- Anticoagulants
- Antiprostaglandins

The use of many medications can affect the skin and can lead to an increased risk of breakdown and delay in healing. Steroids and nonsteroidal anti-inflammatory drugs (NSAIDs) are only a few of the many drugs that affect the skin in older adults. In fact, the use of steroids before or shortly after injury can prolong healing by inhibiting epidermal regeneration and collagen synthesis and decreasing the tensile strength of wound tissues. Not only is the function of fibroblasts and collagen synthesis impaired, but the use of steroids may affect the phagocytic and antibacterial elements of wound repair.[7]

The use of NSAIDs can delay the reepithelialization of the stratum corneum. Oral NSAIDs, which have been shown to reduce the inflammatory response, may have a significant effect on wounds during the acute phase, or on those wounds where inflammation is a desired response.

Narcotics and sedatives can increase the risk for skin disruption simply by decreasing the patient's mental alertness, thus leading to decreased mobility and activities.

Chemotherapy (immunosuppressive agents) is associated with an increased risk of infection and alteration of collagen synthesis, metabolism, and fibroblast and myofibroblast function.[11] The use of immunosuppressive agents may decrease the tensile strength of tissues, as well as negatively influence a patient's response to customary wound care.

Other important drug categories that can affect healing are antineoplastic drugs, anticoagulants, and antiprostaglandins. Complications may also occur as a result of other numerous factors and need to be considered:

- Immunosuppressive diseases
- Cytotoxic cleaners, dressings, agents
- Radiation therapy
- Patient's environment
- Lack of attention to primary etiology of the wound (inadequate pressure relief, inappropriate shoe gear, inadequate compression with venous disease) and poor patient care
- Patient noncompliance
- Inappropriate wound care
- Nutritional state (including obesity or malnutrition)
- Decreased sensation or paralysis
- Altered mental status
- Urinary incontinence
- Hypovolemia
- Physical disability and chronic illness leading to immobility

Diseases of the immune system result in an increased risk of infection. A decrease in hematocrit (red blood cells as a percentage of blood volume) or diminished hemoglobin (red blood cell volume) will decrease the availability of oxygen to the system. Any disease that reduces red blood cell production will lead to anemia. Too many red blood cells will also affect healing due to the predisposition of

blood clot formation. Low platelet counts can increase the risk of bleeding because of the impaired coagulation function.

Diabetes mellitus is not only associated with poor circulation and ischemia from mechanical factors, but this disease is complicated by an impaired immune system. These patients are less resistant to bacteria that can lead to infection. A decrease in perspiration resulting from the autonomic involvement allows the skin to crack and fissure, and increases the vulnerability to infection. Infection can lead to necrosis, gangrene, and amputation.

Chronic venous insufficiency is another problem that increases the risk for infection and is a common medical problem among the elderly. This condition also increases the risk of acute thrombophlebitis with potentially life-threatening results. Arterial insufficiency leads to ulceration due to an insufficient blood supply to the lower extremities. Any of these circulatory conditions can be exacerbated by smoking, diabetes, hypertension, or trauma. There is poor perfusion in the lower extremities with arterial insufficiency leading to claudication and self-restricted activity levels.

Pulmonary diseases reduce the amount of oxygen introduced into the system thereby affecting peripheral perfusion. Neurological disorders not only reduce mobility but also impair sensation and increase the risk of breakdown.

Obesity is a neglected problem in the older adult population. With obesity, adipose tissue is poorly vascularized, decreasing the nutrients' supplies to the various layers of the skin. The increased load places undue stress on the tissues. These patients, though this may not be suspected, are most often malnourished. They consume large amounts of empty calories that do not contain sources of vitamins and minerals.

Converse to obesity is emaciation in the elderly. This clearly will increase vulnerability of tissues, especially over bony prominences, and the likelihood that skin status will be compromised as a result of nutritional deficiencies is great.

Older adults are often plagued with urinary or bowel incontinence. Many elders with incontinence suffer from skin breakdown due to the irritants in excrements and the chronic exposure to moisture. The destruction of the skin's integrity from moisture, combined with bacteria and acidic pH from urine and feces, make the skin more susceptible to infection.

Prolonged hypovolemia can result in reduced venous return and a decrease in cardiac output (see Chapter 13) and can lead to a decrease in leukocyte production and activity and compromise collagen production.[13]

Factors affecting repair of wounds in the older patients include, but are not limited to, delayed cellular activity, decreased wound breaking strength, decreased barrier properties, diminished biosynthetic activity, delayed collagen remodeling and contraction, and decreased vascularity.[12] While caution is suggested in treating the elderly, particularly those with friable skin, not all aged individuals have decreased ability to heal. Variations in medical status and health allow many elderly to heal as well as the younger population. Surgeries are frequently performed on the elderly with no problems with healing. When treating the elderly for healing wounds from any origin:

■ Exercise caution when using adhesives and tapes on friable skin.
■ Avoid frequent scrubs.
■ Avoid irritating and cytotic agents.[12]

Complication of wound repair may occur because of numerous intrinsic and extrinsic factors. It is important for the wound care team to consider the whole of a patient's medical status when dealing with a wound in an elderly person. When a wound shows no response to treatment after two weeks, the patient's medical and wound status should be reevaluated. When there are no new findings regarding medical status, a different wound care approach (product, modality, medication) should be considered.

NUTRITIONAL CONSIDERATIONS IN WOUND CARE

Optimal nutritional status is essential for healing a wound, regardless of the age of a patient.[14] However, protein-calorie, vitamin, and mineral malnutrition, especially in those hospitalized postsurgical elderly patients, occurs in about 50% of older individuals. In fact, it has been determined that nutritional status often deteriorates during a hospital stay.[15] Elderly patients discharged from the hospital with open wounds are likely to have tenuous nutritional status and need careful attention to diet if their wounds are to heal. Nutritionally, the immune system can be bolstered through attention to the diet.

For more information on nutritional considerations in wound care, see CD.

PATIENT AND WOUND EVALUATION

Accurate assessment and evaluation of a wound is very important. Identifying causation problems (positioning, diagnoses, functional capabilities) will assist the clinician in treating the current wound and preventing future wounds from occurring.

Thorough knowledge and assessment of the physical and pathological etiologies of wounds are prerequisites to treating lesions successfully. Patient evaluation should include a comprehensive review of systems, review of medications, prior and current treatment modalities, the patient's awareness of the problem, the external environment that may affect wound care and future prevention, and nutritional status. If possible, the date of wound onset should be established in addition to identifying contributing factors. A history of significant medical diagnoses such as diabetes, hypertension, congestive heart failure, renal disease, COPD, peripheral vascular disease, lymphatic insufficiency, recent weight loss, and other problems that may impact the effective treatment of the wound should be established. A history of previous wounds and the types of treatments and results is also an important area of assessment. Medications that may affect wound healing such as steroids or anticoagulants need to be documented. Identifying allergies to topical medications or whirlpool additives should be determined.

Laboratory findings, especially culture reports of the wound if available, will assist in establishing the direction of intervention. Any malnourished geriatric patient is not at a greater risk for the development of an ulceration, but will require more healing time. Testing the protein and serum albumin levels is crucial to predicting wound healing. A low protein level will impede collagen synthesis, fibroblast proliferation, and wound remodeling. Phagocytosis and the immune response will also be impaired. An elderly patient with a wound will need higher protein sources. Low serum albumin levels respresent late manifestation of protein deficiency. Normal albumin levels are 3.5 to 5.0 gm/dL. A severely compromised albumin level would be less than 2.5 to 3.0 gm/dL.

Laboratory evaluation may also be needed to determine the availability of other nutrients which will expedite wound healing. For example, vitamins A and C assist in collagen synthesis. Vitamin C affects fibroblastic and immune function, while vitamin A promotes re-epithilialization. Minerals such as zinc may increase epithelialization and cell production.

Chapter 13 provides a model for assessing peripheral circulation and central cardiovascular status. Evaluating the presence of pulses, particularly in distal wounds of the lower extremity, will determine the viability of the tissues for healing. Assessing the overall skin integrity including hydration, turgor, and areas of discoloration will provide information on the tissue's nutritional status and the prospect of healing the wound.

Arterial pathologies need to be assessed in an objective manner. It is crucial that the tissue receive oxygen. If blood flow to a wound is impeded, oxygenation and nutrients will be blocked and CO_2 and metabolic by-products will not be removed. Without oxygen, collagen synthesis and fibroblast differentiation will not occur. In the course of the physical exam, beyond assessing dorsal pedis pulse and a posterior tibial pulse, if a portable Doppler is available, this is an objective means of evaluating peripheral circulation. The Buerger-Allen protocol of assessment described in Chapter 13 is also an excellent means of objectifying the status of peripheral circulation.

Venous problems will affect the removal of waste products from the lower extremities and affect the nutritional health of the tissues.[16] Has the patient ever experienced a leg injury? A previous injury often leads to increased venous hypertension, which will progress to lipodermatosclerosis—the visible brown pigmentation and induration of the legs. Edema will keep oxygen and vital nutrients from entering the wound site.

Determine the neurosensory status (e.g., anesthesias, paresthesias, pain, pressure) using the Symmes-Weinstein filaments as described in Chapter 13 to establish the integrity of sensory input. Assessing pain patterns will help to identify symptoms and activities that increase or decrease pain.

Determining mobility status including ADLs, flexibility, strength, locomotion, and self-positioning will be predictive of rate of healing as well as the potential efficacy of preventive interventions. Assess position needs and equipment to promote wound healing. Immobility is the leading cause of pressure ulceration.[16] A healthy individual capable of feeling noxious stimuli over a bony prominence will alleviate pressure by moving that part. On the other hand, elderly patients who are immobilized secondary to illness with sensory deprivation, friable skin, and poor circulation have no comparable defense. Nor do diabetics, who have a diminished protective sensory threshold. If the individual cannot reposition her- or himself or move the affected limb, an ulcer sets in via hypoxia. This is a patient that needs pressure-relieving devices and repositioning on a regular schedule.

The presence of incontinence is another risk factor that increases the potential for skin breakdown by creating a moist environment which, if not attended to, leads to maceration and chemical irritation. If incontinent patients move their extremities in a urine or bowel-soaked environment, shear and friction will easily tear the outer layer of soft wet skin, eventually resulting in a breach in integument and paving the way for the possibility of wound infection.

When evaluating a wound, it is important to augment the assessment by appraising risk factors:

- Is the patient ambulatory?
- Is the patient oriented and able to understand directives?
- Is the patient eating independently or receiving nourishment through other sources (supplements, tube feeding)?
- Does the patient have a sensory deficit, or can pain be felt in the wound area?
- Does the patient have a significant other or caretaker who can assist with care of the wound?
- Are there other contributing factors, such as urinary incontinence, poor nutrition, arterial occlusions, venous insufficiency, or perhaps diabetes?

DOCUMENTATION AND STAGING OF WOUND STATUS

In the present arena of wound care, accurate documentation is critical for securing reimbursement. While the principal rationale for documentation is to legally record information, equally important is communication with other health care professionals and third-party payers. Over time, documentation can also be used as a database for clinical research, outcomes, peer review, and the quality improvement process.

Wound evaluation and documentation includes determination of:

- Etiology and type of wound
- Infection versus contamination
- Size of wound
- Undermining of sinus tracts
- Quality and quantity of exudate
- Underlying structures (muscles, tendons, bones)
- Stage of healing
- Chronicity
- Response to previous treatment

In evaluating the wound, it is important to document the location of the wound and the type of wound (e.g., arterial versus venous insufficiency, vasculitic, pressure ulcer, diabetic ulcer, burn, abrasion, surgical, laceration, shearing, hematoma, stasis). The charting of the size of the wound should include the length, width, depth, presence of undermining, and description of the shape of the wound. The status of the wound bed and the surrounding tissue should be described in a clear and concise manner. Color, odor, and exudate are all indications of wound status. The color of the wound is indicative of the stage of repair. Odor is the best way to determine if the wound is infected. It is helpful to evaluate odor after a wound has been cleansed with sterile water or saline. Foul odor may result from accumulation of wound exudate, necrotic tissue, and dressing by-products, especially after the use of occlusive dressings. Common examples of appearance of wounds are provided in Table 14.2. Necrotic tissue promotes bacterial growth and when left in a wound will slow the formation of granulation tissue and epithelialization, inhibiting angiogenesis.[16]

The presence of the exudate should be recorded and the description of the drainage would include the amount, color, and viscosity (i.e., serous, serosanguineous, sanguineous, or purulent). The condition of the wound tissue includes a description including the presence of granulation, epithelialization, slough, eschar, or hemorrhage. It is also important to note the condition of the surrounding tissue in terms of pain, swelling, tenderness, erythema, discoloration, maceration, inflammation, skin temperature,

TABLE 14.2   Common Descriptions of Wound Appearance in Documentation

Description	Implication
Red-reepithelializing	Bright red with indications of superficial cell migration. Good wound bed and healing well.
Red-granulating	Bright or true red in appearance associated with islands of granulation tissue and good healing.
Red-chronic	Red appearance but no indication of granulation. Poor or delayed healing
Red-dusky	Dull, gray, or dark red in appearance without signs of granulation, with or without signs of localized ischemia. Poor healing with possibility of infection.
Yellow-granulating	Areas of fibrotic tissue (not usually classified as healthy or unhealthy) present in conjunction with areas of granulating tissue. No necrotic tissue present. Delayed healing.
Yellow-chronic	Areas of fibrotic tissue without areas of granulation. Poor healing.
Yellow-ischemic	Fibrotic tissue in conjunction with signs of ischemia or tissue necrosis. Delayed or poor healing.
Black-dry	Dry, desiccated eschar whether black or brown in appearance. Poor healing with tissue death.
Black-wet	Wet gangrenous appearance. Tissue death with progressive infection.
Black-mixed	Areas of necrotic tissue present with areas of yellow and/or red tissue. Tissue death with areas of infection and sporadic areas of healing.

Formulated with information from: Mulder, G.C., Fairchild, P.A., Jeter, K.F. Clinician's Pocket Guide to Chronic Wound Repair. 3rd ed. Long Beach, CA: Wound Healing Institute Publications; 1995.

skin texture, and hair loss. If edema is significant, baseline girth measurements need to be taken.[16]

It is important that the wound be graded in some fashion so that all health care professionals know the nature of the wound they are dealing with. There are many acceptable staging guidelines. Many clinicians use the Wagner's ulcer grade classification system, which is specific to foot ulcerations; others prefer the more general staging system developed by the National Pressure Ulcer Advisory Panel. Both provide a means of objectifying wound status and facilitating consistent communication of the status of the wound.

Wagner's classification[17] was developed to objectively evaluate foot condition and ranks vascular dysfunction in grades of 0 to 5 as follows:

Grade 0: The skin is without ulceration. No open lesions are present, but potentially ulcerating deformities, such as bunions, hammer toes, and Charcot's deformity, may be present. Healed partial foot amputation may also be included in this group.

Grade 1: A full-thickness superficial skin loss is present. The lesion does not extend to bone. No abscess is present.

Grade 2: An open ulceration is noted deeper than grade 1. It may penetrate to tendon or joint capsule.

Grade 3: The lesion penetrates to bone, and osteomyelitis is present. Joint infection or

plantar fascial plane abscess may also be noted.

Grade 4: Gangrene is noted in the forefoot.

Grade 5: Gangrene involving the entire foot is noted. This is not salvageable with local procedures.

The National Pressure Ulcer Advisory Board[16] provides a staging scheme for nonfoot ulcers. This staging is as follows:

Stage I: Nonblanchable erythema of intact skin, heralding lesion of skin ulceration. Dangerous if left unprotected. Often progresses quickly to Stage II or greater.

Stage II: Partial-thickness skin loss involving epidermis and/or dermis. Clinically, the lesion presents as a large blister or abrasion. Displayed most commonly under heels of the elderly due to friction and shear from heel movement, and especially in the immobile elderly following hip surgery.

Stage III: Full-thickness skin loss involving damage or necrosis of subcutaneous tissue, which may extend down to, but not through, underlying fascia. It is imperative to check for undermining or sinus tracts.

Stage IV: Full-thickness skin loss with extensive destruction, tissue necrosis or damage to muscle, bone or supporting structures.

These classification systems assist in describing the severity of the wound. In many cases these staging systems have prognostic value and, in some instances, reimbursement value. Complete description and classification are essential components of the diagnostic and therapeutic process in wound care.

Included in the grading or staging of a wound, the following descriptors should be provided in the initial and ongoing documentation of the wound.

- Location of wound
- Surface dimension of wound
- Color of wound base
- Presence of necrotic tissue (amount and color)
- Depth and tissue layers involved
- Exudate (amount, color, odor)
- Condition of the surrounding skin
- Undermining
- Clinical signs of infection (see the subsequent section on microbiology)

There are several methods that can be used to determine the size and shape of a wound. Whichever method is chosen, it is imperative that the therapist continues to use the same method consistently throughout the healing process, as different methods give different results. The

therapist may wish to use a combination of methods. For example, measuring length and width as well as volume gives an excellent three-dimensional representation of the wound's actual size. As the wound heals, the length and width may actually become larger, yet the total volume of the wound will decrease. It is imperative to document which methods are being utilized, so the same techniques can be followed by other therapists. Therapists must also coordinate measuring procedures with the nursing staff or wound care team members.

It is helpful to keep the time intervals between measurements consistent. A decline in the rate of healing may be the first indication of a need to change treatment approaches.

In the presence of an ulceration, objective documentation of wound size is best accomplished by tracing the wound on sterilized x-ray film or through photographs on a line-graphed film. This is helpful in monitoring improvement or decline in wound status. Some x-ray type films are available with a bull's eye pattern that provides diameter and metric measures. This sort of industry-prepared measuring tool is useful in objectively tracing wound perimeters. Figure 14.3A provides an example of this sort of device.

Tracings, tape measurement guides, volumetric displacement, plain meter, and photographic measurement are all excellent ways of documenting wound status. The combination of measurement techniques employed will be

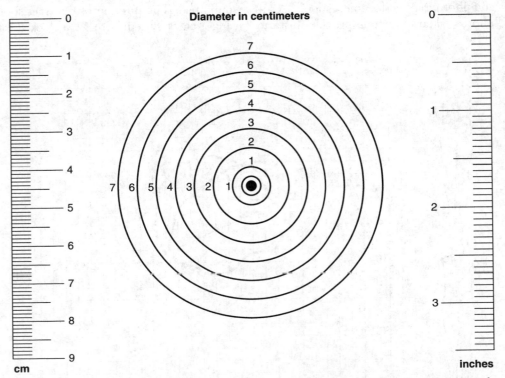

Figure 14.3A   Bull's eye and linear measurement acetate (x-ray) film for tracing and measuring size of wound. Center of bull's eye is placed in center of wound and periphery of wound is traced.

dictated by the patient's individualized status and plan of care. Wounds may be measured in a linear fashion and described as an area (e.g., 6 cm by 4 cm) or traced on an acetate measuring guide as presented in Figure 14.3A. Length and width of a wound to obtain size may be accomplished by using a clear ruler and measuring the longest and the widest aspects of the wound. Tracings on acetate can be transferred to a grid as shown in Figure 14.3B. As depicted in this drawing, the wound is represented by the solid line and the measured area of undermining is represented by the dashed line. Periodic tracing can be superimposed on this graph in varying colors and dated to indicate ongoing status of the wound. This gives a wonderful visual representation of the change in wound size and status. By utilizing graph paper, width and length measures are easy to obtain. Area of the wound can be calculated by counting the number of squares contained within the boundaries of the wound.

If acetate film is not available for tracing, placing two layers of plastic wrap over the wound and using a permanent ink marker to trace the outline of the wound is an inexpensive way of tracing the wound. Dispose of the bottom layer of plastic as infectious waste and photocopy the top layer onto the metric graph paper. Approximate the area within the wound by counting the boxes within the wound's borders (see Figure 14.3B).

Tracings enable more accurate comparison of change in wound perimeter over time. These small acetate (x-ray film) measuring sheets are provided at no charge by numerous companies that provide wound care products. Many clinicians add photographic documentation.[18] A series of accurate photos taken over time provides historic data about the wound and its progress and serves as visual support for written documentation. A photograph of the wound is the most reliable documentation. Serial photographs provide objective evaluation of wound healing as demonstrated in Figure 14.4.

Measuring wound depth can be accomplished by putting a cotton-tipped applicator or tongue depressor into the base of the wound and then placing the acetate or ruler across the wound surface and marking the point it encounters the cotton swab or depressor. This measures the distance from the tip of the swab to where the applicator is even with the intact skin and provides a measure of the depth of the wound.

Undermining, which is defined as skin overhanging a dead space, should be measured with a gloved finger or a cotton-tipped applicator. To measure undermining place a cotton-tipped applicator into the wound to the extent of the undermining. Gently lift the applicator toward the skin surface until the skin is raised slightly. Mark this location with a skin pencil. Repeat at close intervals around the perimeter of the wound. On the grid paper the areas of undermining and their depth can be indicated with dashed lines as indicated in Figure 14.3B. This area, as it is probed, can be traced on the plastic wrap or acetate film as described above.

When sinus tracts are suspected, they should be probed gently with a cotton-tipped applicator or a small red rubber catheter to determine their length. A cotton-tipped applicator is placed into the tract and the distance is measured from the tip of the swab to where the tract enters the wound bed. The position of the tract should be noted by using a clock system with 12 o'clock the head of the pa-

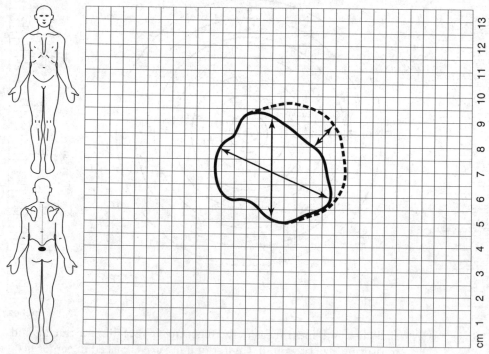

Figure 14.3B   Grid documentation of location and area of a wound.

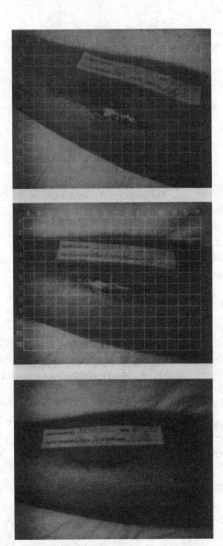

Figure 14.4 Photographic documentation of wound status over time. (*Reprinted with permission from Susan E. Morey. Originally appeared In: Morey, S.E. Photos supplement written documentation. Physical Therapy Products. January–February 1998; 66–67.*)

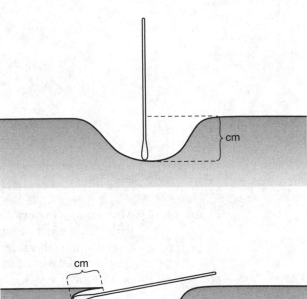

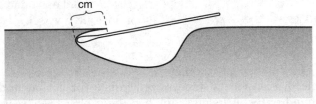

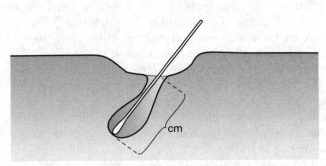

Figure 14.5A Measuring the depth of a wound using a cotton-tipped swab. Measuring the extent of undermining of a wound. Measurement techniques for determining the depth, extent of undermining, and sinus tract of a wound using a cotton swab applicator.

tient, and 6 o'clock the feet. Measurement techniques for depth, sinus track, and undermining are provided in the drawing in Figure 14.5A.

Volumetric measures are also very helpful. By filling the wound with sterile water or saline just to the point of overflowing and then suctioning the water out of the wound using a needleless syringe, the volume of water it takes to fill the wound can be measured in ccs or mLs by reading the syringe markings. This gives an accurate measure of the volume of the wound. (Note: the wound must be in a position that it can be filled without the water spilling out.) Figure 14.5B provides a pictorial demonstration of this technique.

One technique for measuring volume is to use a substance called Jeltrate. This is a hydrocolloid substance that will not adhere to the wound or damage granulation tis-

sue. A word of caution, however: This gel-like substance should not be used in wounds with very small surface openings or with large areas of undermining or tracking. The Jeltrate technique involves adding water to the Jeltrate powder according to the package instructions. Then pour the liquid into the wound and allow it to solidify (takes around five minutes). Remove the mold from the wound and place it into a graduated cylinder partially filled with a premeasured amount of water. Record the amount of water displaced as demonstrated in Figure 14.5C. This water displacement represents the volume of the wound. This mold is also an excellent teaching tool for patients, family members, or nursing staff.

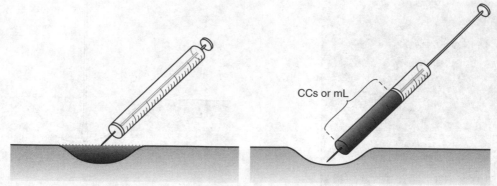

Figure 14.5B   Measuring area of wound using a volume measurement. Fill wound with sterile water or saline to level point. Suction fluid from wound to get volume measure in ccs or mLs. Volumetric measurement using Jeltrate mold of wound and determining displacement of water in a premeasured vessel.

There are many excellent wound assessment tools available that provide a standardized format for documenting wound status. A helpful tool, because it objectively scores each parameter for accurate monitoring of the patient's condition, was developed by Barbara Bates-Jensen. A description of the use of this tool and the tool itself are provided in Figures 14.6A and 14.6B, respectively.[19,20]

Accurate documentation enables critical evaluation of the wound-healing process and helps to inform clinicians of the wound status in an objective way. The key to future research in the pathophysiology of chronic wounds and in therapeutic efficacy depends on precise reporting of incidence and types of chronic wounds and the use of consistent terminology. Documentation can provide the database of healing as well as nonhealing wounds required to establish the need for physical therapy or the database of healing needed to secure reimbursement from intermediaries.

MICROBIOLOGY

Bacteria is often found in chronic wounds. There is a distinction drawn between a contaminated wound and an infected wound. According to Mulder and associates,[12]

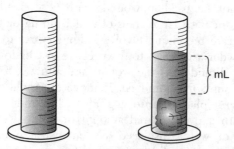

Figure 14.5C   Volumetric measurement using Jeltrate mold of wound and determining displacement of water in a premeasured vessel.

wound appearance can be misleading. The degree of contamination and the distinction between contamination and infection are difficult to determine; other signs of wound infection may need to be assessed.[12]

Indicators of wound contamination may include periwound erythema, inflammation, nonpurulent drainage, malodorous (foul smelling) wound prior to cleansing, and multiple organisms present on swab culture. The same signs are present with infection; however, other established signs of infection are elevated body temperature, cellulitis, purulent drainage, wet gangrene, increased leukocytosis, persistently malodorous wound (even after cleansing), and greater than 10^5 organisms per gram tissue on culture.[12] Other indications of infection might include pain, swelling, redness, inflammation, and heat.

Swab cultures are of questionable value as multiple bacteria are often present in wound fluid and wound surface, particularly when occlusive dressings have been used. Surface organisms do not correlate well with number and type of organisms present in the tissue. Other clinical signs of infection must be present when determining that organisms present on culture are of clinical significance. For the most accurate results, it is important that the wound be thoroughly cleansed prior to culturing. Organisms found need to be coupled with other clinical indicators of infection.

LOWER EXTREMITY ULCERS

Different wound types exhibit different characteristics depending on their underlying etiology and cannot all be treated identically. Combinations of wound types further complicate the identification and treatment of wounds, especially in the elderly. For example, many diabetic ulcers result from pressure. Likewise, many patients with peripheral vascular disease may also be diabetic or have other

NAME: _____

Complete the rating sheet to assess pressure sore status. Evaluate each item by picking the response that best describes the wound and entering the score in the item score column for the appropriate date.

LOCATION: Anatomic site. Circle, identify right (R) or left (L) and use "X" t mark site on body diagrams:

_____ Sacrum & coccyx   _____ Lateral ankly
_____ Trochanter   _____ Medial ankle
_____ Ischial tuberosity   _____ Heal   _____ Other site

SHAPE: Overall wound pattern; assess by observing perimeter and depth.
Circle and *date* appropriate description:

_____ Irregular   _____ Linear or elongated
_____ Round/oval   _____ Bow/boat
_____ Square/rectangle   _____ Butterfly   _____ Other shape

Item	Assessment	Date	Date	Date
		Score	Score	Score
1. SIZE	1 = Length × width <4 sq cm 2 = Length × width 4 – 16 sq cm 3 = Length × width 16.1 – 36 sq cm 4 = Length × width 36.1 – 80 sq cm 5 = Length × width <80 sq cm			
2. DEPTH	1 = Nonblanchable erythema on intact skin 2 = Partial-thickness skin loss involving epidermis &/or dermis 3 = Full-thickness skin loss involving damage or necrosis of subcultaneous tissue; may extend down to but not through underlying fascia; &/or mixed partial- &/or full-thickness &/or tissue layers obscured by granulation tissue 4 = Obscure by necrosis 5 = Full-thickness skin loss with extensive destruction, tissue necrosis, or damage to muscle, bone, or supporting structures			
3. EDGES	1 = Indistinct, diffuse, none clearly visible 2 = Distinct, outline clearly visible, attached, even with wound base 3 = Well defined, not attached to wound base 4 = Well defined, not attached to base, rolled under, thickened 5 = Well defined, fibrotic, scarred or hyperkeratotic			
4. UNDERMINING	1 = Undermining <2 cm in any area 2 = Undermining 2 – 4 cm involving <50% wound margins 3 = Undermining 2 – 4 cm involving >50% wound margins 4 = Undermining >4 cm in any area 5 = Tunneling &/or sinus tract formation			
5. NECROTIC TISSUE TYPE	1 = None visible 2 = White/gray nonviable tissue &/or nonadherent yellow slough 3 = Loosely adherent yellow slough 4 = Adherent, soft, black eschar 5 = Firmly adherent, hard, black eschar			
6. NECROTIC TISSUE AMOUNT	1 = None visible 2 = <25% of wound bed covered 3 = 25% to 50% of wound covered 4 = >50% and <75% of wound covered 5 = 75% to 100% of wound covered			
7. EXUDATE TYPE	1 = None or bloody 2 = Serosanguineous: thin, watery, pale red/pink 3 = Serous: thin, watery, clear 4 = Purulent: thin or thick, opaque, tan/yellow 5 = Foul purulent: thick, opaque, yellow/green with odor			

Figure 14.6A   Pressure Sore Status Tool. (© 1990 Barbara Bates-Jensen. Used with permission.)

Item	Assessment	Date	Date	Date
		Score	Score	Score
8. EXUDATE AMOUNT	1 = None 2 = Scant 3 = Small 4 = Moderate 5 = Large			
9. SKIN COLOR SURROUNDING WOUND	1 = Pink or normal for ethnic group 2 = Bright red &/or blanches to touch 3 = White or gray pallor or hypopigmented 4 = Dark red or purple &/or nonblanchable 5 = Black or hyperpigmented			
10. PERIPHERAL TISSUE ENEMA	1 = Minimal swelling around wound 2 = Nonpitting edema extends <4 cm around wound 3 = Nonpitting edema extends ≥4 cm around wound 4 = Pitting edema extends <4 cm around wound 5 = Crepitus &/or pitting edema extends ≥4 cm			
11. PERIPHERAL TISSUE INDURATION	1 = Minimal firmness around wound 2 = Induration <2 cm around wound 3 = Induration 2–4 cm extending <50% around wound 4 = Induration 2–4 cm extending ≥50% around wound 5 = Induration >4 cm in any area			
12. GRANULATION TISSUE	1 = Skin intact or partial thickness wound 2 = Bright, beefy red, 75% to 100% of wound filled &/or tissue overgrowth 3 = Bright, beefy red, <75% & > 25% of wound filled 4 = Pink &/or dull, dusky red &/or fills ≤25% of wound 5 = No granulation tissue present			
13. EPITHELIALIZATION	1 = 100% of wound covered, surface intact 2 = 75% to <100% of wound covered &/or epithelial tissue extends >0.5 cm into wound bed 3 = 50% to <75% of wound covered &/or epithelial tissue extends to <0.5 cm into wound bed 4 = 25% to <50% of wound covered 5 = <25% of wound covered			
TOTAL SCORE				
SIGNATURE				

PRESSURE SORE STATUS CONTINUUM

1   10   13   15   20   25   30   35   40   45   50   55   60   65

Tissue health   Wound regeneration   Wound degeneration

Plot the total score on the Pressure Sore Status Continuum by putting an "X" on the line and date beneath the line. Plot multiple scores with their dates to see at a glance regeneration or degeneration of the wound.

Figure 14.6A   (Continued)

Instruction for use

General guidelines:

Fill out the attached rating sheet to assess a pressure sore's status after reading the definitions and methods of assessment described below. Evaluate once a week and whenever a change occurs in the wound. Rate according to each item by picking the response that best describes the wound and entering that score in the item score column for the appropriate date. When you have rated the pressure sore on all items, determine the total score by adding together the 13 item scores. The higher the total score, the more severe the pressure sore status. Plot total score on the Pressure Sore Status Continuum to determine progress.

Specific instructions:

1. **SIZE:** Use ruler to measure the longest and widest aspect of the wound surface in centimeters; multiply length × width.

2. **DEPTH:** Pick the depth, thickness, most appropriate to the wound using these additional descriptions:
   1 = Tissues damaged but no break in skin surface.
   2 = Superficial, abrasion, blister, or shallow crater. Even with, and/or elevated above, skin surface (e.g., hyperplasia).
   3 = Deep crater with or without undermining of adjacent tissue.
   4 = Visualization of tissue layers not possible due to necrosis.
   5 = Supporting structures include tendon, joint capsule.

3. **EDGES:** Use this guide:
   Indistinct, diffuse = Unable to clearly distinguish wound outline.
   Attached = Even or flush wound base; *no* sides or walls present; flat.
   Not attached = Sides or wall *are* present; floor or base of wound is deeper than edge.
   Rolled under, thickened = Soft to firm and flexible to touch.
   Hyperkeratosis = Callous-like tissue formation around wound and at edges.
   Fibrotic, scarred = Hard, rigid to touch.

4. **UNDERMINING:** Assess by inserting a cotton-tipped applicator under the wound edge; advance it as far as it will go without using undue force; raise the tip of the applicator so it may be seen or felt on the surface of the skin; mark the surface with a pen; measure the distance from the mark on the skin to the edge of the wound. Continue process around the wound. Then use a transparent metric measuring guide with concentric circles divided into four (25%) pie-shaped quadrants to help determine percent of wound involved.

5. **NECROTIC TISSUE TYPE:** Pick the type of necrotic tissue that is predominant in the wound according to color, consistency, and adherence using this guide:
   White/gray, nonviable tissue = May appear prior to wound opening; skin surface is white or gray.
   Nonadherent, yellow slough = Thin, mucinous substance; scattered throughout wound bed; easily separated from wound tissue.
   Loosely adherent, yellow slough = Thick, stringy, clumps of debris; attached to wound tissue.
   Adherent, soft, black eschar = Soggy tissue; strongly attached to tissue in center or base of wound.
   Firmly adherent, hard/black eschar = Firm, crusty tissue; strongly attached to wound base *and* edges (like a hard scab).

6. **NECROTIC TISSUE AMOUNT:** Use a transparent metric measuring guide with concentric circles divided into four (25%) pie-shaped quadrants to help determine percent of wound involved.

7. **EXUDATE TYPE:** Some dressings interact with wound drainage to produce a gel or trap liquid. Before assessing exudate type, gently cleanse wound with normal saline or water. Pick the exudate type that is predominant in the wound according to color and consistency, using this guide:
   Bloody = Thin, bright red.
   Serosanguineous = Thin, watery, pale red to pink.
   Serous = Thin, watery, clear.
   Purulent = Thin or thick, opaque tan to yellow.
   Foul purulent = Thick, opaque yellow to green with offensive odor.

Figure 14.6B   Instructions for use of the Pressure Sore Status Tool.

8. EXUDATE AMOUNT: Use a transparent metric measuring guide with concentric circles divided into four (25%) pie-shaped quadrants to determine percent of dressing involved with exudate. Use this guide:

None	= Wound tissues dry.
Scant	= Wound tissues moist; no measurable exudate.
Small	= Wound tissues wet; moisture evenly distributed in wound; drainage involves ≤ 25% of dressing.
Moderate	= Wound tissues saturated; drainage may or may not be evenly distributed in wound; drainage involves 25% to ≤ 75% of dressing.
Large	= Wound tissues bathed in fluid; drainage freely expressed; may or may not be evenly distributed in wound; drainage involves >75% of dressing.

9. SKIN COLOR SURROUNDING WOUND: Assess tissues within 4 cm of wound edge. Dark-skinned persons show the colors "bright red" and "dark red" as a deepening of normal ethnic skin color or a purple hue. As healing occurs in dark-skinned persons, the new skin is pink and may never darken.

10. PERIPHERAL TISSUE EDEMA: Assess tissues within 4 cm of wound edge. Nonpitting edema appears as skin that is shiny and taut. Identify pitting edema by firmly pressing a finger down into the tissues and waiting for 5 seconds; on release of pressure, tissues fail to resume previous position and an indentation appears. Crepitus is accumulation of air or gas in tissues. Use a transparent metric measuring guide to determine how far edema extends beyond wound.

11. PERIPHERAL TISSUE INDURATION: Assess tissues within 4 cm of wound edge. Induration is abnormal firmness of tissues with margins. Assess by gently pinching the tissues. Induration results in an inability to pinch the tissues. Use a transparent metric measuring guide with concentric circles divided into four (25%) pie-shaped quadrants to determine percent of wound and area involved.

12. GRANULATION TISSUE: Granulation tissue is the growth of small blood vessels and connective tissue to fill in full-thickness wounds. Tissue is healthy when bright, beefy red, shiny and granular with a velvety appearance. Poor vascular supply appears as pale pink or blanched to dull, dusky red color.

13. EPITHELIALIZATION: Epithelialization is the process of epidermal resurfacing and appears as pink or red skin. In partial-thickness wounds it occurs throughout the wound bed as well as from the wound edges. In full-thickness wounds it can occur from the edges only. Use a transparent metric measuring guide with concentric circles divided into four (25%) pie-shaped quadrants to help determine percent of wound involved and to measure the distance the epithelial tissue extends into the wound.

© 1990 Barbara Bates-Jensen. Used with permission.

Figure 14.6B   (Continued)

chronic disabilities that limit their activity levels, which puts them at greater risk for breakdown as a result of immobility and pressure. The type of pressure causing diabetic ulcers is repetitive, callus-forming pressure, whereas pressure ulcers are an ischemic event. Therefore, identification and treatment of a diabetic ulcer is different from that of a pressure ulcer. The fact that current treatment strategies are based on proper wound classification illustrates the need for the clinician to assess and classify wounds properly, even if a particular wound type is not seen in the clinician's practice setting. Table 14.3 provides five different types of wounds that may be encountered in the clinic and describes characteristics that differentiate each one.[21–25]

Arterial Ulcers

Inadequate blood supply can result in poor oxidative and nutritive status in the tissues and lead to an arterial ulcer. Vascular insufficiency can be the consequence of various diseases such as arteriosclerosis obliterans or atheroembolism. They can also occur when blood supply is restricted because of constriction or pressure that impedes blood flow into an area. Typically these ulcers occur in the distal appendages (lower extremities more than upper extremities) and occur over bony prominences. Clinical manifestations include claudication when walking, rest pain, pain in lower extremities when legs are elevated for extended periods of time, poor quality or absent pulses, atrophic changes, and history of wounds with minor trauma.[4]

Characteristically, individuals with arterial ulcerations will complain of very painful lower extremities, which are often relieved in the dependent position and aggravated by elevation.[26] Wounds present with minimal drainage, are usually superficial, are irregular in shape and borders, are often associated with dry necrotic eschar, and present almost anywhere on the leg, though are most commonly found on the dorsum of the foot or on the toes. The tissues surrounding the wound may be blanched or purpuric in appearance and the peri-wound tissue is often shiny and tight.[12]

Vascular testing is often used to substantiate the presence of hypoperfusion due to arterial insufficiency. The

TABLE 14.3 Differentiating Between Ulcer Types by Characteristics

Type of Ulcer: Ulcer Characteristic	Arterial Ulcer	Venous Ulcer	Diabetic Ulcer	Pressure Ulcer	Vasculitic Ulcer
Predisposing factors/cause	Peripheral vascular disease, diabetes mellitus, advanced age	Valve incompetence in perforating veins, history of deep vein thrombophlebitis and thrombosis, failed calf pump, history of ulcers, obesity, age	Diabetic patient with peripheral neuropathy and/or peripheral vascular disease	Multiple medical diagnoses, age, impaired mobility, poor nutrition, decreased cognitive status, incontinence, impaired circulation	Often accompanied by history of recurrence; almost always accompanied by connective tissue disease and systemic inflammatory conditions
Location and depth	Usually distal to impaired arterial supply, between toes or tips of toes, over phalangeal heads, around lateral malleolus, at sites subjected to trauma or rubbing of footwear; usually relatively shallow, but may be deep	On medial lower leg and ankle, on malleolar area, usually shallow	Any sites on the foot and lower limb subjected to pressure, friction, shear or trauma; plantar aspect, metatarsal heads, great toe, heel; shallow to deep; may have sinus tracking or undermining	On heels, sacrum, coccyx, occiput, any bony prominence subjected to pressure, friction or shear, depth ranges from blanchable erythema of intact skin to deep destruction and loss of tissue	Below malleolus on dorsum of foot; shallow in depth
Wound bed and wound appearance	Pale, gray, or yellow, with no evidence of new tissue growth; gangrene, necrosis, or cellulitis may be present; almost always accompanied by wound bed eschar; often accompanied by exposed tendons	Variable appearance frequently ruddy, beefy red, granular tissue; calcification in wound base is common; a superficial gelatinous fibrinous necrosis may occur suddenly with healthy appearing granulation tissue underneath	Granular tissue unless PVD present; often has deep, dry, necrotic area; cellulitis or osteomyelitis may be present, neuropathic ulcers almost always accompanied by eschar and often accompanied by exposed tendon	Extensive necrotic tissue may be present; extensive undermining, sinus tracts, tunneling may be present (tissue necrosis is usually greater than the external appearance of the epidermal defect)	Typically arise from small reddened areas swhich continue to increase in size; necrotic with marked vascularity; wound bed contains mixed necrotic and red granulation tissue
Exudate/drainage	Minimal exudate	Frequently moderate to heavy exudate	Low to moderate exudate; an infected ulcer may have purulent drainage	Exudate varies	Exudate varies
Wound shape and margins	Smooth, even, regular; shape will conform to injury if caused by trauma; punched out appearance	Tend to be large with irregular margin	Smooth, even; may be small at surface with large subcutaneous abscess, characterized by callus around the ulcer and undermined edges	Usually well-defined; shape frequently is round but will conform to shape of ulcer and may be irregular if large	Irregular, blistering edge; purple-red, hemorrhagic, "angry looking," intense surrounding erythema

(*continued*)

TABLE 14.3   Differentiating Between Ulcer Types by Characteristics

Type of Ulcer:	Arterial Ulcer	Venous Ulcer	Diabetic Ulcer	Pressure Ulcer	Vasculitic Ulcer
Surrounding skin	Pale, blanched, gray, cool, thin; no hair on legs/toes; little or no edema; often accompanied by *livedo reticularis*	Pigmented, edematous, macerated; characterized by hyperpigmentation, dermitis, and lipodermatosclerosis; often accompanied by *livedo reticularis*	Dry, thin, frequently callused	Nonblanchable erythema; clinical infection is indicated by redness, warmth, induration or hardness, swelling	Hyperemic; characterized by *atrophie blanche*, *livedo reticularis*, and *purpura*; often accompanied by hyperpigmentation
Pain	Often accompanied by severe pain at rest and numbness, parasthesias; pain often increases with leg elevation; sudden unset with acute, gradual onset with chronic; claudication relieved by rest; rest pain relieved by dependency; with total occlusion no position gives complete relief	Varies unpredictably; small but deep ulcers around malleoli are typically the most painful; pain often improves with leg elevation; deep muscle pain with acute deep vein thrombosis; mild pain postphlebetically	No sensation, or constant or intermittent numbness or burning; neuropathic ulcers are almost always accompanied by numbness and parathesias	Varies	Often accompanied by severe pain at rest, numbness, parasthesias
Healing	Must have increased blood supply to heal	Epithelialization often fails despite good granulation; healing using compression may take 4 to 6 months, depending on degree of lipodermatosclerosis, and presence of cardiovascular disease	Patient must comply with diet, glucose regulation, exercise, and foot care/wear, aggressive revascularization and appropriate antibiotics may be needed for healing	Must eliminate/reduce pressure, shear, and friction and implement appropriate skin care for healing	Must control the inflammatory process and establish adequate circulation to heal

Table compiled from the following references:
Alvarez, O.M., Gilson, G., Auletta, M.J. Local aspects of diabetic foot ulcer care: Assessment, dressings, and topical agents. In: Levin, M.E., O'Neal, L.W., Bowker, J.H., eds. The Diabetic Foot. 5th ed. St. Louis: Mosby Year-Book; 1993: 259–281.
Falanga, V., Eaglstein, W.H. Leg and Foot Ulcers: A Clinician's Guide. London: Martin Dunitz Limited; 1995.
Hess, C.T. Nurse's Clinical Guide to Wound Care. 2nd ed. Springhouse, PA: Springhouse Corporation; 1997: 28–29.
Holloway, G.A. Arterial ulcers: Assessment, classification and management. In: Krasner, D., Kane, D., eds. Chronic Wound Care: A Clinical Source Book for Healthcare Professionals. 2nd ed. Wayne, PA: Health Management Publications; 1997: 158–164.
Maklebust, J., Sieggreen, M.Y. Pressure Ulcers: Guidelines for Prevention and Nursing Management. 2nd ed. Springhouse, PA: Springhouse Corporation; 1996: 30.
atrophie blanche—a shrinkage and whitening of the skin surrounding the wound
livedo reticularis—a netlike dermatitis
purpura—easy bruising

presence of vascular plaques (arteriosclerotic plaques) is associated with a resistance to blood flow and a decrease in "downstream" pressure. The diagnosis of peripheral arterial disease hinges on a thorough history and physical examination. Laboratory finding are also very important adjuncts in confirmation of arterial insufficiency.[12,26]

Intermittent claudication is a classic symptom of arterial disease. Intermittent claudication is fatigue or pain in the muscles of the lower extremities produced by activity (typically walking) and relieved by rest. Claudication is distinguished from other pain in the extremities because some exertion is always required to produce this symptom and it does not occur at rest.[26] For differential diagnosis, the two conditions that may be confused with claudication are osteoarthritis of the hip or knee and neurospinal compression due to osteophytic narrowing of the lumbar neurospinal canal (spinal stenosis).

When rest pain is present, this is a sign of advanced arterial ischemia, which can lead to gangrene if arterial reconstruction or other interventions (e.g., Buerger-Allen exercises—see Chapter 13) are not implemented. In contrast to claudication, rest pain does not occur in a specific muscle group; rather the patient describes the pain as a burning discomfort most notably confined to the foot. Typically, it is aggravated by elevation of the extremity and relieved by dependency. Rest pain is part of a continuum in arterial vascular disease. It is classically preceded by claudication.

When atherosclerotic disease is present, the distal pulses are usually diminished. If there is an occlusion present the pulse distal to the occluded artery is barely palpable or absent. Bruits may be present and are indicative of turbulent blood flow due to a partially obstructed vessel. It can be heard through a stethoscope and is the loudest during systole.[26]

As described in Chapter 13 in relation to peripheral vascular disease, the pallor of the foot indicates the stage of ischemia. Elevated only slightly, the foot will blanch white and when the foot is dependent it turns a deep red to bluish-purple hue. Rubor is a cyanotic, purple discoloration of the foot on dependency. It appears because, with reduced inflow, blood in the capillary network is relatively stagnant and oxygen extraction is high. Hemoglobin becomes deoxygenated and the capillary blood has an increasing blue hue. In arterial disease, this peripheral discoloration clears on elevation. (Note: In venous insufficiency the discoloration does not resolve with positional changes.)

In an individual with chronic ischemia, the temperature of the skin of the lower extremity decreases and the foot is cool to touch.

Ulcerations due to ischemia are usually very painful and accompanied by ischemic rest pain as described above. The margin of the ulcer is sharply demarcated or punched out, and the base is devoid of healthy granulation tissue. The surrounding skin is pale and mottled, and

signs of chronic ischemia are invariably present. Tissue necrosis first becomes apparent in the distal extremity or at an ulcer site. It stops at the point where blood supply is sufficient to maintain tissue viability.[26] The first stage of necrosis associated with ischemia is dry gangrene. This becomes wet gangrene if infection sets in.[12]

Moderately severe degrees of chronic ischemia produce muscle atrophy and loss of strength in the ischemic zone.[26] Frequently, there is associated decreased joint mobility; subsequent changes in foot structure and gait increase the likelihood that the individual will develop an ulcer.

Chronic ischemia is accompanied by loss of hair growth in the undernourished areas of the lower extremity. The skin becomes frail and transparent and appears dehydrated. Skin appearance is usually shiny and scaly. Poor circulation also leads to thickening of the nails, which become dense and brittle. Due to poor nutritional status, the lower extremity undergoes a pigment change which presents as a darkening (brownish) of the skin in the poorly nourished areas.[12] Simply looking at the foot will be sufficient for identifying significant arterial insufficiency.

Vascular Testing Screening for vascular insufficiency is accomplished through noninvasive vascular testing which may include segmental extremity pressure measures, toe pressures, Doppler waveform analysis, pulse volume recording (PVR), or transcutaneous measurement of oxygen ($TCPO^2$).

An easy way to screen for vascular insufficiency is to measure the resting systolic blood pressure at the brachial artery and at the posterior tibial or dorsalis pedis artery. The ankle/brachial index (ABI) is determined by dividing the pressure obtained at the ankle by the brachial arterial pressure. The ratings of the ratios[12] are as follows:

Ratio	Pathological Implication
> 1.2	Suspect vessel wall calcification, stiffness
1.0–1.2	Normal
0.3–0.9	Claudication
0.0–0.3	Ischemic rest pain, nonhealing ulcers

The ABI is a helpful tool in substantiating the presence of pathology. A ratio greater than 1.2 indicates that the vessel walls are inelastic and stiff. Blood pressure measures are elevated and often the pulses are visible, bounding on the surface without palpation. A ratio of 1.0 to 1.2 is considered normal. The lower ratios indicate poor tissue perfusion. A ratio of 0.3 to 0.9 is associated with claudication, which indicates ischemia on increasing oxygen demands during exercise and activity. Minimal variation between the ankle and the brachial blood pressures results in low ratios (0.0 to 0.3) and would result in ischemic rest pain. The lower the ABI the poorer the rate or possibility of healing.

In addition to the standard ABI, segmental pressures can be obtained at various levels on the leg for localization of occlusive disease. Segmental pressures are performed with the patient in supine and by applying the blood pressure cuff to various levels of the lower extremity (e.g., high thigh, lower thigh, upper calf, ankle). The brachial blood pressure is taken and the highest brachial pressure is used for the denominator. From this, a segmental pressure measurement is obtained. Gradients of more than 20 mm Hg between sites are diagnostic of occlusive disease in the intervening segment.

Another helpful means of testing vascular status is toe pressure. Because of the common finding of inaccurately high ABIs in diabetic patients, measurements of toe pressure is particularly useful. In the normal patient, there is a gradient of 20 to 30 mm Hg between the ankle and the toe, so a correction must be made when toe pressures are being used. Healing of distal wounds can be expected when toe pressures are greater than 40. Healing rarely, if ever, occurs if toe pressures are less than 20 mm Hg, and pressures between 20 and 40 are at risk.

Every clinician has used or at least been exposed to the more commercial form of assessing vascular status, the Doppler waveform analysis. This measurement provides an analog signal that is proportional to the velocity of blood in the vessel being evaluated. The signal is displayed on a screen or recorded for latter analysis. The overall shape of the waveform reflects the status of the vessel proximal to the point studied. In the lower extremity, the normal velocity wave is triphasic, with reverse flow in early diastole. Proximal stenosis first eliminates the reverse flow; and with more severe lesions, there is bunting of the systolic upstroke and increasing flow during diastole.

Another valuable measurement of vascular status is the pulse volume recording (PVR). The blood entering a limb during systole causes an increase in the total volume in the extremity. During diastole, volume returns to normal. This phenomenon results in the pulse pressure oscillation seen with the sphygmomanometer while taking blood pressure. A variety of plethysmograph recorders have been devised using a mercury gauge, water displacement, and impedance. In the 1970s, the pulse volume recorder (PVR) was developed to diagnose peripheral vascular disease.[12] The diagnosis is based on the qualitative evaluation of the PVR waveform. Severe occlusive disease produces a flattened wave with a slow upstroke and downstroke. The absolute amplitude measurements are of limited value from patient to patient because substantial changes result from variations in cardiac output and vasomotor tone. Nonetheless, comparison of amplitudes from one side to the other in the same patient may be very useful for assessing unilateral disease. Like toe pressures, the PVR is particularly helpful when ABIs do not seem accurate.

The transcutaneous measurement of oxygen ($TCPO^2$) can be performed percutaneously using a special instrument. Determination of accurate $TCPO^2$ is fraught with many difficulties in the elderly, however, and requires an experienced clinician, patience, a warm room, and absence of vasoconstriction from other factors. $TCPO^2$ should be measured on the dorsum, not the plantar surface of the foot. Ideally, a reference value is obtained at the chest. Analogous to absolute toe pressures, a $TCPO^2$ value of 40 correlates with good healing. A $TCPO^2$ below 20 mm Hg indicates poor or absent healing, whereas a measurement between 20 and 40 mm Hg places the individual in the at-risk zone.

Venous Ulcers

Venous ulcerations are caused by venous hypertension, valvular incompetence, and generally accompanied by a history of deep vein thrombosis. There are numerous theories that exist regarding the etiology of venous ulcers. The most predominant theories hypothesize that wounds develop because of the failure of the calf and foot muscle pump; that there is damage to the veins secondary to WBC adhesion to capillaries; that poor nutrition and waste removal results from pericapillary fibrin deposition; and that the vein damage leading to ulceration is the result of previous trauma.[27] The veins in the lower extremities lose their tone and become distended allowing for the pooling of blood. Figure 14.7 demonstrates the appearance of the veins damaged by venous pathology. The veins can be damaged by gravitational stresses of prolonged standing, obesity, or pregnancy and become distended. Many veins in the lower extremities have semi-lunar valves that prevent backflow of blood during diastole (as demonstrated in the inset of Figure 14.7) and become frail and unable to prevent blood from being directed toward the heart. The blood pools in the lower extremities, resulting in lower extremity stasis, edema, and visible distention of the veins.

This chronic stasis and edema is the reason tissues become vulnerable to breakdown. Stale blood pools in the lower extremities, waste products are not removed, the provision of oxygen is low, and the toxic effects of accumulating metabolites result in breakdown in tissue health. Under the weight of the edematous lower extremities, the stress on the poorly nourished, vulnerable epithelium results in shallow skin breaks and ultimately venous stasis ulcers.

Characteristic of the venous ulceration is that it is not often painful, and that patients are usually comfortable with their legs elevated. If there is pain in the area of the ulcer, this discomfort is relieved by elevation. Acute deep vein thrombosis (DVT) is often accompanied by severe muscle pain and the arterial pulses are normal. Eczema or stasis dermatitis along with edema and dark pigmentation are generally associated with the presence of venous ulcers.[27]

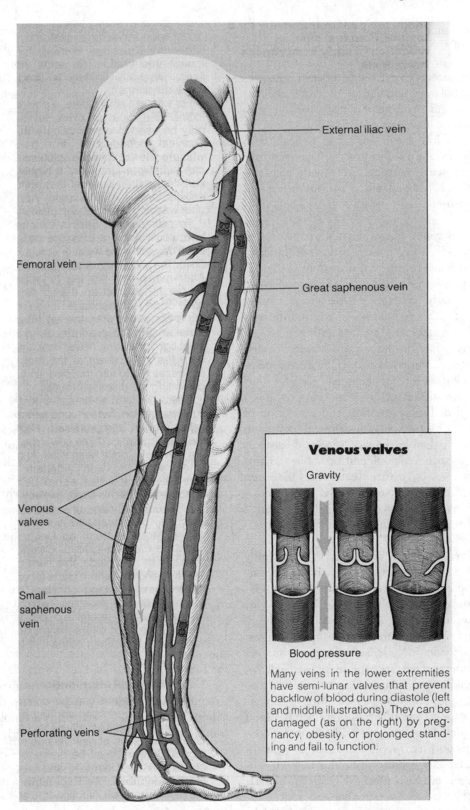

External iliac vein

Femoral vein

Great saphenous vein

Venous valves

Small saphenous vein

Perforating veins

Venous valves

Gravity

Blood pressure

Many veins in the lower extremities have semi-lunar valves that prevent backflow of blood during diastole (left and middle illustrations). They can be damaged (as on the right) by pregnancy, obesity, or prolonged standing and fail to function.

Figure 14.7   Anatomy of a problem: How venous stasis ulcers develop.

The location of these ulcers is usually on the medial aspect of the distal third of the lower extremity and behind the medial malleolus.[12] The so-called gaiter area around the ankle is rich in perforated veins. Venous ulcers occur predominantly in an ambulatory population, though in the elderly, they may be found in nonambulatory patients who spend most of their time in a chair or bed bound.

The appearance of lower extremities in patients with venous ulcers includes a firm (brawny) edema, reddish-brown discoloration with postphlebitic syndrome, evidence of healed ulcers, dilated and tortuous superficial veins, swollen limbs; increased warmth and erythema indicate acute DVT.

Wounds related to venous insufficiency are associated with lipdermatosclerosis. The characteristic appearance of venous ulcers is that they are superficial wounds with periwound and leg hyperpigmentation, lipodermatosclerosis, and a moderate-to-high exudate. These ulcers usually have uneven edges, ruddy granulation tissue, and though, they are superficial, are associated with bleeding.

The clinical signs, etiologic classification, anatomic distribution, physiologic dysfunction tool (CEAP) is a helpful wound assessment scale for venous ulcers.[28] This scoring system of chronic venous dysfunction provides a base for comparison of limb condition and evaluation of treatment outcomes. This tool classifies clinical signs from Class 0 (no visible or palpable signs of venous disease) to Class 6 (skin changes with active ulceration). The remaining three elements each have three categories based on type of venous dysfunction, anatomic extent of the disease, and clinical signs/symptoms of venous dysfunction.[28] Although the grading of symptoms is subjective, the grading of signs is objective.

To rule out arterial disease it is important to carefully assess the patient's vascular status. This can be accomplished by manual palpation of pulses, Doppler examination, and plethysmography.[12] Refer to Table 14.3 for differentiation between arterial and venous ulcers.

Treatment goals in the intervention with venous pathology and ulceration include increasing venous return, decreasing venous stasis and the associated edema, providing compression, and addressing the wound environment. Dressing and pharmacological intervention is dependent on the stage of the ulcer. Generally, in Stage I nonblanchable erythema of the skin with venous ulcers, the use of hydrogels and hydrocolloid dressings or semipermeable foam wafers are used to dress the area. Hydrocolloids and hydrogels are also used for Stages II and III ulcers; however, the dressings are changed more frequently. With the deeper wounds of Stages II and III, the use of calcium alginates is often used to enhance autolysis, especially in a draining wound. Stage IV ulcers are generally treated with hydrogel sheets and hydrogel-amorphous dressings when there is a low level of exudate. In the presence of high exudate wounds, calcium alginates are employed similar to Stage III.

Compression modalities such as stockings, elastic wraps, medicated wraps, and Unna boots are often used to control stasis and edema. Compression modalities vary in the amount of stretch and elasticity, both intrinsically and extrinsically, and in the manner in which they are applied. Correct application is extremely important to product effectiveness. Considerations for the prescription of compression method include the patient's daily activities and her or his tolerance of the chosen modality. Cost, especially in the elderly, is an important variable in choosing the appropriate modality. The presence of a wound and its status will also play a role in the selection of compression intervention.

In the elderly, compression stockings are difficult to apply and often improperly donned, creating constriction and frictional pressures. They may be expensive, especially the custom-fitted stockings. Compression stockings should not be used with arterial disease if there is infection present, weeping dermatitis, or friable tissue. It is also not advisable to use stockings when a wound is present as they are usually nonabsorptive of exudates and do not address the skin status.

Elastic wraps are easy to apply, inexpensive, and available at a local pharmacy. Often, these are compression modalities that, if properly applied, accommodate the older person's need for compression in a more user-friendly manner. The same contraindications apply to Ace wraps as the stockings. They should not be used with arterial disease, severe infection, weeping dermatitis, or friable tissue. One difficulty encountered is the problem of keeping elastic wraps in place. If improperly applied, they may also result in uneven compression. They tend to lose elasticity quickly and require frequent replacing.

Medicated elastic wraps and Unna boots are often used as they protect and medicate the wound. The cost of these devices is moderate.

Pneumatic compression devices are sometimes applied to decrease lower extremity edema. With sequential cuff filling, these devices address the underlying pathology. Pneumatic pumps do not eliminate the need for compression stockings or elastic wraps and should be avoided in the presence of CHF and severe arterial disease.

Wound dressings provide an optimal environment for wound repair, but do not address the problem of increased venous return. They are used to promote re-epithelialization and granulation when the underlying pathophysiology has been treated. Occlusive compression dressings, bandages, wraps, and pneumatic sequential compression devices should not be used in the presence of clinical signs of infection, cellulitis, or severe arterial disease.

Prevention interventions are extremely important. Venous ulcers may reoccur within days after healing if venous disease is neglected after wound closure. Wound closure does not signify resolution of the patient's primary vascular problem. Continued use of compression therapy, particularly stockings and pneumatic compression devices, is helpful for ulcer prophylaxis.

Diabetic Ulcers

Ulceration in the foot in diabetic patients is the most common location and causes serious disability and considerable consumption of scarce resources. The high morbidity and mortality rates associated with diabetic ulcers is attributed to the pathophysiology of the disease and inadequate knowledge of treatment principles for these ulcers.[12] Accurate identification of those patients at particular risk means that ulcers could be prevented. It is important to understand those factors in the diabetic elder that cause ulceration. Figure 14.8 provides a schematic representation of the probable interaction between major factors responsible for diabetic foot ulcerations.

As Figure 14.8 depicts, the pathology of foot ulceration is a multifaceted combination of contributory factors including neuropathy, abnormal blood flow, mechanical stresses, and a suppressed immune system response to infection.

Vascular disease found in diabetics is significantly different from that in nondiabetic patients. Diabetic vascular disease occurs at a younger age and is more accelerated. Occlusion usually involves the multisegmental small vessels (microvascular). Large vessel occlusion is rare.[29]

The classical symptom of arterial circulation impairment, intermittent claudication, occurs more commonly in diabetics compared with nondiabetic individuals.[30,31] In addition to the effects of diabetes, all the usual risk factors for atheroma such as smoking, hypercholesterolemia, and hypertension are as relevant in diabetics as in nondiabetics, and these factors will add to the risk of developing lower limb ischemia and consequent ulceration.

In addition to large vessel atheroma, degenerative arterial changes are also found more distally in diabetes.[30] In the evaluative process, changes similar to those discussed under the section on arterial ulcers will be observed. Care must be taken not to confuse the nocturnal foot pains of ischemia with pain due to peripheral neuropathy. The former is usually associated with absent peripheral pulses and cold feet, while the latter presents with bounding pulses and a warm foot. Absent peripheral pulses, cold peripheries (especially in a warm environment), and slow capillary return are all indicative of peripheral vascular disease and susceptibility to ischemic ulceration. Noninvasive measurement of blood pressure in the peripheral arteries using a Doppler ultrasound provides an objective measurement that is more sensitive to peripheral circulatory changes and not masked by edema. The most commonly used measurement in physical therapy is the ratio of ankle to brachial supine systolic blood pressure (Ankle Pressure Index—API), a value of greater than 0.9 being normal. As long as there is not extensive peripheral vascular calcification, which prevents arterial compression by the sphygmomanometer cuff, a reduced API is a reliable guide to impaired circulation.

Macroangiopathy is associated with the arterial/venous involvement associated with poor peripheral circulation.

Microangiopathy comprising capillary occlusion and nutrition to the extremities is associated with ulceration in the diabetic. Abnormal autoregulation of skin blood flow results in poor perfusion of the tissue and nutritional breakdown of the sensory tissues creating the classic neuropathy. Calcification of the vascular walls is a well-recognized radiological feature in diabetes. It is thought to be related to sympathetic denervation of the blood vessels. Vascular calcification influences blood pressure recordings.[32]

In diabetic individuals, blood flow velocity is increased, possibly owing to arteriovenous shunting. Reduced peripheral perfusion of distal tissues is presumed to result. Clinically, microvascular involvement presents with insensate feet that are warm to touch with distension in the dorsal foot and lower calf veins. Generally an elevated venous pressure can be demonstrated by the height to which the leg needs to be elevated before the veins collapse. Peripheral pulses are bounding, ankle pressure index is high, and venous pO_2 in the dorsal foot veins is high.[33,34]

On evaluation, the typical appearance of the lower extremity with circulatory involvement includes shiny skin, digital redness, dependent rubor, loss of hair growth, delayed superficial venous plexus filling time, and subcutaneous fat atrophy. These are important and classic features that require documentation on initial assessment of the elderly diabetic patient.

Neuropathy generally affects the motor, sensory, and autonomic nerves of the leg and often presents as a stocking-like parasthesia of the foot. Loss of sensation in the diabetic foot results in absence of sensitivity to pain, temperature, and pressure. When trauma occurs, the patient is unaware of tissue damage, inflammation, and infection until an ulcer becomes evident. Neurotrophic ulceration in the feet of patients with peripheral neuropathy but no evidence of occlusive peripheral vascular disease is a familiar problem in diabetes. The primary lesion is often complicated by secondary infection.

Early microvascular and nutritional deficits in peripheral somatic neuropathy in diabetic patients present with complaints of lancinating, stabbing, or burning pains or paresthesia. Such symptoms are very uncommon in patients with neurotrophic foot ulceration due to the sensory loss. On comparative clinical examination stocking-like peripheral sensory loss to pinprick, cold/warm, light touch, and vibration is extensive, and loss of tendon reflexes is greater in patients with neurotrophic ulceration than those with painful early symptoms of neuropathy.[29] Often there is clawing of the toes, indicating motor denervation of the intrinsic foot muscles, which releases an unopposed action of the long extensor tendons. On EMG studies in diabetics, evoked nerve action potentials are exceptionally attenuated, implying a much greater large fiber axonal loss.[29]

A striking feature of diabetic symmetrical sensory polyneuropathy is the concurrent involvement of autonomic nerves. It

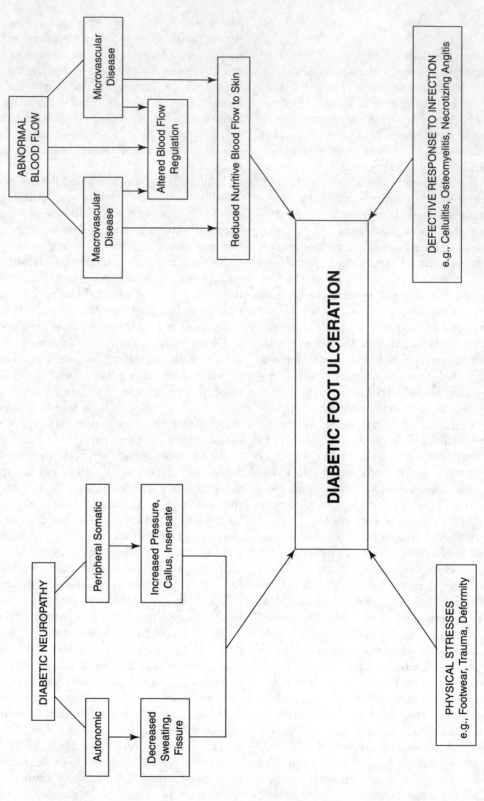

Figure 14.8   Probable interaction between the major risk factors responsible for diabetic foot ulceration.

has been suggested that autonomic neuropathy may be the principal cause of neurotrophic ulceration.[30,31,32] The diabetic foot rarely sweats, suggesting autonomic involvement.

Increased mechanical stresses in the presence of neuropathy places the foot at great risk for breakdown.[35,36] In clinical practice it is often obvious that pressure from inappropriate footwear greatly increases the susceptibility of ulceration. Additionally, the characteristic clawed toe deformity, secondary to motor denervation, exposes the metatarsal heads and toes to increased pressure and trauma.[36] Charcot foot deformity and a high medial plantar arch are important endogenous factors causing areas of increased pressure. Extensive callus formation occurs at sites of increased pressure and intensifies the forces on the subcutaneous tissues.[36] Plantar ulcers frequently result from pressure points, particularly calluses. Predominant areas of occurrence are submetatarsals, distal digits, medial 5th, 2nd metatarsal head, and 1st metatarsophalangeal joint.

Whatever the cause of the initial skin break, infection almost invariably exploits the situation and rapidly becomes an integral component of the clinical lesion. The type (e.g., *Staphylococcus aureus*, *Streptococcus*, anaerobic organisms) and severity (e.g., superficial cellulitis, osteomyelitis, deep abscess, or necrotizing angiitis) of the associated infection is a major determinant of outcome (e.g., healing, chronicity, gangrene).

There is an increased susceptibility to infection in patients with diabetes. It has been found that there is an impairment in neutrophil function in diabetes which is thought to comprise defective vascular adherence/escape and to defective phagocytosis/killing. Defective lectin receptors on macrophages have also been described.[37] All of these abnormalities are related to the prevailing level of hyperglycemia, so that any diabetic patient with poor glycemic control is at greater risk for infection. Infection is also more probable if foot hygiene is poor.

The characteristic presentation of a diabetic foot ulceration[12] includes:

- Round, punched-out lesion with elevated rim
- Periwound hyperkeratosis
- Surrounding hyperkeratosis and anhydrosis
- Eschar and necrotic debris in ulcer base uncommon (unless accompanied by vascular disease or infection)
- Low to moderate drainage (unless infected)

Evaluation of the diabetic patient with ulceration includes the diabetic status, nutritional status, vascular status of affected extremity, neurological status, ulcer status, and footwear. The ulcer evaluation includes the parameters described above: size, precise anatomical location, stage of ulcer (Wagner's Scale is more commonly used in diabetics as it incorporates the level of infection of a wound),[17] appearance of ulcer base, description of amount and type of exudate, periwound appearance, and documentation of exploration for sinus tracts, fistulas, and bone exposure. In addition to Wagner's Scale,[17] the Diabetic Wound Classification System[38] is a tool that grades wound status. This tool, developed at the University of Texas, is based on wound grade and stage to categorize foot wounds in diabetics. Depth is graded 0 (pre- or postulcerative lesion) through grade III (wound penetrating to bone or joint). Within each grade there are four stages (A through D) that take into account infection and peripheral vascular disease.[38]

Treatment of the diabetic ulceration includes pressure relief, debridement, attention to the types of dressings used, total contact casting, treatment of infection, and steps taken toward prevention of future skin breakdown once the ulcer is healed.[39]

Ideal pressure relief for a foot ulcer is no weight bearing at all and bed rest. However, in the elderly who are already at greater risk for the complications associated with inactivity (see Chapter 8), it is crucial that ADL and exercise be incorporated into the daily treatment plan.[40,41] In an ambulatory patient, footwear should be modified to relieve pressure on the ulcer and maintain ambulation. Felt or high-density foam inserts, moldable plastazote or other soft insoles, soft-soled heeling sandals or shoes, or modified shoes may be of benefit. Use of walking aids such as crutches or walkers helps to further decrease trauma to the ulcer during weight-bearing activities. A total contact cast is helpful, not only in providing the best mode of intervention for pressure relief for ambulation but also in providing an ideal healing environment for the wound.[39] The authors recommend fabrication of a total contact cast and subsequent bifurcation to provide a removable splint.[42] This redistributes the forces and protects the wound during weight-bearing activities and allows the wound to be more closely monitored for stages of healing.

Most diabetic ulcers are surrounded by a thick rim of keratinized tissue. Untreated, this will impede healing.[41] Surgical debridement should extend through the callus and expose underlying pink viable tissue. All necrotic tissue needs to be debrided from the wound. Once the wound is debrided surgically, physical therapy and nursing care should maintain the debridement of the wound as needed. Sharp debridement is usually the most effective and efficient form of debridement, but should be done by an experienced clinician. Eschar and fibrotic debris may be removed by enzymatic debriding agents (when minimal debris is present) or by dressings that will be described subsequently. Hydrotherapy (whirlpool) is used for brief periods to soften and loosen eschar and debris and cleanse the wound; however, in the elderly diabetic patient, it is not recommended.

The majority of diabetic ulcers occur on weight-bearing surfaces making it difficult for dressings such as hydrocolloids, hydrogel sheets, and thin film dressings to stay in place. They may be used on non-weight-bearing wounds with minimal drainage. Silver sulfadizine and gauze have been found to be effective in reducing bacterial colonization on all stages of low exudate diabetic ulcers—on both weight-bearing and non-weight-bearing surfaces.[41]

As mentioned before, total contact casting is a below-the-knee cast that limits excessive foot motion and redistributes the body's weight over the entire foot.[39,42] Patient compliance is improved because ambulation is permitted. Casts are padded over all bony prominences to prevent further tissue injury and total relief of pressure is provided surrounding and over the wound. Casts are changed on a seven- to fourteen-day protocol to assess wound status. Often, while contained in the cast, nature does its own healing so that when the cast and dressings are removed, autolysis has occurred. Despite maintenance in a closed environment, the wound often looks healthier after total contact casting then it did when the casting was originally done. Appropriate training from individuals experienced with this technique is mandatory prior to applying contact casts, as these are very different from standard plaster casts. Casts are generally discontinued when re-epithelialization occurs.[39,42]

One of the most common complications of diabetic ulcers is bacterial infection. The presence of hyperglycemia, as mentioned, greatly increases the risk for infection.[37] Because of this, the assessment and evaluative processes become ever more important. Early diagnosis and treatment will reduce the threat of sepsis and limb loss. However, early detection is difficult. The typical symptoms of infection, pain, erythema, and increased skin temperature may be masked by peripheral vascular disease, microvascular pathology, and neuropathy. In fact, the appearance of the wound and surrounding tissues may not verify the presence of infection at all. Hyperglycemia over a prolonged period may actually be the first indicator of infection.[37] Cultures for polymicrobial organisms will also assist in confirming the presence of bacteria.

Complications, such as progressive cellulitis, unresponsiveness to oral antibiotics, systemic signs of infection, abscess formation, and osteomyelitis require aggressive use of IV antibiotics and hospitalization. Osteomyelitis may be difficult to differentiate from diabetic osteopathy and chronic inflammation with either x-ray or bone scan. A bone biopsy is the only definitive diagnostic tool for establishing the presence of osteomyelitis. Surgical debridement of the infected bone followed by IV antibiotics is often required to eradicate the infection.[12] Another complication requiring surgery is an infected diabetic foot ulcer compromised by gangrene.

To summarize, treatment of the diabetic ulcer consists of local wound care and the use of systemic broad-spectrum antibiotics. Nonviable tissue is debrided and the wound and surrounding tissue are protected; once the ulcer is healed, preventive intervention is paramount. Prevention incorporates instruction on daily foot care and appropriate footwear, daily inspection of feet and foot hygiene, regular monitoring of glucose levels and insulin administration, and regularly scheduled checkups with a health care professional.

Pressure Ulcers

The destructive process of epithelial tissue-related ischemia, immobility, inactivity, and poor nutrition can lead to the development of a pressure ulcer. In addition, frictional and shear forces, and moisture damage to the skin contribute to the breakdown of integumentary tissues. An individual's inability to interpret discomfort related to chronic pressure and pathologies that lead to insensate conditions may also add to the risk of developing a pressure ulcer.[43–45]

In an older population prevention is key. Based on the evaluative information already discussed, the risk for developing a pressure ulcer should be determined. The ability to predict the potential for skin breakdown may be the best means of preventing ulceration from occurring. All pressure ulcers are preventable if attention is directed to insensate areas, malnutrition, skin fragility, and the physical or cognitive inability to accomplish pressure relief without guidance or assistance.

On first encounter with an elderly patient, whether it be in the home or in a health care setting, screening to determine risk for pressure ulcers should be done. There are several valuable risk assessment tools which have been proved reliable and valid for the prevention of pressure ulcers. The tools utilized with the geriatric patient population are the Braden scale, the Norton tool, the Knoll Assessment Scale, or the Gosnell scale. The selection of tools is primarily based on the setting of care and the tool that is used by various wound care teams in a given setting.

The Braden scale[46] was developed for an acute-care setting. It is also a useful tool in both the long-term care and home settings. As a result of its versatility, it is the tool this author most frequently utilizes. The Braden scale assesses six risk factor and scores each risk on a scale of 1 to 4 (worst to best scenario). The numerical score provides an objective means of grading risk.

The Norton tool[47] has been found reliable and valid in elderly patients with chronic wounds. This risk assessment tool provides a numerical score based on five areas of risk in patients with a history of long-standing integumentary problems.

Developed in an acute-care setting, the Knoll Assessment Scale[48] addresses variables specific to that care environment (e.g., surgical status, medical complexity, hydration, polypharmacy). This tool is valid and reliable and widely used. The scale has been modified by Aronovitch and co-workers[49] to identify the common elements that require the employment of specialized pressure relief surfaces for pressure reduction.

Last, the Gosnell scale[50] was developed specifically for long-term care geriatric patients. The scale assesses five risk factors and scores these on a best to worst rating scale. It goes a step beyond other tools by providing information on vital signs, skin appearance, fluid intake and output, interventions, and medications. Although useful, this scale has not yet been validated.

Wound assessment in pressure wounds is described above. The National Pressure Ulcer Advisory Panel (NPUAP) staging system, which is based on the Shea staging system originally published in 1975,[51] is pressure-ulcer specific. Ulcers are staged by describing the extent of tissue damage, from I (nonblanchable erythema) to IV (extending through the deep fascia into underlying anatomic structures). Another wound assessment tool which is very helpful is the Sessing Scale.[52] This tool is a seven-point observational scale anchored by verbal descriptions of wound healing. This instrument measures an important domain of healing independent of wound size or depth. The Sessing Scale describes granulation tissue, infection, necrosis, and eschar. It is not designed to measure healing but to predict healing.[52]

Early intervention is also key. If the pressure ulcer is detected and treated in early stages (Stage I OR II) it will take less time to heal and creates fewer, if any, systemic problems. Early intervention includes adequate pressure reduction with frequent reposition and specialized pressure relief surfaces as warranted.[12] Attention to nutritional status and hydration, perineal care if the individual is incontinent, and close monitoring for signs of skin pressure (e.g., redness that doesn't immediately blanch with pressure relief) are important care principles.[43,45] If areas of redness are noted, protective devices such as heel lifts or padding at bony prominences will help in preventing skin breaks and resulting in ulceration.[12]

When a pressure ulcer does occur it is important to address the treatment areas of pressure relief, debridement, a moist wound healing environment, and correction of factors that may be contributing to pressure ulcers (e.g., incontinence, malnutrition).

One of the key areas in wound care management is the ability to remove the source of irritation or pressure to allow normal healing to occur. The areas most likely to break down are those parts of the body where there is little fat between the skin and bone, such as the back of the head, rim of the ears, shoulder blades, spine, coccyx, sacrum, greater trochanter, medial and lateral malleolus, and heels.

Treatment principles inherent in pressure relief include the following:

- Determine what may be the cause of breakdown
  - Pressure over a bony prominence
  - Improper fitting shoes, brace
  - Friction, shearing
  - Immobility
- Incorporate pressure-reducing techniques
  - Inspect skin frequently for signs of redness. Redness normally disappears within fifteen minutes after removing pressure from uninjured skin
  - Maintain clean skin and attempt to prevent maceration from moist environments

- Avoid wrinkles in sheets of bed, chair cushion, and clothing (consider seams of socks and clothing)
- Avoid shearing forces when transferring or moving in bed (using a draw sheet may be recommended)
- Bedridden patients should be repositioned at least every two hours
- Wheelchair patients should perform weight shift every thirty minutes (tilt chair back, lateral and forward weight shift, wheelchair push-up)
- Use positioning and pressure-reducing devices to avoid pressure on wound as warranted
- Patient instruction if appropriate
  - Skin care and self-inspection techniques
  - Weight-shifting techniques
  - Instruction for patients with sensory loss
    ○ Proper shoe gear
    ○ Inspect shoes prior to donning (e.g., shake out sand or other debris that may be in shoes)
    ○ Never walk barefoot
    ○ Always test bath water temperature before taking bath or shower
    ○ Check for wrinkles in socks and clothing
- Once wound is healed
  - Begin subjecting healed area to pressure gradually, checking for signs of pressure and with frequent pressure relief periods
  - Maintain functional scar mobility
- Protect healthy tissue to prevent development of wounds
  - Use a screening tool to identify those who are at risk for development of a pressure sore or other type of wound
  - Educate patient and staff
  - Use position and pressure-reducing devices to prevent pressure ulcer development

When a wound has necrotic tissue, this must be debrided in order to provide a better environment for wound healing and contraction. Debridement can be accomplished by (1) sharp debridement down to the level of viable tissue, (2) debridement through the use of transparent adhesive or hydrocolloid water dressings that adhere to the necrotic tissue and promote autolysis in superficial wounds, or (3) calcium alginates, exudate-absorptive dressings and amorphous hydrogels which absorb necrotic tissue and promote autolysis, especially in dry and low exudate wounds.[12]

For cleansing a wound the use of normal saline or a nonionic surfactant wound cleanser to remove wound debris and dressing material residue is often employed.[12] In the elderly, as in any age patient with a wound, harsh disinfecting agents that are cytotoxic to granulation tissue should not be used in wound care.

Intervention will be dependent on the stage of the wound. Any lesion with black eschar, soft or hard, should not be staged until the eschar has been debrided free from the wound base. Based on the patient's history and risk factors, treatment strategies incorporate debridement as well as the use of modalities and dressings.

In a stage I pressure ulcer, the objective of treatment is to prevent skin breakdown. This can be accomplished by relieving pressure (e.g., elevating heels off the bed, frequent turning, use of pressure-relieving splints or a special support surface). Elderly bed-bound patients who are unable to move and roll must have a mattress for off-loading pressure points evenly. At this stage of ulcer development, transparent film dressing is often used as a protective measure to prevent progression of tissue breakdown beyond stage I.[2,6] There are sprays and gels available that protect and cover the skin, and some clinicians use semipermeable foam in the treatment of stage I ulcers.

Stage II ulcers involve the loss of epidermis and dermis due to friction or pressure. Blister development occurs and there is a break in the tissue. The blister requires debridement and the wound needs to be kept moist to promote healing. The objective of treatment in a stage II ulcer is to cover and hydrate and create a moist environment for healing. Either transparent film, hydrogel, antibiotic, absorption-type, or hydrocolloid dressings are used. In addition to covering, hydrating, and protecting the wound, dressings are chosen for absorption of exudates and insulation. High galvanic electrical stimulation may be employed, especially in the presence of infection. Attention to nutrition is important.

The objectives of treatment of a stage III ulcer are the same as in stages I and II. In addition, prevention of infection is paramount with a stage III ulcer. A primary goal in treatment is to promote granulation and contraction of epithelial tissue. This can be accomplished through the use of modalities, such as high galvanic electrical stimulation or ultrasound, and through the use of dressings. Hydrogel, absorption type, antibiotic, or hydrocolloid dressings, if drainage is low to moderate, are most effective to maintain a moist environment and enhance healing.

The primary goals in the treatment of stage IV ulcerations are to promote granulation and obliterate dead pressure ulcer space. Topical antibiotics, hydrogels, and absorptive type dressing are used to decrease and prevent infection and promote autolysis.

Sometimes saline-soaked, fluffed gauze dressings applied in wet to damp fashion are used to pack a wound and keep it moist. This approach is used in stage II to stage IV wounds. In the elderly, gauze impregnated with silver sulfadiazine may be used in stage III and stage IV ulcers to help decrease the presence of bacteria.

Vasculitic Ulcers

Evaluation and treatment of vasculitic ulcers is the same as other types of wounds. The difference is the etiology of the wound. These types of wounds are due to vasculitis, a term that applies to a diverse group of diseases characterized by inflammation in blood vessel walls. Most of these pathologies are autoimmune diseases—rheumatoid arthritis, systemic lupus erythematosus, systemic sclerosis, tuberculosis, sarcoidosis, and multiple organ dysfunction syndrome—which are complicated by inflammatory vascular conditions. Vasculitic lesions are more frequently found in patients with connective tissue disorders and in patients whose immune system is suppressed (HIV and AIDs).[53] Patients whose immune system has been compromised by medical interventions, such as cancer patients undergoing chemotherapy, are also prone to inflammatory vasculitis, compromised nutritional status, and resultant skin ulcerations.[54]

Blood vessels of various sizes in different parts of the body may be affected causing a wide spectrum of clinical manifestations. The inflammation of the vessels often causes narrowing or occlusion of the vessel lumen and produces ischemia of the tissues. The inflammation may weaken the vessel wall, resulting in aneurysm or rupture with subsequent hemorrhage into the tissues, which impedes nutrient and oxygen exchange. These two problems are most commonly associated with skin breakdown and vasculitic ulceration.

As a consequence, evaluation requires assessment of the medical condition and patient stability, as well as the determination of systemic involvement of disease manifestations. The presence of an ulceration may be only a small reflection of widespread involvement. Major symptoms of small blood vessel vasculitis are skin lesions that are accompanied by fever, malaise, and myalgia.[54] Intervention strategies must take into consideration that within the context of both wound healing and autoimmunity/immune suppression, molecular mechanisms of age-related changes (described in Chapter 2) affect an organism's ability to repair damaged cells and tissues. This impacts on the rate of healing. Vasculitic ulcers often turn out to be chronic, nonhealing ulcers. They are more likely to become infected because of the compromised vascular and immune systems. It is important that vasculitic conditions be identified early so that preventive interventions can be employed to eliminate the need for wound care.

OTHER TYPES OF WOUNDS

Though the most frequently encountered types of wounds in an older population are pressure, arterial and venous, and diabetic ulcers, other types of wounds may occur as well. These wounds include extravasation sites with necrotic tissue, abrasions and skin tears, dehisced surgical wounds, gastrointestinal and gerito-urinary fistulas, and burns from radiation therapy or other causes. This section of the chapter will deal primarily with the treatment approaches utilized in the elderly for care of these wounds.

Extravasation Sites

An extravasation site is a lesion that involves a bleed from a vessel into the surrounding tissues causing a hematoma. An accumulation of blood which becomes dense and stone-like can constrict blood supply to the area and cause breakdown of the tissues surrounding it, often resulting in death of the tissue.[12] The goal of treatment is the removal of the necrotic tissue and steps to facilitate healing. Autolysis, the spontaneous disintegration of necrotic tissue by the action of the patient's own enzymes, is encouraged through the application of transparent nonadhesive dressings or thin transparent hydrocolloid wafer until the necrotic tissue has been eliminated or the wound fluid leaks out. This approach decreases the trauma typically caused by debridement of the necrotic tissues with a sharp instrument. Once the dead tissue has dissipated, the wound can be cleansed and monitored for granulation and re-epithelialization.

Abrasions and Skin Tears

Abrasions and skin tears are very common in an older population. Due to the tissue-like texture of the skin, dehydration, and poor nutritional condition, even a seemingly minor trauma can result in an abrasion or skin tear.[12] The primary goal of treatment is to protect the area from further damage. Transparent nonadhesive dressings, thin transparent hydrocolloid, or semipermeable foam dressings are helpful in facilitating the drainage of fluids from the wounds and for re-epithelialization.

It is important that ADLs be evaluated and that situations that may place an elderly individual at risk for skin tears or abrasions be minimized.

Dehisced Surgical Wounds

Older patients, due to the fragility of the integumentary tissues, may experience the separation of all the layers of an incision or wound.[12] Treatment goals will include the repair, debridement, and healing of the dehisced lesion. For exuding wounds, calcium alginate dressing is often recommended as these products facilitate wound drainage. Once the surgical wound has stopped draining, a hydrocolloid or hydrogel wafer dressing (preferably transparent) or an amorphous hydrogel dressing is recommended for application to the affected area.

The biomechanical components of ADL need to be evaluated in order to prevent the surgical wound from splitting again. Assistive devices such as reaching tools may be helpful in reducing stress to the surgical site.

GI and GU Fistulas

Fistulas may occur from weakening of the gastrointestinal tract, which may result in communication with the external environment creating a wound, or they may be the result of a surgical procedure, such as the implantation of a feeding tube or a colostomy. The importance of maintaining a clean wound bed is very important in a gastrointestinal (GI) or genito-urinary (GU) fistula.[12] Daily evacuation and collecting of wound drainage is usually accomplished through suctioning. Saline or a nonionic surfactant wound cleanser is used to remove debris in the affected area. The most commonly used dressing is the application of a sealant over all intact skin, which is then covered by a transparent adhesive dressing, and finally gauze is applied to the immediate fistulated area.

Radiation Burns

Burns resulting from radiation therapy need to be treated to prevent infection and extensive tissue damage.[12] Pain control is accomplished by keeping the wound moist. The application of amorphous hydrogels to exuding wounds covered by nonadherent dressings is most frequently used. It is important not to use dressings that adhere to the wound or surrounding radiation-damaged skin as this may result in further tissue trauma. Activated charcoal dressings or gauze soaked with chlorophyllin copper complex solution are also used to control odor as well as promote healing. For lightly draining wounds, hydrocolloid or hydrogel wafer dressings, semipermeable foam dressings, or nonadherent dressings are used. For a large wound with profuse drainage, an ostomy-type pouch with a drainage collector may be employed.[55-57]

Burns

Due to a loss in sensation resulting from many pathologies, poor visual acuity, diminished temperature sensation, and decreased cognitive capabilities, elders are at a much higher risk of burns due to accidents (e.g., touching a hot surface, scalding from bathwater that is too hot). The principle of classifying a wound in order to treat it properly extends to understanding the mechanics of burn care and different types of burns. The goals of acute burn wound management are the same as those of managing any wound.[55] All wounds heal differently depending on the depth of the injury. Wounds that extend only into the epidermis or dermis can heal by tissue regeneration. Wounds that extend more deeply through the dermis heal by scar formation and contraction, because structures such as subcutaneous tissue, glands, and hair follicles are unable to regenerate.[56,57]

Burns also heal by different mechanisms depending on depth. Partial-thickness burns (which may involve the entire epidermis but still have intact hair follicles and sweat glands) will experience revascularization within a short period of time following the burn (one to two weeks).[56] However, full-thickness burns (which extend through the entire thickness of the skin with possible involvement of connective tissue, muscle, or bone) experience occlusion of the arterial vascular supply, with revascularization delayed for several weeks, and are incapable of healing by self-regeneration (requiring grafting). Table 14.4 provides

TABLE 14.4   Characteristics of Wounds Causes by Burns and the Variations in Healing.

Type of Burn: Characteristics	Superficial	Superficial Partial-Thickness	Deep Partial-Thickness	Full-Thickness	Subdermal
Predisposing Factors/Cause	Sunburn, ultraviolet exposure, minor flash	Brief exposure to flash flame, liquid spills; brief exposure to dilute chemicals	Hot liquids or solids; flash flame, direct flame; intense radiant energy, chemicals	Prolonged contact with flames, hot liquids, steam, chemicals, high-voltage electrical current	Electrical injury
Location and depth	Only minimal epithelial (epidermis) damage	Damage to epidermis, with minimal to dermis	Entire epidermis and more dermal involvement than superficial partial-thickness burn (epidermis, papillary dermis, and reticular dermis); intact hair follicles and sweat glands	Entire thickness of skin through reticular dermis to subcutaneous (epidermis, dermis, epidermal appendages, portion of subcutaneous fat; possible involvement of connective tissue, muscle, or bone)	Damage extends beneath dermis to subcutaneous tissue
Wound bed and wound appearance	Red or pink	Moist, bright pink or red color; large, intact blisters; brisk capillary refill when skin is blanched	Mix of red and waxy white; sluggish capillary return when skin is blanched	Mosaic of colors, including black, tan, red, white, pale yellow, brown; reddened area stays red when pressure is applied	Mummified and devitalized appearance
Exudate/drainage	Dry or with small blisters	Large amounts of exudate when blisters rupture or are removed	May have large amounts of exudate	Tissue is leathery, rigid, and dry	Dry
Swelling and capillary refilling	Some swelling, particularly if eyes are involved	Brisk capillary refill when skin is blanched	Massive swelling can cause problems with range of motion; slow, sluggish capillary return when skin is blanched	Swelling below eschar but not in area of eschar; reddened areas stay red when pressure is applied; poor circulation to distal area of full-thickness injury	Little swelling; thrombosed blood vessels

Pain	Delayed pain	Extremely painful	Generally dull pain; decreased pinprick sensation, but pressure sensation intact	Insensate areas from nerve destruction	Insensate areas
Healing	Spontaneous healing in 3 to 5 days; generally no scar	Spontaneous healing in less than 21 days, usually 7 to 10 days; minimal scarring	Spontaneous healing in 2 to 3 weeks, possible conversion to fullthickness injury; hypertrophic scarring and scar contracture likely	Incapable of self-regeneration; requires skin graft to heal; scarring around periphery of wound between skin grafts	Incapable of selfregeneration; requires skin graft or flap to heal; neurologic involvement possible; muscle paralysis possible; scarring around periphery of wound or between skin grafts

Table compiled from information in the following references:
Greenfield, E., Jordan, B. Advances in burn wound care. Critical Care Nurs Clin North Amer. *1996; 8(2):203–215.*
Staley, M., Richard, R. Management of the acute burn wound: An overview. Adv Wound Care. *1996; 10(2):39–44.*
Yarbrough, D.R. Pathophysiology of the burn wound. In: Wagner, M.M., ed. Care of the Burn-Injured Patient. Multidisciplinary Involvement. *Littleton, MA: PSG Publishing Company; 1981: 19–31.*

a summarization of the characteristics of wounds causes by burns and the variations in healing expected from each type of wound.[55–57]

With burns in the elderly, like with any burn victim, emphasis needs to be placed on hydration, nutrition, and the maintenance of mobility. Pain is often a limiting factor in accomplishing activities of daily living. Occupational therapy often will provide splinting to maintain proper joint and extremity alignment, as well as determining the assistive devices that may facilitate independence while allowing for a decrease in pain experienced during those activities.

WOUND MANAGEMENT

Because advanced age is associated with delayed wound healing and repair, prevention remains the cornerstone of wound care in the older population. Healing is complicated by the increased prevalence in older patients of conditions that predispose them to pressure ulcers, such as malnutrition, immobility, and systemic disease. If preventive measures fail, there are treatments available to minimize surface contact at pressure points and therapeutic agents to promote wound healing.[2] These treatment approaches include physical modalities, debridement, incontinence care, topical dressings that create an optimal healing environment, specially designed support surfaces, growth factor topicals, and nutritional interventions that can increase the proliferation, migration, and protein biosynthesis of cells in the wound bed.

Electrical Stimulation

Numerous research articles are available on the effects and benefits of electrical stimulation on healing. Electrical stimulation used as an adjunct to other interventions has been found to be effective.[58–61] The use of electrical stimulation, particularly high galvanic, is the modality of choice in elderly with chronic wounds.[58,59,61]

Electrical stimulation works by enhancing the body's bioelectric system on a cellular level. When the skin is wounded, it conducts a current generated between the surface skin (a negative current) and the inner tissues (a positive current) in an attempt to attract healing cells, which are responsible for releasing growth factors that are involved in the process of collagen synthesis.[60] This process is referred to as the "current of injury" and continues until the injury has healed.

A moist environment is required for the body's bioelectrical system to function properly. There must be a medium to conduct "natural" current. If the wound is dry then that medium is lost. Lack of current, or current disruption, is suspected to be one of the reasons why chronic wounds do not heal without outside stimulus to jumpstart the healing process. The rationale for applying elec-

trical stimulation is that it mimics the natural current and initiates or accelerates the wound-healing process.[58–60]

The wound-healing process, which includes the inflammation, proliferation, epithelialization, and remodeling phases, is enhanced with electrical stimulation. Electrical stimulation facilitates these steps via an electrical current which transfers energy to a wound through the electrodes.[58–60] One electrode is placed on the external skin a distance away from the wound and the other in the wound bed to assist the flow of current for healing.

Although there are many waveforms available for electrotherapy, high-voltage (galvanic) electrical stimulation, the most commonly used current for wound healing is a monophasic twin-peaked high-voltage pulsed current that gives the cells an interrupted type of stimulus at a high frequency and causes the body to respond to the stimulation by laying down collagen.[61] High galvanic stimulation also allows for the control of the polarity and variation in pulse rates, which are both important to the healing process.[58,59]

As uninjured skin has a negative potential which shifts to positive when the skin is injured, the use of polarization (e.g., placing the negative lead over the wound) increases the rate of epithelialization.[61] There is strong evidence that a negative polarity increases protein, DNA, and collagen synthesis and fibroblast proliferation. A theoretical effect of high-voltage current is that it accelerates soft tissue healing by elevating tissue temperature and stimulating cellular metabolism.[58–60] It also increases cutaneous circulation, which promotes wound healing and improves the oxygen and nutritional exchange. It cannot be assumed that high galvanic electrical stimulation causes similar wound reactions as continuous low-voltage direct current. Low-volt current has bactericidal and sclerosing effects at the cathode (negative electrode), and anode (positive electrode) respectively. High galvanic current does not deliver enough charge on the skin to alter skin pH or cause electrochemical reactions, compared with low-voltage direct current.[58,59]

Contraindications to the use of high-voltage pulse current include osteomyelitis, malignancy, pacemakers, and electrical current should not be used over topical agents with metal ions (e.g., zinc-containing substances and the like). The recommended pulse rate/voltage is 100 pps/high voltage (100 V) or above. Daily frequency of intervention is recommended with a length of therapy ranging from 30 to 60 minutes. The coupling agent is usually a lead (sterilized product lead or aluminum foil with an alligator clip) over a sterile saline-soaked gauze placed directly in the wound.

Polarity will vary based on the intent of the therapy. The positive electrode will enhance autolysis and epithelialization, The negative lead promotes granulation and is used for infection or inflammation.

Generally, high galvanic current is utilized with the deeper stage II, III, and IV wounds. Although the specific means by which electrical stimulation may promote healing is still being explored, more and more evidence exists to support the hypothesis that electrical current creates the proliferation of connective tissue and decreases the inflammatory response. There is a modification of endogenous electrical potentials of tissue; stimulation of cellular biosynthesis and replication occurs; there are antibacteriacidal effects, enhanced circulation, and the generation of a cellular electrophyiological effect.[58–61] Electrochemical effects at electrode sites, such as increased cell temperature, changes in pH, or release of ions from the electrodes, may possibly occur during low-voltage electrical stimulation, though these reactions have not been substantiated in high-voltage current interventions.[58–61] Nonetheless, the rate of healing is decreased when high galvanic current is employed as a wound-healing agent.[58,61] Ulcers treated with high galvanic pulsed current demonstrate a significantly greater rate of wound contraction (measured by a decrease in wound size)[58] and ultimately the healing time is reduced.[58,61]

Ultrasound

Ultrasound is used as a physical therapy modality for the treatment of soft tissue trauma, hematosis and inflammation, and induration. Therapeutic benefits are well documented.[62–65] Ultrasound has been purported to benefit healing by increasing O_2 transport, decreasing pain, expediting tissue repair and wound closure, increasing angiogenesis, and decreasing edema.[62]

Ultrasound works in two ways, dependent on the variable of continuous versus pulsed delivery. Continuous ultrasound is primarily utilized to heat the tissues, whereas pulsed ultrasound produces a nonthermal effect.[65] It is the nonthermal effect that stimulates wound healing by causing changes in cell membrane, which in turn stimulate tissue repair. However, the heating effects of continuous ultrasound are also beneficial as circulation to the wound is improved, which enhances oxygen and nutrient availability to the healing tissues.

Dyson[65] has demonstrated that when soft connective tissues are injured, platelets and mast cells become activated and release chemotactic agents, which attract leucocytes and monocytes to the site of injury. Ultrasound can stimulate the release of histamine and enhance calcium transport, thereby stimulating metabolic activity and furthering the production of these chemotactic agents.[65] The primary role of leucocytes is to remove debris and pathogens from the wound, while monocytes develop into phagocytic macrophages, which release growth factors essential for the development of new connective tissue. Therefore, it is proposed that this is one of the mechanisms by which ultrasound promotes wound healing.[62–65]

Not only does ultrasound appear to have an impact on cellular activity during the inflammatory phase of healing, during the proliferation phase it has been demonstrated that fibroblasts exposed to therapeutic levels of ultrasound can be stimulated to synthesize collagen. The entry of calcium ions is also increased and facilitates reparative responses.[65] When ultrasound is applied to a wound, the rate of contraction can be accelerated, presumably because of direct or indirect effects on the myofibroblasts during the proliferative stage.[65]

The increase in collagen formation has also been determined to increase the strength of scar tissue in addition to normalizing the cross-linking fiber pattern of repair, so that scar tissue following ultrasound is more elastic and stronger.[65]

Contraindications to the use of ultrasound include acutely infected wounds, malignancies, pacemakers, deep vein thrombosis or emboli, and osteomyelitis. The chosen frequencies are 3 Mhz for superficial wounds and 1 Mhz for deep wounds with an intensity of 0.5 to 1.0 w/cm. Treatment frequency will depend on setting, however; it is recommended daily for acute wounds and a minimum of three times per week for chronic wounds. Coupling agents might include hydrogel dressings, degassed water, and ultrasound gel pads.

Whirlpool

The use of whirlpool, in the elderly, to immerse an extremity should be used sparingly. Long periods of time spent with the extremity soaking in water will result in emaciation and sloughing of healthy tissues. If the whirlpool is used, it should be used for brief periods of time (less than 10 minutes) to soften necrotic tissue for debridement, remove exudate, and provide a way of vigorously cleansing and rinsing the wound. Short periods of immersion in a warm whirlpool bath with the turbulent and agitated water massaging the extremity will increase cutaneous vasodilatation and oxygen transport, ease discomfort associated with the wound, and decrease muscle spasm.[66] The use of whirlpool prior for debridement is particularly helpful when there is necrotic tissue present or when preparing burn patients for wound debridement. Whirlpool intervention should be discontinued as a mode for cleansing the wound once the ulcer no longer requires debridement.[67]

Whirlpool intervention is contraindicated in elders with moderate to severe cardiac or pulmonary dysfunction, recent skin grafts, acute febrile conditions, advanced arterial disease, tendency for hemorrhaging, gangrene, venous insufficiency, and in the presence of a comatose or persistent vegetative state. If total or half-body immersion is employed, urinary incontinence and incontinence of bowel are also considerations.

If the goal of treatment is to keep the wound hydrated (which in most cases it is), soaking in water may actually result in dehydration.[21] Additionally, good granulation tissue may be damaged with agitation of the water. Temperature of the water should not exceed 115° to avoid skin burns; in a hypertensive patient, the temperature should not exceed 104° as this may cause a sustained elevated blood pressure.

Debridement

Sharp debridement is the removal of necrotic tissue utilizing scissors, tweezers, forceps, and scalpels. Blunt debridement is mechanically removing necrotic tissue by gently cleansing the wound surface with gauze, Q-tips, or other blunt materials.

Debridement of the wound is typically done by medical personnel, including physical therapists, that have been specifically trained in the skill of debridement. The goal of debridement is to provide a clean wound bed to enhance healing. The frequency and duration of debridement is based on the amount and pace of necrotic tissue formation. While debridement of the entire eschar down to viable tissue is the most efficient means of gaining healthy tissue, it may not be a reasonable alternative for some chronic wounds.

Great caution needs to be employed when debridement is performed in a patient with diabetes, sensory loss, or exposed tendons, ligaments, or bone. If there is excessive bleeding at the wound site, debridement should be curtailed until bleeding is controlled. Sharp debridement must be avoided in patients who have low platelet counts or in those taking anticoagulants.

Hyperbaric Oxygen Therapy

Hyperbaric oxygen therapy (HBO) has been advocated for selected nonhealing wounds and anaerobic wound infections. Patients are treated in chambers that provide O_2 to an isolated spot or to an entire extremity. In fact, treatment of ischemia in elderly subjects has been found to significantly enhance wound healing.[68]

There are topical oxygen bandages and plastic chambers for extremities that deliver oxygen to the wound; however, these are not considered hyperbaric. Their value in treating chronic wounds is questionable and the cost of treatment is expensive.[12]

Incontinence Care

Elderly patients who are incontinent and immobile are at a greater risk for skin breakdown and the development of pressure ulcers. Both fecal and urinary incontinence have been positively associated with the development of ulcers.[67] Skin care, focusing on maintaining a dry environment, thorough cleaning following an accident, moisturizers, barrier creams, ointments, and films are often recommended to prevent ulceration.

Frequent toileting is important in the older patient who requires assistance with bed mobility, ambulation, transfers, and managing clothing. (See Chapter 5.) It is also important to provide proper cleaning using perineal washes with surfactants and humectants to decrease bacterial growth. Soaps and cleaning agents with detergents, such as sodium laurel sulfate or alcohol, should be avoided. These substances cause drying and irritation of the skin, which could lead to bacterial infection and breakdown.

Lotions to moisturize the skin assist in maintaining the viability of the skin surface. Moisturizing products should not contain alcohol, which will create excessive drying of the skin and may lead to skin dehydration, cracking, and subsequent ulceration.

Often, water-repellent barrier creams, ointments, or films are used if a patient is continually wet from incontinence or wound drainage. Patients with occasional incontinence may benefit from a perineal wash and moisturizer; however, others with continuous drainage may require a barrier to moisture. Powder may be used to absorb surface moisture followed by the application of a barrier cream or medicated ointment.

If an older individual, exposed to organisms in the urine or feces, develops a fungal infection, a rash will develop. Generally a prescription antifungal agent will be required. These medicinal substances come in powders or creams. There are also OTC antifungal powders which are used preventively for patients on antibiotics and those with mild rashes characterized by redness and itching.[12]

SURGICAL INDICATIONS

Topical treatment that provides a moist healing environment will encourage but not guarantee a successful cascade of wound-healing events. Debridement continues to be important in the healing process. It accelerates healing by removing necrotic debris and can be accomplished autolytically, chemically, mechanically, or surgically. For example, a venous ulcer covered with fibrinous necrotic tissue may heal faster if the fibrinous tissue is debrided to reveal healthy granulation tissue underneath. When necrotic tissue is deep and extensive, debridement is usually a surgical procedure.

The most important goal in wound care is rapid and lasting closure. Surgery is indicated in nonhealing ulcers. Skin grafts are indicated when spontaneous healing is compromised by the size and depth of the wound and when inadequate perfusion of the skin decreases the likelihood of healing.[69] The problem of compromised healing is even greater in diabetic patients if neuropathy and/or vasculopathy is present.[70] Surgical grafting of cultured autologous skin grafts is complemented by rehabilitation involvement inclusive of immobilization of the area with a removable cast or splint, and biostimulation with pulsed electrical fields.[71]

The following acrostic developed by Mulder and associates[12] delineates guidelines warranting surgical evaluation and potential surgical intervention:

N = necrotic tissue

O = osteomyelitis

H = hidden sinus tracts and tunnels

E = eschar (unresponsive to minor sharp debridement or dressing)

A = abscess and arterial insufficiency

L = large defects too big to close by secondary intervention

I = ischemia

N = nonhealing wound after 30 to 45 days' treatment

G = graft-ready wound beds and wound beds with tendon and bone exposed

Several different companies have attempted to develop materials that will act as temporary skin coverings. These materials contain any combination of cultured keratinocytes, fibroblasts, collagen, and synthetic materials.[72] The products are used with burns and chronic wounds. Skin replacements may be the wound dressing of the future, replacing current synthetic and semisynthetic dressings. Skin equivalents with dermal and epidermal layers have been found to be useful on full-thickness wounds when surgically applied.[71,73]

Conservative healing without the need of surgery and anesthesia is preferable in the elderly patient. Combined innovative approaches to wound care that incorporate noninvasive interventions such as growth hormones, biosynthetic dressings, electrical stimulation, and other modalities are the preferred methods in the older patient.

SUPPORT SURFACES

By controlling the parameters of friction and pressure it is possible to prevent pressure ulcers from forming and to treat stage I and II ulcers successfully with conservative measures. A major consideration in such treatment is the selection and use of effective support surfaces such as wheelchair cushions and mattresses.[74] In this regard, the perfect support surface would have the following characteristics:

- Minimizes the pressures under the bony prominences
- Controls the pressure gradient in the tissue
- Provides stability
- Allows weight shifts
- Allows ease of transfer
- Controls the temperature at the skin interface
- Controls the moisture at the skin interface
- Is lightweight
- Has a low cost
- Is durable and easy to clean
- Meets required infection control standards

Although a number of products have been introduced to the market, the perfect support surface does not exist. Many of the support products fulfill some criteria of the perfect support surface, but none seems to provide maximum protection for all individuals. As a result, provision of support surfaces needs to be an adjunct of intervention.[74]

As an adjunctive intervention special support surfaces play a key role in the prevention and treatment of pressure ulcers. The best support surface, as described above, needs to have properties that include interface pressure, friction and shear characteristics, moisture vapor transmission rate, thermal insulation properties, indentation load deflection, density, ease of use, safety, and patient comfort.

Interface pressure is the most commonly used measure when comparing support surfaces. Interface pressure is a measure of the force the support surface applies to the tissue it is supporting. Interface pressure measures are in millimeters of mercury (mm Hg) and are described as pressure relief and pressure reduction. Pressure relief is defined as pressure below 25 to 32 mm Hg.[12] Pressure reduction is defined as the reduction of interface pressures to 26 to 32 mm Hg.[12] While somewhat useful in objectively evaluating support surfaces, interface pressures are not the precise standard that would be ideal for managing patient care. They should not be used as the sole parameter in evaluating the efficacy of the surface in determining pressure relief and reduction.

The choice of support surfaces will also depend on the following variables:

- Patient's diagnosis
- Number of hours the patient uses the support system
- Types of activities performed
- Usage environment (climate, continence, etc.)
- Living arrangements (independent, varying levels of assistance, residential facility)
- Tissue history (history of ulcers, decreased sitting tolerance, surgery to repair ulcers)
- Body build
- Pressure magnitude and distribution

For both mattress and seating products available for support surfaces, Table 14.5 provides the advantages and disadvantages of various pressure-reducing materials used in these products.

Though this chapter is not the forum for a thorough review of every available support surface, it is important that the reader explore the many invaluable resources available for determining the best product for individual patients.[5,12,74] The selection of a support surface, whether for the bed, chair, or wheelchair, is a complex multifactorial process. It is evident that no single device serves all elderly persons with the multiplicity of system involvement seen with advancing age. Furthermore, even the most sophisticated devices will not prevent tissue breakdown.

TABLE 14.5   Advantages and Disadvantages of Pressure-Relieving Products

Product	Advantages	Disadvantages
Air-Filled Products	Lightweight	Subject to puncture
	Easy to clean	Not easily repaired
	Effective with many patients	Inflation must be checked frequently
		User instability
Liquid-Filled Flotation Devices	Easy to clean	Subject to puncture
	Effectiveness	Heavy
Gel-Filled Devices	Adjusts to body movement	Heavy
	Easy to clean	
Foam Products	Availability	Wears out quickly
	Many variations/densities	Not easily cleaned
	Inexpensive	Properties change with time
	Lightweight	Can support combustion
	Can be easily modified	

Support surfaces are part of the total pressure management regimen that must be individualized for each older person.

WOUND CARE PRODUCTS

There are numerous wound care products required for appropriate healing beyond support surfaces. These include cleansers and moisturizers, pharmaceutical, agents, and various types of dressings. Mulder and associates provide a comprehensive list of these products in the *Clinicians' Pocket Guide to Chronic Wound Repair.*[12] Wound products include:

- Wound cleansers
- Skin moisturizers
- Ointments
- Skin sealants
- Lubricating sprays, ointments, and dressings
- Enzymatic debriding agents
- Transparent adhesive dressings
- Hydrocolloid wafer dressings
- Hydrocolloid paste, granules, and powder dressings
- Exudate absorptive dressings
- Exudate absorptive dressings with antimicrobial activity
- Calcium alginates
- Semipermeable foam dressings
- Hydrogels

- Impregnated gauzes
- Nonadherent dressings
- Composites (island dressings)
- Contact layers
- Specialty absorptive dressings
- Activated charcoal dressings
- Wound pouches

Pharmaceutical Agents[12]

Wound cleansers are applied directly into the wound for purification. Moisturizers add moisture to the epidermis and assist in maintaining the intact skin. Ointments provide a petrolatum-based barrier or water-resistant cream against bodily secretions or chemical injury.[75]

Skin sealants provide some degree of protection from mechanical and chemical injury by providing a copolymer film on the skin. These sealants usually contain alcohol and need to be cautiously used in the treatment of the elderly. Due to the problem with dehydration in older adults, the alcohol may exacerbate this condition. Extra emphasis on adequate hydration and moisturization of the wound bed is important in conjunction with the use of skin sealants.

Lubricating sprays, ointments, and dressings provide a protective dressing and add moisture to the epidermis.[75]

Enzymatic debriding agents are pharmaceutical agents, which assist in obliterating necrotic tissue, exudates, and denatured collagen.[75] The destructive process is accomplished through proteolytic enzyme action. Some enzymatic debriding agents are provided in dressing products.[12]

Dressings[12,75]

Historically, wound dressings were used in order to protect the wound from the external environment. It is now understood that dressings play an active, not passive, role in wound management. Dressings create an environment that will optimize the wound-healing process. Key to this is maintaining moisture in the wound. Extensive research has demonstrated that healing of normal wounds is significantly enhanced in a moist environment compared to those allowed to dry.[1,2,8,67]

Dressing choice will be influenced by the wound's stage in its healing process. A wound in the inflammation stage must be treated differently from one with significant epithelialization. Since a wound is constantly in a state of change, dressing choices must periodically be reevaluated.[75]

Transparent adhesive dressings provide a semipermeable, sterile, thin film that creates a moist environment. This type of dressing is nonabsorptive and enables autolysis of devitalized tissue. Transparent adhesive dressings protect the skin and wound against friction and are referred to as "second skin."

Dressings that interact with the wound environment and contain pharmaceutical agents are helpful in enhancing healing.[75] These include calcium alginates, as well as certain hydrocolloid and hydrogel wafer dressings that can deliver substances to the wound to stimulate healing.[12]

Hydrocolloid wafer dressing and hydrocolloid paste, granules, and powder dressings are commonly used in the treatment of wounds in the elderly.[12] Wafers contain hydroactive, absorptive particles that interact with the wound exudate to form a gelatinous mass, which then can be debrided with dressing removal. They provide minimal to moderate absorption (depending on the product) and enable autolysis of devitalized tissue. These dressings are contraindicated where anaerobic infection is suspected.[12] In the elderly, the hydrocolloid dressings are preferred for use in the coccyx area as they require no secondary dressing (which could add to frictional stresses and moisture) and cover and protect the area similar to the transparent adhesive second skin dressings.

Exudate absorptive dressings absorb draining exudate and fill dead space.[75] They conform to the wound surface and keep the wound surface clean and moist. Exudate absorptive dressings enable autolysis of devitalized tissue.[12] These dressings often come with pharmaceutical agents with antimicrobial activity. These dressings absorb exudate and reduce bacterial load in the wound.[75] The disadvantage of use of the antimicrobial absorptive dressings is that they require a secondary dressing.

Calcium alginates are highly absorbent and provide an interactive pharmaceutical dressing. These dressings convert into a viscous hydrophilic gel after contact with exudate. Trapped fibers in the wound are biodegradable and the meshing of the dressing with the wound makes possible the autolysis of devitalized tissue.[12]

Semipermeable foam dressings absorb exudate while maintaining a moist wound surface. The outer layer of the foam dressings is hydrophobic, which helps to maintain moisture in the wound. These dressings also permit autolysis of devitalized tissue.[75]

Hydrogel dressings maintain a clean and moist wound surface. They are oxygen-permeable, allowing for oxygenation of the wound. The hydrogels cool the surface and are often refrigerated to enhance the cryotherapeutic effects of reducing pain and inflammation.[75] The hydrogel dressings absorb minimal exudate. Some products require a secondary dressing. These dressings enable the autolysis of devitalized tissue on removal.[12]

Impregnated gauzes are nonadherent fine or open mesh gauze that enable autolysis of devitalized tissue.[12] Nonadherent dressings, or more appropriately termed low adherent, are used on dry or lightly exudating wounds to provide absorptive and autolytic properties in the treatment of a healing wound. Composite dressings, also called island dressings, are nonadherent absorbent dressings with a pad located in the center. They provide absorption of minimal exudate and are bacteria- and moisture-resistant adhesive dressings. Contact layers are also classed as nonadherent dressings and are used on wounds under absorbent cover dressings.[12] Specialty absorptive dressings are low-adherent dressings used on dry or lightly exudating wounds and are often used as a secondary dressing.[75]

Activated charcoal dressings absorb exudate and reduce the concentration of wound odor. They are frequently used with high exudate wounds. Enzymatic debriding agents embedded in gauze dressings are designed to destroy necrotic tissue, exudate, or denatured collagen through proteolytic enzyme action.[12]

Wound pouches, which look like ostomy pouches, have attached skin barriers and can be cut to fit the wound shape and size. Hinged caps allow for treatment or inspection and can be adapted for continuous drainage.[12]

Living skin equivalents (synthetic approximations) are also used as temporary skin coverings. These materials contain any combination of a number of substances including cultured keratinocytes, fibroblasts, collagen, and synthetic materials.[12] Substances such as hyaluronic acid, which is a naturally occurring lubricant and a component in the synthesis of connective tissues, has been found to be effective in enhancing healing of chronic wounds.[73,75]

Growth Factors

Several growth factors that stimulate wound healing have been isolated. Autologous growth factors can be harvested from a patient's blood and applied to the patient's nonhealing wound.[76] Genetic recombinant growth factors are being researched in many centers with promising results.

During coagulation and inflammation, platelets, neutrophils, macrophages, and lymphocytes are the predominant cell types as they function to kill bacteria and clear the wound site of cellular debris and foreign material prior to the reparative phases. This type of cells, especially platelets, also acts to initiate and sustain the proliferative and remodeling stages of wound repair by synthesizing and releasing growth factors that serve to regulate healing.[76]

Besides serving as an important source of several growth factors, fibroblasts serve other vital functions—making them the most important cell type during this phase of healing. They produce matrix proteins, of which collagen is the most important, providing strength and integrity to the healed wound. Also, fibroblasts convert into myofibroblasts within the granulation tissue of the open wound, leading to contraction and healing. Other cells, such as keratinocytes and vascular endothelial cells, are active in producing granulation tissue and restoring the epithelium and vascular integrity.

Continuous synthesis and degradation of collagen characterize the remodeling phase, which relies on a balance between factors that promote synthesis of extracellular matrix components and enzymes that degrade these components. Growth factors, which are synthesized and released locally at the wound site, regulate the functions of each of the cell types. The growth factors include platelet-derived growth factor, transforming growth factor–beta (TGF-β), and epidermal growth factors.[76]

At the molecular level, chronic wounds may result ultimately from a deficiency in growth factors or inhibition of their function. This deficiency may be partly the result of elevated levels of proteinases that act to degrade growth factors and extracellular matrix components at the wound site. It has been demonstrated that the healing response can be induced in chronic wounds by either adding exogenous growth factors or inhibiting proteinase activity at the wound site.[76] Recently developed pharmaceutical dressings containing growth factors are being utilized with successful results in elderly populations.

Nutritional Agents

Scientists have discovered that a multipurpose protein found in several bodily fluids has another important function; it can promote the healing of abnormal skin wounds, which are a significant problem in the elderly. Researchers demonstrated that the protein, called secretory leukocyte protease inhibitor (SLPI), plays a critical role in normal wound healing and enhances healing in wounds that are slow to heal.[77,78] SLPI is found in fluids that bathe mucosal surfaces such as bronchial fluids, cervical fluids, and saliva, and is a remarkably versatile substance. It has anti-inflammatory, antiviral, antifungal, and antibacterial prop-

erties. In recent years, investigators demonstrated that SLPI found in saliva blocks HIV-1 infection.[78,79]

Many elderly patients that have delayed healing processes lack the SLPI gene, and this is demonstrated markedly by impaired wound healing with an increase in inflammation and the activity of the enzyme elastase, which destroys tissue.[77,79] Without the presence of SLPI to act as a molecular brake, a cascade of events occurs that results in the destruction of tissue and impaired wound healing. However, the topical application of SLPI actually reverses the abnormal response and enhances the rate of healing.[77] Researchers believe that SLPI has three major functions in wound healing. It inhibits elastase, controls the activation of leukocytes, and reduces TGF-β activation. SLPI appears to be a component of innate or natural host defense mechanisms that maintain a balance between protective inflammation responses and overzealous or uncontrolled inflammation that can lead to tissue destruction and failure to heal.[77–79] Interestingly, the fact that animals tend to lick their wounds may be nature's way of delivering SLPI to the wound site via saliva.

With aging, the skin is thinner, more fragile, and more susceptible to injury. Progressive normal and pathological aging changes increase the risk for chronic health problems that may lead to open wounds and delayed healing. Optimum care of chronic wounds supports the older person's specific health and care needs, progresses to cleansing and debridement of the wound, then uses appropriate nutrition, modalities, coverings, and protective interventions to promote healing.

ALTERNATIVE MEDICINE AND WOUND HEALING

Alternative and complementary medicine includes a vast array of wound care modalities which requires at least mention in this chapter. Many elderly individuals, disenchanted with the outcomes of allopathic care, seek these forms of treatment for chronic wounds. Some alternative and complementary therapies may offer benefits for patients with wounds and wound pain. These therapies include acupuncture, energy healing, guided imagery, hypnosis, prayer, and relaxation techniques.[80] Although we will not go into wound healing and each alternative intervention, it is important that the therapist be aware of the complement of state-of-the-art wound care practices in wound care clinics. In some studies these interventions have been shown to effectively heal wounds and provide relief of wound pain during the healing process.[80]

References

1. Goodson WH, Hunt TK. Wound healing and aging. *J Invest Dermatol.* 1979; 73(1):88–91.

2. Reed MJ. Wound repair in older patients: Preventing problems and managing healing. *Geriatrics.* 1998; 53(5):88–94.

3. Irion G. *Physiology: The Basis of Clinical Practice.* Thorofare, NJ: Slack; 2000: 181–189.

4. McCulloch JM, Kloth LC, Feedar JA. *Wound Healing: Alternatives in Management.* 2nd ed. Philadelphia: FA Davis; 1995.

5. Sussman C, Bates-Jensen BM. *Wound Care: A Collaborative Practice Manual for Physical Therapists and Nurses.* Gaithersburg, MD: Aspen Publishers; 1998.

6. Boynton PR, Jaworski D, Paustian C. Meeting the challenges of healing chronic wounds in older adults. *Nurs Clin North Am.* 1999; 34(4):921–932.

7. Eaglstein WH. Wound healing and aging. *Dermatol Clin.* 1986; 4(3):481–484.

8. Van Rijswijk L. General principles of wound management. In: Gogia PP, ed. *Clinical Wound Management.* Thorofare, NJ: Slack; 1995.

9. Wong RA. Chronic dermal wounds in older adults. In: Guccione A, ed. *Geriatric Physical Therapy.* St Louis: Mosby; 2000: 376–398.

10. Myer AH. The effects of aging on wound healing. *Top Geriatr Rehabil.* 2000; 16(2):1–10.

11. Stotts N, Wipke-Tevis D. Co-factors in impaired wound healing. In: Grasner D, Kane D, eds. *Chronic Wound Care: A Clinical Source Book for Healthcare Professionals.* Wayne, PA: Health Management Publications; 1997.

12. Mulder GC, Fairchild PA, Jeter KF. *Clinicians' Pocket Guide to Chronic Wound Repair.* 3rd ed. Long Beach, CA: Wound Healing Institute Publications; 1995.

13. Jones P, Millman A. Wound healing and the aged patient. *Nurs Clin North Am.* 1990; 25(1):263–277.

14. Campbell S. *Pressure Ulcer Prevention and Intervention: A Role for Nutrition.* Westerville, OH: Ross Products; 2001.

15. Nicolle LE, Huchcroft SA, Cruse PJ. Risk factors for surgical wound infection among the elderly. *J Clin Epidemiol.* 1992; 45(4):357–364.

16. Grossman MR. Treating pressure ulcers in the geriatric patient. *Podiatry Today.* July–August 1996; 66 73.

17. Wagner FW. The dysvascular foot: A system for diagnosis and treatment. *Foot Ankle.* 1981; 2(1):64–69.

18. Morey SE. Photos supplement written documentation. *Physical Therapy Products.* January–February 1998; 66–67.

19. Bates-Jensen BM, Vredevoe DL, Brecht ML. Validity and reliability of the Pressure Sore Status Tool. *Decubitus.* 1992; 5(6):20–28.

20. Bates-Jensen BM, McNees P. Toward an intelligent wound assessment system. *Osteotomy Wound Manage.* 1995; 41(7A):80–87.

21. Alvarez OM, Gilson G, Auletta MJ. Local aspects of diabetic foot ulcer care: Assessment, dressings, and topical agents. In: Levin ME, O'Neal LW, Bowker JH, eds. *The Diabetic Foot.* 5th ed. St Louis: Mosby Year-Book; 1993: 259–281.

22. Falanga V, Eaglstein WH. *Leg and Foot Ulcers: A Clinician's Guide.* London: Martin Dunitz Limited; 1995.

23. Hess CT. *Nurse's Clinical Guide to Wound Care.* 2nd ed. Springhouse, PA: Springhouse Corporation; 1997: 28–29.

24. Holloway GA. Arterial ulcers: Assessment, classification and management. In: Krasner D, Kane D, eds. *Chronic Wound Care: A Clinical Source Book for Healthcare Professionals.* 2nd ed. Wayne, PA: Health Management Publications; 1997: 158–164.

25. Maklebust J, Sieggreen MY. *Pressure Ulcers: Guidelines for Prevention and Nursing Management.* 2nd ed. Springhouse, PA: Springhouse Corporation; 1996: 30.

26. McCulloch J, Hovde J. Treatment of wounds due to vascular problems. In: Kloth L, McCulloch J, Feedar J, eds. *Wound Healing: Alternatives in Management.* Philadelphia: FA Davis; 1990: 177–195.

27. Phillips T, Machado F, Trout R, Porter J, Olin J, Falanga V. Prognostic indicators in venous ulcers. *J Am Acad Dermatol.* 2000; 43(4):627–630.

28. Beebe HG, Bergan JJ, Bergqvist D. Classification and grading of chronic venous disease in the lower limbs: A consensus statement. *VASA.* 1995; 24(4): 313–318.

29. Young RJ, Zhou YQ, Rodriguez E, Prescott RJ, Ewing DJ, Clarke BF. Variable relationship between peripheral somatic and autonomic neuropathy in patients with different syndromes of diabetic polyneuropathy. *Diabetes.* 1986; 35(2):192–197.

30. Levin M. Diabetic foot wounds: Pathogenesis and management. *Adv Wound Care.* 1996; 10(2):24–30.

31. Steed DL. Diabetic wounds: Assessment, classification and management. In: Krasner D, Kane D, eds. *Chronic Wound Care: A Clinical Source Book for Healthcare Professionals.* 2nd ed. Wayne, PA: Health Management Publications; 1997: 72–177.

32. Edmonds ME, Morrison M, Law JW, Watkins PJ. Medial arterial calcification and diabetic neuropathy. *Brit Med J.* 1982; 284:928–930.

33. Boulton AJM, Hardisty CA, Betts RC, et al. Dynamic foot pressure and other studies as diagnostic and management aids in diabetic neuropathy. *Diabetes Care.* 1983; 6:26–33.

34. Corbin DOC, Morrison DC, Young RJ, et al. Blood flow in the diabetic foot: Analysis of Doppler ultrasound waveforms by the Laplace transform damping method. *Diabetes Res Clin Prac.* 1985; 9:S109–S110.

35. Edmonds ME, Nicolaides KH, Watkins PJ. Autonomic neuropathy and diabetic foot ulceration. *Diabetic Med.* 1986; 3(4):344–349.

36. Nawoczenski DA, Birke JA. Management of the neuropathic foot in the elderly. *Top Geriatr Rehabil.* 1992; 7(3):36–48.

37. Matthews DM, Glass EJ, Stewart J, Collier DA, Clarke BF, Weir DM. Impairment of human monocyte "lectin-like" receptor activity in insulin dependent diabetics. *Diabetic Med.* 1986; 3(4):358–366.

38. Lavery LA, Armstrong DG, Harkless LB. Classification of diabetic foot wounds. *J Foot Ankle Surg.* 1996; 35(6):528–531.

39. Birke JA, Patout CA. The contact cast: An update and case study report. *Wounds.* 2000; 12(2): 26–31.

40. American Diabetes Association. Position statement: Office guide to diagnosis and classification of diabetes mellitus and other categories of glucose intolerance. *Diabetes Care.* 1992; 15(Suppl 2):4.

41. Gambert SR: *Diabetes Mellitus in the Elderly: A Practical Guide.* New York: Raven Press; 1999.

42. Bottomley, JM. A conservative approach in the treatment of a foot ulceration in a homeless diabetic patient: A case report. (unpublished)

43. Allman R. Epidemiology of pressure sores in different populations. *Decubitus.* 1989; 2(2):30–33.

44. Bennett L, Lee B. Pressure versus shear in pressure sore causation. In: Lee B, ed. *Chronic Ulcers of the Skin.* New York: McGraw-Hill; 1985: 39–56.

45. Kosiak M. Prevention and rehabilitation of ischemic ulcers. In: Kottke F, Stillwell G, Lehman J, eds. *Krusen's Handbook of Physical Medicine and Rehabilitation.* 3rd ed. Philadelphia: WB Saunders; 1982: 881–888.

46. Bergstrom N, Braden BJ, Laguzza A, Holman A. The Braden scale for predicting pressure sore risk. *Nursing Research.* 1987; 36:205–210.

47. Norton D, McLaren R, Exton-Smith AN. *An Investigation of Geriatric Nursing Problems in Hospitals.* London: Churchill-Livingston; 1975.

48. Rubin CF, Dietz RR, Abruzzese RS. Auditing the decubitus ulcer problem. *Am J Nurs.* 1974; 74(10): 1820–1821.

49. Aronovitch S, Millenbach L, Kelman GB, Wing P. Investigation of the Knoll Assessment Scale in a tertiary care facility. *Decubitus.* 1992; 5(3):70–76.

50. Gosnell DI. An assessment tool to identify pressure sores. *Nursing Research.* 1973; 22(1):55.

51. Shea JD. Pressure sores: Classification and management. *Clin Orthop Relat Res.* 1975; 112:89–100.

52. Ferrell BA, Artinian BM, Sessing D. The Sessing Scale for assessment of pressure ulcer healing. *J Amer Geriatr Soc.* 1995; 43(1):37–40.

53. Hunder GG. Vasculitic syndromes: An update on diagnosis and management. *J Musculoskel Med.* 1993; 10(1):50–60.

54. Kudravi SA, Reed MJ. Aging, cancer, and wound healing. *In Vivo.* 2000; 14(1):83–92.

55. Greenfield E, Jordan B. Advances in burn wound care. *Critical Care Nurs Clin North Amer.* 1996; 8(2): 203–215.

56. Staley M, Richard R. Management of the acute burn wound: An overview. *Adv Wound Care.* 1996; 10(2):39–44.

57. Yarbrough DR. Pathophysiology of the burn wound. In: Wagner MM, ed. *Care of the Burn-Injured Patient. Multidisciplinary Involvement.* Littleton, MA: PSG Publishing Company; 1981: 19–31.

58. Griffin JW, Tooms RE, Mendius RA, Clifft JK, Zwaag RV, El-Zeky F. Efficacy of high voltage pulsed current for healing of pressure ulcers in patients with spinal cord injury. *Phys Ther.* 1991; 71(6): 433–444.

59. Jaskoviak PA, Schafer RC. High voltage therapy. *Amer Chiropractor.* 1986; 12:68–84.

60. Sussman C. Electrical stimulation. In: Sussman C, Bates-Jensen BM, eds. *Wound Care: A Collaborative Practice Manual for Physical Therapists and Nurses.* 2nd ed. Gaithersburg, MD: Aspen Publishers; 2001.

61. Feedar JA, Kloth LC, Gentzkow GD. Chronic dermal ulcer healing enhanced with monophasic pulsed electrical stimulation. *Phys Ther.* 1991; 71(9): 639–649.

62. Sussman C. Ultrasound. In: Sussman C, Bates-Jensen BM, eds. *Wound Care: A Collaborative Practice Manual for Physical Therapists and Nurses.* 2nd ed. Gaithersburg, MD: Aspen Publishers; 2001.

63. Nussbaum EL, Biemann I, Mustard B. Comparison of ultrasound/ultraviolet-C and laser for treatment of pressure ulcers in patients with spinal cord injury. *Phys Ther.* 1994; 74(9):812–823.

64. Byl NN, McKenzie A, Wong T, West J, Hunt TK. Incisional wound healing: A controlled study of low and high dose ultrasound. *JOSPT.* 1993; 18(5): 619–628.

65. Dyson M. Mechanics involved in therapeutic ultrasound. *Physiotherapy.* 1987; 73(3):116–120.

66. Sussman C. Whirlpool. In: Sussman C, Bates-Jensen BM, eds. *Wound Care: A Collaborative Practice Manual for Physical Therapists and Nurses.* 2nd ed. Gaithersburg, MD: Aspen Publishers; 2001.

67. Feedar JA, Kloth LC. Conservative management of chronic wounds. In: Kloth LC, McCulloch JM, Feddar JA, eds. *Wound Healing: Alternatives in Management.* Philadelphia: FA Davis; 1990.

68. Quirinia A, Viidik A. The impact of ischemia on wound healing is increased in old age but can be countered by hyperbaric oxygen therapy. *Mech Ageing Dev.* 1996; 91(2):131–144.

69. Leung PC, Hung LK, Leung KS. Use of the medial plantar flap in soft tissue replacement around the heel region. *Foot Ankle.* 1988; 8(3):327–330.

70. Cevera JJ, Bolton LL, Kerstein MD. Options for diabetic patients with chronic heel ulcers. *J Diab Complic.* 1997; 11(3):358–366

71. Faglia E, Manuela M, Gino M, Quarantiello A, Signorini M. A combined conservative approach in the treatment of·a severe Achilles tendon region ulcer in a diabetic patient: A case report. *Wounds.* 1999; 11(5):105–109.

72. Campoccia D, Doherty P, Radice M. Semisynthetic resorbable materials from hyaluronan esterification. *Biomaterials.* 1998; 19:2101–2127.

73. Harris PA, Di Francesco F, Barisoni D, Leigh IM, Navsaria HA. Use of hyaluronic acid and cultured autologous keratinocytes and fibroblast in extensive burns. *Lancet.* 1999; 353(1):35–36.

74. Krouskop TA, Garber SL, Cullen BB. Factors to consider in selecting a support surface. In: Krasner D, ed. *Chronic Wound Care: A Clinical Source Book for Healthcare Professionals.* King of Prussia, PA: Health Management Publications; 1990: 142–151.

75. Ovington LG. Dressings and adjunctive therapies. AHCPR Guidelines revisited. *Ostomy Wound Management.* 1999; 45(Suppl 1A):94S–106S.

76. Perricone N, Kerstein MD, Kirsner RS, Norman RA, Phillips TJ. How to approach acute and chronic wound healing in the elderly. *Wounds.* 1999; 11(6): 145–151.

77. Wahl SM, Arend WP, Ross R. The effect of complement depletion on wound healing. *Am J Pathol.* 1974; 75(1):73–89.

78. Schmidtchen A. Degradation of antiproteinases, complement and fibronectin in chronic leg ulcers. *Acta Derm Venerol.* 2000; 80(3):179–184.

79. Barron LG, Meyer KB, Szoka FC. Effects of complement depletion on the pharmacokinetics and gene delivery mediated by cationic lipid-DNA complexes. *Hum Gene Ther.* 1998; 9(3):315–323.

80. Papantonio C. Alternative medicine and wound healing. *Ostomy Wound Manage.* 1998; 44(4):44–50.

15

Establishing Community-Based Screening Programs

Pearls

- Prevention strategies can improve the quality of life and conserve health resources.

- "Successful aging" is a combination of good lifestyle and behavioral habits, including exercise, diet, and socioeconomic well-being.

- Resiliency of the human being is incredible.

- There is a need to change the health care approach from curative to preventive interventions. It is important to convince third-party payers through research efforts of the efficacy of preventive approaches.

- Primary, secondary, and tertiary prevention are the three levels of health intervention.

- Eighty-six percent of those aged 65 and older have at least one chronic disease.

- "We must protect what we can't replace."

Introduction

The prevention of disease or mitigation of disability can improve a person's quality of life at any age. Anyone can benefit from gains in function, fewer periods of acute illness, more days free of disability, and less need for long-term care.[1] Prevention strategies can also conserve health resources. In 2000, those over age 65 years represented 12.4% of the population, but they accounted for more than 30% ($200 billion) of public health care costs.[2] Health care expenditures by older people totaled an average of $6,299 per person.[2,3] Since the older age group is the fastest growing segment of the population, these health care cost estimates signal the need to examine strategies that might lower expenditures, such as health promotion and disease prevention, for those over age 65 years. In the next 25 years, the number of people over the age of 60 years will double; and those over 85 years are projected to increase more than any other age group.[4,5]

Nearly $1 of every $4 spent on health care each year can be attributed to behavioral factors, including crime, drug abuse, and the use of alcohol and tobacco; therefore, behavior accounts for $171 billion of the $666 billion

Americans spend on health care.[2] The health care crisis cannot be successfully resolved unless damaging patterns of behavior are altered. Twenty-two billion dollars in annual health care costs are attributable to cigarette smoking and other forms of tobacco use, and alcohol abuse may add another $85 billion a year. Other behavioral cost factors include failure to use technology like seat belts and smoke detectors, failure to have routine medical checkups that could expose cancer and other treatable conditions, and participating in dangerous recreational activities.

There are many factors that contribute to the concept of "successful aging,"[6] the most important of which is optimal health. The human being's resiliency is incredible. It allows many elderly individuals to function adequately with considerable degrees of disability because of their inconceivably large amount of reserve. A person's ability to function independently is closely associated with optimum health status because it impacts the ability of the elderly person to successfully reside in the community at the highest possible level of independence rather than being institutionalized. Other factors that directly impact an individual's ability to maintain independence in the community are adequate financing and the individual's support system (e.g., significant others such as family, kin, friends, or church).[7] In a report published by the US Department of Health and Human Services, this conclusion was reached:

> Many analysts of the Medicaid program argue that one of the major problems of both Medicare and Medicaid is the total reliance on institutional care, acute hospital care, and long-term nursing home care. Presently under Medicaid, approximately 70 percent of total program dollars are spent on institutional care: 33 percent in hospitals, 37 percent in long-term care facilities. According to these analysts, both forms of institutional care are some of the more expensive available options. The critics of Medicaid's heavy reliance on institutional care argue that Medicaid incorrectly emphasizes curing the ills of the elderly as opposed to preserving the health of the elderly. They state that in order to increase the preventive aspects of Medicaid, both the federal and state government should encourage the growth of community-based alternatives to institutional care. They argue that in many cases people who could live on their own with very little help with shopping, cooking, or medical care are inappropriately placed in nursing homes.[8]

The allocation of resources focuses on long-term care in an institutional setting like nursing homes rather than on preventative care, a costly alternative. There is a gap in the system between the income support provided to the "well" elderly and the intense health care provided to the "sick" elderly. There is nothing in between. Physical and occupational therapists have a unique opportunity to demonstrate innovation and leadership in the development of community screening programs that combine health care, personal care, and social maintenance; maximize effective preventive approaches; use the special knowledge of physical rehabilitation potentials to reduce unnecessary institutionalization; and ensure proper use of limited resources. This chapter focuses on screening programs that are community based and enhance the elderly individual's ability to maintain the highest level of physical functioning and independence.

Physical problems affecting the older adult are often undetected until they cause a debilitating loss in the person's capability to independently maintain activities of daily living (ADLs) and functional ambulation. The complications of many chronic diseases can be minimized or prevented by early detection through community based screening programs, regular medical care, environmental adaptations to facilitate function, and fitness programs that promote independence and the overall well-being of the elderly. Few elders have annual physical checkups, and rarely, if ever, are functional limitations directly addressed. In light of this, preventive screening programs have the triple benefit of identifying high-risk individuals, detecting medical and physical problems, and preventing them from progressing into a loss of functional independence.

PREVENTION/HEALTH PROMOTION

Interventions, such as exercise, diet, stress reduction, and smoking cessation, have been shown to positively affect the musculoskeletal, cardiovascular, cardiopulmonary, sensory, and neuromuscular systems. These preventive modalities can lead to corrective and ameliorative changes that have the potential of delaying the onset of pathologies, as well as preventing the disabling effects of existing chronic disease(s).[9–11] Even in the oldest-old population, those 85 years of age and older, research reveals that improvements can be made in every system of the body through exercise.[12] Proper attention to diet significantly modifies the onset of certain disease processes,[13] and the implementation of dietary control in combination with exercise has the potential of reversing, if not avoiding, some pathological manifestations, such as diabetes[14,15] and coronary artery disease.[16] Stress reduction and exercise also have positive effects on hypertension.[17] It is never too late to stop smoking. For example, a study by Rogers and associates[18] showed a significant improvement in cerebral blood flow in elderly subjects who stopped smoking and this improvement happened in a matter of three to five days. In a relatively short period of time, the abstinence from cigarettes also significantly improves cardiovascular and cardiopulmonary circulation and perfusion.[19] In terms of the quality of life for the elderly, preventive interventions can have a substantial impact on health care needs and days free of disability.

Types of Prevention

There are three levels in preventive health care: primary, secondary, and tertiary. Primary aging is the maturation of an organism exclusively attributable to the passage of time. Primary prevention is the prevention of any ill effects that may occur as a result of microtrauma during that maturation process. The goal of primary prevention is to avoid or delay the onset of debilitating pathologies and functional disabilities. An example would be a fitness program for the well elderly that included aerobic as well as stretching and strengthening exercises to enhance the cardiovascular, musculoskeletal, and neuromuscular systems. Primary prevention is synonymous with health promotion and seeks to prevent disease in susceptible individuals by reducing the exposure to risk factors. The basic interventions include better diet, more exercise, smoking cessation, better sanitation, and accident prevention. Primary prevention uses education to encourage individuals to modify behaviors.

Secondary aging relates to systemic or organ-specific changes associated with either acute or chronic disease. Secondary prevention is the implementation of therapeutic interventions at the earliest possible time within the acute phase of an illness. For instance, with pneumonia, the early intervention with chest physical therapy and the early resumption of ambulation and exercise avoids the debilitating effects of bed rest and increases the individual's ability to ward off the infection.[20] Secondary prevention in chronic illness deals with the earliest possible intervention to reverse or maintain existing impairments and prevent further deficits from impeding maximal functional capabilities of the elderly individual. Screening programs are the hallmark of secondary prevention at the community level.

Tertiary aging refers to functional impairments that have already progressed to the level of disability (see Chapter 9) and impede ADLs. Tertiary prevention attempts to minimize the ill effects of diseases once they have occurred and to rehabilitate the elderly individual's residual capacities. Functional activities and therapeutic interventions, such as proprioceptive neuromuscular facilitation (PNF) and Bobath techniques, in addition to strength and endurance training, are all important elements in restoring function and preventing further decline in chronic illnesses.

Webster[21] states, "It is increasingly clear that what was previously accepted as normal primary aging actually relates much more to unappreciated secondary or tertiary influences." Preventive measures that address the most prevalent diseases, such as heart disease, cancer, and cerebral vascular accidents, are particularly applicable in the elderly population. There is a correlation between healthful interventions like diet and exercise and the development of disease, and there is compelling evidence that suggests that the control of risks, such as smoking, an unhealthy diet, high blood pressure, physical inactivity, and exposure to toxic substances in the environment, could significantly diminish the prevalence of the three leading causes of death in the United States.[10]

HEALTH PROBLEMS IN THE ELDERLY/SYMPTOM PREVALENCE

Studies estimate that of the US population who are 65 years of age and older, 86% have at least one chronic disease that limits their functional activities and decreases the number of "disability-free" days progressively with advancing age.[22] Chronic diseases that affect older adults are sometimes misidentified as normal age changes and can go untreated for years.

Heart disease, cancer, and cerebral vascular disease cause almost 70% of deaths in the United States.[10] According to the National Center for Health Statistics, the elderly population is afflicted (in decreasing order of frequency) by arthritis (48%), heart disease (40%), hypertension (39%), cataracts (36%), diabetes (28%), cancer (26%), osteoporosis/hip fracture (16%), and stroke (9%).

Comorbidites are common, and the frequency of these disorders increases with advancing age.[23]

The major causes of frailty and disability in the elderly relate to the broad functional problems of immobility and instability. Intellectual impairment is also a major component of functional decline. Confounding factors with the elderly include depression and transient dementias, isolation, urinary and bowel incontinence, sexual dysfunction, immune deficiency and infections, malnutrition, sleep disorders, impairment of sensory abilities, and iatrogenesis. Many of the health problems of the elderly are especially well suited for preventive efforts. For instance, impaired mobility, injuries, sensory loss, adverse drug reactions, deconditioning due to lack of exercise, depression, malnutrition, alcohol abuse, hypertension and cardiovascular disease, cancers, osteoporosis, urinary incontinence, and abuse and neglect are all preventable or can be postponed as a result of screening programs that identify these problems and follow-up intervention to address each individual's risk factors.

SCREENING CONCERNS IN THE ELDERLY

Planning preventive care packages and counseling approaches for older people requires special considerations. Most older people suffer from one or more chronic diseases or syndromes and total risk increases as a function of the number of individual risk factors.[24]

Screening tests and lab standards have not been developed or adapted specifically for the elderly.[25] "Aging, even without disease, changes physiology, which can alter lab test results."[26] Most of the normal lab values are based on 20- to 40-year-old subjects. This makes it difficult to determine what is abnormal in terms of a test result in the elderly. Aside from lab values, normal physiological changes of aging and the use of medications to treat chronic diseases may mask the symptoms of other physical problems.

Some diseases and conditions, such as coronary heart disease, may manifest themselves differently in older patients than in younger.[27] For example, an elevated serum cholesterol level becomes less predictive of heart-related morbidity in an older individual. In fact, a low serum cholesterol level is a predictor of mortality in people of advanced age,[28] because they are associated with an increased risk of cancer and hemorrhagic stroke.

Some chronic conditions common in old age have competing risk factors. For example, obesity is a major risk factor for heart disease, diabetes, and other chronic diseases, but modest obesity is protective for osteoporosis.[29] Conversely, low body weight is a significant risk factor for hip fracture.[30]

In older individuals, functional disabilities associated with chronic diseases become as important as preventing the onset of disease.[31] Of the population aged 65 years who live independently, 24% have some degree of functional impairment, 15% are unable to perform major activities, and 11% are less impaired. Of those who are dependent on others for daily care, 6% are in nursing homes and 14% are homebound.[22]

What to Screen For

Many diseases can be prevented or forestalled by identifying and avoiding high-risk behaviors, while others can be treated in the early stages, thereby reducing the risk of disability or death. Yearly physical assessments are the preferred method for identifying problems; however, the majority of people 65 years of age and over do not seek medical attention on an annual basis. As a result of initiatives implemented by the Surgeon General in the early 1980s, many agencies now offer preventive health programs, including screening for high-risk behaviors and the presence of disease. The costs associated with the treatment of chronic disease are clearly not desirable in today's malnourished economy. Health screening and early detection of disease processes can reduce costs substantially.

Screening programs for the elderly need to address behavior patterns, such as smoking, level of activity, dietary habits, living environment, health care needs such as dental and foot care, and immunization history. These programs aim to determine what the problems are and how to address them from an educational perspective. Ideally, screening programs should have a follow-up mechanism or referral sources for evaluating and treating physical or medical problems identified during the screening. Screening programs for the elderly can be holistic, and screen all systems of the body, or they can be system or disease specific (e.g., blood pressure screening, diabetes screening, cholesterol screening, or dental screening).

Primary prevention screening programs include immunizations, accident prevention, exercise programs, posture and flexibility assessment, nutritional modifications, and smoking and alcohol cessation. Secondary prevention screening focuses on early detection and treatment and is particularly applicable in disorders such as hypertension, vision and hearing impairments, musculoskeletal problems, neuromuscular involvement, depression, and iatrogenic adverse drug affects. Tertiary preventive screening focuses on functional assessment and maximizing physical potential and environmental efficiency to prevent the progression of functional decline.

The United States Preventive Services Task Force[32,33] has identified screening interventions that successfully alter the outcomes of various diseases, and emphasizes the importance of educating the elderly population in high-risk behavior modification. For instance, the Task Force advised that elderly individuals be provided with educational material regarding the benefits of physical activity in disease prevention and that guidance in establishing appropriate exercise levels and selected modes of exercise be provided on an individual basis to each person screened. Other components of the Task Force's recommendations include smoking cessation programs; dietary modification to prevent diseases associated with dietary excesses or imbalances (e.g., osteoporosis, heart disease, some cancers, cerebral vascular accidents, or dental diseases); alcohol cessation programs when abuse is identified; home modification screening to reduce the potential for accidental injuries; vaccination programs for pneumococcal, influenza, and tetanus immunization; and screening for preventive "chemoprophylaxis" programs, such as low-dose aspirin therapy (325 mg every other day) for those at risk for cardiovascular diseases and estrogen replacement therapy for women who are at increased risk of developing osteoporosis.

Prescreening for High-Risk Populations

Before a comprehensive community based screening program is initiated, it is valuable to prescreen the community served to identify groups within the older population that would benefit from specific health screening procedures. Health questionnaires or interviews are helpful tools in identifying subgroups within the elderly population that may require special attention (e.g., diabetes mellitus, cardiovascular or pulmonary problems, a decrease in functional ADLs, or foot problems). There are some particularly valuable prescreening tools available. For instance, the Self-Evaluation of Life Function questionnaire developed by Linn and Linn[34] includes questions about health behaviors, existing diseases, symptoms, level of basic and instrumental ADLs, medication use, cognitive status, and socioeconomic well-being.

Another useful tool for prescreening the community elderly is the Health Hazard Appraisal (HHA), which is used in many preventive health care programs in both the United States and Canada[35] to determine high-risk populations for screening in community based settings. Safer[35] demonstrated that through the use of the HHA prescreening tool, Milwaukee residents reduced their health risk by 32% as a result of the health screening, follow-up counseling, and interventions that were employed to address the health care needs determined by the prescreening. The HHA prescreening is based on the assumption that "an individual's response to health threats depends on how he or she feels physically rather than on a rational calculation of health benefits and risks." The HHA is a valuable educational tool. By questioning elderly individuals and generating a "health hazard score," it informs people about how their health habits and lifestyles affect their probability of dying within 10 years from potentially preventable causes. The HHA also helps to target the population that are most likely to benefit from health screening and follow-up counseling and intervention programs. See the Evidence-Based Medicine Box below.

**Prevention of Falls in the Elderly Trial:
A Randomised Controlled Trial;
by Close; *Lancet*; 1–99[36]**

- 182 patients who presented to the emergency room after a fall
- Intervention group =
  - medical and OT assessment
  - 1×—home evaluation and Barthel Index
  - education on home modifications
  - referral—as needed
- Falls = control = 510, 183 in experimental group

Secondary Prevention Screening Tests

Screening and assessments necessary for health promotion in the elderly should include the evaluation of the presence of chronic diseases; symptoms that may suggest the presence of disease; health habits including nutrition, exercise and activity levels, smoking, medication use, and substance abuse; the evaluation of musculoskeletal, neuromuscular, and sensory deficits; safety; and mental status.

Cardiovascular Disease

Routine monitoring of blood pressure is an important component in controlling and reducing high blood pressure. Individuals with diagnosed high blood pressure need to be counseled regarding appropriate exercise levels, weight reduction, dietary sodium reduction, and alcohol consumption. Periodic screening with the finding of persistent high blood pressure (e.g., greater than 140/90 mm Hg) may direct the health care professional to refer the individual for possible drug therapy to control excessively high blood pressure. Routine monitoring of the ECG is recommended in individuals who are symptomatic (e.g., had a previously positive ECG, angina, or dyspnea on exertion), but it is not recommended for those elderly who are asymptomatic. Though somewhat controversial, total serum cholesterol measurements are often employed to determine the presence of elevated blood cholesterol levels that have also been shown to place an individual at a higher risk for the development of cardiovascular diseases.

Cardiovascular screening should also include weight monitoring, and in those individuals who are 20% overweight by the height/weight standards, appropriate dietary and exercise counseling should be implemented as a preventive measure. Additionally, information on transient ischemic attacks, the presence of diabetes mellitus, cardiac arrhythmias, claudication, and any musculoskeletal limitations that place the individual at a high risk of developing problems associated with inactivity should be recorded and monitored. Peripheral vascular status and skin condition are important to evaluate, especially in the diabetic or someone with known peripheral vascular disease.

Cancer

There is little agreement as to the efficacy of screening for cancer in the elderly, and conflicting data exist regarding the accuracy and efficiency of the screening strategies in all ages (e.g., breast exams, mammography, and Papanicolaou [Pap] testing). Because certain cancers are more easily treated if diagnosed early, the consensus is that regular screening for cancer is recommended until more substantial evidence is presented that negates the value of the screening strategies in question. In the *Summary of Current Guidelines for the Cancer-Related Checkup: Recommendations*,[37] the recommendations for cancer screening are:

- Annual Pap smears and pelvic examinations for all women who are sexually active or are 18 years of age or older. After three consecutive normal annual examinations, Pap tests may be performed less frequently or at the discretion of the physician.
- Endometrial tissue samples at menopause for women who are at high risk.
- Baseline mammogram between 35 and 39 years of age. Repeat every two years from age 40 to 49 and annually thereafter.
- Breast physical examination every three years for women between 20 and 40 years of age and yearly thereafter.
- Breast self-examination monthly for all women 20 years and older.
- Stool guaiac slide test every year for men and women over 50.
- A sigmoidoscopic examination every three to five years for men and women over age 50.
- Yearly digital/rectal examination for men and women over age 40 to screen for prostate and rectal cancer.
- Cancer examination and health counseling every three years after age 20 and yearly after age 40.

The second most common neoplasm in the United States is colorectal cancer, and it also has the second highest mortality rate.[37] Sigmoidoscopy and fecal occult blood testing are important in the early detection of this disease, especially in a known high-risk population (e.g., family or personal history of cancer, colonic polyps, or inflammatory bowel disease). High-risk patients include those with ulcerative colitis involving the entire colon with a duration of seven or more years, a past history of an adenoma of the colon, or a past history of colon cancer or female genital cancer.[38] Early detection is particularly important in colorectal cancer as the survival rate in asymptomatic patients is 90% compared to 43% in those with more advanced disease.[38] Once symptoms of colorectal cancer occur, the disease is usually in an advanced and nonlocalized stage, which decreases the likelihood of successful surgical removal. There are home screening tests for occult blood that are reliable and available through a pharmacist; however, the tests require several stool smears over a three-day period with dietary restrictions and are difficult to accurately accomplish when elders have physical or cognitive deficits. Cost-effectiveness studies clearly indicate that the early detection of colorectal cancer significantly reduces the overall medical costs and improves survival.[39]

Breast cancer is the second leading cause of cancer deaths in women, and of those deaths, 50% occur in women over the age of 65 years,[40] and 75% of all breast cancers occur in women over the age of 50 years.[41] There is some controversy regarding the accuracy of both self-breast exams and mammography; however, it is recommended that breast examination be taught to all women, especially to those over the age of 50, and that a breast self-examination be done monthly. After the age of 40, the American Cancer Society recommends that women have a breast examination by a physician and a mammogram annually.[37]

Cervical cancer is accurately detected by a Pap test; however, many older women do not have Pap smears on a regular basis. For the most part, women diagnosed with cervical cancer after the age of 65 years are usually in the advanced stages of the disease, and 41% of all deaths from cervical cancer occur in women over the age of 65 years. Yearly screening using the Pap smear for three consecutive years is recommended by the American Cancer Society.[37] If the test is negative for three years it is recommended that Pap tests be done at the discretion of the physician or at least once every five years thereafter.

Digital rectal examination is the best way to screen for prostate cancer in men. The American Cancer Society recommends that men receive a yearly screening for prostate cancer after the age of 40, and every three to five years after the age of 50 as the greatest incidence of this form of cancer occurs in the age range of 40 to 50 years.

A total skin examination is an important part of the routine physical examination. Inspection of the mouth is also recommended for those who are known smokers and for those who use excessive amounts of alcohol. Seventy-five percent of deaths from oral cancers occur in individuals 55 years of age and older.[42] Screening for oral cancer can be done routinely during periodic dental care; however, many elderly individuals do not go to the dentist on a regular basis, and it is recommended that oral screening be done by the physician or other health care personnel at community based screening clinics and health fairs since it is a noninvasive assessment.

Diabetes Mellitus

Over 8.6 million people in the United States over the age of 65 have diabetes mellitus.[43] Diabetes has been found to contribute to cardiovascular diseases, end-stage renal failure, amputations, blindness, and peripheral neuropathies.[43] The American Diabetes Association[43] recommends that periodic serum glucose measurements be taken in the elderly population as the incidence of diabetes mellitus increases exponentially with increasing age. In known diabetics, the recommendations include periodic testing for asymptomatic bacteriuria, hematuria, and proteinuria by urinalysis screening.

Osteoporosis

The elderly population, particularly white females over the age of 60, have the highest risk for developing osteoporosis. Subtle changes in posture related to the breakdown of vertebral body height directly affect the individual's flexibility and strength. The person may report that he or she is "shrinking," or that he or she has pain in the cervical, thoracic, or lumbar region(s) of the back. Because height changes are frequently the first clinical indication of osteoporosis, regular screening should include height measurement. Reed and Birge[44] found that 75% of the elderly that they screened who had a two-inch loss in height had osteoporotic changes on x-ray. Measuring height is a reliable, inexpensive, and noninvasive screening tool for osteoporosis.

Other valuable screening information for the evaluation for osteoporosis includes nutritional information and dietary habits (e.g., calcium intake, excessive caffeine or soda consumption, or excessive protein intake), level of activity or inactivity, family history of osteoporosis, and alcohol and tobacco consumption. All of these factors have been found to have a contributory effect toward the development of osteoporosis. Low estrogen levels in women have also been found to influence the integrity of bone.[45] It is particularly important in postmenopausal women that height measurements be taken periodically to screen for osteoporotic changes. Since osteoporosis contributes to more than 1.5 million fractures in people over the age of 65 years annually,[45] screening becomes a vital component in the identification of risk factors and the prevention of accidental injury.

Health Habits

Nutrition, exercise levels, smoking, substance abuse, and medication use need to be considered when screening the elderly. Optimal health is the key factor in maintaining an independent and productive life. Health promotion and disease prevention activities have the potential of interrupting or slowing the progression of aging and disease before pathological changes become irreversible. The expected outcome of health promotion must reach beyond longevity toward an acceptable quality of life without debilitating physical or mental disabilities.[23,46] Preventive measures seek to detect the precursors that allow for early intervention and risk factors for disease that can be modified,[47] because modification of personal health habits could have a potential impact on disease outcomes. For instance, smoking cessation improves physical stamina and lessens susceptibility to infections, while it reduces the risk of lung cancer and heart disease.[10]

To meet the needs of the elderly population, health care practitioners involved in screening strategies should educate individuals on ways to promote good health by adopting better lifestyle habits and a safer local environment; assist people to identify their own genetic/familial predispositions and risk factors for specific diseases; and promote public awareness of the myths, as well as the realities, pertaining to good health.[29]

One of the most significant advances in the past decade has been the convergence of opinion on what constitutes a "proper diet." Two documents, the 1988 *Surgeon General's Report on Nutrition and Health*[48] and the 1989 National Research Council's *Report on Diet and Health*,[49] summarize the consensus of the scientific community and make dietary and health recommendations for the general public,[50] including reducing dietary fats and cholesterol; limiting salt intakes; limiting the use of alcohol; maintaining adequate but not excessive protein intakes; eating more fruits, vegetables, and complex carbohydrates; balancing caloric intake with expenditure to maintain a healthy weight; and avoiding the use of dietary supplements in excess of the NRC's recommended dietary allowances (RDAs). Both documents caution against unsafe dietary practices, health fads, and outright health fraud, much of which is directed at older persons.[48] Screening for nutritional problems is best accomplished by a registered dietitian; however, if this is not feasible, the collection of information on socioeconomic status, food supply, eating patterns, and self-perceived nutritional and dietary status is valuable in establishing the need for further counseling and education.

The effects of inactivity mimic the effects of aging.[51] Almost 50% of the functional decline attributed to aging may, in fact, be related to inactivity.[52] Increasing energy expenditure through exercise appears to influence mortality and morbidity through a number of complex physiological mechanisms (see Chapter 13).

Despite these benefits, there has been some reluctance in recommending fitness programs for the elderly because exercising too intensely may injure muscles or joints, provoke heart attacks and irregular heart rhythms, increase blood pressure, and increase fall-related fractures.[53] Regular exercise training can increase protein turnover (37% higher muscle catabolism) in the elderly. As a result, elderly individuals prescribed an exercise program should be advised to increase their protein intake.[54] Some elderly are unable to maintain high-intensity training programs because of weight reduction's association with the loss of lean muscle mass.[55] Therefore special attention to the dietary needs of the exercising elder need to be considered

when prescribing a fitness program. It is important to determine the intensity, duration, and frequency of physical training to delay declines in functional capacity. These variables vary from one elderly individual to the next.

Combined with a calorie-appropriate diet, regular physical activity maintains a reasonable body weight, delays loss of lean muscle mass, and promotes good physical performance. A high activity level can predict survival for both institutionalized and people living in the community aged 60 to 80.[56,57] High-intensity training appears to decrease fat cell hypertension, increase insulin resistance, and slow the rate of decline of VO2 max in older persons.[58-60]

Exercise programs designed for the elderly can reduce bone loss and strengthen skeletal muscle in both men and women of very advanced age,[58-61] thus decreasing the risk of falls and fractures.[62,63] For example, a group of sedentary men and women aged 86 to 96 years, including those with a past history of falling, increased the strength in the knee extensors by as much as 167% to 180% after an eight-week course in weight-lifting exercise.

It is never too late to quit smoking. At any age, cigarette smoking imposes higher risks of coronary heart disease, lung and mouth cancers, stroke, and osteoporosis.[64] Smoking cessation results in a decline of body nicotine within 6 months, a reduced risk of sudden heart attack in 1 to 2 years, and a lowered risk of cancer in about 15 years. Smoking combined with low-calorie intakes can also compromise vitamin C status, which is essential in wound healing, infection, and maintenance of the connective tissue health. Smokers take two to three times longer to heal wounds, require longer to recover from acute illnesses such as pneumonia, and are twice as likely to die prematurely of coronary artery disease.[64]

The use of medications is another risk factor to look for when screening an elderly population. The 1991 National Disease and Therapeutic Index indicates that 42.7% of all prescription drugs are doled out to people 60 years of age and older in the United States. The average number of prescriptions per elderly American is 15.7, and there are over 9 million adverse drug reactions in people over the age of 65 years each year.[65] Normal aging results in changes in the way older adults absorb, metabolize, distribute, and excrete medications. The half-life of drugs is longer in the elderly and the cumulative effects of drugs last longer. Because the elderly are often existing on polypharmacy, they are more likely to overdose and experience adverse effects when medication combinations are inappropriate. Falls and fractures can be related to drug effects; for instance, beta-blockers often induce an orthostatic hypotensive response on standing. Certain drugs actually induce neurological symptoms, such as tardive dyskinesia and parkinsonism, and many drugs create mental impairment. These drugs are discussed more thoroughly in Chapter 7. Additionally, noncompliance has been found to be a problem in close to 50% of the elderly.[65] Wolf and co-workers[65] found that the factors related to older persons not taking their medications were financial difficulties, language barriers, sensory deficits, accidental overdoses, and cognitive impairments.

Pharmacists often evaluate and monitor medication problems that may occur, but the elderly do not always go to the same pharmacy. Over 13% of all expenditures for medications by the elderly are for over-the-counter medications, which makes monitoring that much more difficult.[66] Screening and education for medication use often takes the form of health education programs combined with a review of current medications by a pharmacist or nurse in a community screening program.

According to Maddox[67] over 5% of the elderly population abuse alcohol. Late-onset alcohol-related problems occur in less than 1% of the elderly, however, because most were abusers before reaching the age of 65 years.[67] In addition, as an individual ages the alcohol tolerance diminishes: less alcohol is required to produce intoxication in the elderly, so dependency may develop at a level of drinking that would not cause addiction in a younger individual. Willenbrig and Spring[68] have developed a screening tool that contains four questions and is accurate for identifying alcohol abuse 95% of the time. One question is designed to elicit subtle defensiveness while the other three directly ask about drinking habits and patterns. While individual screening by health care professionals is recommended, mass screening is not because of the low incidence of late-onset alcoholism and the fact that the screening has not been shown to lead to a decrease in morbidity or mortality.[28]

Drug abuse is not an issue in the elderly population. It can be expected, however, that as those individuals who use substances such as cocaine, heroin, marijuana, and so forth, age, drug abuse may become a significant problem.

Sensory Deficits

Visual acuity testing in asymptomatic older adults should be done routinely. Although many older persons maintain nearly normal vision, their eyesight is subject to various changes and disabilities as discussed in Chapters 3 and 5. Yearly eye exams are recommended to detect the presence or progression of presbyopia, as well as the presence of disease. Three disorders—cataracts, glaucoma, and senile macular degeneration—are commonly found through screening.[28]

Anyone with impaired hearing should receive an otoscopic examination and audiometric testing. Between 30% and 60% of people over age 65 and up to 90% of nursing home residents in that age group are estimated to suffer from some degree of hearing loss.[69] Screening for hearing loss can range from a thorough history and interview of family members to testing by a clinical audiologist. A tuning fork is a wonderful screening tool. According to

Alpert,[70] if the health care provider can hear the fork's hum when the client can no longer hear it and visual inspection of the ear shows no gross pathology (e.g., cerumen, serous otitis), then there is a hearing deficit. With a suspected hearing deficit, a more definitive audiometric screening by a trained individual can be easily employed in a community setting.

Psychological Problems

Elderly individuals should be specifically screened for depression and the potential for suicide. This screening needs to include a family history of depression/suicide, the presence of a chronic illness, recent loss (real or perceived), problems with sleep disorders, the presence of multiple somatic complaints, recent divorce or separation, unemployment, alcohol abuse, living alone, and the presence of prolonged bereavement. Depression is more prevalent in the older population than any other age group. White men, in particular, are at the highest risk for suicide. Alpert[70] recommended the Beck Depression Inventory as a reliable test in elderly populations.

Dementia

The Mental Status Questionnaire, Fact-Hand Test, and Dementia Rating Scale are frequently used along with screening for other mental, neurological, and physical deficits to determine if patients are suffering from dementia. In the early stages, however, it is difficult to distinguish true dementia from depression, the adverse effects of medication, and other mental and physical illnesses. Screening can determine only whether or not a problem exists, not what the underlying cause is. Magaziner and associates[71] were able to show that a shortened version of the Mini-Mental Status Examination could be used as a reliable predictor of scores on the longer version of the test. The shortened version makes screening easier and more cost effective.

Urinary Incontinence

Urinary incontinence affects a significant number of elderly persons. In fact, urinary incontinence contributes to nursing home admission in nearly half of the elderly admitted to long-term care facilities. Women have a weakening of the muscles of the pelvic floor and abdomen following pregnancy, which can be treated with Kegal exercises. In addition, birth injuries, hormonal changes, infections, tumors, or side effects of medications may cause urinary incontinence. Men develop urinary incontinence most often because of bladder or prostate disease. Causes of urinary incontinence need to be determined to prevent the need for institutionalization.

Safety

Elderly individuals account for almost 30% of all accidental deaths and about 15% of all hospitalized accident victims. Baker and Harvey[72] report that for every fall that results in a hip fracture, the incidence of mortality is higher. Decreased mobility, reduced independence, and a higher incidence of illness are common after a hip fracture. Impaired hearing and eyesight, slower physical reactions, poor balance and coordination, circulatory changes, orthostatic hypotension, and decreased physical stamina are among the reasons for the high accident rate in elders. For these reasons it is important to assess the older adult's risk for falls as well as the presence of fall hazards in the home. The US Consumer Product Safety Commission has developed a "Home Safety Checklist for Older Consumers" to help spot possible safety problems in the home. These were distributed through Area Agencies on Aging (AAAs) to senior centers, public health departments, and other community groups. Copies may be obtained from the US Consumer Safety Commission, Washington, DC, 20207. See Evidence-Based Medicine Strategies below.

Occupational Therapy for Independent-Living Older Adults; by Clark; *JAMA*; 10–97[74]

- Significant benefits for the OT preventative treatment group were found across various health, function, and QOL domains.
- Program = didactic teaching and direct experience:
  - community safety and transportation
  - joint protection, energy conservation, adaptive equipment
  - exercise and nutrition

Embedding Health-Promoting Changes into the Daily Lives of Independent-Living Older Adults: Long-Term Follow-up of OT; by Clark; *J Gerontol*; 1–01[75]

- A 9-month preventative OT program showed significant gain in functioning that was retained for at least 6 months after termination.
- RCT with treatment and social activity (weekly), nontreatment.
- OT group:
  - transportation, safety, social relationships, transportation, and finances
  - didactic presentation, peer exchange, direct experience, personal exploration

---

A Geriatric Experience in the Acute Care Hospital; by Landi; *Am J Phys Med Rehab*; 1–97[75]

- Set up comprehensive preventative rehab programs.
- Findings: experimental group improved in:
  - locomotion
  - eating
  - personal hygiene
- 77.5% of experimental group was discharged to home versus 58.3% of control.

PRIMARY PREVENTION

Advancing primary prevention for those over the age of 65 requires a change in attitude that accepts the growing proof that individuals of any age may benefit from adopting health-promoting behaviors.[27] The attitude that diseases of old age are irreversible and inevitable needs to be dismissed. Life expectancy has been extended, accounting for the growth in population of those over the age of 85. In fact, those who are presently age 65 years can expect to live an average additional 17 years (19 years for women and 14.5 years for men).[22]

Primary preventive efforts directed at personal health practices are among the most effective interventions available to health care practitioners caring for older adults. Traditional clinical activities, such as routine unfocused testing, are generally of less value in preventing disease than is counseling. Although demonstrated advantages of preventive services for older people are limited, emerging research is quite convincing. For instance, research on cancer etiology suggests that a 10- to 20-year latent period exists between events that may induce some cancers and the clinical expression of disease. Based on an average 15-year latency period, cancer detected after age 70 could have begun between ages 55 and 60 years. Therefore, many of the quarter of a million cancers induced in people after age 60 might have been prevented by primary prevention measures, such as smoking cessation and dietary changes.[76] Comprehensive screening strategies should be tailored to the individual risk profile of each elderly person. See EBM below.

Older individuals are more susceptible to acute diseases and episodes, such as infections, pneumonia, food poisoning, and orthostatic hypotension with resulting falls and injury.[77] Most of these conditions are preventable with proper intervention to maintain optimum health, thereby warding off these acute episodes. The growth of community "wellness" services or activities for older people signals a growing commitment to postponing disease and disabilities in older persons. Using Title IIIB grants from the federal government in response to Surgeon General Koop's efforts, 37 states had initiated community wellness programs for the elderly by 1985.[77]

Over the past 20 years, some of the major causes of morbidity and mortality in old age have declined, although the extent to which health promotion efforts are responsible has not been determined. Over these two decades, stroke deaths declined 55%, heart attacks decreased by 40%, and substantial progress had been made in hypertension control.[1] Evidence indicates that those who reach old age in good health tend to stay healthy until shortly before death, often well into the seventh or eighth decade of life.[78]

A COMMUNITY BASED SCREENING PROGRAM/MODEL PROJECT

Screening for Foot Problems

Many systemic diseases manifest themselves in the lower extremity, including diabetes, peripheral vascular disease, heart and kidney disease, arthritis, and nutritional deficiencies.[79–81] Many orthopedic conditions, arising from long-standing biomechanical imbalances, ill-fitting shoes, or both, plague the elderly patient and interfere with functional mobility. The most common foot disorders in individuals over the age of 65 years include pes planus (flat feet), excessive calluses, hallux abducto valgus, painful bunions, and toe deformities.[81,82] With advancing age the plantar fat pads atrophy,[83] resulting in increased stress on and microtrauma to the underlying soft tissue and osseous structures. Degenerative joint diseases compromise the articular surfaces of the joints of the foot, interfering with weight bearing and leading to decreased mobility. Circulatory changes further compromise the integrity of the tissues of the foot. Elders may not even be aware of losses in sensation to pain, pressure, and temperature. The loss of "protective sensation" to shoe pressures, wrinkles in the socks, or foreign objects in the shoe may be the beginning of a pressure point that may quickly become a callus or an open sore, which, if let untreated, may develop ulceration, infection, or gangrene, and lead to eventual amputation.[82–85] Routine foot screenings can help eliminate small problems and keep them from becoming larger.

Foot problems are the fourth leading cause of complaint in institutionalized elderly individuals.[80] Lack of ambulation and the ability to independently get to the bathroom are often reasons for admission to nursing homes. Individuals who are mobile and ambulatory in their own homes and community retain their dignity and generally live longer than those who are immobilized or institutionalized.[79,84]

Low-income elders are particularly at risk for poor foot care, because podiatric services are not covered by insurance companies. Elders who are on a fixed pension or receive a small social security check cannot afford out-of-pocket visits to have toenails cut. Medicare will not cover the cost of protective shoe gear for the diabetic person at risk for amputation, but it will cover the cost of shoes following an amputation (as part of the prosthetic costs). Complications from foot problems are the cause of 20% of all diabetic admissions to hospitals, and 50% of all nontraumatic amputations is enormous. Inpatient hospitalization, surgical procedures, and rehabilitation programs including prostheses, result in costs of $10,000 to $30,000.[86] Both the personal and financial impacts of foot problems in diabetic patients are of serious magnitude. Findings from the Medicare Shoe Demonstration Project strongly supports the cost benefits of providing protective foot gear to diabetic patients.[85,87]

Low-income elders often wear shoes that are inadequate, ill-fitting, and therefore dangerous. Ill-fitting shoes may create excessive pressure to the foot or repetitive pressures leading to foot lesions that are difficult to heal in the diabetic. Ill-fitting shoes increase the likelihood of falling and hip fractures are a major factor in the morbidity of elders.[88]

Medicare's lack of reimbursement for routine foot care forces elders to attempt self-care of the feet. Limited limb mobility, decreased eyesight, diminished sensation, and unsteady hands may lead to wounds that fail to heal and result in eventual amputation.

Foot care is a unique medical specialty that contributes to the physical, psychological, and social health of the elderly individual. Delivery of a comprehensive foot care program reduces the problems associated with foot pain and discomfort, lower extremity fatigue, and the secondary problems associated with lack of ambulation.

The "Community Foot Care Project" servicing low-income elders in fourteen communities in Central Massachusetts was inspired by the nonambulatory status of patients that were being admitted to hospitals and nursing homes. In one nursing home, 72% (based on an unpublished clinical data collection at Cushing Hospital in Framingham, Massachusetts) of the patients returned to an ambulatory status after receiving foot care, shoes, and orthotics. Preventing foot problems was key to keeping the community elders from becoming institutionalized elders. The foot care program was developed to screen low-income elders in the community for foot and medical problems, provide education on foot care, and dispense orthotics and free shoes.

The Foot Care Project uses an interdisciplinary team of a community coordinator, social worker, podiatrist, and physical therapist who work together to provide eighteen community clinics held yearly in fourteen different communities. The community coordinator schedules the clinics at community senior centers, and the social worker takes a detailed medical history on the eighteen to twenty patients seen at each clinic. A podiatrist renders free nail cutting and debridement of excessive calluses, and the physical therapist evaluates the elder person for lower extremity problems and specific foot dysfunction using the screening tool shown in Figure 15.1. After the initial evaluation in the community setting, if the screening reveals

Foot Screening Tool

Date _____

Name _____

Address _____

Phone ( ) _____

Sex _____ DOB _____

Language or Communication problems: ☐ No

☐ Yes (describe) _____

Primary Doctor/Podiatrist _____

Address _____

Phone ( ) _____

SUBJECTIVE DATA

Medical History: _____
_____

1. Do you have:
   - ☐ Arthritis _____
   - ☐ Circulatory Problems_____
   - ☐ Heart Disease _____
   - ☐ Diabetes Mellitus _____
   - ☐ Kidney Problems _____
   - ☐ High Blood Pressure _____
   - ☐ Foot Problems _____
   - ☐ Eye Problems _____
   - ☐ Thyroid Problems _____
   - ☐ Hearing Problems _____
   - ☐ Vertigo _____
   - ☐ Dizziness _____
   - ☐ Fx hip _____

2. Did you have an injury in the:

		Left Leg		Right Leg	
		Sprain	Fx	Sprain	Fx
No					
Yes	hip				
	knee				
	ankle				
	foot				
	back				

3. Are you experiencing any leg pain?

	Left Leg	Right Leg
No		
Yes Hip		
Knee		

If yes, describe:

Night cramps		
Claudications		
Radiating		

Continued

Figure 15.1

Continued from previous page

4. Are you experiencing any foot pain?

	Left Leg	Right Leg
No		
Yes Aching		
Burning		
Stabbing		
Nail pain		
Shoe pain		
Met heads		
Toes		

Pain increased:	Left Leg	Right Leg
When standing		
When walking		
When wearing shoes		
In the morning		
In the afternoon		
At other times (describe)		

OBJECTIVE DATA

1. Ambulates without assistance?   ☐ No   ☐ Yes

2. Ambulates with assistive devices?   ☐ No   ☐ Yes

cane	
walker	
crutches	
other	

3. Falls? ☐ No ☐ Yes   describe _____

4. Distance ambulated?   ☐ Home   ☐ 1 block   ☐ 2 blocks   ☐ 5 blocks
                            ☐ 1 mile   ☐ Unlimited

5. Regular exercise?   ☐ No   ☐ Yes

Continued

— Continued from previous page —

6. Examination of Feet (Removing shoes and stockings)

	Left Foot		Right Foot	
	Unacceptable	Acceptable	Unacceptable	Acceptable
Cleanliness of foot?				
Socks/stockings a good fit?				
Proper fitting shoes?	☐ Short		☐ Short	
	☐ Long		☐ Long	
	☐ Narrow		☐ Narrow	
	☐ Worn down		☐ Worn down	
Shoe Wear: Heel				
Sole				
Lateral Counter				

7. Problems

☐ Bunions

	Left Foot	Right Foot
HAV		
Taylor		

		Left Foot					Right Foot				
		I	II	III	IV	V	I	II	III	IV	V
☐ Calluses	Spin										
	Pinch										
	IPK										
	Sub										
	Shear										
☐ Corns	Met Heads										
	Heloma Molle										
	Heloma Durum										
☐ Involuted Nails											
☐ Ingrown Toenails											
☐ Nail Trophic Changes											

— Continued —

───── *Continued from previous page* ─────

	Left Foot					Right Foot				
	I	II	III	IV	V	I	II	III	IV	V
☐ Circulatory Problems										
	DPP: ☐ 0 PTP: ☐ 0					DPP: ☐ 0 PTP: ☐ 0				
	☐ 1+ ☐ 1+					☐ 1+ ☐ 1+				
	☐ 2+ ☐ 2+					☐ 2+ ☐ 2+				
	☐ 3+ ☐ 3+					☐ 3+ ☐ 3+				
☐ Toe Clubbing										
☐ Toe Deformities Hammer										
Claw										
Mallet										
Crossing										
Hallux										
	I	II	III	IV	V	I	II	III	IV	V

	Left Leg	Right Leg
☐ Foot/Ankle Deformities		
☐ Dermatitis/[PI]Fungus Infection		
☐ Dry, Scaly Skin		
☐ Edema Foot		
Ankle		
Extremity		

☐ Infection (Describe) _____

☐ Other _____

ASSESSMENT

_____
_____
_____
_____
_____
_____
_____
_____

───── *Continued* ─────

—*Continued from previous page*—

Recommend:　☐ None
　　　　　　☐ Refer to orthotics clinic　　　　Date: _____　Time: _____
　　　　　　☐ Refer for shoes _____
　　　　　　☐ Refer to pediatrist
　　　　　　☐ Refer to podiatrist
　　　　　　☐ Educated in _____
　　　　　　☐ Orthotics fabricated　　Date: _____　Time: _____

　　　　　　_____
　　　　　　_____

　　　　　　2-month follow-up:　　　Date: _____　Time: _____
　　　　　　6-month follow-up:　　　Date: _____　Time: _____

Comments:

_____
_____
_____
_____
_____
_____
_____
_____
_____
_____
_____
_____
_____
_____
_____
_____
_____
_____
_____
_____
_____
_____
_____
_____
_____

foot dysfunction or biomechanical problems leading to functional losses, the patient is scheduled for an outpatient clinic visit for orthotic fabrication and shoe distribution by the physical therapist and physical therapy intervention as needed for musculoskeletal/biomechanical problems. Patients return to the outpatient clinic for two- and six-month reassessments. Foot care is taught to family members when patients are unable to care for themselves. Knowledge of foot care (Figure 15.2) is assessed by a questionnaire before and after treatment. Guidelines for foot care by the patient and family are provided and explained at the first visit (Figure 15.3). This project is funded by a Federal III B grant from the Massachusetts Baypath Area Agency on Aging. Over 100 letters were drafted and sent to area stores and manufacturers of shoes asking for donations, which yielded 1500 pairs of shoes. Research projects were also established, with area shoe manufacturers donating 36 to 50 pairs of shoes for each of these projects. Shoe drives among hospital employees also yield numerous pairs of adequate shoes.

Goals for any community foot care program should be to promote pain-free ambulation, restore maximum function, maximize foot care knowledge and safety awareness, and decrease hospitalizations related to foot problems.

To meet these goals the following methods are proposed:

1. Offer foot care at community centers close to home for the greatest possible participation. (Greater participation was seen when the foot care team went to the patients rather than having them attend a hospital or outpatient-based clinic. For many, lack of transportation was a major deterrent to seeking help and needed foot care.)

2. Establish an easy screening tool that is reliable and highly reproducible.

3. Determine whether the foot dysfunctions are complications associated with tissue changes, biomechanical abnormalities, or chronic disease processes.

4. Provide easy-to-read literature and offer corrective treatment so that the elders can participate in community and personal activities.

5. Arrange the details for getting the patient to the outpatient clinic for orthotic fabrication and treatment.

6. Have local radio or newspaper spots explaining the service.

7. Team up with agencies conducting screening clinics (i.e., the American Diabetic Association) so that patients can be identified and treated within the same clinic appointment.

Resources for meeting these objectives are provided in Figure 15.4. It is evident from the remarkable response to the program that a desire for foot care and a willingness to participate in order to remain an active and useful member of the community was enhanced.

SPECIAL CONSIDERATIONS IN SCREENING PROGRAMS

The majority of elderly adults are highly motivated to seek out strategies for improving their health. Annual physical examinations provide screening for problems in the older adult; however, screening procedures are often not paid for by third-party payers, and regular checkups become an out-of-pocket expense for the elderly. In many cases they are abandoned. Older adults seek acute care much more frequently than do younger people.[22] This may be the result of insidious symptoms left unchecked by the lack of annual physical examinations. Additionally, many older adults, especially the groups at highest risk, such as minorities (who make up 10% of the total elderly population) and those living at or below the poverty level (who make up 20% of the elderly population),[89] do not have their own physicians and are treated only on an acute-care basis through clinics and emergency rooms.

These problems need to be addressed through an interdisciplinary approach using a variety of community service settings. Groups, such as public health and social services departments, senior centers, and area agencies of aging (AAAs), need to come together to identify potential barriers to the provision of health promotion, screening, and assessment programs. The collaborated effort will enable health care practitioners to pool information and resources and provide the most successful and well-attended programs for screening in the elderly.

Foot Care Knowledge Questionnaire

Name: _____

Date: _____

1. Do you inspect your feet
   A. Once a month
   B. Once a week
   C. Once a day

2. Do you wash your feet
   A. Daily
   B. Two times a week
   C. Weekly

3. When you wash your feet do you use
   A. Cool water
   B. Lukewarm water
   C. Hot water

4. At night do you walk·around barefoot
   A. Never
   B. Sometimes
   C. Always

5. Daytime, do you walk around barefoot
   A. Never
   B. Sometimes
   C. Always

6. How often do you change your socks
   A. Every day
   B. Twice a day
   C. Less than three times a week

7. Do you buy shoes that
   A. Are tight and need to be broken in
   B. Just fit
   C. Are a little big

8. Do you
   A. Trim your toenails straight across
   B. Trim your toenails in a curve
   C. Never trim your toenails

9. Do you treat your own corns/calluses
   A. With a razor blade
   B. With medicine to dissolve them
   C. Wait for the podiatrist or other doctor

10. If you have a blister, do you
    A. Open it up
    B. Keep it covered so it does not pop open
    C. Ignore it

Figure 15.2

Self-Care Guidelines: Recommended Foot Care

1. Inspect feet daily for swelling, sores, cracks, reddened areas or cuts. Observation of bottom of feet can be done with a mirror.

2. Wash feet daily. Use mild soap and lukewarm water. Rinse thoroughly. Dry carefully and gently with clean, soft towel, especially between the toes.

3. If skin is dry, apply lanolin or other lubricating lotions or creams. Do not put lanoline or other preparations between toes or around the toenails. Avoid excess of lanolin or other preparations. Polysorb Hydrate, Carmol, or Nivea can be used.

4. Powder or cornstarch can be used when feet tend to perspire.

5. Do not go barefoot. Always protect feet, especially when on the beach or in swimming. Sharp stones, glass, cans, ringworm, ticks, chiggers, staples, pins are hazardous for feet.

6. Wear clean stockings or socks at all times. Avoid socks or elastics that constrict legs (i.e., knee socks with tight tops).

7. Break in new shoes gradually (wear for a few hours each day). Recommended heel height: 1/2" for men, 3/4" for women. No tapered or pointed shoes.

8. Check shoes before putting them on. Shake them to make sure nothing is in them.

9. Do not use hot water bottles or heating pads on feet.

10. Do not soak feet.

11. Never perform bathroom surgery. Go to your doctor or podiatrist about corns, calluses, ingrown toenails, bacterial and fungal infections, abscess, and lacerations.

12. Trim your toenails frequently. Cut them straight across and not too short.

13. Care of your feet should include doing exercise several minutes a day to speed up blood flow. Bend feet up and down and side to side, and move feet in circles at the ankle. When sitting, place your feet as high as your chair and NEVER CROSS YOUR LEGS!

14. When buying shoes you should have 1/2" space in front of your longest toe and shoe shape should fit the contour of your foot. The best shoe is a tie shoe with a wide and deep toe box and strong heel counter.

15. Smoking constricts the blood vessels. Smoking is discouraged.

Figure 15.3   (Courtesy of Jennifer M. Bottomley, Ph.D, M.S., P.T. and Holis Herman, M.S., P.T. Department of Physical Therapy, Cushing Hospital.)

Patient Educational Resources

Krames Communications
312 90TH Street
Daly City, CA 94015-1898

Pamphlets:
1. The Foot Book (#1078)
2. Foot Owner's Manual (#1005)
3. Ankle Owner's Manual (#1073)
4. Foot Surgery (#1119)
5. Laser Foot Surgery (#1321)
6. Walking For Fitness (#1263)
7. Running (#1117)
8. Diabetes and Your Feet (#1372)

Thermal-Moldable Shoes, Inc
100 DeVille
Williamsville, NY 14221-4408

Pamphlet:
1. For Diabetics On the Go
2. For Arthritics On the Go
Thermold Shoes

P.W. Minor and Son, Inc
3 Treadeasy Avenue
P.O. Box 678
Batavia, NY 14021-0678

   Extra Depth Shoes

The Langer Foundation
1011 Grand Blvd
Deer Park, NY 11729

Pamphlets:
1. Walking As an Exercise
2. "Facts for Runners and Other
   Athletes"
3. When Your Feet Hurt You Hurt
   All Over

Channing L. Bete Co., Inc
Scriptographic Booklet
South Deerfield, MA 01373

Pamphlet:
1. About Foot Care
2. Fun, Fitness and Your Feet

The Arthritis Foundation
Massachusetts Chapter
Parker Building
124 Watertown, MA 02172

Pamphlet:
1. Arthritis Surgery Information to
   Consider
2. Arthritis Basic Facts
3. Arthritis—Exercise and Your
   Arthritis
4. Arthritis—A Serious Look At the
   facts

Fund for Podiatry Education and Research
9312 Old Georgetown Road
Bethesda, MD 20814

Newsletter
"Foot News"

US Department of Health, Education, and Welfare
US Government Printing Office
Washington, DC 20402

Pamphlet:
Feet First—A Booklet About Foot Care

PAL Health Technologies, Inc
293 Herman Street
Perkin, IL 61554

Pamphlets:
1. Maybe You Need Orthotics
2. What Is Pronation?
3. Oh My Aching Feet!
4. Foot Surgery
5. Walking—Make It Easy On Yourself
6. Running . . . and Jogging
7. Skiing—Your Feet . . .
8. Ice Skating/Roller Skating

Department of Public Health
Center for Health Promotion
150 Tremont Street
Boston, MA 02111

Pamphlet:
Walking—A Lifetime Activity

Figure 15.4

References

1. Dominick AL, Ahern FM, Gold CH, Heller DA. Relationship of health-related quality of life to health care utilization and mortality among older adults. *Aging Clin Exp Res.* 2002; 14(6):499–508.

2. Health, United States. Expenditures for health care and prescribed medicine according to selected population characteristics: United States, selected years 1987–99. Health, United States, 2003.

3. NCHS Health Statistics on Older Persons. United States, 1986: *Analytical and Epidemiological Studies.* Series 3. NCHS: Washington, DC: US Department of Health and Human Services; 1987. Publication No. 25 (PHS):87–1409.

4. Sundwall D. Health promotion and Surgeon General's workshop. *Surgeon General's Workshop on Health Promotion and Aging.* Washington, DC: US Department of Health and Human Services; 1988.

5. Nicastri, C Fields S. Health promotion/disease prevention in older adults—An evidence-based update. Part II: Introduction and screening. *Clin Geriatr.* 2004; 12(11):17–25.

6. Fields S., Nicastri C. Health promotion/disease prevention in older adults—An evidence-based updated. Part II: Counseling, chemoprophylaxis, and immunizations. *Clin Geriatr.* 2004; 12912:18–26.

7. Shore H. Therapeutic strategies and institutional care. In: Lesnoff-Caravaglia G, ed. *Handbook of Applied Gerontology.* New York: Human Sciences Press; 1987: 447–452.

8. US Department of Health and Human Services. *Recent Medicaid Cutbacks: Shocking Impacts on the Elderly.* HHS Pub. 148; 1992.

9. Wallack SS, Tompkins CP, Gruenberg L. A plan for rewarding efficient HMOs. *Health Affairs.* Summer 1988; 80–96.

10. Havas S. Prevention of heart disease, cancer and stoke: The scientific basis. *World Health Forum.* 1987; 8:344–351.

11. Frame PS. Clinical prevention in primary care: The time is now! *J Fam Pract.* 1989; 29:150–156.

12. Liarson EG, Bruce RA. Exercise and aging. *Ann Intern Med.* 1986; 105:783–785.

13. Chernoff R. *Geriatric Nutrition: The Health Professional's Handbook.* Rockville, MD: Aspen Publishers; 1991.

14. Bogardus C, Ravussin E, Robbins DC, et al. Effects of physical training and diet therapy on carbohydrate metabolism in patients with glucose intolerance and non-insulin-dependent diabetes mellitus. *Diabetes.* 1984; 33:311–318.

15. Helmrich SP, Ragland Dr, Leung RW, et al. Physical activity and reduced occurrence of non-insulin-dependent diabetes mellitus. *N Engl J Med.* 1991; 325: 147–152.

16. Astrand, PO. Exercise physiology and its role in disease prevention and in rehabilitation. *Arch Phys Med Rehabil.* 1987: 68:305–311.

17. Paffenbarger RS, Hyde RT, Wing AL, Hsieh CC. Physical activity, all-cause mortality and longevity of college alumni. *N Engl J Med.* 1985; 314:605–613.

18. Rogers R, Meyer J, Judd B, et al. Abstention from cigarette smoking improves cerebral perfusion among elderly chronic smokers. *JAMA.* 1985; 253 (20):2:970–974.

19. McGinnis JM, Nestle N. The Surgeon General's report on nutrition and health: Policy implications and implementation strategies. *Am J Clin Nutr.* 1989; 49(1):23–28.

20. Gladman JRF, Barer D, Venkatesan P, et al. The outcome of pneumonia in the elderly: A hospital survey. *Clin Rehab.* 1991; 5:201–205.

21. Webster JR, Prevention, technology, and aging in the decade ahead. *Top Geriatr Rehab.* 1992; 7(4): 1–8.

22. National Center for Chronic Disease Prevention and Health Promotion. *Healthy Aging: Preventing Disease and Improving Quality of Life Among Older Americans.* www.cdc.gov; 2004.

23. Center for Disease Control. *Web-based Injury Statistics Query and Reporting System* (WISQARS) [Online]. 2001 National Center for Injury Prevention and Control, Center for Disease Control and Prevention (producer). Accessed October 16, 2002, from www.cdc.gov/ncipc/wisgars.

24. Tinetti ME, Speechley M, Ginter SF. Risk factors for falls among elderly persons living in the community. *N Engl J Med.* 1988; 319(26):1701–1707.

25. Celentano D, Klassen A, Weisman C, et al. Cervical cancer screening practices among older women; results from the Maryland Cervical Cancer Case-Control Study. *Clin Epidemiology.* 1988; 41(6):531–541.

26. Garner B. Guide to changing lab values in elders. *Ger Nurs.* 1989; 10(3):144–145.

27. Ory MG. Considerations in the development of age-sensitive indicators for assessing health promotion. *Health Promotion.* 1988; 3(2):139–149.

28. Frame PS. A critical review of adult health maintenance: Part 4. Prevention of metabolic behavioral and miscellaneous conditions. *J Fam Pract.* 1985; 23(1):2939.

29. Koop CE. *Keynote Address, March 2023, 1988: Surgeon General's Workshop on Health Promotion and Aging.* Washington, DC: US Department of Health and Human Services; 1988: 1–4.

30. Pruzansky ME, Turano M, Luckey M, et al. Low body weight as a risk factor for fracture in both black and white women. *J Orthop Res.* 1989; 7(2): 192–197.

31. Fried LP, Bush TL. Morbidity as a focus of preventive health care in the elderly. *Epidemiol Rev.* 1988; 10:4864.

32. Woolf SH, Kamerow DB, Lawrence RS, et al. The periodic health examination of older adults: The recommendations of the US Preventive Services Task Force. *J Am Geriatr Soc.* 1990; 38:871823.

33. Woolf SH, Kamerow DB, Lawrence RS, et al. The periodic health examination of older adults: The recommendations of the US Preventive Services Task Force. *J Am Geriatr Soc.* 1990; 38(part II): 933–942.

34. Linn M, Linn B. Self-Evaluation of Life Function (SELF) scale: A short, comprehensive self-report of health for elderly adults. *J Gerontol.* 1984; 39(5): 603–612.

35. Safer M. An evaluation of the Health Hazard Appraisal based on survey data from a randomly selected population. *Pub Health Rep.* 1982; 97(1):3137.

36. Close J, Ellis M, Hooper R, Glucksman E, Jackson S, Swift C. Prevention of falls in the elderly trial (PROFET): A randomised controlled trial. *Lancet.* 1999; 353:93–97.

37. American Cancer Society. *Summary of Current Guidelines for the Cancer-Related Checkup: Recommendations.* Atlanta, GA: American Cancer Society; 1988. Pamphlet No. 334701PE.

38. Winawer S. Screening for colorectal cancer: an overview. *Cancer.* 1980; 45(5 suppl):1093–1098.

39. Allison J, Feldman R. Cost benefits of hemocult screening for colorectal carcinoma. *Dig Dis Sci.* 1985; 30(9):860–865.

40. Verbrugge LM. Long life but worsening health? Trends in health and morbidity of middle-aged and older persons. *Milbank Memorial Fund Quarterly/Health and Society.* 1989; 82:475–519.

41. Hayward R, Shapiro M, Freemen A, et al. Who gets screened for cervical and breast cancer? Results from a new national survey. *Arch Intern Med.* 1988; 148(5):1,177–181.

42. American Cancer Society. *Cancer Facts and Figures.* New York: American Cancer Society; 1985.

43. American Diabetes Association. www.diabetes.org; 2004.

44. Reed A, Birge S. Screening for osteoporosis. *J Gerontol.* 1988; 14(7):18–20.

45. National Osteoporosis Foundation. www.nof.org; 2004.

46. Walker SN. Health promotion for older adults: Direction for research. *Am J Health Promotion.* Spring 1989; 3(4):47–52.

47. National Institutes of Health. Nutrition Coordination Committee, Program in Biomedical and Behavioral Research and Training, 11th Annual Report of the National Institutes of Health. Washington, DC: US Department of Health and Human Services; 1987: 111.

48. Surgeon General's Report on Nutrition and Health. *Dietary Fads and Frauds.* US Public Health Service. Washington DC: US Government Printing Office; 1988. US Department of Health and Human Services Publication No. 88-50210; Stock No. 017-001-00465-1.

49. Commission on Life Sciences, National Research Council. *Report on Diet and Health.* Washington, DC: National Academy Press; 1989.

50. McGinnis JM. *Promoting Health-Preventing Disease: Year 2000 Objectives for the Nation.* Office of the Assistant Secretary for Health, Office of Disease Prevention and Health Promotion. Washington DC: US Government Printing Office; 1989.

51. Drinkwater BL. *The Role of Nutrition and Exercise in Health. Continuing Dental Education.* Seattle, WA: University of Washington; 1985.

52. Nieman DC. *The Sports Medicine Fitness Course.* Palo Alto, CA: Bull Publishing; 1986.

53. Peck WA, Avioli LV. Physical exercise and bone health. In: *Osteoporosis the Silent Thief.* Washington, DC: American Association of Retired Persons; 1988.

54. Suominen H, Heikkinen E, Liesen H. Effect of 8 weeks endurance training on skeletal muscle metabolism in 56–70 year old men. *Eur J Appl Physiol.* 1987; 37:173–180.

55. Shepard RJ. *Physical Activity and Aging.* 2nd ed. Rockville, MD: Aspen Publishers; 1987.

56. Kaplin GA, Seeman TE, Cohen RD, et al. Mortality among the elderly in the Alameda County study: Behavioral and demographic risk factors. *Am J Pub Health.* 1987; 77(3):307–312.

57. Stones MJ, Dornan B, Kozma A. The prediction of mortality in elderly institution residents. *J Geriatr Psychol Sci.* 1989; 44(3):72–79.

58. Evans W. Exercise and muscle metabolism in the elderly. In: Hutchinson ML, Munro HN, eds. *Nutrition and Aging.* Orlando, FL: Academic Press; 1986.

59. Craig BW, Garthwaite SM, Holloszy JO. Adipocyte insulin resistance: Effects of aging, obesity, exercise, and food restriction. *Am Physiol Soc.* 1987; 62(1):95.

60. Wang JT, Ho LT, Tang KT, et al. Effect of habitual physical activity on age-related glucose tolerance. *J Am Geriatr Soc.* 1989; 37(3):203–209.

61. Smith EL, Gilligan C, Smith PE, et al. Calcium supplementation and bone loss in middle-aged women. *Am J Clin Nutr.* 1989; 50:833–842.

62. Tinette ME, Speechley M. Prevention of falls among the elderly. *N Engl J Med.* 1989; 320(16): 1055–1059.

63. Blake AJ, Morgan K, Bendall MJ, et al. Falls by elderly people at home: Prevalence and associated factors. *Age Ageing.* 1988; 17(6):365–372.

64. Hemenway D, Coldtz GA, Willet WC, et al. Fractures and lifestyle: Effects of cigarette smoking, alcohol intake and weight on risk of hip fracture in middle-aged women. *Am J Pub Health.* 1988; 78: 1554–1558.

65. Wolf S, Fugate L, Halstrand E, et al. *Worst Pills, Best Pills.* Washington, DC: Public Citizen Health Research Group; 1988.

66. Gibson R, Waldo D. National health expenditures. *1980 Health Care Financing Rev.* 1981; 3:1–54.

67. Maddox G. Aging, drinking, and alcohol abuse. *Generations.* 1988; 12(4):14–16.

68. Willenbrig M, Spring W. Evaluating alcohol use in elders. *Generations.* 1988; 12(4):27–31.

69. Kart C, Metress E, Metress S. *Aging, Health and Society.* Boston: Jones & Bartlett; 1988.

70. Alpert M. Health screening to promote health for the elderly. *Nurse Pract.* 1987; 12(5):42–44, 48–51, 54–58.

71. Magaziner J, Bassett S, Hebel J. Predicting performance on the Mini-Mental Status Exam: Use of age and education specific equations. *J Am Geriatr Soc.* 1987; 35(11):996–1000.

72. Baker S, Harvey A. Fall injuries in the elderly. *Clin Ger Med.* 1985;1(3):501–512.

73. Clark F, Azen SP, Zemke R, Jackson J, Carlson M, et al. Occupational therapy for independent-living older adults. *JAMA.* 1997; 278(16):1321–1326.

74. Clark F, Azen SP, Carlson M, Mandel D, LaBree L, Hay J, Zemke R, et al. Embedding health-promoting changes into the daily lives of independent-living older adults: Long-term follow-up of occupational therapy intervention. *J Gerontol.* 2001; 56B(1):60–63.

75. Landi F, Zuccala G, Bernabei R, Cocchi A, Manigrasso L, Tafani A, de Angelis G, Carbonin P. A geriatric experience in the acute care hospital. *Am J Phys Med Rehab.* 1997; 76(1).

76. Sorenson AW, Seltser R, Sundwall D. Primary cancer prevention as an attainable objective for the elderly. In: Yancik R, ed. *Perspectives on Prevention and Treatment of Cancer in the Elderly.* New York: Raven Press; Raven Press Aging Series: 1983: 24.

77. Maloney S. Healthy older people. In: *Surgeon General's Workshop on Health Promotion and Aging.* Washington, DC: US Department of Health and Human Services; March 1988.

78. Munro HN. Aging and nutrition: A multifaceted problem. In: Hutchinson ML, Munro HN, eds. *Nutrition and Aging.* Orlando, FL: Academic Press; 1986.

79. Collet BS. Podiatry and public health: A systematic approach. *Cur Podiatry.* 1979; 28:32–37.

80. Collet BS, Katzew AB, Helfand AE. Podiatry for the geriatric patient. *Ann Rev Gerontology/Geriatrics.* 1984; 4:221–234.

81. Evanski PM. The geriatric foot. In: Jahss M, ed. *Disorders of the Foot.* Philadelphia: WB Saunders; 1982: 964–978.

82. Gould N, Schneider W, Ashikaga T. Epidemiological survey of foot problems in the continental United States: 1978–1979. *Foot Ankle.* 1980; 1:8–10.

83. Helfand AE. *Clinical Podogeriatrics.* Baltimore: Williams and Wilkins; 1981.

84. Helfand AE. Common foot problems in the aged and rehabilitative management. In: Williams TF, ed. *Rehabilitation in the Aging.* New York: Raven Press; 1984: 291–303.

85. Soulier SM. The use of running shoes in the prevention of plantar diabetic ulcers. *J Am Podiatric Med Assoc.* 1986; 76(7):395–400.

86. Bessman AN. Foot problems in the diabetic. *Comprehensive Ther.* 1991; 8(1):32–38.

87. Mathmatica. *The Medicare Shoe Demonstration Project: Preliminary Findings.* Summary for HCFA, unpublished document; October 1990.

88. Jette AM, Harris BA, Cleary PD. Functional recovery after hip fracture. *Arch Phys Med Rehabil.* 1987; 68:735–740.

89. American Association of Retired Persons (AARP). *A Profile of Older Americans.* Washington, DC; 1988. AARP pamphlet No. PF3049 (1228)-D996.

16

Communication

Pearls

- Changes in the major structures of the ear establish three main types of hearing loss: conductive (which can be reversed), sensorineural (which cannot be reversed), and mixed (which can be partially reversed).
- Detecting hearing loss in a physical therapy setting can range from the use of cues to screenings to more formal tests, such as the Hearing Handicap Inventory.
- Simple interventions, such as changes in the mode of communication and environment (i.e., speaking slowly in a noncompeting environment), will enhance communication.
- All five major senses tend to decline with old age, and yet they are needed to enhance communication; therefore, physical therapists should bring in the other senses as much as possible.
- The voice of an older person changes with age because of reduced respiratory efficiency and changes in the oral and laryngeal cavities. Nevertheless, these changes have little impact on the older person's ability to communicate.
- Accuracy, completeness, timeliness, and honesty are the keys to effective note writing.
- To motivate older persons, the therapist must first assess the person's internal motivation (i.e., values and experience) and then assess and appropriately modify the external factors of motivation (i.e., the physical and social environment).

Introduction

A patient gets better, a child graduates from college, a pain is felt, a new idea comes to mind, and yet this information is unable to be communicated. Why? Is it old age? Is it because the recipients of the information do not understand? Is there some pathological process that is going on that is impairing the communication process?

This chapter will discuss ways that communication may be different with age. The first section will explore the older individual in terms of normal and pathological changes with age that impact communication. A special section discusses the ethnic influences on aging and communication. Impediments and enhancements to communication with the health professional will also be examined. The final sections of this chapter will explore writing skills and the important topic of compliance and motivation.

Normal Changes with Age Affecting Communication

Hearing

Normal Changes with Age Affecting Hearing. Hearing loss is third only to arthritis and hypertension as the most common physical complaint of the aged.[1] Statistics show that between 25% and 40% of persons over the age of 65 suffer from hearing loss.[1] In addition, with each consecutive decade after 70, the prevalence of those affected increases dramatically.[1]

Changes in the major structures of the ear establish the three main types of hearing loss: conductive, sensorineural, and mixed. Conductive hearing loss is a result of changes in the outer or middle ear that blocks the acoustic energy. The changes in the external and middle ear follow.

Changes in the external ear

1. Decreased sensation that causes the patient to be unaware of a buildup of wax.
2. Excess hair growth in the outer ear, especially in men, that can aid in the accumulation of wax.
3. A decrease in the wax-producing glands and a subsequent tendency for the wax to become drier.

Changes in the middle ear

1. The tympanic membrane becomes more rigid and translucent with age.
2. Negative pressure in the middle ear as a result of a decrease in the elasticity and displacement of tissue in the nasopharynx causes the eustachian tube to resist opening.[2]

Sensorineural hearing loss occurs because of changes in the inner ear. These changes follow.

Changes in the inner ear

1. Death of hair cells in the cochlea.
2. Damage to the basilar membrane within the cochlea.[2]

Mixed disorders are a combination of sensorineural and conductive. In general, conductive hearing disorders may be reversed, sensorineural disorders cannot, and mixed disorders can be partially reversed.

A common term used to describe the hearing loss of old age is presbycusis. This general type of hearing loss is sensorineural and, therefore, not reversible. The characteristics of presbycusis are

1. A reduced sensitivity to high-pitched sounds, such as sh, s, t, z, v, f, ch, and g.
2. Bilaterally the hearing loss is equal.
3. Men are more affected than women.
4. A decreased hearing of pure tones.[3]

The hearing loss often associated with old age is usually insidious. It gradually appears, and often patients do not realize that they are misinterpreting communications. For example, when an older person with presbycusis is asked, "How old are you?" The answer may be "fine." This inappropriate response may lead to frustration on the part of the patient, family, and health professional. In addition, the older person with hearing loss may feel depressed, isolated, and angry.[4]

Pathological Changes with Age Affecting Hearing. The classification, manifestation, and approach to the pathological changes with age affecting hearing are similar to the normal changes already listed. In conductive hearing loss, some of the common causes might be infection and osteosclerosis.[2] In the area of sensorineural changes, some causes may be drug toxicity, brain tumor, or Meniere's disease.[2] Finally, in mixed disorders, a foreign body or an infection can cause the problem.

Evaluation. For both normal and pathological changes in hearing with aging, thorough screening is imperative to delineate the cause and type of hearing loss. Table 16.1 lists several signs of hearing impairment.

In addition, once a person is suspected of having a hearing loss, the "Hearing Handicap Inventory" can be administered. This test evaluates the person's response to the hearing loss emotionally and socially. Figure 16.1 is a sample hearing handicap test.

TABLE 16.1   Clues to Detecting Hearing Impairment

The person states that words are difficult to understand.
The person is unable to hear high-pitched sounds (a faucet dripping, high notes of a violin).
The person may complain of a continuous hissing or ringing background noise.
The person ceases to enjoy concerts, TV programs, and social get-togethers because he or she is unable to understand much of what is being said.
The person understands a conversation that takes place in a quiet room, but misunderstands most of the conversation when the room is noisy.
The person can participate in a conversation with one other person but has difficulty if two or more conversations are going on.
You may need to get the person's attention before speaking to him or her.
The person understands you when you are speaking face to face but is confused when your back is turned or your mouth isn't clearly visible. This person may be "speech-reading" (watching lips, facial expressions, and gestures) to understand the message.
The person becomes angry and frustrated when he or she misunderstands something.
The person may attempt to blame hearing loss on outside factors. He or she may accuse you of talking too fast or of mumbling, or may say, "It's too noisy in here."
The person becomes irritable and tires easily during conversation, because listening is hard work.
The person may become annoyed when spoken to loudly (recruitment). This occurs commonly with presbycusis.

Reprinted with permission from Dwyer, B. Detecting hearing loss and improving communication in elderly persons. In: Focus on Geriatric Care & Rehabilitation. Rockville, MD: Aspen Publishers; 1987: 1(16)3–4.

The Hearing Handicap Inventory for the Elderly

The purpose of this scale is to identify the problems your hearing loss may be causing you. Answer YES, SOMETIMES, or NO for each question. *Do not skip a question if you avoid a situation because of your hearing problem.* If you use a hearing aid, please answer the way you hear *without* the aid.

		YES (4)	SOME-TIMES (2)	NO (0)			YES (4)	SOME-TIMES (2)	NO (0)
S-1.	Does a hearing problem cause you to use the phone less often than you would like?	☐	☐	☐	E-14.	Does a hearing problem cause you to have arguments with family members?	☐	☐	☐
E-2.	Does a hearing problem cause you to feel embarrassed when meeting new people?	☐	☐	☐	S-15.	Does a hearing problem cause you difficulty when listening to TV or radio?	☐	☐	☐
S-3.	Does a hearing problem cause you to avoid groups of people?	☐	☐	☐	S-16.	Does a hearing problem cause you to go shopping less often than you would like?	☐	☐	☐
E-4.	Does a hearing problem make you irritable?	☐	☐	☐	E-17.	Does any problem or difficulty with your hearing upset you at all?	☐	☐	☐
E-5.	Does a hearing problem cause you to feel frustrated when talking to members of your family?	☐	☐	☐	E-18.	Does a hearing problem cause you to want to be by yourself?	☐	☐	☐
S-6.	Does a hearing problem cause you difficulty when attending a party?	☐	☐	☐	S-19.	Does a hearing problem cause you to talk to family members less often than you would like?	☐	☐	☐
E-7.	Does a hearing problem cause you to feel "stupid" or "dumb"?	☐	☐	☐	E-20.	Do you feel that any difficulty with your hearing limits or hampers your personal or social life?	☐	☐	☐
S-8.	Do you have difficulty hearing when someone speaks in a whisper?	☐	☐	☐	S-21.	Does a hearing problem cause you difficulty when in a restaurant with relatives of friends?	☐	☐	☐
E-9.	Do you feel handicapped by a hearing problem?	☐	☐	☐	E-22.	Does a hearing problem cause you to feel depressed?	☐	☐	☐
S-10.	Does a hearing problem cause you difficulty when visiting friends, relatives, or neighbors?	☐	☐	☐	S-23.	Does a hearing problem cause you to listen to TV or radio less often than you would like?	☐	☐	☐
S-11.	Does a hearing problem cause you to attend religious services less often than you would like?	☐	☐	☐	E-24.	Does a hearing problem cause you to feel uncomfortable when talking to friends?	☐	☐	☐
E-12.	Does a hearing problem cause you to be nervous?	☐	☐	☐	E-25.	Does a hearing problem cause you to feel left out when you are with a group of people?	☐	☐	☐
S-13.	Does a hearing problem cause you to visit friends, relatives, or neighbors less often than you would like?	☐	☐	☐					

FOR CLINICIAN'S USE ONLY: Total Score: _____

Subtotal E: _____

Subtotal S: _____

Figure 16.1   (Reprinted with permission from Ventry, I., Weinstein, B. The hearing handicap inventory for the elderly: A new tool. In: *Ear Hear.* Baltimore: Williams & Wilkins; 1982: 128–134.)

After the hearing-impaired person completes this test, the caregiver totals the numerical value of the responses for a total score and two subscores delineating values for the emotional and social/situational areas. Patients who avoid social encounters and are becoming emotionally isolated are identified by a high "S" score value. Persons whose emotional supports are weak would score high points in the "E" category.

A rough estimate of total scores is as follows:[2]

- 0–16 The individual does not have a perceived handicap due to hearing loss. This person either has little objective hearing loss or enjoys adequate coping skills.
- 17–42 The person has a mild-to-moderate self-perceived handicap. This person requires evaluation for other stressors and may need help with realistic goal setting, defining needs, and following through with care.
- 43+ The person's coping skills are extremely limited. This person requires concrete direction in terms of self-care and seeking proper assistance for the hearing loss.

Interventions. Interventions for hearing loss range from specific rehabilitation programs to appropriate assistive devices (i.e., hearing aids). In addition, the health team can keep in mind measures and aids to communication (Tables 16.2 and 16.3).

Vision and the Other Senses

Hearing obviously impacts communication. Nevertheless, changes in the other senses also impact communication. The major, but normal, change with age in vision, called presbyopia, begins as early as the fourth decade. (For specific information on presbyopia and vision changes, see Chapter 3.) Most vision deficits normally caused by aging can be managed by changes in lenses.[5] In addition, environmental modifications can enhance communication as well as ensure safety.[6]

The literature also notes a decline in the senses of touch, taste, and smell.[7] Lack of information in these areas can alter normal communication. Suggestions for health professionals in this area are:

1. Try to use touch as much as possible to enhance communications.
2. Bring in the other senses as much as possible. For example, describe the smell of the bread the patient is making or the roses he or she just received.
3. Instruct the family or staff in methods of seasoning food to enhance the sense of taste (i.e., different healthy seasonings).
4. Make a mental checklist to include the other senses in a treatment session (for example, show the patient the menu for the day, and discuss the taste and smell of the food).

TABLE 16.2   Communicating with the Hearing Impaired

Keep the following measures in mind.

Get the person's attention by calling his or her name but do not shout or touch the person first, since this may startle him or her.

Keep your conversation focused and introduce the topic (for example, "Mr A, I'd like to talk with you about your family"). The person then can focus on ideas and key words. Let the person know when you are going to change topics.

If the person does not understand you, phrase your thought differently rather than repeating the same statement over and over. Repetition only leads to frustration.

Face the person directly during conversations. A distance of 3 to 6 feet is ideal. In group situations, no speaker and listener should be more than 6 feet apart.

Your face should be visible to the listener. Do not eat, chew gum, or smoke while talking to hearing-impaired persons.

Do not speak to hearing-impaired persons from another room or while they are concentrating on an activity, such as reading or watching television.

Speak at a slightly greater than normal loudness and at a normal rate.

Do not overarticulate. This distorts the sounds of speech and the speaker's face, thus limiting the use of cues from facial expression.

Reduce the amount of background noise when carrying on conversations. Turn off the radio or TV. If there are other conversation nearby, move to a quieter area.

Be certain that hearing-impaired persons wear their eyeglasses and hearing aids, if they have these devices.

Use body language, facial expressions, and gestures to help convey what you have to say.

Never speak directly into the person's ear. Although this amplifies the sound of your voice, it decreases clarity, and the listener is unable to make use of visual cues.

Provide a public address system for group situations or meetings. Many elderly persons complain that they enjoy meetings, but for various reasons the speaker avoids using a microphone.

Reprinted with permission from Dwyer, B. Detecting hearing loss and improving communication in elderly persons. In: Focus on Geriatric Care & Rehabilitation. *Rockville, MD: Aspen Publishers; 1987: 1(6):6.*

Voice Changes with Age

A person's ability to vocalize is another important variable in communication. Studies on voice cues alone have shown that older speakers tend to be negatively rated as compared to younger speakers.[8,9] There are normal changes that occur with age in the voices of men and women; however, they do not cause significant problems with communication. Men, according to Honjo and Isshiki,[10] experience a higher fundamental frequency due to "vocal fold atrophy." Women, on the other hand, experience a lower frequency due to a slight hoarseness and vocal fold edema.[10]

Normal aging changes can affect voice production. A list of the changes with age in the human body that can affect speech follows.

1. Reduced respiratory efficiency caused by
   a. Degeneration of vertebral discs (senile kyphosis).[11]
   b. Decreased elasticity of the rib cartilages, as well as ossification, and calcification of these cartilages.[12]
   c. Reduced recoil and elasticity of the lungs[13] resulting in lower frequencies, decreased loudness, and shortening of the length of utterances per breath.[14]

2. Changes in the oral cavity caused by
   a. Changes in the structure of the lower jaw.
   b. Loss of dentition.
   c. Weakening and loss of sensitivity of the pharyngeal muscles.
   d. Reduced activity of the salivary glands.[15]
   e. Atrophy of the lips and tongue[16] resulting in an alteration in resonance, increased nasality, and reduced articulatory accuracy.

3. Changes in the laryngeal cavity caused by
   a. The laryngeal cartilages undergoing ossification and calcification.
   b. Drying out of the laryngeal mucosa.
   c. Reduced vascular supply to the mucosa.
   d. Progressive thinning and shortening of the vocal folds resulting in vocal tremors, roughness, breathiness, and hoarseness.[17]

As mentioned earlier, the changes listed essentially have minimal effect on communication, however, pathological causes, such as dysarthria, apraxia, aphasia, dementia, laryngectomy, and chronic obstructive pulmonary disease (COPD), can cause significant impairment in communication (Table 16.4).

Evaluation of pathologies of the voice should be done by a trained speech and language professional. The treatment, however, cannot be done solely by these professionals. To maximize the benefits of treatment, the family, staff, and rehabilitation team must become involved. Table 16.5

TABLE 16.3 Aids to Communication

The following tips are for hearing-impaired individuals, who by definition experience difficulty communicating.

Do not strain to hear or to read lips. A combination of hearing and seeing enables you to understand most speakers better.

Watch the speaker carefully so that you can observe the lips, as well as other body language.

Look for ideas rather than isolated words. As you become familiar with the rhythm of a person's speech, you will pick up key words that will help you put together what the speaker is trying to communicate.

Position yourself directly across from the speaker. Avoid facing a bright light.

Try to determine the subject under discussion as quickly as possible. Ask your friends to give you a lead, such as "We are talking about the housing situation."

Remember that conversation is a two-way affair. Do not monopolize it in an attempt to control it. Listening takes more energy, but you learn more.

Don't be afraid that people will think you are staring at them while you are trying to understand what they are saying. It is always polite to look at the person who is talking to you.

Tell the speaker what part of what he or she said that you don't understand. Merely saying, "I didn't understand," does not provide the necessary information to correct your problem. Let speakers know that they are talking too softly, that their hand is in front of their mouth, and so on.

If you don't understand something, ask the speaker to rephrase the statement. If you have understood some part of what has been said, use those words in your question, asking the speaker to supply the words you have missed.

Don't get into the habit of allowing anyone else, such as your spouse of friends, to speak or listen for you.

Everyone needs time to relax. At such times, a person simply does not listen. Allow yourself the luxury of withdrawing at times, but do not confuse this with your hearing loss.

Reprinted with permission from Dwyer, B. Detecting hearing loss and improving communication in elderly persons. In: Focus on Geriatric Care & Rehabilitation. *Rockville, MD: Aspen Publishers; 1987: 1(6):6.*

TABLE 16.4 Pathological Causes of Impaired Communication

Name	Characterized By	Disease Associated	Speech Muscles	Communications
Flaccid dysarthria	Damage to the peripheral nervous system Cranial nerve Motor muscle Spinal or cranial nerve axons Myoneural junctions	Bulbar palsy Myasthenia gravis Muscular dystrophy Polymyositis	Weak Hypotonic	Slurred Slow Breathy Weak Hypernasality
Spastic dysarthria	Damage to central nervous system Bilateral upper motor neuron lesions	Multiple cerebrovascular accidents (CVA) Multiple sclerosis (MS) Traumatic brain Injury	Hypertonicity Disintegration of movement	Slow Labored Low pitch Imprecise consonants Monopitch Hypernasality
Ataxic dysarthria	Damage to cerebellum or its tracts	CVAs Tumors MS Toxic or metabolic disorders Encephalitis	Uncoordination of force, speed, timing, range, and direction	Imprecise consonants Inconsistent nasality Scanning speech Vocal tremor Loudness variation
Dyskinetic dysarthria	Damage to extrapyramidal motor system Hypokinetic Hyperkinetic	Parkinson's disease Epilepsy Tics Chorea Ballism Encephalitis	Rigidity Reduced range of force Tremor at rest Abnormal Interrupted	Monopitch loudness Breathy or hoarse Short rushes of speech Difficulty initiating speech Erratic changes in pitch and loudness Intermittent hypernasality Harshness
Mixed dysarthria	Damage to multiple lesions in the central nervous system	Multiple strokes Tumors Head trauma Degenerative disease—ALS or MS	Combination of hypokinetic and hyperkinetic depending on motor system affected	Combination of hypokinetic and hyperkinetic depending on motor system affected
Wernicke's aphasia	Damage to the left cerebral hemisphere (posterior lesion of temporal lobe)	CVA Brain tumor Cerebral trauma Cerebral infection Intracranial surgical procedures		Impaired auditory comprehension Fluent, flowing verbal output, low in information Word substitution

TABLE 16.4 Pathological Causes of Impaired Communication (Continued)

Name	Characterized By	Disease Associated	Speech Muscles	Communications
Broca's aphasia	Damage to the left cerebral hemisphere (anterior lesion of frontal lobe)			Restricted vocabulary and grammar Word retrieval difficulties Slow, labored, halting
Verbal apraxia	Same—coexists with Broca's aphasia			Impairment in motor programming, not muscle function Difficulty initiating speech Inconsistent articulation errors
Right hemisphere	Damage to right hemisphere (non-dominant side of brain)	CVA		Attention and perceptual deficits Unable to comprehend emotional and perceptual tone Flat effect, monotone
Dementia	Progressive degeneration to central nervous system	Hydrocephalus Alzheimer's Vitamin deficiency Multi-infarct dementia Endocrine disorders Pick's disease (See Chapter 4 for further listing.)		**Initial stage** Fluent conversation with elaborate detail Reduced attention and memory Disorientation Repetition and blame **Mid stages** As above plus word-finding deficits Perservative responses Self-correction absent **Advanced** Unable to communicate or understand Echolalia
Laryngectomy	Surgical removal of larynx due to cancer	Cancer	No muscles of speech in larynx	No voice—person communicates with facial expression and writing Uses esophageal muscles to speakRestricted loudness and pitch range Chronic hoarseness
COPD	Chronic airflow obstruction with reversible or irreversible components	Emphysema Bronchitis Asthma		Difficulty with energy expenditure of talking

TABLE 16.5 Strategies for Improving Communication

Aphasia

1. Be familiar with the person's level of comprehension and adjust rate, length, and complexity of language to a level at which the person can respond with success.

2. Use concrete, familiar vocabulary in short, clear sentences.

3. Use gesture and facial expression to augment what is said, or demonstrate the information you are trying to convey.

4. Provide written and visual cues.

5. Phase questions for short responses, multiple choice, or yes/no responses.

6. Rephrase a message if not understood initially.

7. Give the person adequate time to respond.

8. Encourage the aphasic person to use gestures, facial expressions, and writing, if appropriate, to augment what is said.

9. Let the person know that you have understood the message by repeating it back conversationally.

10. Be patient and supportive to reduce any stress associated with communicating.

11. Treat the person as an adult at all times.

Right Hemisphere Dysfunction

1. Minimize external distractions in the environment.

2. Position yourself and any materials within the person's visual field if he or she has a left visual field defect.

3. Establish eye contact to ensure attention to the conversation.

4. Provide orienting materials like clocks and calendars.

5. Provide structured activities.

6. Help the person structure responses by cueing with relevant details; if the person goes off on a tangent, cue him or her back to the topic at hand.

7. Be concrete and direct in language use; avoid figurative language and sarcasm.

8. This person may not understand lengthy, complex directions, so repeat and rephrase to assure understanding of important details.

Dementia

1. Establish eye contact prior to addressing the person to ensure attention.

2. Use short, grammatically simple, and concrete input. Avoid the use of pronouns.

3. Keep to one topic at a time. Be redundant; repeat and rephrase critical information.

4. Provide multisensory input, both visual and tactile, to enhance comprehension. For example, provide illustrations or photographs, write down key words, or use gesture and demonstration.

5. Ask yes/no and either/or questions.

6. Provide external orientation and memory aids, such as name bracelets, reminder signs, and calendars.

7. Share successful communication techniques with the patient's caregivers.

Dysarthria

1. Communicate in a quiet, nondistracting environment.

2. Encourage the person to speak at a slower rate.

3. Have the person exaggerate production of consonants and separate syllables within words.

4. Encourage the use of shorter utterances compatible with breath support and meaning.

5. Provide honest feedback about the intelligibility of the message.

6. Provide appropriate feedback about loudness level.

7. Become familiar with the person's alternate or augmentative communication methods, such as language boards and gestures.

TABLE 16.5   Strategies for Improving Communication (Continued)

Laryngectomy

1. Talk in a quiet environment.

2. Consider facial expressions, gestures, speech-reading cues, and situational and linguistic context, if you have difficulty understanding the person.

4. Provide support and encouragement for the use of the new voice.

Chronic Obstructive Pulmonary Disease

1. Encourage short utterances compatible with breath supply.

2. Encourage a reduced rate of speech.

3. Do not engage in conversation while the person is involved in physical activity.

Reprinted with permission from Cherney, L. Aging and communication. In: Lewis, C., ed. Aging: The Health Care Challenge. Philadelphia: FA Davis; 2002.

provides a list of strategies for improving communication for the various pathologies already noted.[3]

Ethnicity

How can a person's origins, rules, and contrasts affect communication between the person, family, and health professional? Is cultural diversity a major concern when looking at the demographics in the United States? In the year 2000, an estimated 30% of the population was Asian, Hispanic, Native American, and African American.[18] Often, people tend to overgeneralize or overemphasize cultural differences and therefore miscommunicate. Table 16.6 provides a list of possible verbal and nonverbal miscommunication sources between cultural groups.[19]

So how does one work most effectively with cultural differences? Like other areas of human intervention, the therapist must make an appropriate evaluation of the situation. Table 16.7 provides examples of assessment categories for ethnic behavior.[20]

The therapist should consider this checklist when working with older adults; however, prior to implementing any intervention the therapist should rank its importance. In a study done by Chee and Kane,[21] the priority of ethnic factors was addressed. They discovered that Japanese-Americans highly rated ethnic factors in a nursing home, such as similar ethnic background of staff, ethnic foods, programming activities, and community involvement.[21] The blacks in this study placed more emphasis on access to family than on the ethnic considerations.[21]

The key to ethnic considerations in communications with older persons is to evaluate effectively the needs of the patient, become more sensitive to their concerns, and to provide modifications in the environment commensurate with the needs identified.

The Team

Why place the team in the middle of a chapter on communication? There are two reasons: first, to explore the method in which the team interacts with itself and its effectiveness in this effort; and second, to examine the team or the individual on the team's ability to communicate with the older patient.

What is the role of the team in geriatric rehabilitation? There is no definitive answer to this question. In the studies to follow, the team is a constantly changing variable. It can simply be a doctor and a nurse, or it can be expanded to include a social worker, dietitian, occupational therapist, speech-language pathologist, physical therapist, leisure services professional, psychologist, or dentist.[22]

Is the team more effective in delivering care to the older person? The results of several studies on this subject follow.

1. The use of a geriatric consultation team resulted in a comprehensive view of the elderly and reduced early recurrent readmissions.[23]

2. The geriatric consultation service improves awareness of functional problems, and increases use of rehabilitative services, but does not decrease the rate of readmission.[24]

3. The geriatric consultation team was unable to alter the degree of functional decline.[25]

4. The geriatric consultation team in the acute care hospital caused a 21% decline in the census of older patients.[26]

5. The patients who received consultation from the geriatric team fared similarly to the control group.[27]

TABLE 16.6   Some Possible Verbal and Nonverbal Sources of Miscommunication between Cultural Groups

African Americans	Opposing View	Hispanics	Opposing View
• Touching of one's hair by another person is often considered offensive.	• Touching of one's hair by another person is a sign of affection.	• Hissing to gain attention is acceptable.	• Hissing is considered impolite and indicates contempt.
• Preference for indirect eye contact during listening, direct eye contact during speaking as signs of attentiveness and respect.	• Preference for direct eye contact during listening and indirect eye contact during speaking as signs of attentiveness and respect.	• Touching is often observed between two people in conversation.	• Touching is usually unacceptable and usually carries a sexual overtone.
• Public behavior may be emotionally intense, dynamic, and demonstrative.	• Public behavior is expected to be modest and emotionally re strained. Emotional displays are seen as irresponsible or in bad taste.	• Avoidance of direct eye contact is sometimes a sign of attentiveness and respect; sustained direct eye contact may be in terpreted as a challenge to authority.	• Direct eye contact is a sign of attentiveness and respect.
• Clear distinction between "argument" and "fight." Verbal abuse is not necessarily a precursor to violence.	• Heated arguments are viewed as suggesting that violence is imminent.	• Relative distance between two speakers in conver sation is close.	• Relative distance between two speakers in conversation is farther apart.
• Asking "personal questions" of someone one has met for the first time is seen as improper and intrusive.	• Inquiring about jobs, family, and so forth of someone one has met for the first time is seen as friendly.	• Official or business conversations are preceded by lengthy greetings, pleasantries, and other talk unrelated to the point to business.	• Getting to the point quickly is valued.

		Asians	Opposing View
• Use of direct questions is sometimes seen as harassment (e.g., asking when something will be finished is seen as rushing that person to finish).	• Use of direct questions for personal information is permissable.	• Touching or hand-holding between members of the same sex is acceptable.	• Touching or hand-hold ing between members of the same sex is considered as a sign of homosexuality.
• Interruption during conversation is usually tolerated. Access to the floor is granted to the person who is most assertive.	• Rules of turn-taking in conversation dictate that one person has the floor at a time until all points are made.	• Hand-holding/hugging/ kissing between men and women in public looks ridiculous.	• Hand-holding/ hugging/kissing between men and women in public is acceptable.

TABLE 16.6   Some Possible Verbal and Nonverbal Sources of Miscommunication between Cultural Groups (Continued)

		Asians	Opposing View
• Conversations are regarded as private between the recognized participants. "Butting in" is seen as eavesdropping and is not tolerated.	• Adding points of information or insights to a conversation in which one is not engaged is seen as being helpful.	• A slap on the back is insulting. • It is not customary to shake hands with persons of the opposite sex. • Finger beckoning is used only by adults to call little children and not vice versa.	• A slap on the back denotes friendliness. • It is customary to shake hands with persons of the opposite sex. • Finger beckoning is often used to call people.
		Native Americans	**Opposing View**
• Use of expression "you people" is seen as pejorative and racist. • Accusations or allegations are general rather than categorical and are not intended to be all-inclusive. Refutation is the responsibility of the accused.	• Use of expression "you people" tolerated. • Stereotypical accusations or allegations are all-inclusive. Refutation or making exception is the responsibility of the person making the accusation.	• Personal questions may be considered prying • Gushing over babies may endanger the child.	• Personal questions are acceptable particularly when establishing case history information • Gushing over babies shows admiration of the child.
• Silence denotes refutation of accusation. To state that you feel accused is regarded as an admission of guilt.	• Silence denotes acceptance of an accusation. Guilt is verbally denied.	• A bowed head is a sign of respect. • It is acceptable to ask the same question several times, if you doubt the truth of the person.	• Lack of eye contact is a sign of shyness, guilt, or lying. • It is a sign of inattention if the same question is asked several times.

Reprinted with permission from Cole, L. E Pluribus Unum: Multicultural Imperatives for the 1990s and Beyond. *Rockville, MD: American Speech-Language-Hearing Association; September 1989: 69.*

It appears from these results that the efficacy of the geriatric team is not completely proven in controlled studies. Some of the negative outcomes may be a direct result of poor communication among the team. To improve this communication, Lee, Pappius, and Goldman[28] suggest

1. Direct communication (preferably face-to-face or by phone).
2. Frequent follow-up notes.
3. Agreement on the reason and roles of the team's intervention.
4. Limited suggestions to other team members.[28]

Finally, Blumenfield and associates[29] suggest providing a complete educational program prior to implementing the geriatric team in an acute hospital.[29]

The most important member of the team, and one that is classically left out of studies of the type listed, is the patient. Patients desire information. However, they do not engage in information-seeking behavior when communicating with doctors.[30] Beisecker and Beisecker's study[30] in this area provides five important points to consider when working with patients (Table 16.8).

In addition, health professionals tend to spend less time with older patients as is evidenced by the startling results of Radecki and co-authors' study[31] on the amount of time physicians spent with older patients. In this study, the authors found that internists and cardiologists spend more time with patients (approximately 18 minutes), as compared to general practitioners (approximately 12 minutes). All types of physicians studied spent less time with the older patient (2 to 3 minutes less).[31]

TABLE 16.7   Assessment Categories with which to Elicit Rituals, Beliefs, and Symbols of Care Activities

Sleep

Condition of room/environment: Occupancy of rooms and bed/sleeping surface, kind of bed/sleeping surface and other furniture, condition of room (temperature, lights, doors and windows open or closed, other artifact/symbols in room).

Kinds of covering, comforting materials: Pillow/head support (height/number of supports used, type, positioning); covering (blanket type, sheet type, other).

Sleepwear: Covering on head, body, legs, feet (type and variation by season or event).

Care of bed linen: Kind of cleaning, frequency, how, by whom.

Bedtime ritual: Time, tasks, others involved, food or liquid consumed, sensory stimulation, symbols/icons used.

Rules for sleeping: When, with whom, how, in what positions, where, beliefs related to rules.

Rules for awakening: By whom/what, how, mechanisms used.

Awakening rituals: Time, tasks, others involved, food or liquid consumed, sensory stimulation, symbols/icons used.

Personal Hygiene

Tending one's body: Rituals for mouth care (tools and substances used, time, who can assist); rituals for body and hair care (how, when, where, how often, substances used, taboos, gender rules, symbols, beliefs associated with aspects of ritual).

Associations with health/illness: Care associated with body fluids/excretions, symbolism, body temperature, activities of tending one's body, substances used in rituals, seasonal/climate taboos, kinds of activities, time of day/year, gender rules, beliefs.

Eating

Kinds of foods: Preferences, dislikes, specific to an event, ritual, specific to time of day/week/month/year, seasonal, rules or taboos for hot foods, cold foods, rules for amount, type, composition, beliefs, and symbolism associated with specific foods.

Schedule of foods: Rules for when/when not to eat; amount related to time of day; healthy/ill status; associated with certain rituals, beliefs, symbols; before/after meal rituals, symbols/icons used/present.

Environment for eating: Place, people, position, taboos/rules, symbols/icons used/present.

Implements/utensils: Kind, number, rules for use of each, taboos, utensils as symbols.

Reprinted with permission from Rempusheski, V. The role of ethnicity in elder care. Nurs Clinics N Am. *September 1989; 24(3).*

TABLE 16.8   Patient Information-Seeking Behavior when Communicating with Doctors

1. Patients express a uniformly strong desire for medical information.
2. Patients are much less willing to assume responsibility for medical decision making, preferring to delegate that responsibility to doctors.
3. Patients, on the average, exhibit relatively low rates of information-seeking behavior when interacting with doctors.
4. Situational variables explain information-seeking communication behavior for all types of patients better than do patient attitudes and sociodemographic characteristics.
5. Patient attitudes toward medical decision making are related to patient information-seeking communication behaviors only for patients with long interactions with physicians.

Reprinted with permission from Beisecker, A., Beisecker, B. Patient information-seeking behaviors when communicating with doctors. Med Care. *January 1990; 28(1):19–28.*

Finally, in communicating with this valuable member of the team, what is an appropriate label to use? According to Barbato and Feezel,[32] the only terms rated positively by both young and old were "retired person," "mature American," and "senior citizen." All other terms were rated negatively.[32]

The key to communicating effectively with the older patient is best described by Purtillo in *The Allied Health Professional and the Patient: Techniques of Effective Interaction.*[33] Table 16.9 summarizes simple steps to more effective communication.

TABLE 16.9   Simple Steps to more Effective Listening

- Be selective in what you listen to.
- Realize that words are only symbols—we impose our meanings on others' words.
- Concentrate on central themes rather than isolated statements.
- Judge content rather than style or delivery.
- Listen with an open mind—do not focus on emotionally charged words.
- The average person can listen four times faster than he or she can speak—use extra time to summarize.

Reprinted with permission from Walker, R. Effective listening. Am J Med Technol. *1969; 35:8–10.*

The success of verbal communications depends on (1) the way material is presented—the vocabulary used, the clarity of voice, and the organization; (2) the attitude of the speaker; (3) the tone and volume of his or her voice; (4) the degree to which both speaker and receiver are able to listen effectively.[33]

WRITING

The topic of writing is adequately covered in numerous books and articles.[34–41] This section will define the different types of writing and give suggestions for the specialist to improve them.

The first major type of writing for communication is clinical documentation, which is composed of initial, progress, daily, and discharge note writing. For both legal and reimbursement purposes, the keys to effective note writing are:

1. Accuracy: State exactly what you plan to do and did.
2. Completeness: Provide all necessary information and avoid extraneous comments.
3. Timeliness: Chart as close to the time of interaction as possible.
4. Honesty: Tell exactly what happened, do not assume, appear, or seem.

Table 16.10 provides a list of dos and don'ts for charting.[42]

> For sample initial, progress, and discharge notes, see CD.

Another important area of writing is professional writing. Professional writing includes articles for publication and business letters. Even though this area of communication is not formally taught in school, therapists can choose to hone their skills in this area.[34,35]

> For two excellent articles on how to start writing, see CD.

COMPLIANCE AND MOTIVATION

The final areas to be discussed in this chapter are compliance and motivation. Motivation is an inner urge that moves a person to action.[43] Compliance is following orders and doing what is instructed.[44] As important as all the skills used in evaluation and treatment are in the rehabilitation realm, a person's drive and ability to follow through with a program may be just as important as the actual program itself.

Motivation may be broken up into internal and external motivations. Internal motivation is made up of the

TABLE 16.10   The Dos and Don'ts of Charting

Do

Chart concisely, completely, and accurately.

Be objective and avoid tentative or vogue statements.

Chart promptly.

Be neat and legible.

Make entries in sequence, beginning with the most important data.

Use standard abbreviations and those approved by the agency.

Sign all timed entries with written signature and credentials.

On flow sheets, include as much routine data as possible.

Record problem-focused client information.

Make corrections appropriately.

Omit unnecessary words like "client" when the meaning is clear.

Include refusals of or omissions in care with the reason for the refusal or omission.

Don't

"Block" time on the chart.

Skip lines or leave white space.

Use ditto marks to repeat information.

Erase or use correct fluid over a notation.

Chart before the fact.

Use pencil or colored pens other than black or dark blue.

Make personal comments, argue, or complain on the medical record.

Reprinted with permission from Ignatevicius, D. Documentation. Focus on Geriatric Care and Rehabilitation. *Rockville, MD: Aspen Publishers; 1988: 2(4).*

person's past values and experiences (desire, fear, thirst, and hunger).[43] The therapist can gain insight into a person's internal motivation by learning as much as possible about them. Table 16.11 provides a checklist to assist the therapist in gathering this information.

External motivation is characterized by the factors in the person's physical and social environment. Some of these factors are privacy, rewards, expectations from others, lighting, and temperature.[43] It is obvious that the therapist can influence external factors with a well-designed environment and appropriate interaction with the patient.

Additional compliance and motivation factors can be described by various models. One of the most widely accepted models for health behavior is the Health Belief Model by Becker,[45] which is illustrated in Figure 16.2. Its

TABLE 16.11   Hints to Gaining Insight into Patients' Internal Motivating Factors

- Read the case history with care.
- Talk with the client about his or her history.
- Ask the client about his or her current and past expectations about performing activities of daily living.
- Ask family members about their performance expectations for the client.

Stay alert for past experiences and value that could affect motivation. Listen and look for

- Successful past motivators.
- Cultural factors that could influence behaviors.
- Past experiences of pain.
- Need for approval.
- Need for independence.
- Need for control.
- Fear.
- Depression.

Reprinted with permission from Duchene, P. Motivation of older adults. Focus on Geriatric Care and Rehabilitation. *Rockville, MD: Aspen Publishers; 1990: 3(8):2.*

main benefit in understanding patient behavior is isolating factors in individual patient compliance.

Orem's Self-Care Model is a particularly useful model for the rehabilitation of older patients. It differentiates between self-care (a patient's choice to act in a way that promotes health) and compliance (the patient's choice to follow instruction).[46] Figure 16.3 is a visual representation of the Orem model.[47] To use this model, the therapist must assess and contrast the person's assets and liabilities along the following dimensions: cognitive, psychological, and physical; and the therapist must design a strategy based on these findings.[46]

The Pinkston Behavioral Model is another useful model for geriatric rehabilitation, especially for patients with cognitive impairments. It requires mutual participation of caregiver and patient, the use of behavioral reinforcement, and continued caregiver involvement.[46] Table 16.12 lists Pinkston's behavioral interventions for self-care behaviors, and Figure 16.4 provides an example of Pinkston's behavioral record. Besides models, various lists have been generated to help the practitioner in the area of motivation (Tables 16.13 and 16.14).

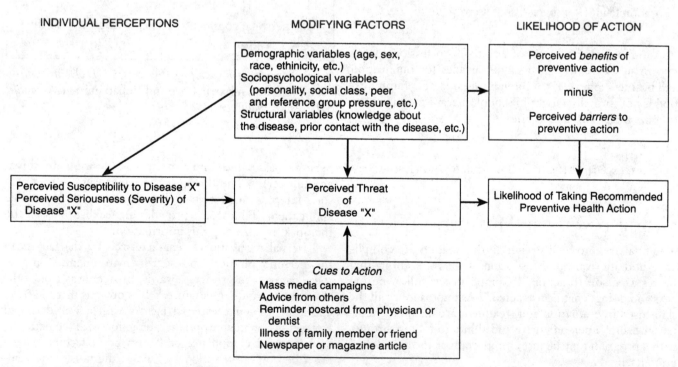

Figure 16.2   Health belief model. (*Reprinted with permission from Becker, M.H., et al. A new approach to explaining sick-role behavior in low-income populations.* AJPH. *March 1974; 64(3):206.*)

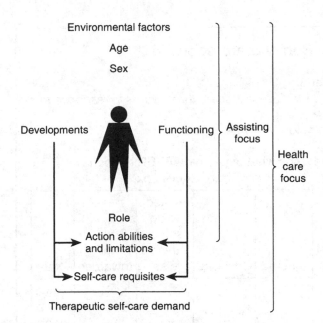

Environmental factors

Age

Sex

Developments — Functioning } Assisting focus

Health care focus

Role

Action abilities and limitations

Self-care requisites

Therapeutic self-care demand

Figure 16.3   Orem's self-care model. (*Reprinted with permission from Orem, DE.* Nursing: Concepts of Practice. *3rd ed. New York: McGraw-Hill; 1985.*)

The final concept in compliance and motivation, and a thoughtful end to this discussion of communication, is an exploration of the Advocacy Model as it relates to compliance and motivation as discussed by Guccione.[48] In this model, the therapist acts on behalf of the patient based on the patient's desires. Getting to this point, however, takes five steps.

1. Provide the patient with all the information, so he or she is able to fully exercise free choice.
2. Assist the patient in determining which information is relevant to the decision.
3. Disclose personal views, so the patient realizes that the clinician may have a personal as well as professional bias.
4. Assist the patient in clarifying his or her own values.
5. Ascertain how patients comprehend their individuality.[48]

TABLE 16.12   Pinkston's Behavioral Interventions into Self-Care Behaviors

Step	Implementation
1. Defining desired behavior	Select specific behavioral outcome (i.e., client will dress in underwear, slacks, shirt, shoes, and socks; client will wash face 3 times a day; client will use washroom 4 times a day).
2. Setting and using a schedule	Designate a time to begin and end each occurrence of self-care.
3. Providing response opportunity	Arrange or ask client to arrange materials (e.g., clothing, soap, and towel) so that they are usable and within easy reach.
4. Prompting correct behavior	Have the support person prompt the client to go through each step of the task in the correct order. If there is no response, the prompt is repeated once or twice, then 2 minutes later if necessary.
5. Allowing time for behavior to occur	If the client is attempting to complete a self-care task, instruct the caregiver to wait until the task is completed. This should occur within 5 minutes.
6. Praise appropriate behavior	If the client is able to complete the task, the caregiver offers praise or touching (food, token, or point on the recording form may also be used) and then prompts the client to go on to the next step.
7. Assistance if the behavior does not occur	If the client does not respond to the prompt within 30 seconds, the caregiver guides the older person through the various steps required. The caregiver provides help with any items the client is unable to complete because of physical impairment or pain.
8. Ignoring inappropriate behavior	If the client engages in inappropriate behavior, such as complaining, arguing, or any behaviors that serve to bring about an unnecessary delay in the process, the caregiver should remove his or her attention from the client until the behavior ceases. Caregiver then returns to step 4.
9. Recording	Behavior is recorded on recording form.

Reprinted with permission from Pinkston, E.M., Linsk, N.L. Behavioral family intervention with the impaired elderly. Gerontologist. *1984; 24:576–583.*

An Example of Pinkston's Behavioral Record

Name: Mr. Green   Date: Wednesday, November 3

Behavior: *Conversation—Communication or talking where Mr. G says at least three words in response to questions or statements by another family member.*

Please note when the behavior occurs and what happens before and after.

TIME		BEFORE	DURING	Describe what others did AFTER the behavior occurred. Check box.					
start	stop	What happened before the behavior occurred?	What happened when the behavior occurred?	Did not notice	Ignored	Criticized	Asked to do something else	Praised or rewarded	Other
9:00	9:03	Sitting at table	Asked for more breakfast	☐	☐	☐	☐	X	Gave more eggs
9:05	9:07	Asked what will do today	Said he would like to go for a walk	☐	☐	☐	☐	X	☐
10:30	10:33	Returned from walk	Complained about cold	☐	☐	☐	X	☐	☐
TOTAL			3				1	2	

Figure 16.4   (*Reprinted with permission from Pinkston, E.M., Linsk, N.L.* Care of the Elderly: A Family Approach. *Elmhurst, NJ: Pergamon Press; 1984: 30.*)

TABLE 16.13   Motivation List

The following is a list suggested by Dr. Raymond Harris to assist a leader (or therapist) to motivate an older individual to participate in the physical exercise program.

1. Recognition that the approach requires mental, emotional, and physical engagement.
2. Individualization of the program to the group or to the person.
3. Satisfaction of some of the participant's basic psychic needs.
4. Provision of choice elements and alternatives.
5. Social support and reinforcement.
6. Continuous productive measurement certifications from the beginning by assessment devices.
7. Incorporation of creative opportunities, such as novelty, change of pace, or improvisations.
8. Engagement of recreational elements, such as play and game qualities.
9. Personal projections of the leader as a concerned, interested, competent, and helpful person.
10. Attention to the aesthetics of the environment and the propitious atmosphere.
11. Counseling to some degree as an adjunct.

Reprinted with permission from Harris, R., Frankel, L. A Guide to Fitness After Fifty. New York: Plenum Press; 1977.

TABLE 16.14   Your Client and Motivation for Self-Care

- Learn what the client believes is important and identify the client's priorities.
- Set mutual goals together.
- Recognize that your client's goals are more important than the staff's or institution's goals.
- Incorporate the individual's past experiences in the goal determination process.
- Help your client to have realistic expectations by discussing program goals.
- Stress that increasing independence in self-care is often a long, slow process.
- Reinforce positive and independent behaviors by giving concrete feedback on goal attainment.
- Use concrete, visible, and personally significant rewards.
- Involve the family in the goal-setting process whenever possible.

Use contracts as motivators

- Establish a contract with the client emphasizing choices based on realistic short-term goals.
- Include a realistic plan and time frame for goal accomplishment.
- Be certain to include reinforcers for goal attainment.
- Encourage the individual to agree verbally or consent to the contract.
- Have the contract signed by the individual and the health care providers.

Reprinted with permission from FOCUS on your client and motivation for self-care. In: Focus on Geriatric Care and Rehabilitation. Rockville, MD: Aspen Publishers; 1990.

References

1. Hills, G. The changing realm of the senses. In: Lewis C, ed. *Aging: The Health Care Challenge.* Philadelphia: FA Davis; 2002.
2. Dwyer B. Detecting hearing loss and improving communication in elderly persons. *Focus Ger Care Rehab.* November–December 1987; 1(6).
3. Cherney L. Aging and communication. In: Lewis C, ed. *Aging: The Health Care Challenge.* Philadelphia: FA Davis; 2002.
4. Heller B, Gaynor E. Hearing loss and aural rehabilitation of the elderly. *Clin Nurs.* 1981; 3:1.
5. Boone D, Bayles K, Koopmann C. Communication aspects of aging. *Otolaryngol Clin N Am.* May 1982; 15(2)
6. Cullinan TR, Silver JH, Gould ES, et al. *Lancet.* 1979; 24:1642–1644.
7. Hills G. The changing realm of the senses. In: Lewis C, ed. *Aging: The Health Care Challenge.* Philadelphia: FA Davis; 2002.
8. Ryan EB, Capadano HL. Age perceptions and evaluative reactions toward adult speakers. *J Gerontol* 1978; 33:98–102.

9. Stewart MA, Ryan EB. Attitudes toward younger and older adult speakers: Effects of varying speech rates. *J Lang Social Psych*. 1982; 1:91–109.

10. Honjo I, Isshiki N. Laryngoscopic and voice characteristics of aged persons. *Arch Otolaryngol*. 1980; 106:149–150.

11. Kahane JC. Anatomic and physiologic changes in the aging peripheral speech mechanism. In: Beasley DS, Davis GA, eds. *Aging: Communication Processes and Disorders*. New York: Grune & Stratton; 1981: 21–46.

12. Noback GJ. Correlation of stages of ossification of the laryngeal cartilages and morphologic age changes in other tissues and organs. *J Gerontol*. 1949; 4(abstract):329.

13. Lynne-Davies P. Influence of age on the respiratory system. *Geriatrics*. August 1977; 57–60.

14. Meto M. Aging and motor speech production. *Top Geriatr Rehabil*. July 1986; 1(4).

15. Massler M. Oral aspects of aging. *Postgrad Med*. 1971; 49:179–183.

16. Cohen T, Gitman L. Oral complaints and taste perception in the aged. *J Gerontol* 1959; 14:294–298.

17. Mysak E, Hanley T. Aging processes in speech: Pitch and duration characteristics. *J Gerontol* 1958; 13:309–313.

18. Meadows J. Cultural diversity. *Community Health Section Newsletter*. 1993.

19. Cole L. *E Pluribus Unum: Multicultural Imperatives for the 1990s and Beyond*. Rockville, MD: American Speech-Language-Hearing Association; September 1989; 69.

20. Rempusheski V. The role of ethnicity in elder care. *Nurs Clin N Am*. September 1989; 24(3).

21. Chee P, Kane R. Cultural factors affecting nursing home care for minorities. *J Am Geriatr Soc*. February 1983; 31(2).

22. Maguire G. *Care of the Elderly: A Health Team Approach*. Boston: Little, Brown; 1985.

23. Berkman B, Campion E, Swagerty E. Geriatric consultation team: Alternate approach to social work discharge planning. *J Geriatr Social Work*. Spring 1983; 5(3):77–87.

24. Campion E, Jette A, Berkman B. An interdisciplinary geriatric consultation service: A controlled trial. *J Am Geriatr Soc*. December 1983; 31(12):792–796.

25. McVey L, Becker P, Saltz C, et al. Effect of a geriatric consultation team on functional status of elderly hospitalized patients. *Ann Intern Med*. January 1989; 110(1):79–84.

26. Barker W, Williams F, Zimmer J, et al. Geriatric consultation teams in acute hospitals: Impact on back-up of elderly patients. *J Am Geriatr Soc*. June 1985; 33(6):422–427.

27. Gayton D, Wood-Dauphinee S, deLorimer M, et al. Trial of a geriatric consultation team in an acute care hospital. *J Am Geriatr Soc*. August 1987; 35(8): 726–736.

28. Lee T, Pappius E, Goldman L. Impact of interphysician communication on the effectiveness of medical consultation. *Am J Med*. January 1983; 74: 106–112.

29. Blumenfield S, Morris J, Sherman F. The geriatric team in the acute care hospital. *J Am Geriatr Soc*. October 1982; 30(10):660–664.

30. Beisecker A, Beisecker B. Patient information-seeking behaviors when communicating with doctors. *Med Care*. January 1990; 28(1):19–28.

31. Radecki S, Kane R, Solomon D. Do physicians spend less time with older patients? *J Am Geriatr Soc*. August 1988; 36(8):713–718.

32. Barbato C, Feezel J. The language of aging in different age groups. *Gerontologist*. 1987; 27(4):527–532.

33. Purtillo R. *The Allied Health Professional and the Patient: Techniques of Effective Interaction*. Philadelphia: WB Saunders; 1973.

34. Lynch B, Chapman C. *Writing for Communication in Science and Medicine*. New York: Van Nostrand Reinhold; 1980.

35. Piotrowski M. *Rewriting Strategies and Suggestions for Improving Your Business Writing*. New York: Harper & Row; 1989.

36. Aslanian M, Manalio G, Taylor C. The joys of paperwork: Care plans really can work. *Caring*. October 1986; 92–94.

37. Lewis C, Jackson S. Medicare documentation: The paperwork challenge. In: Lewis C, ed. *Aging: The Health Care Challenge*. Philadelphia: FA Davis; 2002.

38. Bouchard MM, Shane HC. Use of the problem-oriented medical record in the speech and hearing profession: Special Reports. *ASHA*. March 1977; 157–159.

39. Griffith J, Ignatavicius D. *The Writer's Handbook*. Baltimore: Resources Applications; 1986.

40. Lewis C. *Documentation and Functional Assessment*. Akron, OH: Great Seminars and Books: 2004.

41. Murphy J, Beglinger JE, Johnson B. Charting by exception: Meeting the challenge of cost containment. *Nurs Man*. 1988; 19:2,56–72.

42. Ignatavicius D. Documentation. *Focus Geriatr Care Rehabil*. September 1988; 2(4):1–8.

43. Duchene P. Motivation of older adults. *Focus Geriatr Care Rehabil*. February 1990; 3(8):1–8.

44. Ransdem E. Compliance and motivation. *Top Geriatr Rehabil*. April 1988; 3(3):1–15.

45. Becker MH, McVey LJ, Saltz CC, et al. A new approach to explaining sick-role behavior in low-income populations. *AJPH*. March 1974; 64(3):206.

46. Thibodaux L, Shewchuk R. Strategies for compliance in the elderly. *Top Geriatr Rehabil*. April 1988; 3(3):21–34.

47. Orem D. *Nursing: Concepts of Practice*. 3rd ed. New York: McGraw-Hill; 1985.

48. Guccione A. Compliance and patient autonomy: Ethical and legal limits to professional dominance. *Top Geriatr Rehabil*. April 1988; 3(3):62–74.

PART III

Administration and Management

17

Attitudes and Ethics in Gerontology

Pearls

- The shift in modern medicine from a paternalistic role toward giving the patient more responsibility in decision making may be threatening to the aged who are more comfortable with traditional roles.

- Rehabilitation therapists should practice beneficence in medical decision making and not be a neutral party. They should encourage acceptance of an appropriate treatment, being careful not to coerce or deceive the patient.

- Ombudsmen funded by Medicare are available to provide information regarding patient rights and protection in long-term care facilities.

- In informed consent, therapists are obliged to provide information in language a patient can understand regarding risks, benefits, and alternate treatment options, except when the

- therapist exercises therapeutic privilege (e.g., withdrawing information that the therapist feels will cause the patient direct harm as a result of knowledge).

- The common types of elder maltreatment include caregiver and self-neglect, emotional and psychological abuse, fiduciary exploitation, and physical abuse.

- Advanced directives, such as a living will, are documented desires of medical management used to ward off unwarranted care and promote death with dignity.

- The American Geriatric Society opposes active euthanasia and feels that while lethal injections may be appropriate for a few patients suffering from unrelenting pain, there is too much at risk for abuse for frail, disabled, and economically disadvantaged elderly.

INTRODUCTION

In the past, the medical treatment of a patient was primarily humanistic due to the paucity of scientific knowledge. Patients were treated spiritually rather than the disease being treated. Given the rapid advances in medical science, there is a great concern that spiritual treatment or meeting the patient's emotional needs will take a backseat to more technologically oriented treatments.[1] As this concern grows, the ability to meet the emotional needs of the elderly has also diminished, which has been a natural consequence of the increased specialization in medical technology.[1] An older person with multiple problems may have several different physicians and therapists to care for his or her different needs. With the demise of the general practitioner, the intimate relationship between clinician and patient likewise ceases.

In addition to technological changes, attitudes are changing and a concern for patients' "rights" is growing. The *Miranda* decision,[2] which required that people ac-

cused of a crime be informed of their rights under the law, has dramatically changed the legal institution. Likewise, an analogous development is occurring in the health care system with more of an emphasis placed on informing patients of their rights. Medicine is shifting away from a paternalistic role to giving the patient more responsibility in decision making, and this may be threatening, especially to the elderly who may be more comfortable with traditional roles.[3] This chapter will discuss many controversial issues ranging from allocation of resources to patient rights, death, and abuse.

Ethics and Managed Care and Medicare

Changes in health care in the form of shrinking economic resources, increased patient participation in decision making, and ongoing professional turf battles are dilemmas facing practitioners. Managed competition and care are mechanisms that function to varying degrees to limit access to rehabilitation therapists in choice of treatment and number of visits. Under managed care, there is the potential for therapists to be "double agents" with contractual obligations to the managed care plan and professional fiduciary responsibilities to the patient. These competing needs of differing groups (e.g., consumer, provider, insurer, and purchaser of care) affect therapists' clinical decision making in a managed care environment. Therapists must be able to analyze clinical cases and use moral reasoning and ethical judgment in deciding on resource allocation and distribution of justice. While every professional educational program in rehabilitation must teach some content in ethics, the degree to which ethics is integrated into clinical practice and part of professional development varies. Under the managed care model of care, practicing the ethics of care becomes increasingly difficult, especially in the area of geriatrics.

The United States has focused attention on the rising costs of health care coincident with the increasing age of the population. Arguments have been made to overtly ration care to older persons; however, general acceptance of the need to ration scarce resources, whether or not such a policy is actually formalized, can lead to covert rationing. Overt rationing under managed care has already occurred. Some of the data put forth to justify that rationing must be challenged, and ethical principles should be applied to provide appropriate and perhaps less costly care.[4] Because the concept of managed care is involved with medicine, a moral enterprise, public and private policy enters the ethical arena.[5–7] Health care costs have risen steadily for many years as a result of an inflationary reimbursement system, technological advances, an aging population, and increasing patient expectations. This has accelerated the growth of managed care organizations in an attempt to control costs. Medicare has evolved toward the managed care model of health care delivery through the implementation of prospective payment systems and capitation on many services, inclusive of rehabilitation.

PERSONAL ATTITUDES

How the aged are dealt with depends on how they are viewed. When negative stereotypes exist and therapists have a negative view of the elderly, the health care the individual receives is compromised.

Most studies of attitudes toward the elderly have focused on gender, contact, race, and socioeconomic status. Even though labels are an important descriptive tool, attitudes may develop toward a group as a whole that ignores individual differences.[8,9] Increased contact with the elderly allows people to view them on a more personal level rather than generalizing or stereotyping about the meaning of being old. Harris and Fiedler[10] demonstrated that the more contact preadolescents had with the elderly, the more positive their attitude was to that population. Preadolescent attitudes are important to examine since ac-

cording to Piaget, preadolescence is a transitional stage between concrete and formal operations, as well as the beginning of attitude judgments and stereotyping.[10]

At a very young age, people learn that all old people must be looked after and attribute personality traits to them, such as childishness, irritability, incapability of reasoning or of learning new information, and inability to make important decisions about their lives. If the rehabilitation therapist makes these generalizations regarding the elderly, he or she may fail to notice or investigate personality changes that have recently occurred, such as confusion. It may be assumed that the patient has been confused for a long time because he or she is old, when in reality the onset of confusion was a week prior to contact and due to physiological or pharmaceutical causes.[11]

Society also tends to believe that body image is not important to an older person and does not view the elderly as sexual beings. It is easy, therefore, to overlook the emotional needs of an 85-year-old woman who has just had a mastectomy and fail to explain the prosthetic options that are available.[11]

MEDICAL DECISION MAKING

One of the basic ethical principles that guides health care providers in making decisions is called *beneficence*. This involves providing benefits to the patient, including preserving life. When a clear medical picture is present, the clinician and patient usually agree on the decisions that must be made; however, when it is not present, "defensive medicine," which does not necessarily benefit the patient but instead builds evidence against malpractice, is often practiced.[12]

The paradigm of good decision making is properly informing competent patients of their care options, and the possible outcomes and risks of treatments so they can decide the course of treatment, which should be limited only by the clinician's availability and willingness to provide the treatment.[13] The clinician should not be a neutral party and should take an active role in encouraging acceptance of an appropriate treatment, but the patient must not be coerced or deceived.[14]

An important consideration in medical decision making is the individual's value system. What constitutes quality of life to the patient may be very different from the clinician's philosophical beliefs, and when making decisions, the *self-determination* or *autonomy* of the patient should always prevail.[12] Decisions in rehabilitation therapy treatment, which have usually been based on scientific knowledge and professional experience, can be deficient since the moral aspect of the treatment may have been ignored. The value system of the patient must be considered, especially with regard to goal setting. What may be considered functional by the therapist may not meet the goals the patient has set.[15]

Decisional capacity must be assessed by the health provider before intervention is implemented and should be based on the individual's mental status, judgment, and short-term memory. The greater the risk of the treatment, the more carefully the decisional capacity must be evaluated. Many elderly people who are not capable of making their own decisions are treated as if they are, because they nod their head and agree with everything the clinician says. Elderly patients are denied the right to choose proper medical care if they are not properly evaluated by the health care team.[14]

If it is determined that an elderly patient is no longer able to make his or her own decisions, the first appeal should be to any specific documents of empowerments executed while the patient was capable. These empowerments or advanced directives, which include power of attorney and living wills, make it possible for health care professionals to determine the wishes and values of the patient and will be covered in depth later.

If the patient is unable to make medical decisions and advanced directives are not present, a surrogate decision maker must be chosen. This surrogate is usually a spouse or, as is often the case with the elderly, a son or daughter. For the elderly who have outlived all family and friends, the only alternative may be a court-appointed guardian. In special cases where the court feels the patient is unable to make medical decisions but the clinician and family feel the patient is capable, both the patient and the court-appointed surrogate must agree on a course of treatments.[14]

Conflicts regarding medical decisions may exist within the elderly patient, such as retaining a normal appearance versus attaining the best cure possible, or deciding whether to spend one's life savings on a costly treatment knowing it will be a financial burden to the rest of the family. In these cases, the patient should be the one to resolve the dilemma with the help and support of the clinician. The responsibility of the clinician is to present the facts regarding the treatment choices, but it may be more helpful to supply information about others who have been through similar experiences.[13]

Professional conflicts may be present that affect decision making by placing the patient's needs in competition with the clinician's interests. For example, a therapist may want a patient to reach a normal, functional status but also hopes the patient will need his or her services for a long period of time to financially support the practice. In this case, the clinician must obviously serve the needs of the patient and disregard his or her own incentives.[13]

Other difficult situations arise when a competent patient has poor judgment regarding his or her ability to function at home or in society (such as driving a car), in which case the clinician is responsible for weighing the risks of performing these activities and must act to preserve the safety of the patient and others. In such cases, the therapist must not act in ways that would be only moderately beneficial to the patient but would also be detrimental to society or the patient's overall safety.[13]

Insufficient legal focus has been placed on discharge planning, which has become more of an issue with the formation of diagnostic related groups (DRGs). It has been determined, however, that if a patient is capable of making decisions, it is illegal to place that patient in a residential facility against his or her will. The family would have to petition the court for guardianship in order to override the patient's discharge preference.[14]

ALLOCATION OF RESOURCES

The growth of the elderly population, especially of that over the age of 85, poses economic and ethical dilemmas due to the rapid increase in the demand for health care services at a time when resources are scarce. Some important questions are: (1) how should these resources be rationed; (2) who should be responsible for allocating these resources; and (3) how should the scarcity of these resources affect medical policy decisions.[4]

Allocation of resources is commonly based on need and the belief that society should take care of its members. The disproportionate amount of medical care the elderly needs makes this group particularly vulnerable when it comes to rationing resources. Critics of Medicare view the program as "overgenerous and unwarranted" for people who do not have the need for this special help. Some feel that the dispensing of Medicare funds should be based on financial need rather than on medical need. Public opinion on this topic is indicated in a state poll showing moderate support (36%) for age criteria in health care, and the feeling that resources should be given to people who will receive the most long-term benefit from the treatment, which can exclude the elderly.[2,16]

Clinicians have always felt age is an important consideration when making medical decisions, but they are unclear about the ethical and moral implications of their actions. Sometimes it is felt that it is better to allocate resources to the young, who have their whole lives ahead of them, rather than the elderly, who have already experienced life, since the young are more capable of adjusting to handicaps and will be able to repay the costs with future contributions. Productivity has always been a criteria of need, which is ironic because elderly people are forced out of the workplace due to mandatory retirement and are, therefore, considered less productive. However, one must also consider that the elderly have contributed to society and that society has a responsibility to take care of them.[8,9,16,17]

One difficulty in basing medical decisions on age is the uncertainty of the prognosis in determining how long a person will live, particularly for an older person who is suffering from multiple illnesses. Another important factor that age criteria fail to recognize is that each person's life is important to him or her, and a longer life is not more valuable than a shorter one. Society must be careful not to devalue the life of an older individual, particularly one who is dependent, since this may lead to abusive discrimination of the elderly. Each person has an equal right to life no matter how old the individual is, and the quality of life should be evaluated by the patient only and not the clinician.[14,16]

When limited resources exist obviously not everyone will be entitled to every possible medical benefit, but the question remains of how rationing should be implemented. Should health care be distributed according to ability to pay or is it a social obligation to supply care regardless of financial ability? Ideally, everyone should have the right to proper health care, which should not be considered a luxury but a basic need. Conflicts arise when people use resources without replenishing them by either paying personally or having insurance that will pay. When this occurs, society is harmed because other people, in addition to not receiving the services, will have to replenish the funds.[18,19]

Who should be responsible for distributing these scarce resources? If the therapist is given the chore of making funding decisions the trust between the patient and the practitioner may be jeopardized. Patients trust that the physical therapist will provide the treatment needed regardless of financial concerns. Controlling expenditures are counterbalanced by the ethical obligations of the practitioner and negligence laws that demand that maximum effort should be made to cure the patient.[14]

With the growth of the health maintenance organization (HMO) industry, clinicians are given the new role of "gatekeeper" and, given the limited resources, must face the situation where resources spent on one patient will mean fewer resources for another. When a patient's health provider or insurance policy does not provide payment for health care services, the clinician should respect the right of the patient to limit treatment he or she does not value if it involves using personal funds. Conflicts for the clinician arise when the patient wants the treatment more than the provider and will pay for the care with personal funds. In this scenario, the clinician must consider that even though financial resources will not be compromised, access to resources (space and equipment) may hinder other patients from receiving care who need it more.[3]

In the past, the patient had to be cautious because reimbursement policies encouraged clinicians to provide unnecessary treatment. Today with the change in public policy and the addition of DRGs, the patient's rights are in danger of being violated due to incentives to limit treatment, decreasing the role of the clinician as the patient's advocate. The presence of these DRGs will affect the elderly the most since treatment will be discontinued prematurely for individuals with long-term illnesses. When economic incentives provided to clinicians lead them to deny beneficial care, there is a direct threat to the requirement that clinical decisions be competent and respect the patient's decision-making autonomy. For example, one cost-control method is rewarding an institution for offering a treatment at a lower cost. Hospitals that deliver treatment for less than the DRG rate can keep the difference. As a result, hospital administrators are examining the decisions of the clinicians to use resources and are applying pressure to physicians to deny beneficial treatment and the patient's right to choose that treatment.[9,18]

Another new medical policy that creates a conflict of interest is the addition of case managers to insurance companies because the managers' dominant measure of success is keeping costs low even though they want the patients to be satisfied with their care. If the patient's interests were always served, obviously the cost-saving goal would not be achieved. Therefore, formal ethics do not provide the answer. One suggestion is to give the balancing responsibility to the direct-care provider who is given incentives to conserve costs, but also possesses the moral and professional desire to meet the needs of the patient. This, however, creates a conflict of interest for the clinician, who is left with a situation in which the balance between the benefit for the patient and the cost to the system is unclear: to deny the patient the resource without informing him or her about the denial is ethically wrong. Providers have an obligation to inform patients regarding care options, even though they are denied these options by the system.[13]

Because of all these conflicts regarding allocation of resources, one can see that health care professionals will become frustrated with not being able to supply quality treatment unless they become more directly involved with health care policy formation and evaluation. The true challenge for the medical care system in the future will be learning how to balance the increasing medical needs of the elderly with the financial limitations of the system.[8,13]

CAREGIVER STRESS

Contrary to what many people believe, a majority of elderly people are being cared for at home by family members.[4] Studies show that family members who provide care to disabled relatives experience emotional, physical, and social strain. They also suffer from higher rates of depression, perceived burden, social isolation, family discord, and poor physical health than people who do not have this responsibility. A study done by Rabins and associates[20] of a small sample of elderly chronically ill individuals revealed family caregivers underwent some adaptations over a two-year period. It was found that anger and anxiety toward their situation decreased but guilt and depression persisted.[20]

Two reasons physical or occupational therapists would naturally involve the family of an elderly patient is that they are a valuable source of information and they will provide care for the patient. However, the practitioner should be aware that the plan of care worked out by the patient and the clinician may be a burden on family members, and there are limits to the burdens of care that should be placed on the family. This creates a conflict of interest between the patient and the family.[3]

If the care of the elderly patient places a financial burden on the family, there is an ethical obligation to allow the family to participate in decision making. Conflicts arise when the decisions of the family and the patient differ, putting pressure on the two parties and possibly compromising the autonomy of the patient. Problems also occur when the family underestimates the difficulty or cost to them of the proposed patient care, which may lead to harm to all parties. Caring for an elderly relative at home impairs the freedom, independence, and satisfaction of others in the home, and responsibilities fall more on the functional family members, which causes resentment. In this case, it is the moral obligation of the clinician as well to help the family evaluate the responsibility they are undertaking.[3]

ELDER ABUSE

Identification and the subsequent reporting of elder abuse is an unfortunate circumstance to which many health care providers are exposed to in geriatrics. As the practice of rehabilitation involves the development of an ongoing relationship with patients during the course of treatment, and may also include frequent contact with the patients' families, it is critical that physical and occupational therapists know how to identify and effectively intervene in situations of suspected abuse.

Elder abuse occurs most commonly in residential rather than institutional settings, and the most likely perpetrators are known by the victim.[21,22] Although a defined set of risk factors has not yet been developed, careful questioning and assessment can help determine whether a patient is at increased risk. Some potential risk factors for mistreatment of older people include age, race, low income, functional or cognitive impairment, a history of violence, and recent stressful events.[21,23] Both depression and dementia have been identified as particularly strong risk factors associated with abuse of the elderly.[24,25] There is little information in the literature concerning the clinical profile of mistreated older people.

The common types of elder maltreatment include caregiver and self-neglect, emotional and psychological abuse, fiduciary exploitation, and physical abuse.[23] Assessment consists of comprehensive physical examination, including scrutiny of the musculoskeletal system, neurologic and cognitive testing, and detailed social and sexual histories.[26] Clues that cannot be explained medically may signal elder abuse. To properly intervene, clinicians should be familiar with state laws governing reporting procedures and patient privacy.[27,28]

Though as clinicians we are less likely to explore abuse beyond the physical, psychological, and cognitive realms, there is a dearth of literature on financial exploitation of elderly persons.[29] In fact, financial abuse accounts for up to one-half of all types of elder abuse in the United States, accounting for over 500,000 victims. Psychological abuse, including deception, intimidation, and threats, always accompanies financial exploitation.[29] Despite the devastating emotional and financial losses incurred, rehabilitation professionals are reluctant to recognize, diagnose, and assist impaired elderly victims of financial exploitation. This type of abuse, if suspected, should provoke a referral to a social worker or legal consultant by the rehabilitation professional.

PATIENT DIGNITY

Elderly people should be able to live out their lives with dignity, security, and independence. The tendency in American society is to place the elderly in nursing homes where they lose their identity, self-esteem, and individuality instead of encouraging and helping them to spend their remaining years in the dignity of their own homes. The readiness to place the elderly in these institutions stems from a negative basic attitude toward the elderly in this country. In Scandinavia, there is a system called "open care" where the elderly are not dependent on the charity and patience of relatives: Older people in this system retain their independence through programs that allow them to live in their own homes safely with outside help. The cost of this expensive program is paid for by the Scandinavian people through extremely high taxes. This basic attitude, that it is the responsibility of society to take care of its elderly, differs from the United States, which tends to be motivated by politics and would not consider advocating the costly care the Scandinavians have chosen.[30]

Principle I of the American Physical Therapy Association (APTA) Code of Ethics states that physical therapists must respect the rights and dignity of all individuals.[31] Likewise, Principle 2 of the American Occupational Therapy Association (AOTA) states that occupational therapy personnel shall respect the rights of the recipients of their services (autonomy, privacy, confidentiality).[32] This must be considered when implementing medical intervention because to ignore this principle is to treat the individual as less than human. When the therapist is not able to see the older person as an individual, treating the patient with dignity is compromised.[8]

One way the clinician can maintain the dignity of patients is to respect their autonomy and right to make decisions regarding their care. The health care professional must remember that even though elderly persons may be in a dependent state, the individuals have had a whole lifetime of self-determination that should not cease because they are temporarily or permanently disabled. This includes their right of confidentiality with respect to family members at the onset of treatment. This does not preclude the clinician from exploring the reasons the patient desires this confidentiality, especially when bad feelings are present, but ultimately the desires of the patient should prevail.[3]

There is also a tendency for health care professionals to treat the elderly, given their dependent state, like children, which is an assault on the individual's self-esteem and dignity. Because of this view, the clinician may assume that sons and daughters of the elderly should assume a parenting role, and important decisions will be discussed with the patient's children rather than with the patient. The health care provider may treat the older patient like a child on a smaller scale, such as assume the patient may be addressed by his or her first name, placing bows in an elderly woman's hair, or referring to an elderly man or woman as "cute," all of which compromise a patient's dignity.[11]

The main way to promote self-esteem and dignity in the elderly population is to change the attitude that society has toward growing old. Given the difficulty of changing this global problem, it may be a start to at least change the way rehabilitation therapists feel toward the elderly.[11]

PATIENTS' RIGHTS

The rehabilitation therapist is responsible for the maintenance of the basic rights of human beings during their illnesses, such as independence of expression, decision, and action. The APTA House of Delegates has adopted rights* for the individual referred or admitted to the physical therapy service that include but are not necessarily limited to:

1. The selection of a physical therapist of one's own choosing to the extent that it is reasonable and possible.
2. Access to information regarding practice policies and charges for services.
3. Knowledge of the identity of the physical therapist and other personnel providing or participating in the program of care.
4. Expectation that the referral source has no financial involvement in the service. If this is not the case, knowledge of the extent of any financial involvement in the service by the referring source must be explained.
5. Awareness of the physical therapy goals, desired outcomes, and procedures that are being rendered.

6. Receipt of information necessary to give informed consent prior to the initiation of services.
7. Participation in decisions involving the physical therapy plan of care to the extent reasonable and possible.
8. Access to information concerning his or her condition.
9. Expectation that any discussion or consultation involving the case will be conducted discreetly and that all communications and other records pertaining to the care, including the source of payment for treatment, will be treated as confidential.
10. Expectation of safety in the provision of services and safety in regard to the equipment and the physical environment.
11. Timely information about impending discharge and continuing care requirements.
12. Refusal of physical therapy services.
13. Information regarding the practice's mechanism for the initiation, review, and resolution of patient complaints.[33]

The AOTA[†] has established a similar set of statements regarding the rights of patients when referred for occupational therapy:

1. Occupational therapy personnel shall collaborate with service recipients or their surrogate(s) in determining goals and priorities throughout the intervention process.
2. Occupational therapy personnel shall fully inform the service recipients of the nature, risks, and potential outcomes of any intervention.
3. Occupational therapy personnel shall obtain informed consent for subjects involved in research activities indicating they have been fully advised of the potential risks and outcomes.
4. Occupational therapy personnel shall respect the individual's right to refuse professional services or involvement in practice, research or educational activities.
5. Occupational therapy personnel shall protect the confidential nature or information gained from educational, practice, research, and investigational activities.[34]

There is a particular need to safeguard the rights of elderly individuals in nursing homes. Ombudsmen funded by Medicare are available to provide information regarding patient rights and protection in long-term care facilities.[14] Task forces have also been formed consisting of nursing home staff members and administrators; government officials; and medical, legal, and social service pro-

---

*Patients' Rights reprinted with permission of the American Physical Therapy Association.

†Patients' Rights reprinted with permission of the American Occupational Therapy Association.

fessionals to help protect the rights of elderly people in long-term care facilities. One accomplishment of the task force was to determine when it is appropriate for a patient to receive "supportive care" in a facility by setting up recommendations and guidelines. In the past, nursing homes abused patients by placing them on supportive care orders regardless of their health status.[35] Sometimes supportive care is taken to mean "no care necessary," leading to neglect of the elderly patient's basic needs. The task force defines supportive care as "care that is intended not to prolong life but to promote the dignity of the patient, minimize pain, preserve hygiene, and support the psychological, social, emotional, and spiritual needs of the patient and family."[36,37]

The Right to Refuse

One right that has the interest of lawyers and ethicists but has not been focused on by health professionals is the right to refuse. One may wonder if a refusal is due to the patient's denial of his or her illness or even to suicidal desires, or if it is a result of a well-thought-out balancing of the risks and benefits of a particular treatment. The courts have distinguished between a suicide and refusal of care that may or may not prolong life and protect the rights of the individual to refuse treatment. When dealing with the elderly where chronic irreversible and debilitating conditions are present for which there is often no cure, limited treatment may be desired by the patient. One reason for this is that although the care is meant to prolong life, it is actually prolonging death. The American Medical Association's (AMA) Council on Ethical and Judicial Affairs states that competent patients have the moral and legal right to refuse treatment whether it is life sustaining or not. This may be overridden in the case where the refusal of treatment affects another person, particularly minor children.[14,37]

One important fact the clinician must remember is that a refusal does not mean the patient is incompetent or crazy, and it has been suggested that for some groups of chronically ill patients, refusal should be offered as an option before treatment is initiated.[35] The single greatest reason for refusal of care is misunderstanding or miscommunication of the treatment involved.

A study by Applebaum and Roth[37] concluded that many patients refuse treatment as a way to find out more information regarding their care. When psychological factors were implicated in reasons for refusal, it was usually due to the distinctive way that individual deals with stress; the denial of illness was not commonly a direct cause.[14,37]

Often the clinician did not investigate the reason why the patient was refusing and, therefore, did not respond accordingly. For example, if a patient refused because he or she misunderstood the treatment plan, the response of the clinician would not be to offer clearer information since the reason for the refusal was not sought. Forced treatment by health professionals as a response to refusal was not uncommon but was usually limited to patients who were incompetent and unable to make their own decisions. Substitute consent was not usually obtained in these cases before treatment was started. When dealing with competent patients, there were responses of what was termed "forceful persuasion," where patients were told they had no choice if the treatment was considered essential by the clinician.[37]

In rehabilitation therapy, refusal of care can be as obvious as refusing treatment or as subtle as not performing the prescribed home exercise program. These patients are typically labeled noncompliant, and it is usually assumed that this problem exclusively lies with the patient, and the only solution is the person's compliance. The patient's right to autonomy over his or her body is not recognized, and the right of the patient not to comply with the advice of the physical therapist is not acknowledged. In a long-term care facility, noncompliance is often the only way a patient can exert control over his or her life, particularly in a rehabilitation setting. Reasons for the patient's noncompliance should be sought with the intention of understanding the rationale for nonparticipation. When a clinician places the problem of noncompliance totally on the patient, it is easy for therapists to avoid examining their own behavior or the influence of the health care setting on the patient's nonparticipation. The therapist can enhance compliance by taking the time to explain routine procedures, listening to the patient's concerns and fears, and involving the patient in goal setting. Although persuading the patient with clear and accurate information is encouraged, the autonomy of the patient must always be respected, even when the patient chooses to continue noncompliance.[38]

The rehabilitation therapist must also be wary of patients who unquestioningly follow every directive of the clinician and should not assume these patients understand the treatment being implemented. Often, this behavior is motivated out of fear of the health professional or fear of a bad medical outcome. The need to evaluate the decision-making capacity of a compliant patient is easy to miss because it is patients who refuse care who are usually having their competency challenged. From a moral point of view, therefore, unquestioned compliance may be as much of a problem as noncompliance.[38]

Rights of Patients with Dementia

In order to respect the rights of patients with dementia, their wishes regarding medical intervention must be documented when they are still in a competent state. Often family understanding of the patient's wishes or prior values without specific documentation is not sufficient to make decisions about life-sustaining treatment. Given the difficulty of determining what best serves the interests of a severely demented patient, the court system recommends that the individual state specific preferences before the onset of disability. Discontinuing treatment that would prolong severe pain in the patient is clearly permissible according to the courts, because it is universally accepted that death is preferable to living with unrelenting pain. The clinician must also consider the pain and suffering that is present when treatment is forced on the incompetent patient against his or her wishes. An incompetent patient often can have strong preferences regarding treatment even though these preferences are not based in reality, and forcing unwanted treatment may cause the patient to experience a painful and humiliating violation.[39,40]

As previously mentioned, when it has been determined by careful evaluation that a patient is unable to make his or her own decisions regarding medical care, a surrogate decision maker must be chosen. It is believed that, to the extent possible, the rights of the incompetent patient should be an extension of the rights of the competent; and respect, self-determination, and promotion of well-being should be observed.[17]

For the clinician, it is clear that one must yield to the wishes of a competent patient, but dealing with a surrogate who may be acting in bad faith or have conflicts of interest is more complicated. For example, if the surrogate demands treatment that the clinician deems unnecessary, the clinician must make it clear that treatment is not indicated. If the family member still insists on the treatment, a court order must be obtained. This is an expensive and time-consuming process and tends to discourage a family member acting out of guilt or self-serving motives. Only the court can authorize a plan of care that is opposed by an incompetent patient's next of kin. If the health care professional has concerns regarding the decision made by the surrogate, the surrogate appointment should be reviewed by an ethics committee or consultant but can be legally changed only by the court system. Even though the surrogate should be more limited in his or her decision-making power than a competent patient, the family members should have some range of discretion so that they are not just carrying out the desires of the clinician.[13]

When considering the ability of the mentally impaired to make medical decisions, a precise mental evaluation is critical since the legal system has customarily taken an all-or-nothing approach to this decision. Either an individual is capable of making all decisions or he or she is declared incompetent and denied the right to make any decisions at all.[41–43] Elderly patients with fluctuating mental abilities need to be carefully evaluated before they are judged incapable of making medical decisions. "Windows of lucidity" may exist in patients where, in their more lucid moments, they are able to understand information that is given to them and consequently make clear decisions. An elderly person may experience what is called "sundowning" in which he or she experiences increased confusion at night and may need to be evaluated at different times of day in

order to evaluate his or her ability to understand information.[14,42]

General mental status exams may be a good assessment for impairments when cognition is already severely compromised, but they are not adequate in assessing gradations of decision-making capacity.[44] In assessing competence, the most important part of the formal evaluation should be testing of the patient's ability to understand his or her medical situation. For example, the patient may not know what day it is but appears to understand the benefits of physical therapy and, therefore, is capable of making decisions even though disorientation is present.[12]

It is often assumed that preconceived beliefs about the elderly, as well as the paternalistic patterns of medical practice, may lead clinicians to underestimate the decisive capabilities of the older patient. However, in a study done by Fitten and associates[44] it was found that when clinicians rely on brief medical evaluations, test of recall, and their own judgment, they are most likely to assume incorrectly that the decision-making capacity of the patient is intact. The outcome of this research stresses the importance of a systematic evaluation that directly probes the patient's understanding of the issues involved and the reasoning underlying his or her treatment decisions.[44]

Future scenarios for the prevention and delay of Alzheimer's disease (AD) draw attention to a variety of ethical issues that need to be considered. The determination through genetic susceptibility testing in asymptomatic persons at high risk for AD, may eventually prove accurate enough to be of use in identifying at-risk individuals decades before probable onset (see Chapter 2). The ethical dilemmas created by both genetic testing and the genome projects in altering genetic makeup present a number of value-based issues for many clinicians, public policy makers, and insurers. Early identification of genetic susceptibility could lead to the application of pharmacologic and lifestyle interventions that delay onset of the disease and maximize preventive efforts.[45] By delaying or preventing the onset of AD, the patients may ultimately die of unrelated ailments of old age before they lose their capacity to communicate and to recognize loved ones. The other side of the coin is that the early identification of the possibility of developing AD could bias insurers in coverage for such benefits as long-term care insurance or rehabilitation.

INFORMED CONSENT

The legal and ethical foundation of informed consent is self-determination and autonomy, or, in other words, the right to decide what is done to one's body. Medical professionals are obligated to provide information regarding the risks and benefits of the recommended treatment plan in a language and style that the patient can understand, as well as to inform the patient about alternate treatment options. By giving the patient proper and clear information the health professional is allowing the patient to execute his or her right to choose.[14]

All states have a combination of statutes, common laws, and regulations that require that the informed consent of a competent patient must be obtained before treatment is started. Some states do recognize *therapeutic privilege*, which is an exception to the informed consent process and allows a physician to withhold information if, in the opinion of the physician, the patient would suffer direct harm as a result of the knowledge. This doctrine is not usually appropriate.[14]

The perception of the elderly as being too old to learn new information can compromise their right to be informed. The health professional must remember that learning is a lifelong process, even though age-related changes can affect learning and comprehension. Some variables that may affect learning in the older patient are alterations in sensory perception, motivation, response time, memory, and sleep-wake cycles, all of which require modified teaching strategies in order to enhance the comprehension of information (see Chapter 18). One of the major factors in the learning process is sensory perception, such as sight and hearing, and because this is often compromised in the elderly, it should be evaluated and compensated for, if needed, before the clinician begins to present information. One can compensate for the increased response time that may be present in an older person by decreasing the rate and amount of information presented. Creating a relaxed, private atmosphere may be necessary to decrease anxiety and increase the client's capacity to comprehend.[46] The clinician must take responsibility to implement these strategies in order to ensure that elderly patients can understand what medical treatments are being considered and can exercise their right to be informed.

Informed consent is generally recognized as necessary when providing potentially dangerous treatment, such as chemotherapy, blood transfusions, and surgery. However, in treatments like physical therapy, which is considered noninvasive, the necessity of consent is often overlooked. From a moral point of view obtaining consent to perform "harmless" treatment is just as important as for hazardous treatment. Physical or occupational therapy may be considered routine; however, rehabilitation can be considered extremely invasive considering the amount of time patients need to dedicate to it and the impact it has on their lives.[38,42]

It is felt that it is the therapist's responsibility to ensure that information presented to the patient is understood and to be sensitive to cues regarding the patient's level of understanding. Purtilo feels it is better to give the patient too much rather than too little information.[8] Those who do not believe informed consent is appropriate feel patients cannot possibly understand the complexity of the

medical situation and are, therefore, incapable of making decisions. However, what these individuals fail to recognize is that it is not necessary for the patient to understand every detail but only the major issues.[47]

Therapists are also in a special situation regarding informed consent since their main focus is management of disability and pain control. Patients who are experiencing pain, changes in lifestyle, and anxiety may agree to anything that could possibly make their situation better. The clinician should not take this eagerness for granted and should always properly explain what is being implemented.[47] Informed consent should not simply be obtained for legal or malpractice reasons but to protect the patient's right to know and preserve patient autonomy.

DEATH ISSUES

Advances in medical technology that tend to prolong the dying process have created a new group of ethical issues regarding patient autonomy and death.[48] Dying at home has become rare; it now occurs most frequently in hospitals and long-term care settings that are dominated by professionals and their use of technology. Medical management is usually geared toward promoting life at all costs, which often can overlook the value systems and desires of the individuals involved.

Advanced directives, which are documented desires of medical management, can be used to ward off unwarranted care and promote death with dignity. Specificity is important in order for advanced directives to be as effective as possible. The documents should include a statement that the person has presence of mind and is able to make decisions regarding specific possible medical events of the future. A list of interventions that is undesired in the event of certain illnesses should also be included. A competent individual can delegate decision rights to someone else by giving that person power of attorney. Legally, in order for that power to continue after the onset of incompetence, a durable power of attorney must be obtained.[42]

Living Wills

A living will is one example of an advanced directive in which a competent adult expresses his or her wishes regarding medical management in the event of incapacitation. In November 1990, President Bush signed the *Patient Self-Determination Act*, which was created to increase patient involvement regarding decisions involving life-sustaining equipment and encourage more patients to prepare documents, such as living wills, in advance by providing them with the proper information. The *Patient Self-Determination Act* requires hospitals and skilled nursing facilities to develop written policies regarding advanced directives as a condition of Medicare and Medicaid payment. These facilities are required to ask all new patients whether or not they have prepared these documents, as well as to provide written information regarding facility policy and patient rights under the law. In December 1991, requirements went into effect that provide immunity to physicians and other health professionals when they are carrying out the wishes of the patient.[49]

The importance of clear, advanced directives was demonstrated in the US Supreme Court decision of *Cruzan v. Director of Missouri Department of Health*, the first case in which a high court considered termination of life-prolonging measures for an incompetent patient. The court upheld the Missouri decision not to remove the feeding tube of Nancy Cruzan, who was in a vegetative state, at the request of her parents since there was no "clear and convincing" evidence that the patient, if competent, would want it removed.[50]

There are many shortcomings regarding living wills that can make the document ineffective. For example, a living will is applicable only for the terminally ill, and there are limitations on the types of treatments that can be refused by the patient. There is also no penalty for the health provider who refuses to honor the document, and there is a tendency for physicians to make medical decisions based on their interpretation of the living will. For this reason it is important to accompany the document with a durable power of attorney to make it mandatory for the clinician to discuss treatment options with an individual selected by the patient.[51]

Durable power of attorney is present in every state and was primarily developed in order to manage financial matters of incapacitated individuals. Additional proxy laws are being developed state to state that specifically deal with health care. These laws would give an agent named by the patient the same authority for decision making as the patient would have if competent. The decision of the agent prevails when disagreements among family members are present regarding medical management. Since the physician may have difficulty honoring a living will over the objections of the family, the presence of this agent is essential to ensure that the wishes of the patient are respected.[43,51]

Euthanasia

According to *Webster's Dictionary*, euthanasia is defined as the action of inducing the painless death of a person for reasons assumed to be merciful. A moral distinction is made, which is accepted by most physicians, between passive and active euthanasia in which it is considered acceptable to remove life-sustaining treatment but it is unacceptable to actively terminate another person's life. A statement adopted by the House of Delegates of the AMA in 1973 considered "mercy killing" to be contrary to the medical profession's ethical position. On the other hand,

the opinion of the AMA was that ceasing extraordinary treatment that prolongs the life of a body when death is imminent is the decision of the patient, family, or both, with the aiding advice of the physician.[52]

Controversy is centered around active voluntary euthanasia that, for instance, would allow the physician at the request of the patient to administer a lethal medication. The concept that killing someone is morally worse than letting a patient die is one reason why people believe there is a moral difference between active and passive euthanasia. However, this belief does not account for the patient who is in severe unrelieved pain with days to live and who desires to terminate his or her own life. According to the AMA doctrine, the physician is permitted to stop treatment that prolongs the pain thereby causing the patient to suffer more than if direct action were taken.[52,53]

The American Geriatric Society (AGS) opposes active euthanasia and feels that while lethal injections may be appropriate for the few patients suffering from unrelenting pain, there is too much of a risk for abuse of frail, disabled, and economically disadvantaged members of society. The AGS is also concerned that legalized active euthanasia would weaken the motivation of society to develop solutions for proper care of the dying, such as hospice programs and that, given our fiscally obsessed society, active euthanasia may be viewed as a way to contain medical costs.[53]

The mental anguish caused by having to face another day waiting to die may be a growing reason for requests for voluntary active euthanasia. The presence of intractable pain is no longer as widely used as a justification for active euthanasia given the presence of anesthetic levels of pain-relieving medications. The psychological suffering of the patient would be minimized if the individual were able to legally choose the time and place of their death.[54] It has also been argued that making these choices regarding death is fundamental and honors the autonomy of the patient.[55]

If patients were legally given the choice of active euthanasia, the question is how many patients would pursue it. Hospice physicians report that although the topic of active euthanasia frequently arises in passing conversation, only a few patients seriously and persistently pursue its implementation.[55–57]

The debate regarding legalizing voluntary active euthanasia is far from over, and the degree to which supportive services for the dying should be made available must be addressed. Society must develop policies for the dying that will benefit the patient and enhance autonomy but not lead to potential abuses of the weaker members of society.

Cardiopulmonary Resuscitation

In the health care setting cardiopulmonary resuscitation (CPR) is considered a routine procedure administered to patients suffering cardiopulmonary arrest. It has always been assumed that consent to perform CPR is present since the patient is incapacitated and inaction will lead to death. The practice of performing CPR on any patient experiencing cardiac arrest regardless of the state of his or her illness and chances for survival is a cause of concern.[42,58] The right of the patient to refuse treatment also applies to the use of resuscitation, and a patient may express in advance that this procedure be withheld.[59]

The right of the patient to have do not resuscitate (DNR) orders placed in his or her medical chart is established, but the question is how involved is the patient in the decision making? One study revealed that 95% of a group of physicians believed that patients should be involved in resuscitation decisions, but only 10% discussed this issue with their patients. Another study showed that only 20% of the patients with DNR orders in their chart discussed their preferences with their physician prior to the initiation of the orders.[59] Even though decreased mental capacity may be one reason preferences were not discussed, the difficulty both physicians and patients have with discussing death may be another reason for inadequate patient participation. However, the need for this discussion is essential in order for the patient to participate in the decision-making process. In order to assist physicians in managing patients who are not appropriate for CPR, guidelines have been established by the Council on Ethical and Judicial Affairs.[59]

Another concern is that the presence of DNR orders will affect other therapeutic care given to the patient. A study done by Zimmerman and co-authors[60] showed that within 1.7 days of placement of a DNR order in the chart the patient either died or was discharged from the ICU. These results suggest that even though DNR orders specify only withholding of CPR, other therapeutic limits may accompany the order.[60]

A difficult situation arises when the patient, family, or both insist on CPR orders even when the procedure would clearly be futile. Inappropriate resuscitation may even cause harm by producing a chronic vegetative state. Patients and their families may insist on resuscitation out of guilt or fear, as well as out of unrealistic hopes for a cure. In this situation patient autonomy cannot be the only guide and does not allow a patient to demand treatment that is nonbeneficial and potentially harmful.

However, in this scenario, the question arises as to what is the point of offering the patient the choice in an attempt to preserve his or her rights of autonomy if these wishes are later denied. For this reason some physicians believe CPR should not be offered to this type of patient since the choice represents a potential for benefit when there is none.[58]

The issue of CPR in the nursing home setting is a complex one. The benefits are difficult to assess given the degree of debilitation in individuals present in a skilled nursing facility. Furthermore, the violence of the procedure and its small likelihood of success argue against it.

However, to withhold lifesaving therapy from a certain population just because they are dependent can be construed as discriminatory. A limited study done by Finucane and co-workers[61] demonstrated that there is an implicit policy by most nursing homes to withhold CPR from their residents.

The debate on proper policies regarding performing CPR in nursing homes continues, and like other treatments that tend to prolong the life of an already debilitated individual, it is difficult for the clinician to balance patient autonomy with supplying a treatment that is considered nonbeneficial.[62]

Terminal Care

Terminal care is geared toward providing a protective, nurturing, and homelike environment in which there is a large involvement of the health care team in decision making for the patient.[62] Since the elderly resident is dependent on the staff for personal hygiene, meals, and medication, the resident assumes a subservient role by trading his or her autonomy and dignity for the attentive care received.[3]

The older person's own home has a certain therapeutic value that is often not recognized. Home health care is, therefore, receiving new recognition. In this setting, individuals will be more likely to exercise their right to make decisions. There is, however, a danger of a patient becoming overconfident and having unrealistic views regarding his or her capacity to care for him- or herself, which the home care provider must be careful in assessing.[3]

Unlike an acute care setting, the treatment in a long-term care facility is routine and repetitive, making violations of the individual's autonomy more probable. Older people often may have the power to decide but are unable to carry out their personal decisions without the aid of the staff. Without this assistance their freedom to decide is useless and their autonomy infringed on.[63]

Value systems are important to examine when considering the long-term care setting. An individual may be placed in a facility that does not share his or her values and goals, or the patient's status may change while in the facility, making the setting no longer appropriate. It is important for the primary care physician to manage this and prevent or resolve ethical mismatches.[3] For example, the elderly resident in a nursing home may not share the enthusiasm of the rehabilitation therapist to participate in an exercise program.

Although nursing home residents vary in age, degree of function, and levels of cognition and interests, a common denominator is the difficulty in exercising choice. In order to enhance patient autonomy in long-term care facilities, increased staff, space, and resources are needed. Society is responsible for making the decision whether or not this should be a priority. The changes that do not require extra funds should of course be investigated first, and efforts should be made to find out the preferences of nursing home residents themselves.[64,65]

Hospice

The question of how society should deal with their dying population has always represented a void in the health care system that, in the past two decades, has been filled with the fast growth of the hospice. The growth of the hospice setting has received widespread support in the United States, sparking the interest of the health professional specializing in geriatrics, since approximately 66% of the patients in hospices are over 65.[66]

In the hospice, health care and service is provided for the patient and the family and is available at all times. Care is planned and provided by a medical interdisciplinary team, as well as by using family and volunteers to provide physical, emotional, and spiritual care to the patient with an emphasis on palliative care. The hospice is sensitive to needs of the family who obviously experience stress with the patient's terminal illness and also provides follow-up care after the patient dies.[66]

The focus of the hospice is to help the dying patient live the remaining time as fully as possible instead of concentrating on the disease process itself. The care is directed primarily at symptom and pain control to improve quality of life rather than disease control. There are major philosophical differences between hospices and the traditional health care setting, with hospice rules and regulations being extremely flexible to enhance the life of the dying patient.[67]

The rehabilitation therapist does play a palliative role in the hospice setting, using pain control modalities, but more importantly he or she functions as an educator for both the patient and the family. As in a home care setting, the physical or occupational therapist teaches the patient functional and safe tasks, and the family is present to learn as well. Each member of the hospice health care team, including the physical therapist, assumes the role of counselor, which demands good listening and communication skills. The involvement of the therapist is dependent on the resources available as well as the desires of the patient and family.[67]

Suicide

The suicide rate of older people is double that of any other age group.[68] These rates are most likely underestimated, given that the probability of not reporting suicides is highest in the elderly population. Older people are also more likely to complete the task of suicide, use a more violent means, and have a greater male-to-female ratio than any other age group. Conwell and co-authors[68] found that older suicide victims had a lower incidence of psychopathy and were responding to physical illness and loss.

Ethical debate regarding suicide and the elderly leaves health care providers confused about what their response should be. One question is whether suicide in the elderly should be treated like suicide in any other age group with an attempt to prevent it or to respect the right of the older person to choose to die. Health professionals desiring to prevent suicide rarely view it as a rational act well-thought-out by the individual but as a symptom of depression and mental dysfunction. It is equally important to discuss whether or not killing oneself for reasons of old age alone without the presence of terminal illness is ethically justified.[11]

Arguments against the concept of a justifiable suicide are dominated by the belief that killing one's self is a terrible act regardless of the circumstances. Clinicians concerned with suicide prevention may argue that the state of mind of the older person may be temporary and, though circumstances may be bad, they may get better in the future. However, elderly individuals who have deliberated about suicide over a long period of time are not experiencing a passing mental state and, unlike their younger counterparts, the future of an older person is more predictable and less bright.[11]

There is a great desire to promote both "death with dignity" and the right to choose one's own destiny; however, there is a concern that society, as well as the elderly, will view suicide as a solution to problems associated with aging. Taking this a step further, elderly people who do not choose suicide may be viewed as selfish for not committing the act in order to remove their presence as a burden to society.[11]

The issue of suicide and the elderly is complicated by desires to preserve patient autonomy, as well as the fear that making suicide acceptable in the elderly will contribute overall to the reprehensible attitude that the older person is a burden and should be removed. Perhaps these ethical issues will become clearer when the young and old are able to come to terms with their own aging process and mortality.

RESTRAINTS

Restraint issues arise frequently in the practice of rehabilitation therapy in geriatric settings and create many ethical, as well as legal, ramifications. In 1987, Congress passed the *Omnibus Reconciliation Act* (OBRA) to reform the use of physical and chemical restraints in nursing homes in the United States. OBRA prohibits nursing homes from inappropriately using physical and chemical restraints on nursing home residents for nonmedical purposes. Before OBRA, many nursing homes used restraints for the convenience of nursing home staff. For example, if an individual wandered, the staff did not have to watch that individual if the resident were simply tied to a chair. OBRA sought to stop this kind of abuse.

Nursing homes may not use "as needed" or PRN orders for nursing home residents' restraint use under

OBRA. OBRA allows the use of restraints only as a last resort after the facility completes a comprehensive assessment of the resident and determines that less restrictive alternatives have failed. Even if the nursing home facility proves that alternatives have failed, numerous other rules apply to protect residents from being restrained indefinitely. Ongoing assessment and attempts to remove restraints are required.

According to OBRA, that assessment should include input from the therapists involved in care of the residents in the facility. The "Interpretive Guidelines on Physical Restraints," which was implemented in October 1990, state that "a facility must have evidence of consultation with appropriate health professionals, such as occupational or physical therapists in the use of less restrictive supportive devices, *prior to* using physical restraints as defined in this guideline for such purposes."

The physical and occupational therapists are the most qualified health professionals in effectively assessing the necessity for restraining devices, especially in the mobility impaired group. There are clear benefits associated with improving function and stability with the goal of aiding these patients in maintaining their quality of life. Assessing the risk of falls and decline in function if physical restraints are applied are primary parameters in the evaluation of restraints for elderly patients (see Chapter 10 for assessment tools).

From an ethical perspective, to tie or not to tie the elderly is a difficult question. Understaffed nursing homes are fearful of guidelines that may cause an increase in the responsibilities of overburdened and underpaid staff. In addition, the possibility of increased legal pressure has been a source of apprehension regarding nonadherence to the guidelines. The proponents of untying the elderly, however, are advocating unassailable issues in the area of quality of life that must be considered in a comparison of risks and benefits.

The issues of freedom, dignity, self-choice, and enhanced function and mobility are very important ethical issues that arise regarding the choice not to use restraining devices. The physical and occupational therapists are extremely important players in allaying the fears of nursing home staff, improving functional capacity and stability, as well as helping to ensure that the least restrictive and most freedom enhancing environment for older persons is established.

Minority Issues and Ethics

Demographically, the number of different ethnic groups in the United States has grown considerably in the past two decades.[69,70] Inherent in a discussion of attitudes and ethics, it is important to introduce the cross-cultural and diversity phenomena affecting health care. Individuals from different ethnic groups will have grown up and been socialized in accordance with their various cultures. As a result, their health beliefs and practices may be considerably different from the traditional beliefs regarding health care in our western civilization.[71,72] Minorities often assume a subgroup within society and maintain their own "neighborhoods." Assimilation into the common culture may not occur, and it is important that the health care professional respect ethnic diversity by identifying, acknowledging, and accepting cultural beliefs and tendencies.

Cultural expectations are important to consider. The stronger the ties to the old-country practices, language, and rituals, the more likely it is that the individual will not share the beliefs and values of contemporary US health care. It is worthwhile to discuss with each elderly patient and his or her family their perspectives on aging, health and wellness, and what it is they perceive to be the proper practice for care in their condition (a herb, a ritual?).[73]

"Cultural pluralism emphasizes mutual respect between various groups that allows minorities to express their own culture without suffering prejudice or hostility."[74]

The rehabilitation professionals have been culturalized through whatever professional educational program they have experienced. Yet, what they have been taught may not be the way an elderly individual from a different ethnic background sees things. Perhaps their thought is that they are old, they've served their community, and now it is time for them to be served—so, "Why is it important to do these exercises?" We as clinicians need to respect that view. In order to practice effectively, cognizant of the ethics of care,[31,32] it is also important that ethnic considerations and respect for the different beliefs and values be the centerpiece in the care of our elderly patients with diverse cultural backgrounds.

Advocacy: The Role of the Rehabilitation Team

This chapter presents a lot of information that may be seen as extraneous to the role of rehabilitation, but it is not. This information is vital for continuing to improve the quality of life of older persons. To end, we would like to examine and provide additional references on three areas in which a member of the rehabilitation team may become more involved. The first area is becoming a liaison with an Ombudsman Program.[75] These programs are designed to advocate for the sake of older persons. The rehabilitation professional can serve as a consultant to such groups, an information source, or the rehabilitation professional may want to work for or start a group.[78]

The second area is in the area of abuse screening, for which tools are available. Fulmer, in *The Journal of the American Geriatric Society*, reviewed the most current screening and assessment instruments for health professionals in the area of mistreatment.[76] The rehabilitation must always be sensitive to and prepared to identify and report abuse in any setting. The third area is through interdisciplinary training and community outreach.[77] The rehabilitation professional can take the lead in designing programs in this area.

CASE STUDIES: ETHICAL DILEMMAS

Case Study 1

A childless, 78-year-old woman was admitted to the hospital on July 14, 2001, because of weight loss and fever. Her husband died in 1999 and after his death she became depressed, refused to eat, and lost weight. An ileostomy tube was inserted for feeding purposes. It was successful, and the patient gained weight. Psychological interviews revealed her to be well oriented but possibly slightly demented because of her simple answers, and she did not show interest in or awareness of events happening around her. She lost the ability to ambulate and developed multiple contractures. She also developed anemia secondary to poor nutrition. On November 30, 2001, when she was transferred to another facility, she still had the ileostomy, which had not been used for feeding for some time. The patient often complained about the tube and stated she would like it removed. On or around April 27, 2002, the end of the "J tube" broke off and the remaining portion appeared to be "flush" with the surface of the skin. On April 28, 2002, the tube slipped inside, causing the physician to maintain a close observation of her status. The physician believed the tube would pass through the rectum in the feces, which it did several days later. The patient then stated she thought she was going to die and appeared quite depressed. The ethical question in this case is: Should the tube have been removed at the request of the patient given her presumed competence?

Case Study 2

A 95-year-old woman living independently at home with diabetes and congestive heart failure was hospitalized after developing gangrene of one foot. While hospitalized she refused amputation but consented to continue management of her other medical problems, including medication and localized treatment for her foot. She became unpopular with the hospital staff and other patients because of the foot's odor and the related infection control hazards. The house staff on her case expressed that she must be crazy since she refused life-sustaining treatment. The physician and a psychologist experienced in competency assessment evaluated the patient and determined that the patient's cognitive abilities were intact. The evaluation also concluded that the patient refused the surgery due to personal values of not wanting to continue life at her age without her foot even if death without intervention was imminent. Presentation of positive examples of life as an amputee did not change her position. In order to pacify the concern of the staff regarding infection and odor, the ward was visited frequently by in infection control specialist and the patient received whirlpool treatments of the foot. The patient died several weeks later with her wishes respected.[12] The ethical question here: Should surgery have been performed to prolong life?

Case Study 3

An 83-year-old woman whose status postoperatively included a right cerebral vascular accident, was admitted to a nursing home directly from the hospital. At the time of admission, the patient was extremely dependent and could ambulate only short distances with the maximum assistance of two people. She refused to use an assistive device. A mental evaluation performed by the nursing home staff physician revealed the patient was not oriented to time or place but was aware of her medical condition and recognized her daughter who visited her frequently. The physician and the patient's daughter agreed it was important to continue the physical therapy that was initiated in the hospital in order to promote restoration of function as well as independence. When the transporter arrived to take the patient to her first physical therapy session, the patient verbally refused, but she was placed in the wheelchair by the transporter under the direction of the nurse in charge on the floor. In the physical therapy department, the patient expressed the desire to return to her room repetitively and reluctantly cooperated during the evaluation performed by the therapist. Even after a great deal of coaxing and encouragement the physical therapist was unable to convince the patient to ambulate with a walker or a quad cone. In spite of the patient's verbal refusals, she was brought to physical therapy daily where she ambulated short distances with the assistance of two people but refused to perform any other exercises. The ethical question: Should this individual's refusal to participate in therapy have been respected given her cognitive status?

References

1. Braunack-May AJ. What makes a problem an ethical problem? *J Medical Ethics.* 2001; 27:98–103.
2. *Miranda v. Arizona.* 384 U.S. 436 (1966).
3. Talar GA, Waymack MH. Ethics and the elderly. *Primary Care.* 1989; 16:529–541.
4. Blanchette PL. Age-based rationing of health care. *Hawaii Med J.* 1995; 54(4):507–509.
5. Gonsoulin TP. Ethical issues raised by managed care. *Laryngoscope.* 1997; 107(11 pt 1):1425–1428.
6. Rodwin MA. Conflicts of interest and accountability in managed care: The aging of medical ethics. *J Am Geriatr Soc.* 1998; 46(3):338–341.
7. Evans JG. Economic, political and ethical implications of aging. *Aging.* 1998; 10(2):141–142.
8. Purtilo RB. Ethical considerations. In: Jackson OL, ed. *Therapeutic Considerations for the Elderly.* New York: Churchill Livingston; 1987: 173.
9. Purtilo RB. *Ethical Dimensions in the Health Professions.* 3rd ed. Philadelphia: WB Saunders; 1999.
10. Harris J, Fiedler CM. Preadolescent attitudes toward the elderly: An analysis of race, gender, and contact variables. *Adolescence.* 1988; 23:335–340.
11. Werner RM, Alexander GC, Fagerlin A, Ubel PA. The hassle factor: What motivates physicians to manipulate reimbursement rules? *Arch Intern Med.* 2002; 162(10): 1134–1139.
12. Goldstein NIK. Ethical care of the elderly: Pitfalls and principles. *Geriatrics.* 1989; 44:101–106.
13. Lynn J. Conflicts of interest in medical decision-making. *J Am Geriatr Soc.* 1988; 36:945–950.
14. Dubler NN. Legal issues. *Merck Manual.* Rahway, NJ: Merck, Sharp, and Dohme Research Laboratories; 1990: 1142–1161.
15. Coates R. Ethics and physiotherapy. *Aust Physiotherapy.* 1990; 36:84–87.
16. Kilner JF. Age criteria in medicine. *Arch Intern Med.* 1989; 149:2343–2346.
17. Barondess JA, Kalb P, Weil WB, et al. Clinical decision-making in catastrophic situations: The relevance of age. *J Am Geriatr Soc.* 1988; 36:919–937.
18. Daniels N. Why saying no to patients in the United States is so hard. *N Engl J Med.* 1986; 314: 1380–1383.
19. Eddy DM. The individual vs. society: Is there a conflict? *JAMA.* 1991; 265:1446–1450.
20. Rabins PV, Fitting MD, Eastham J, et al. Emotional adaptation over time in care-givers for chronically ill elderly people. *Age Ageing.* 1990; 19:185–190.
21. Marshall CE, Benton D, Brazier JM. Elder abuse. Using clinical tools to identify clues of mistreatment. *Geriatrics.* 2000; 55(2):42–44, 47–50, 53.
22. Jogerst GJ, Dawson JD, Hartz AJ, Ely JW, Schweitzer LA. Community characteristics associated with elder abuse. *J Am Geriatr Soc.* 2000; 48(5):513–518.
23. Collins KA, Bennett AT, Hanzlick R. Elder abuse and neglect. Autopsy Committee of the College of American Pathologists. *Arch Intern Med.* 2000; 160 (11):1567–1568.
24. Dyer CB, Pavlik VN, Murphy KP, Hyman DJ. The high prevalence of depression and dementia in elder abuse or neglect. *J Am Geriatr Soc.* 2000; 48(2): 205–208.
25. Anetzberger GJ, Palmisano BR, Sanders M, et al. A model of intervention for elder abuse and dementia. *Gerontologist.* 2000; 40(4):492–497.
26. Gray-Vickery P. Recognizing elder abuse. *Nursing.* 1999; 29(9):52–53.
27. Ciolek DE, Ciolek CH. *Guidelines for Recognizing and Providing Care for Victims of Elder Abuse and Neglect.* Alexandria, VA: Section on Geriatrics—American Physical Therapy Association; 1999.
28. Wolf RS, Li D. Factors affecting the rate of elder abuse reporting to state protective services program. *Gerontologist.* 1999; 39(2):222–228.
29. Tueth MJ. Exposing financial exploitation of impaired elderly persons. *Am J Geriatr Psychiatry.* 2000; 8(2):104–111.
30. Szulc T. How we can help ourselves age with dignity. *Parade.* May 29, 1988; 4–7.
31. Bottomley JM, ed. *Quick Reference Dictionary for Physical Therapy.* Thorofare, NJ: Slack; 2000: 237.
32. Jacobs K, ed. *Quick Reference Dictionary for Occupational Therapy.* 2nd ed. Thorofare, NJ: Slack; 1999; 229.
33. American Physical Therapy Association. *Code of Ethics.* Alexandria, VA: American Physical Therapy Association; 2005.
34. American Occupational Therapy Association. *Code of Ethics.* Bethesda, MD: American Occupational Therapy Association; 2005.
35. Marcus EL, Berry EM. Refusal to eat in the elderly. *Nutr Rev.* 1998; 56(6):163–171.
36. Moon MA. Task force to protect rights of nursing home patients. *Intern Med News.* 1983; 16:23.
37. Appelbaum PS, Roth LH. Patients who refuse treatment in medical hospitals. *JAMA.* 1983; 215: 1296–1301.
38. Coy JA. Autonomy-based informed consent. Ethical implications for patient noncompliance. *Phys Ther.* 1989; 69:826–833.
39. Arras JD. The severely demented, minimally functional patient: An ethical analysis. *J Am Geriatr Soc.* 1988; 36:938–944.
40. Jones DG. Aging, dementia and care: Setting limits on the allocation of health care resources to the aged. *NZ Med J.* 1997; 110(1057):466–468.

41. Gunn AE. Mental impairment in the elderly: Medical-legal assessment. *J Am Geriatr Soc.* 1977; 25: 193–198.

42. Scott RW. *Professional Ethics: A Guide for Rehabilitation Professionals.* St. Louis: Mosby Year-Book; 1998.

43. Scott RW. *Promoting Legal Awareness in Physical and Occupational Therapy.* St. Louis: Mosby Year-Book; 1997.

44. Fitten LJ, Lusky RL, Hamann C. Assessing treatment decision-making capacity in elderly nursing home residents. *J Am Geriatr Soc.* 1990; 38: 1097–1104.

45. Post SG. Future scenarios for the prevention and delay of Alzheimer disease onset in high-risk groups. An ethical perspective. *Am J Prev Med.* 1999; 16(2): 105–110.

46. Rendon DC. The right to know, the right to be taught. *J Gerontol Nurs.* 1986; 12:33–37.

47. Simm J. Informed consent: Ethical implications for physiotherapy. *Physiotherapy.* 1986; 72:584–587.

48. Gadow S. Aging as death rehearsal: The oppressiveness of reason. *J Clin Ethics.* 1996; 7(1):35–40.

49. Greco PJ, Schulman KA, Lavizzo-Mourey R, et al. The patient self-determination act and the future of advance directives. *Ann Intern Med.* 1991; 115: 639–643.

50. Malloy DW, Clametle RM, Braun EA, et al. Decision making in the incompetent elderly: "The daughter from California syndrome." *J Am Geriatr Soc.* 1991; 39:396–399.

51. Annas GJ. The health care proxy and the living will. *N Engl J Med.* 1991; 324:1210–1213.

52. Rachels J. Active and passive euthanasia. *N Engl J Med.* 1975; 292:78–80.

53. AGS Public Policy Committee. Voluntary active euthanasia. *J Am Geriatr Soc.* 1991; 39:826.

54. Kane RS. The defeat of aging versus the importance of death. *J Am Geriatr Soc.* 1996; 44(3):321–325.

55. Teno J, Lynn J. Voluntary active euthanasia: The individual case and public policy. *J Am Geriatr Soc.* 1991; 39:827–830.

56. Loewy EH. Living well and dying not too badly: Integrating a whole life into a tolerable death. *Wien Klin Wochenschr.* 2000; 112(9):381–385.

57. Muller MT, Kimsma GK, van der Wal G. Euthanasia and assisted suicide: Facts, figures and fancies with special regard to old age. *Drugs Aging.* 1998; 13(3):185–191.

58. Blackhall LJ. Must we always use CPR? *N Eng J Med.* 1987; 317:1281–1285.

59. Council on Ethical and Judicial Affairs, American Medical Association. Guidelines for the appropriate use of do-not-resuscitate orders. *JAMA.* 1991; 265:1868–1871.

60. Zimmerman JE, Knaus WA, Sharpe SM, et al. The use and implications of do not resuscitate orders in intensive care units. *JAMA.* 1986; 255:351–356.

61. Finucane TE, Boyer JT, Bulmash J, et al. The incidence of attempted CPR in nursing homes. *J Am Geriatr Soc.* 1991; 39:624–626.

62. Iris MA. The ethics of decision making for the critically ill elderly. *Camb Q Healthcare Ethics.* 1995; 4(2):135–141.

63. Collopy BJ. Ethical dimensions of autonomy in long-term care. *Generations.* 1990; XIV:9–12.

64. Kane RL, Kane RA. Long-term-care financing on personal autonomy. *Generations.* 1990; XIV:86–94.

65. Hoehner PJ. Ethical decisions in perioperative elder care. *Anesthesiol Clin N Am.* 2000; 18(1):159–181, vii–viii.

66. Greer DS. Hospice: Lessons for geriatricians. *J Am Geriatr Soc.* 1983; 31:67–70.

67. Toot J. Physical therapy and hospice, concept and practice. *Phys Ther.* 1984; 64:665–671.

68. Conwell Y, Rotenber M, Caine ED. Completed suicide at age 50 and over. *J Am Geriatr Soc.* 1990; 38:640–644.

69. Leavitt RL. Introduction. In: Leavitt RL, ed. *Cross-Cultural Rehabilitation: An International Perspective.* Philadelphia: WB Saunders; 1999: 1–7.

70. Luckman J. *Transcultural Communications.* Canada: Delmar Thomson Publications; 2000.

71. Betancourt JR. Becoming a physician: Cultural competence—Marginal or mainstream? *N Eng J Med.* 2004; 351(10):953–955

72. Mouton CP, Johnson MS, Cole DR. Ethical considerations with African-American elders. *Clin Geriatr Med.* 1995; 11(1):113–129.

73. Fadiman A. *The Spirit Catches You and You Fall Down. A Hmong Child, Her American Doctors, and the Collision of Two Cultures.* New York: Farrar, Straus and Giroux; 1997.

74. McDonald H, Galgopal P. Conflicts of American immigrants: Assimilate or retain ethnic identity. *Migration World Mag.* 1998; 127(4):14–19.

75. Estes CL, Zulman DM, Goldberg SC, Ogawa DD. State long-term care ombudsman programs: Factors associated with perceived effectiveness. *Gerontologist.* 2004; 44(1):104–115.

76. Fulmer T, Guadagno L, Dyer CB, Connolly MT. Progress in elder abuse screening and assessment instruments. *J Am Geriatric Soc.* 2004; 52:297–304.

77. Hamel P. Interdisciplinary perspectives service learning, and advocacy: A nontraditional approach to geriatric rehabilitation. *Top Geriatr Rehabil* 2001; 17(1):53–70.

78. Nelson HW, Hooker K, DeHart KN, Edwards JA, Lanning K. Factors important to success in the volunteer long-term care ombudsman role. *Gerontologist.* 2004; 44(1):116.

18

Education and the Older Adult: Learning, Memory, and Intelligence

Pearls

- Learning is defined as the acquisition of a new skill or information through practice and experience, whereas remembering is the retrieval of information that has been stored in memory.
- Encoding and retrieval problems are the cause of memory difficulties in older adults, and instruction in organizing, slower pacing, and verbal and visual associations can improve performance.
- Problem-solving ability appears to decline with age and may be due to education level and fluid intelligence. Training can improve older patients' problem-solving abilities; however, they may not transfer these strategies to problems encountered in real life.
- Memory performance of healthy elderly can be improved through memory training.
- Variables that positively influence learning for the older person are:

- Orderly environment.
- A supportive approach by the therapist with much positive reinforcement.
- Highly organized presentation of material. Simple, concrete, step-by-step information presentation.
- Appropriate rate of presentation of information.
- Choosing meaningful tasks.
- Use of memory strategies.
- Ample time for repetition and practice.
- Depression, anxiety, and motivation will influence learning and memory abilities.
- One is never too old to learn.

INTRODUCTION

Elders of the tribe were once considered teachers, the founts of wisdom. Today, little respect is given to the experiences of a lifetime, and myths perpetuate the notion that learning abilities and memory capabilities decline with age. On the contrary, in our society, elderly individuals must learn new skills as new technology alters basic systems of communication, transportation, finance and recreation on nearly a daily basis. As values change, societal rewards change, and new learning is required.

Learning means the acquisition of information or skills, and it is usually measured by looking for improvements in task performance. When people improve their performance at a given intellectual or physical task, we say that they have learned. Studies of performance in elderly individuals indicate a decline with age. Clearly, there are a number of factors other than learning ability that affect performance. Some of these include physiological responses, physical health status, pathology, depression and motivation. In practice, it is extremely difficult to separate the components of performance in order to examine the influence of learning ability, although a number of studies have attempted to do so. Despite evidence that other factors contribute to the decline in task performance, most researchers still attribute part of this decline to a diminished ability to learn new tasks or acquire new information with age.[1–6]

All age groups can learn. Older individuals just require more time. Tasks that involve manipulation of distinct and familiar symbols or objects, unambiguous responses, and low interference from prior learning are particularly conducive to good performance by older individuals.[7-9]

At various points in time, different approaches to the study of learning and memory have been dominant. In the 1960s, the associative view of learning was most popular. In the 1970s, theories on information processing or conceptual learning were established as the mode for learning and memory. Now, a growing emphasis in learning theories concerns a contextual approach.[10] Thus, it is important to briefly review research on learning and memory from each of these approaches.

Learning and memory are closely related concepts. People must learn before they can remember, and learning without memory has limited utility. Learning is often assessed by memory tasks. "How much have you learned?" is translated to "How much do you remember?" Learning is defined as the acquisition of a new skill or information through practice and experience. Remembering is defined as the retrieval of information that has been stored in memory.[10]

The general learning/memory system involves three processes: acquisition, storage, and retrieval. Memory is often discussed in terms of information: how you put information into the system, how you store it, and how you retrieve it. This is the approach of modern information processing theories, and in this view, learning is part of memory; that is, the acquisition, registration, or encoding phase.

When adding the dimension of age, there are many questions that arise. How do learning abilities change? How does memory change? Does it fade? Do old people forget new things and remember the past? How do societal demands affect learning and memory?

Associative Learning

Based on the assumption that learning and memory involve the association of ideas or events that occur together in time, the associative learning theory involves a stimulus-response bond, and paired association is the most commonly employed mode for testing memory using this theory. The task is to learn an association between two commonly unrelated items, such as basket–therefore, or orange–until. The subject is first presented with two unrelated words, and the subsequent task is to give a correct response to each stimulus word as it appears alone. The ability to recall a paired stimulus represents the contents of memory. There are several factors that appear to influence the amount of information that can be processed with increasing age, including the pace of learning and the environment in which learning occurs, which may be influenced by cautiousness, anxiety, and interference from previously learned information.

The pace of learning is the speed with which a task is performed and is one variable known to affect older learn-

ers more than young ones. The pace of learning can be manipulated in two ways. The anticipation interval is the time allotted for a response. Older subjects perform poorly when this interval is short and do much better when they are given more time to respond.[3,11] Younger subjects also improve as the anticipation interval increases but less than older subjects. If a method called "self-pacing" is permitted (i.e., if learners are allowed as much time as they want), older subjects improve in the number of correct responses they are capable of giving. The second element of pacing in paired associative learning is the time the pair of items is presented for study. This period is referred to as the study time or inspection interval. Increasing the study time also improves performance by older learners, although old and young subjects have been shown to benefit equally from more time.[2,12] Again, if self-pacing is allowed, older subjects benefit more than younger subjects.[13]

The ability to perform associative learning tasks may be affected by variables such as cautiousness, anxiety, and interference. These factors are often associated with errors of omission (not responding) or errors of commission (responding incorrectly). Errors of omission occur most often in fast-paced associative learning situations (rather than errors of commission). Errors of omission are reflective of cautiousness or a reluctance to venture a response unless one is absolutely certain of its accuracy. It has been suggested by researchers that the poorer performance of older adults, as reflected in omission errors, is a function of their being more cautious.[10,13]

To overcome cautiousness, or test this hypothesis, experimenters have requested or demanded responses be made, even if they are wrong. This failed to improve the learning rate of older subjects or to reduce the number of errors of omission.[14] However, in another test of the cautiousness hypothesis, a small monetary reward was given for each correct response and each incorrect response was also rewarded at a slightly lower value, and the absence of a response received no reward. In this situation older learners significantly reduced the number of errors of omission,[15] which suggests that older learners could do better if they took a few more chances.

Another hypothesis regarding the poorer performance of the elderly on paired associative learning suggests that anxiety affects performance. Eisdorfer and associates[16] tested this theory by introducing a drug that blocked physiological arousal. This resulted in significantly fewer errors in older subjects on associative learning tasks compared to elders given a placebo.

A final hypothesis suggests that in some instances of associative learning, older adults are more susceptible to the effects of interference from prior learning. When one word is frequently associated with another word in everyday situations, such as dark–light and water–ocean, the pair is said to have high associative strength. When one word is infrequently associated with another, such as dark–fast and water–book, the pair has low associative strength. If the associative habits of older individuals are more established through a greater number of years of experience, it follows that the age-related difference should be least for high associative pairs.[13] This appears to be the case. In a comprehensive study, Botwinick and Storandt[17] found no age-related differences in performance on an easy list but marked age-related differences in performance on moderate to high difficulty lists. The older adults appear to be more handicapped when learning and recall involve forming associations that are contrary, or in competition with, previously learned verbal associations.

Salthouse[13] conducted studies to determine the mechanisms by which processing speed contributes to the relations between adult age and associative learning. The results of these studies indicated that increased age was related to poorer associative learning largely because of a failure to retain information about previously correct responses. This in turn was related to the effectiveness of encoding briefly presented information in an associative memory task, which was related to measures of processing speed. It was suggested that age-related decreases in speed of processing lead to less effective encoding or elaboration, which results in a fragile representation that is easily disrupted by subsequent processing.[13]

Judging from studies of associative learning, the rate of learning slows gradually through the adult years. Only after the age of 65 does one's learning become demonstrably poorer than that of young adults. The nature of the age deficit remains unclear. Older subjects profit from a slower pace of learning much more than do young adults. Moreover, the older learner may get too anxious or cautious, or may encounter interference from previously learned associations.

INFORMATION PROCESSING

How information is processed has to do with the older adult's learning style, which is unique to each learner. Information processing has to do with the typical manner in which an individual receives, retains, and retrieves information, as well as how the individual responds emotionally in a learning experience. The term "information processing" as a means of learning grew from analogies with computer operations and has become a prominent theory in discussions of memory and perception. It involves associative, conceptual, and contextual learning. Information processing is the mechanism through which an individual processes, stores, and remembers events, tasks, lists, and the like. It involves the wiring of the human hard drive, the brain.

In an interesting study by Spitzer and associates,[18] functional magnetic resonance imaging (MRI), in conjunction with carefully designed, psychometrically optimized stimulation procedures (e.g., word pairs, lists of words, color discrimination tasks), was used to investigate the relationship between brain activation and the processing of word associations. A semantic discrimination task of word-pair similarity selectively activated the left frontal and left frontotemporal areas. Cortical activation was decreased during language activities but highly active when an individual was performing a color similarity task. A similar study[19] used functional MRI to identify cortical areas involved in category learning by prototype abstraction. Elderly participants studied forty dot patterns that were distortions of an underlying prototype and were asked to make yes or no category judgments regarding the objects depicted by the dot patterns. Activity in four cortical areas correlated with the category judgment task. A sizable posterior occipital cortical area exhibited significantly less activity during processing of the categorical patterns than during processing of noncategorical patterns. Significant increases in activity during processing the categorical patterns were observed in left and right anterior frontal cortex and right inferior lateral frontal cortex. Decreases in activation of the visual cortex when categorical patterns were being studied suggest that these patterns could be processed in a more rapid or less effortful manner after the prototype had been learned. The researchers suggest that increases in prefrontal activity associated with processing categorical patterns could be related to any of several processes involved in retrieving information about the learned exemplars.[19]

Performance of complex motor tasks, such as rapid sequences of finger movements or lower extremity sequencing activities, can be improved in terms of speed and accuracy over several weeks by daily practice sessions.[5] This improvement does not generalize to a matched sequence of identical component movements, nor to the contralateral extremity. In a study by Karni and colleagues,[5] the underlying neural changes of learning of complex motor tasks was studied using functional magnetic resonance imaging of local blood oxygenation level–dependent signals evoked in the primary motor cortex (M1). Before training, a comparable extent of M1 was activated by both upper and lower extremity sequences. However, two ordering effects were observed: repeating a sequence within a brief time window initially resulted in a smaller area of activation (habituation), but later in a larger area of activation (enhancement), suggesting a switch in M1 processing mode within a fast learning session. By week 4 of training, concurrent with asymptotic performance, the extent of cortex activated by the practiced sequence enlarged compared with the unpracticed sequence, irrespective of order (slow learning). These changes persisted for several months. The results suggest a slowly evolving, long-term, experience-dependent reorganization of the older adult M1, which may underlie the acquisition and retention of the new motor skill.[5]

Cortical functions concerned with the execution of skilled movements can also be studied through complex interactive tasks. The learning of skilled performance tasks (SPT) offers the greatest amount of information about the electrophysiological components reflecting pre-programming, execution of the movement and control of the results. Overall, these components are indicated as movement-related brain macropotentials (MRBMs). Among them, Bereitschaftspotential (BP) reflects cerebral processes related to the preparation of movement, and skilled performance positivity (SPP) reflects control processes on the result of performance. There is some evidence supporting a training effect on MRBMs, but less clear is whether long-term practice of a skilled activity could modify learning strategies of a new skilled task.[20] Fattapposta and associates[20] recorded MRBMs in elderly subjects trained for a long time to perform a highly skillful activity (i.e., sequencing dancing steps) and compared electrophysiological brain activity to a group of elderly control subjects without any former experience in these skilled motor activities. Their findings demonstrated the existence of a relationship between preprogramming and performance control, as suggested by decrease in the BP amplitude and an increase of the SPP amplitude in the presence of high levels of performance. Long-term practice seems to develop better control models on performance that reduce the need of a high mental effort in preprogramming a skilled action.[20]

CONTEXTUAL LEARNING

Associative learning is often supported by the individual placing some contextual meaning to lists of words, activities, or other learning endeavors. For example, if an important piece of information is presented in **bold** type, it is more likely to be perceived as important because its importance has been stressed through visual intonation. In other words, learning occurs because the information has been presented in context.

In a study by Naveh-Benjamin and Craik,[21] memory for words and the font in which they appeared (or the voice speaking them) was compared in younger and older persons to explore whether age-related differences in episodic word memory are due to age-related differences in memory for perceptual-contextual information. In each of the experimental sessions, young and old participants were presented with words to learn. The words were presented in either one of two font types, or in one of two male voices, and participants paid attention either to the fonts or voices or to the meaning of the words. Subjects were tested on both work and font or voice memory. The results showed that younger participants had better explicit memory for font and voice memory and for the words themselves but that older participants benefited at least as much as younger people when perceptual characteristics of the words (e.g., *italics*, **bold,** tone of voice) were utilized. This study concluded that there was no evidence of an age-related impairment in the encoding of percep-

tual-conceptual information.[21] This is an important finding for geriatric rehabilitation professionals. Much of the printed or spoken information we provide for our elderly patients/clients could conceivably be learned better if it were presented in a perceptual-contextual format.

In a study by Spencer and Raz,[22] age-related differences in memory for facts, source, and contextual details were examined in healthy young (18- to 35-year-old) and old (65- to 80-year-old) volunteers. In all tested memory functions, decline over time was greater in the elderly than in the young. A time-dependent increase in the prevalence of source amnesia errors was clearly associated with old age. Contrary to other studies, measures of frontal lobe functions did not predict source memory.[22] Nevertheless, some of these putative frontal function measures were related to memory for contextual details. The number of perseverative responses on testing was inversely related to performance on both factual and contextual memory tests, but the association with contextual memory was stronger. Difficulties with response selection predicted poor contextual memory in young but not in old adults.[22]

In a subsequent study, Spencer and Raz[23] reviewed the evidence of age differences in episodic memory for content of a message and the context associated with it. Specifically, the authors tested a hypothesis that memory for context is more vulnerable to aging than memory for content. In addition, the authors inquired as to whether effort at encoding and retrieval and type of stimulus material moderate the magnitude of age differences in both memory domains. The results confirmed the main hypothesis: age differences in context memory are reliably greater than those in memory for content. Tasks that required greater effort during retrieval yielded larger age differences in content but not in context memory. The greatest magnitude of age differences in context memory was observed for those contextual features that were more likely to have been encoded independently from content.[23] The possible mechanisms that may underlie age differences in context memory, as suggested by these researchers, are attentional deficits, reduced working memory capacity, and/or a failure of inhibitory processing. The findings of the Spencer and Raz studies[22,23] are substantiated by numerous other studies.[24–27] The major clinical implication of these findings is that elderly humans overwhelmingly seek, create, or imagine context in order to provide meaning when presented with information. The importance of this will be discussed further in a subsequent section of this chapter in relationship to teaching strategies for the elderly.

HUMAN MEMORY

There are many myths about the effects of aging on memory. For example, people are supposed to forget things they've recently learned, but memories from the distant past are supposed to be clear and vivid, sometimes startlingly so. Early learning also appears to have a significant impact on an elderly individual's resourcefulness for both verbal and physical skills in later life. [1,8,9]

Memory is closely related to both intelligence and learning, since remembering is part of the evidence of learning and learning is part of the measurement of intelligence. For example, if a person does not learn, that person has nothing to remember. Conversely, if the individual cannot remember, there is no sign of that person's having learned. [28]

There are essentially four types of memory. Short-term or immediate memory involves recall after very little delay (as little as five seconds up to thirty seconds). Recent memory involves recall after a brief period (from one hour to several days). Remote memory refers to recall of events which took place a long time ago but which have been referred to frequently throughout the course of a lifetime. Old memory refers to recall of events that occurred a long time in the past and which have not been thought of or rehearsed since. [9]

Regardless of type, there are three stages of memory: registration (encoding), retention (storage), and recall (retrieval). Registration refers to the recording of learning or perceptions, and is more commonly referred to as encoding. In concept, it is analogous to the recording of sound on a tape recorder. Retention refers to the ability to sustain registration over time. Recall is retrieval of material that has been registered and retained. Obviously in any type of memory, a failure at any one of these stages will result in no measurable memory. See Figure 18.1 and 18.2.

For more information or memory, see CD.

PROBLEM SOLVING

Many of the learning and memory tasks described in previous sections involved relatively simple problems. Another type of cognitive activity, problem solving, is more complex and may involve aspects of learning and memory not previously discussed. Problem solving requires that a person assess the present state of a situation, define the desired state (or goal), and find a way to transform the present state to the desired state. [29]

The process of solving a problem has been broken down into four steps. [30] The first step is to understand the problem, which involves gathering information on the problem and identifying its important elements. The second step is to devise a plan, using past experience for guidance. The use of a relevant strategy would ensure that one devises an efficient plan. The third step is to carry out the

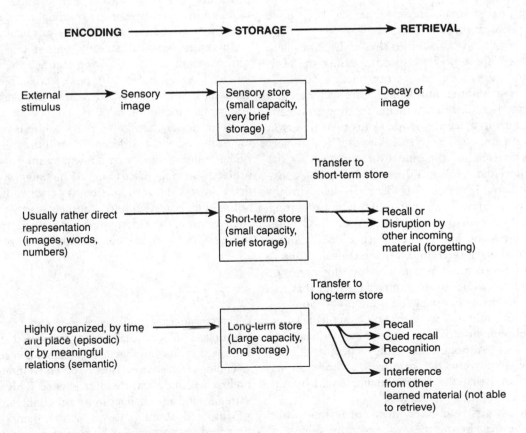

Figure 18.1

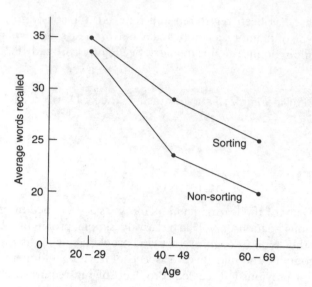

Figure 18.2   Average number of words learned as a function of age. Prior to learning, about half of the subjects carried out a sorting task designed to aid in organizing word lists; the rest of the subjects performed a task that did not involve sorting. (*Reproduced with permission from Hultsch, D. Adult age differences in free classification and free recall. Dev Psych. 1971; 4:338–342. ©1971 American Psychological Association.*)

plan, and the final step is to review what has been done (i.e., was the problem solved?).

There are many types of studies that address problem solving from a "laboratory" perspective (using prefabricated laboratory situations that do not necessarily duplicate problems encountered in real life). One such mode of testing is termed concept attainment. In concept attainment tasks, items in a set are divided into two subsets in accordance with some characteristics or rule. The subject demonstrates mastery of the rule by distinguishing the items that reflect the rule from those that do not. An example of this would be "choose the red circle; do not choose the green circle." Another example is presenting meal content lists with the rule that certain food types may induce illness and having the subjects identify those meals that would make them ill following consumption. A number of studies of this type, in which performance of younger and older adults were compared, found that the old solved fewer problems than the young.[31–33] Some of the difficulties encountered were that older subjects failed to ignore irrelevant information and tended to fixate on useless hunches.[33] Although the elderly people do not spontaneously employ effective strategies, several training studies have found that their performance could be improved with brief training procedures.[34,35]

"Twenty questions" is another means of testing problem-solving abilities. In this type of task, the subject is presented with an array of pictures or words, only one of which is the correct choice. The task is to determine the correct choice by asking less than twenty questions that can be answered with a "yes" or "no." The most efficient strategy is to ask questions that are constraint-seeking (e.g., "Is it a vegetable?"), each of which eliminates a set of possible answers. Asking questions that refer to only one item is inefficient. Again, the elderly tend to do less well on these tasks than younger groups,[36] but their performance improved significantly after training in the use of constraint-seeking questions.

Piagetian theory has been applied to problem-solving measurement as well. Piagetian theory assumes that concrete operational abilities (the ability to think logically about concrete or tangible problems), such as classification and conservation (the recognition that the amount of matter does not change when it is rearranged), develop during middle childhood and that formal operational abilities (the ability to think logically about hypothetical situations or problems) are achieved in adolescence. Do these abilities decline in old age? One hypothesis suggests that operational abilities decline in reverse of the order in which they develop.[9,37,38] In other words, formal operational thought would decline before conservation. Studies of performance by elderly persons on various Piagetian tasks have yielded mixed results. Some show that the elderly do less well than younger people;[39] others find no age differences in formal operational tasks.[40] Success is positively correlated with higher levels of education and higher intelligence scores. Training has been shown to improve performance by the elderly as well.

In summary, these studies suggest that there are age differences in problem-solving abilities and the elderly do less well on a number of types of tasks. Several explanations have been offered. It may be that problem-solving ability is a function of educational level, fluid intelligence, or both, rather than aging per se. These factors, in turn, may reflect cohort differences. Additionally, brief educational training has been shown to improve all types of problem solving discussed.[41] This suggests that the elderly possess the competence to perform the tasks but do not spontaneously employ the necessary strategies. Even after training, the elderly may not transfer the use of these strategies to the problems encountered in real life.

INTELLIGENCE

When considering intelligence, a potential and actual ability are implied. In practice, however, measured ability is always dealt with. Thus, intelligence, as it is studied conceptually by psychologists, has three aspects: potential intelligence, actual intelligence, and measured intelligence. This discussion will center around age changes in measured intelligence.

Measured intelligence is actual mental ability (i.e., measured performance of basic cognitive abilities) defined in terms of responses to items on a test. Yet no matter how extensive or well-prepared a test is, there is always a margin of error in its measurement of actual mental ability. The most frequently used test in studies of adult intelligence and age-related changes is the Wechsler Adult Intelligence Scale (WAIS).

Intelligence quotient (IQ) is a test score that is compared with the normal or average score of 100. When the WAIS is used for adults aged 20 to 75 and older, there is an age factor built into the determination of what is normal. In Figure 18.3, the heavy black line indicates the mean raw scores on the WAIS by age. Note that measured performance peaks about age 25 and declines thereafter, particularly after age 65. In scoring measured performance, a handicap or advantage is built into the WAIS IQ score to control for age. There could be a 40-point difference between the score at age 25 and the score at age 75, and yet the IQ score would be the same. The importance of this is that the most frequently used test of mental ability incorporates an assumption that a 40-point drop in score from age 25 to age 75 is normal.

In practical terms, however, the average decline with age in WAIS scores masks a large amount of individual variation. Any given older person might have an extremely high IQ even when compared to the young. In fact, the correlation between age and IQ is not particularly high, only around −0.40. This means that if the odds against predicting the IQ score were 10 to 1, then knowledge of age would reduce these odds to 6 to 1, not a particularly stunning reduction.

Intelligence testing does not measure a single ability, but rather a set of abilities. Broadly, the WAIS yields separate scores for verbal and performance IQ. The WAIS includes subtests measuring information, vocabulary, comprehension, arithmetic, similarities, digit span, picture completion, object assembly, block design, picture arrangement, and digit symbol tasks.[42] Elderly subjects do best on the information subtest and worst on the digit symbol subtest. The subtests can be broken into two sets; one set dealing with verbal ability and the other dealing with performance ability. Older people consistently do better on the verbal tests than they do on the performance tests. Subtest patterns on the WAIS indicate that stored information and verbal abilities are sustained in old age at a much higher level than are psychomotor-perceptual-integrative skills.[42,43] Of relevance here is that most of the performance subtests are timed while many of the verbal subtests are not. Timed tests may be influenced by reaction time which shows an age-related decline.

There are a number of factors which influence age changes in IQ. Perhaps the most important is the individual's initial level of function. People with scores in the 95th percentile (i.e., with scores high enough that 95 percent of all scores fall below theirs), show a leveling off in vocabulary scores between the ages of 20 and 30. Thereafter, these individuals scores show a plateau or a slight rise with advancing age.[44] On the other hand, people in the 25th percentile show a marked decline in vocabulary scores after the age of 30. This suggests that those with a stronger verbal base to begin with continue to acquire verbal intelligence as the years progress, and those with a weaker verbal foundation initially show a progressive decline in ability as the years go by.

Performance on an intelligence test is closely related to such factors as motivation, anxiety, and cooperation. An environment producing anxiety, or a poorly motivated or uncooperative individual, will prevent accurate measurement of what that individual is actually capable of accomplishing intellectually.

Another factor that has great influence on performance on an intelligence test is the level of education: the higher the educational level, the higher the test scores. It is difficult to determine whether intelligence or education comes first, but they are highly correlated.

IQ is also affected by the health status of the individual being tested. Suboptimal levels of health have been shown to have a negative influence on performance on IQ tests. In fact, it has been hypothesized that rapid declines in IQ after the age of 65 could very likely be the result of poor health. Arteriosclerosis has been correlated to markedly decreased scores.

Most studies of intelligence and age compare test scores of people of different ages using a cross-sectional study model and assume that the only variable is age. This assumption is obviously difficult to defend. Older people have lived through a different era and developed a different body of "symbols" than younger people. Life experience is likely to be a strong influencing variable. The studies discussed measured age differences as opposed to age changes in intelligence. The most accurate study design in the examination of age changes in intelligence would be a longitudinal study following the individual

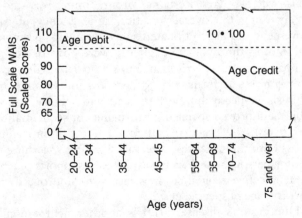

Figure 18.3   Full scale WAIS scores as a function of age. (*Reproduced with permission from Botwinick, J. Cognitive Processes in Maturity and Old Age. New York: Springer; 1967: 3.*)

through life with periodic measures of intelligence. Such studies have been conducted and have shown the same patterns of changes noted above except that the declines observed in overall scores were much smaller. This would suggest that at least part of what appears to be the decline in intelligence of older people is actually a change in skills that are being emphasized by the culture.

Memory is also a factor influencing an older individual's performance on intelligence tests. Studies have shown that short-term memory tends to lose efficiency with advancing age, as previously discussed. Since perceptive and integrative skills depend heavily on short-term memory, and vocabulary and information skills depend mainly on long-term memory, these findings may account for much of the observed difference in IQ test performances between older and younger individuals.

MOTOR LEARNING

Beyond the cognitive components of learning (e.g., memory, intelligence), motor learning is a very important part of therapeutic interventions with the elderly. Considerable age-related changes in the neuromuscular and sensory systems, as described in Chapter 3, paint a picture of progressive decline; however, practicing movement patterns has been found to be very effective in reestablishing ease of movement patterns and postural control.[45–47] Motor learning can occur at any age. Many of the declines in functional capabilities are the result of compensation for muscle imbalances, postural changes, and pain. Rehabilitation efforts that address these compensatory problems will result in relearning of sequential movements.

Recent studies of the improvement of perceptual performance as a function of activity training (i.e., perceptual learning) have provided new insights into the neuronal substrates of this type of skill learning in the adult brain. Issues such as where in the brain, when, and under what conditions practice-related changes occur have been investigated.[48] Karni and Bertini[48] suggest that a behaviorally relevant degree of plasticity is retained in the older adult cortex, even within early, low-level representations in sensory and motor-processing streams. The acquisition and retention of skills may share many characteristics with the functional plasticity subserving early-life learning and development. While the specificity of learning provides localization constraints, an important clue to the nature of the underlying neuronal changes is the time course of learning or relearning activity in a healthy older adult.[48] If, however, a neuromuscular pathology exists, learning is often impaired.

Prior studies have shown that procedural learning is severely impaired in patients with diffuse cerebellar damage (cortical degeneration) as measured by the serial reaction time task (SRTT). Gomez-Beldarrain and associates[49] hypothesized that focal cerebellar lesions can also have lateralized effects on procedural learning. They studied elderly patients with single, unilateral vascular lesions in the territory of the posterior-inferior or superior cerebellar artery, and compared the study group to age- and sex-matched controls. The results of their intervention showed that the study group did not acquire procedural knowledge when performing a task with the hand ipsilateral to the lesion, but showed normal learning with the contralateral hand. This suggests a critical role for the cerebellum and crossed cerebellar-prefrontal connections, or both, in this type of motor learning.[49]

Evidence suggests that patients suffering from Parkinson's disease (PD) demonstrate less sequence learning in the SRTT. One of the problems with this task is that it is motor-intensive and, given the motor difficulties which characterize Parkinson's disease (e.g., tremor, impaired facility of movement, rigidity, and loss of postural reflexes), there is the possibility that patients with PD are capable of sequence learning but are simply unable to demonstrate this because of a decrease in reaction time. Westwater and colleagues[50] examined the performance of patients with PD and healthy controls matched for verbal fluency, on a verbal version of the SRTT where the standard button-pressing response was replaced by a spoken response. The PD group demonstrated less sequence learning than the controls and this was independent of age and severity of illness. These results add support to other studies that have found impaired sequence learning in PD patients.[50]

Individuals with PD have difficulty initiating and performing complex, sequential movements. Practice generally leads to faster initiation and execution of movements in healthy adults; however, whether practice similarly improves motor performance in patients with PD remains controversial. To assess the effects of practice on motor performance, Behrman and associates[51] compared patients with PD to control subjects doing rapid arm-reaching tasks with different levels of movement complexity for 120 trials over two days. Response programming was studied by analyzing the overall reaction time latency of each movement and its fractionated subcomponents, premotor, and motor time. Practice effects were investigated by comparing pretest performance to immediate and delayed retention test performances (10 minutes and 48 hours rest intervals, respectively). Both patients with PD and control subjects improved speeded performance of sequential targeting tasks by practice and retained the improvement across both retention test intervals. Finding a learning effect for persons with Parkinson's disease supports practice as an effective rehabilitation strategy to improve motor performance of specific tasks.

Huntington's disease (HD) is another neuromuscular disease where learning, both cognitive and motor learning, can be compromised. Skill learning in early stage HD patients was compared with that of normal controls on two perceptual-motor tasks, rotary pursuit and mirror tracing, in a study by Gabrieli and associates.[52] HD patients demonstrated a dissociation between impaired rotary pursuit and intact mirror tracing skill learning. These results suggest that different forms of perceptual-motor skill learning are mediated by separable neural circuits. A striatal memory system may be essential for sequence or open-loop skill learning but not for skills that involve the closed-loop learning, of novel visual response mappings. It is hypothesized by these researchers that working memory deficits in HD result from frontostriatal damage and account broadly for intact and impaired long-term learning and memory in HD patients.[52]

TEACHING STRATEGIES FOR THE ELDERLY

Life is an educational process. Some education occurs in formal settings, such as schools, but most learning occurs informally through everyday experiences. It has been shown that adults of all ages benefit from education and that formal educational experiences can assist the older adult to prepare for career changes and retirement. Learning environments are also useful in compensating for deficits in sensory input, memory, and physical changes that may occur with aging.

Though the research previously reviewed indicates that older adults may have more difficulty in the acquisition or encoding of information and in retrieving stored information, these age differences have been found to be quite minimal. Clearly, adults of all ages, in the absence of pathology, have no difficulty in learning.[53] Most of the studies on memory training involve encoding of information into long-term store and focus on training older learners in encoding strategies. Older adult learners do not automatically employ encoding strategies,[54] although when instructed in their use, elderly learners utilize these techniques effectively.

Face-name recall (i.e., remembering people's names) is one of the most common memory problems. Yesavage,[55] in a series of studies, examined the effectiveness of imagery in name-face recall. Elderly subjects were taught to form associations using visual imagery,[55,56] and those subjects who learned this technique were found to have significantly improved face-name recall. In a subsequent study, pretraining in muscle relaxation techniques reduced performance anxiety and significantly improved learning in the same subjects using imagery.[56] These imagery studies used elderly subjects living in the community, which raises the question, "Can similar procedures in memory training be used to improve functioning of elderly individuals with dementia?" So far, the evidence is not very encouraging. In a study examining the effectiveness of visual imagery training among subjects with cognitive declines, subjects improved somewhat in tests given immediately following the training; however, there was

no latency or long-term retention and these improvements were not maintained.[57] However, with intensive memory training in subjects with retrograde and anterograde amnesia and head injury patients, Wilson and Moffat[58] found some improvement in both immediate and latent recall.

It appears that memory performance of healthy elderly people can be improved through memory training.[59] Whether this improvement is maintained over time has not been well documented. It is also not evident that the elderly spontaneously employ these training strategies in everyday situations. Rehearsal of encoding strategies is effective in keeping information in short-term memory, but for encoding information into long-term memory, organizational strategies, mnemonics, and imagery are more useful. Likewise, in prospective memory (i.e., remembering an appointment), using of time monitoring strategies, like calendars or timing devices, has been shown to be particularly effective. Most of the research on memory focuses on the use of internal memory aids (encoding strategies). As most people, young or old, generally use external aids, such as making lists, it would be helpful for future research to examine external strategies for improving memory in the elderly.[60–63]

The elderly do just as well as younger people on recognition tasks but have more difficulty with verbatim recall.[64] They are adept at retaining the gist of a text but have difficulty remembering the details. These findings are important when developing a means of assessing learning in the elderly. For example, multiple-choice or true/false items may be more effective procedures, since both involve recognition memory. Short answer or fill-in-the-blank questions, on the other hand, would be difficult because they require recall of specific information. Providing sufficient time for recall is also important.[62]

When teaching the elderly, it must be kept in mind that there may be some loss of vision or hearing. Compensation for these losses could facilitate processing of the information. Aids, such as larger print, avoidance of rapid speaking, seating the hearing impaired near the speaker to facilitate lip reading, and repetition of the main points, are helpful in assisting the elderly in learning tasks and retaining information. The capacity to pay attention may decline with age,[62] and repetition ensures the learners can grasp a point even if they were inattentive when it was first presented.

Many principles of learning amplify the information-processing model of learning: people learn best in pleasant surroundings; they are most likely to repeat activities which they experience as pleasant; overlearning allows task performance to be accomplished automatically; and people are most likely to remember those tasks in which they have been actively involved (i.e., "doing" influences the depth of encoding and storage). In addition, if individuals "forget" something they once knew, they relearn it faster than if they'd never learned it before.[10]

TEACHING IN THE THERAPEUTIC SETTING

In the process of implementing treatment, allied health professionals consistently function in the role of "teacher." It is important for them to be knowledgeable not only about the content of the information they are conveying but also, even more importantly, about the capability of the elderly individual for learning. Therapists must understand the developmental changes that occur in older persons that ultimately affect their learning capabilities, and adapt instructional sessions to enhance the learning process.

Documented changes in sensory function can limit or distort reception, perception, monitoring, feedback, and transmission of incoming stimuli. A general slowing of neural processes seems to occur with age as demonstrated by decreased conduction over multisynaptic pathways.[65] There is also progressive age-related changes in response to cutaneous, proprioceptive, vestibular and other stimuli.[65] There are reported visual declines in acuity, accommodation, field luminance factors, color sensitivity, perception of ambiguous figures and illusions, figural aftereffects, serial learning, figure ground organization, closure, spatial abilities, and visual memory.[66] Some of these variables have been considered in the IQ and memory research reviewed, though not comprehensibly in any one study. If all of these factors are not considered, then these sensory variables may be confounding with cognitive variables.

Aging changes also occur in the outer ear, the inner ear, and central auditory processing that are reflected in a decreased ability to inhibit background noise and other irrelevant signals, and which decrease auditory acuity and perception of high-frequency sounds. The older person's ability to hear and understand speech in less than ideal listening environments is particularly affected.[67] Attentional deficits further compromise the accuracy of input and registration of stimuli. Inaccuracies in the first stage of learning (input and registration) affect the subsequent stages of information processing. Stimuli which is not adequately registered cannot be effectively encoded (stored) or retrieved.

A marked slowing in learning ability in the elderly is reported whether a simple motor movement or a complex cognitive process is involved. Older adults benefit from having longer periods of time for inspection and response. Self-paced learning leads to the best performance.[68] The elderly tend to make more errors of omission than errors of commission.[69] Concrete information is learned more accurately and efficiently than abstract information,[70] and concept learning is also better when information is conveyed in concrete (as opposed to abstract) language.[69] When the opportunity to practice psychomotor tasks is given, learning and performance improve, regardless of the difficulty of the task.[71] When unlimited numbers of trials are given for the mastery of a task, the elderly can

recall information as effectively as younger persons; however, more trials are required by elderly, to attain this goal.[69] Elderly who are given verbal feedback concerning their performance improve significantly on subsequent related problems. As a general rule, they perform best when instructions are given in a supportive manner.[69] These factors that influence older adult information aquisition should be considered if learning is to be accomplished in the therapeutic setting.

In considering age-related changes in learning, it becomes clear that health care professionals who interact with the elderly must be particularly sensitive to learner needs and diligent in structuring teaching settings to maximize and individualize learning. For example, some people are auditory learners, and some are visual learners, while others need kinesthetic input and learn by doing. Some tasks are better taught by demonstration and some by verbal instruction.

The learning environment determines and influences the educational experience. An environment that is conducive to learning promotes the process, and as a general rule, an environment that is familiar to the learner is the preferred environment for learning new skills. Familiar settings induce a sense of security in which pertinent new information can be attended to. Learning in the natural environment (i.e., the home or work environment) eliminates the need for the client to transfer or generalize information to a home or work setting. In unfamiliar settings, the learner is more likely to be attracted by, and responsive to, novel environmental stimuli. When unfamiliar treatment environments must be used, they should be structured to simulate the natural environment whenever possible and to diminish the number of competing stimuli. Once a new skill is learned, practice in a variety of environments will assist in generalizing its use.

Environments and procedures that are orderly and organized enhance the learner's ability to process information in an orderly and organized fashion. A cluttered or busy environment creates irrelevant, distracting stimuli in the learning environment and impedes the learning process.

Physical and psychological comfort are also important to consider in the treatment setting. Noise levels, color schemes, adequate lighting, ventilation, and comfortable room temperature should all be considered. Glossy, highly waxed floors and work surfaces that distort and reflect light should be avoided. Comfortable chairs and proper table heights are also recommended. Background noises (e.g., computers, air conditioners, running water, and other appliances) should be eliminated so they don't interfere with foreground sound perception. Most kitchen and bathroom settings compromise hearing; the lack of carpeting, drapes, and padded furniture impose additional noise and reverberating sounds.

The persona of the therapist is also an important source of psychological comfort for the elderly learner. A calm, patient, unhurried, interested, knowledgeable and assured health care provider can decrease situational stress and promote a climate of acceptance and reassurance. Conveying verbally and nonverbally that the elderly individual is a valued person with valuable ideas to contribute and that experimentation and failure are important processes in learning new skills enhances the environment. Positive reinforcement for good efforts, as well as good performance, is crucial in facilitating the learning process in an elderly person.

Teaching methods and techniques in the therapeutic setting include all those behaviors employed by instructors to communicate particular pieces of information to the learners.[69] Variables that influence learning include: the organization of material, the rate of presentation, the choice of task, the mode of presentation, and covert strategies.[62]

Organization of Information

New information needs to be presented in a highly organized fashion. Visual displays should be simple configurations that explicitly demonstrate a few salient points. Verbal instructions and directions must emphasize the most important information in a simple manner. Written instructions need to be clearly written in large print with section headings and with emphasis on the major points. Only information relevant to the task at hand should be presented. Differences and similarities between new and old tasks need to be identified. Whole-part-whole learning is a recommended strategy with the elderly. With this technique the entire task and anticipated goal are introduced, then the parts are identified, and each is related to the preceding steps and to the whole. For instance, the person whose end goal is independent meal preparation has to accomplish many component steps in the process of reaching that goal. The individual will have to understand the importance of each step (e.g., mobilizing joints and strengthening particular muscle groups or increasing fine motor coordination and endurance) and how each step relates to the end objective.

Rate of Presentation

Information should be presented at a rate compatible with the learner's ability to comprehend and respond. Generally, this rate will correspond with the complexity of concepts and tasks being taught. Simple, concrete tasks require less time to learn. When instructing the elderly, directions should be presented slowly and ample time for practice provided. If fatigue or confusion occurs, the instructional sessions should be kept shorter.

Task Choice

It is important that the choice of task be directed toward attainment of a preestablished, desirable goal. The task should allow the learners to express and fulfill their own personal needs (e.g., creativity, socialization, mastery). Tasks that interest the learner should be selected, if possible. A preliminary development of an interest inventory will identify what is important to the individual learner. In other words, activities chosen need to be relevant and meaningful to the learner, and the purpose for learning each task needs to be clear. Self-care tasks seem to have the greatest relevance for most elderly individuals. Goals such as transfer training, eating, and dressing are concrete and usually experienced as meaningful. Practice of self-care tasks in a familiar environment is best for obtaining follow-through of the learned tasks. Activities such as mat exercises or fine hand coordination exercises may not seem relevant to the older learner. In these cases, it is important to relate the activities to the established treatment goals. Explain and demonstrate the mobility and strengthening components of mat activities as they relate to functional goals. This will help in making the activities more concrete and necessary for accomplishing the end goal.

Tasks should be sufficiently challenging but easy enough to assure successful experiences. Building on past successes will promote advancing toward the treatment goals. A knowledgeable, enthusiastic therapist can help to motivate learners to engage in the necessary tasks to be learned.

Presentation of Information

Instructions for the older learner should to be concrete, simple, clear, and one step at a time. The learner should be given the opportunity to practice each step before subsequent steps are introduced. Demonstrations, which are carefully planned, are also helpful modes of education. With a good demonstration, the learner is given the opportunity to initiate the exact movement until each step has been completed. It is also advised that demonstrations be done in the same position as the learner will be doing the task. For demonstration to be effective in influencing the learner, it requires skillful observation and visual memorization of the teacher's movements, followed by a transfer of the complex visual information to an opposite orientation. This can be frustrating for the older learner.

To accommodate for hearing loss, the instructor needs to be within ten feet of the listener, use a low pitched speaking voice with a moderate volume (shouting distorts sound in the presence of hearing losses), and find a position so that the listener can see the speaker's mouth. Since much information is communicated by facial expression, gestures, and body language, these should be acknowledged as important facilitators for conveying information. Verbal and nonverbal language need to be congruent, because understanding is enhanced when nonconfusing visual stimuli accompany auditory information.

To compensate for some of the aging changes in vision with aging, use a large, bold print on a solid background for printed material. The use of a visual aid, such as a magnifying glass, may be used when large print is not available. Lighting is also important. Too much light can create glare, and too little light will diminish the older learner's ability to see anything.

Motor learning may be enhanced by physically guiding the learner's extremities through the desired patterns of movement. It is preferable for the teacher to stand behind the learner so that the learner can concentrate on the sensation of movement. Movements should be repeated several times without any alteration in the motion. The learner is eventually weaned from guided patterning and asked to perform the movement without the teacher's tactile, proprioceptive, and motoric assistance.

Covert Strategies

Older adults tend not to spontaneously use organized methods or ploys to enhance learning and memory, as previously discussed. They do, however, benefit from instructions in memory strategies. The use of memory strategies is a means of compensating for real or anticipated deficits in memory.

It is important to optimize overall health status by implementing the concept of independence. The more one can do for oneself, the more one is capable of doing independently. The more that is done for an aged individual, the less capable that person becomes of functioning on an optimal independent level and the more likely the progression of a disability. The advancing stages of disabilities increase an individual's vulnerability to illness, emotional stress, and injury. Aged persons' subjective appraisal of their health status influences how they react to their symptoms, how vulnerable they consider themselves, and when they decide they can or cannot accomplish an activity. Often an aged person's self-appraisal of health is a good predictor of the rehabilitation clinician's evaluation of the individual's health and functional status, but such assessments may also differ in many ways. In older persons, perceptions of their health may be determined in large part by their level of psychological well-being and by whether or not they continue in rewarding roles and activities.[72]

As older persons' perception of their health status is an important motivator for their compliance with a rehabilitation program, it is important to discuss this further. One notable study showed that even when age, sex, and health status (as evaluated by physicians) were controlled for, perceived health and mortality from heart disease were strongly related.[73] Those who rated their health as poor were two to three times as likely to die as those who rated their health as excellent. A Canadian longitudinal study of persons over 65 produced similar results.[74] Over three years, the mortality of those who described their health as poor at the beginning of the study was about three times the mortality of those who initially described their health

as good, regardless of their actual (or measured) health status.

Despite this awareness among older persons of their actual state of health, the aged are known to fail to report serious symptoms and wait longer than younger persons to seek help. It is with this in mind that rehabilitation professionals need to listen carefully to their aged clients. It appears that, contrary to the popular view that older individuals are somewhat hypochondriacal, the aged generally deserve serious attention when they bring complaints to their caregivers. Their perceived level of health will greatly impact the outcomes of functional goals in the geriatric rehabilitation setting whether it be acute, rehabilitative, home, or chronic care.

Rosillo and Fagel[75] found that improvement in rehabilitation tasks correlated well with patients' own appraisal of their potential for recovery but not very well with others' appraisal. Stoedefalke[76] reports that positive reinforcement (frequent positive feedback) for older persons in rehabilitation greatly improved their performance and feelings of success. This indicates that aged persons can improve in their physical functioning when modifications in therapeutic interventions provide more frequent feedback. Some research indicates that older persons with chronic illness have low initial aspirations with regard to their abilities to perform various tasks.[77] As situations in which they succeeded or failed occurred, their aspirations changed to more closely reflect their abilities. Older persons may have different beliefs about their abilities compared to younger persons.[78] When subjects were given an unsolvable problem, younger subjects ascribed their failure to not trying hard enough, while older subjects ascribed their failure to inability. On subsequent tests, younger individuals tried harder and older subjects gave up. These age differences indicate a variation in the perceived locus-of-control. This holds extreme importance in the rehabilitation potential of an aged person. If the cause of failure is seen as an immutable characteristic by the person, then little effort in the future can be expected.

Aged individuals may have a higher anxiety level in rehabilitation situations because they fear failure or are afraid of looking bad to their family or therapist.[79] Eisdorfer[79] found that if anxiety is high enough, then the behavior is redirected toward reducing the anxiety rather than accomplishing the task. Weinberg[80] found that subjects set their own goals for task achievement even if they are directed to adopt the therapist's goals. In another study, Mento, Steele, and Karren[81] reported that the best performance at difficult tasks (as many rehabilitation tasks are) occurs when the aged person sets a very specific goal, such as walking ten feet with a walker. If the person simply tries to do better, then performance is not improved as much.

Depression also plays a big role in learning and memory. King and associates[82] compared the verbal learning and memory of elderly patients with major depression and nondepressed control participants. Except for verbal retention, the depressive group had deficits in most aspects of performance, including cued and uncued recall and delayed recognition memory. As well, there were interactions between depression effects and age effects on some measures such that depressives' performance declined more rapidly with age than did the performance of controls. The results indicate that the integrity of learning and memory are compromised in the presence of late-life depression. Depression of an elderly individual in a rehabilitation setting needs to be addressed as a part of a comprehensive therapeutic intervention. Failure to do so will result in poor learning capabilities for new activities, and failure at a task could further exacerbate the depression.

These are important motivational components to keep in mind when working with an aged client, because the therapeutic approach of the clinician may have the greatest impact on the successful functional outcomes in a geriatric rehabilitation setting.

References

1. Zauszniewski JA, Martin MH. Developmental task achievement and learned resourcefulness in healthy older adults. *Arch Psychiatr Nurs.* 1999; 13(1):41–47.
2. Vakil E, Agmon-Ashkenazi D. Baseline performance and learning rate of procedural and declarative memory tasks: younger versus older adults. *J Gerontol B Psychol Sci Soc Sci.* 1997; 52(5):P229–P234.
3. Norman GR. The adult learner: A mythical species. *Acad Med.* 1999; 74(8):886–889.
4. Woodruff-Pak DS, Finkbiner RG. Larger nondeclarative than declarative deficits in learning and memory in human aging. *Psychol Aging.* 1995; 10(3):416–426.
5. Karni A, Meyer G, Jezzard P, Adams MM, Turner R, Ungerleider LG. Functional MRI evidence for adult motor cortex plasticity during motor skill learning. *Nature.* 1995; 377(6545):155–158.
6. D'Eredita MA, Hoyer WJ. An examination of the effects of adult age on explicit and implicit learning of figural sequences. *Mem Cognit.* 1999; 27(5):890–895.
7. Gardner DL, Greenwell SC, Costich JF. Effective teaching of the older adult. *Top Geriatric Rehabil.* 1991; 6(3):1–14.
8. Hodgson C, Ellis AW. Last in, first to go: Age acquisition and naming in the elderly. *Brain Lang.* 1998; 64(1):146–163.
9. Rubin DC, Rahhal TA, Poon LW. Things learned in early adulthood are remembered best. *Mem Cognit.* 1998; 26(1):3–19.
10. Merriam SB, Cafferella RS. *Learning in Adulthood.* San Francisco: Jossey-Bass; 1991.
11. Arenberg D and Robertson-Tchabo EA. Learning and aging. In: Birren JE, Schaie KW, eds. *Handbook of the Psychology of Aging.* New York: Van Nostrand Reinhold; 1977.
12. Canestrari RE. Age changes in acquisition. In: Talland, GA, ed. *Human Aging and Behavior.* New York: Academic Press; 1968.
13. Salthouse TA. Aging associations: Influence of speed on adult age differences in associative learning. *J Exp Psychol Learn Mem Cogn.* 1994; 20(6):1486–1503.
14. Taub HA. Paired associates learning as a function of age, rate and instructions. *J of Genetic Psych.* 1967; 111:41–46.
15. Leech S and Witte KL. Paired-associate learning in elderly adults as related to pacing and incentive conditions. *Dev Psych.* 1971; 5:174–180.
16. Eisendorfer D, Nowlin J, Wilkie F. Improvement of learning in the aged by modification of autonomic nervous system activity. *Science.* 1970; 170:1327–1329.
17. Botwinick J and Storandt M. *Memory, Related Functions and Age.* Springfield, IL: Charles C Thomas; 1974.
18. Spitzer M, Bellemann ME, Kammer T, et al. Functional MR imaging of semantic information processing and learning-related effects using psychometrically controlled stimulation paradigms. *Brain Res Cognit Brain Res.* 1996; 4(3):149–161.
19. Reber PJ, Stark CE, Squire LR. Cortical areas supporting category learning identified using functional MRI. *Proc Natl Acad Sci USA.* 1998; 95(2):747–750.
20. Fattapposta F, Amabile G, Cordischi MV, et al. Long-term practice effects on a new skilled motor learning: An electro physiological study. *Electroencephalogr Clin Neurophysiol.* 1996; 99(6):495–507.
21. Naveh-Benjamin M, Craik FI. Memory for context and its use in item memory: Comparisons of younger and older persons. *Psychol Aging.* 1995; 10(2):284–293.
22. Spencer WD, Raz N. Memory for facts, source, and context: can frontal lobe dysfunction explain age-related differences? *Psychol Aging.* 1994; 9(1):149–159.
23. Spencer WD, Raz N. Differential effects of aging on memory for content and context: A meta-analysis. *Psychol Aging.* 1995; 10(4):527–539.
24. Sekiya H, Magill RA, Sidaway B, Anderson DI. The contextual interference effect for skill variations from the same and different generalized motor programs. *Res Q Exerc Sport.* 1994; 65(4):330–338.
25. Lee YS. Effects of learning contexts on implicit and explicit learning. *Mem Cognit.* 1995; 23(6):723–734.
26. Bernasconi J, Gustafson K. Contextual quick-learning and generalization by humans and machines. *Network.* 1998; 9(1):85–106.

27. Koutstaal W, Schacter DL, Johnson MK, Gallucio L. Facilitation and impairment of event memory produced by photographic review in younger and older adults. *Mem Cognit.* 1999; 27(3):478–493.

28. Fisher J and Pierce RC. Dimensions of intellectual functioning in the aged. *J Gerontol.* 1967; 22:166–173.

29. Reese HW, Rodeheaver D. Problem solving and complex decision making. In: Birren JE, Schaie KW, eds. *Handbook of the Psychology of Aging.* 2nd ed. New York: Van Nostrand Reinhold; 1985.

30. Polya G. *How to Solve It: A New Aspect of Mathematical Method.* 2nd ed. Princeton: Princeton University Press; 1971.

31. Crovitz E. Reversing a learning deficit in the aged. *J Gerontol.* 1966; 21:236–238.

32. Offenbach SI. A developmental study of hypothesis testing and cue selection strategies. *Dev Psych.* 1974; 10:484–490.

33. Hartley AA. Adult age differences in deductive reasoning processes. *J Gerontol.* 1981; 36:700–706.

34. Sanders JA, Sterns HL, Smith M, Sanders RE. Modification of concept identification performance in older adults. *Dev Psych.* 1975; 11:824–829.

35. Sanders RE, Sanders JA, Mayes GJ, Sielski KA. Enhancement of conjunctive concept attainment in older adults. *Dev Psych.* 1976; 12:485–486.

36. Denney NW. Task demands and problem-solving strategies in middle-age and older adults. *J Gerontol.* 1980; 35:559–564.

37. Papalia D, Bielby D. Cognitive functioning in middle and old age adults: A review of research based on Piaget's theory. *Hum Dev.* 1974; 17:424–443.

38. Muhs PJ, Hooper FH, Papalia-Finlay DE. An initial analysis of cognitive functioning across the life-span. *Int J Aging Hum Dev.* 1980; 10:311–333.

39. Rubin KH. Decentration skills in institutionalized and noninstitutionalized elderly. Proceedings of 81st Annual Convention, American Psychological Association; 1973; 8(part 2):759–760.

40. Papalia-Finley DE, Blackburn J, Davis E. Training cognitive functioning in the elderly—Inability to replicate previous findings. *Int J Aging Hum Dev.* 1980; 12:111–117.

41. Willis SL. Towards an educational psychology of the older adult learner: intellectual and cognitive bases. In: Birren JE, Schaie KW, eds. *Handbook of the Psychology of Aging.* 2nd ed. New York: Van Nostrand Reinhold; 1985.

42. Ackerman PL, Rolfhus EF. The locus of adult intelligence: Knowledge, abilities, and nonability traits. *Psychol Aging.* 1999; 14(2):314–330.

43. Hulicka IM. Age changes and age differences in memory functioning. *Gerontologist.* 1967; 7(2, part II): 46–54.

44. Jones HE. Intelligence and problem-solving. In Birren JE, ed. *Handbook of Aging and the Individual.* Chicago: University of Chicago Press; 1959: 700–738.

45. Wolf SL, Barnhart HX, Ellison GL, Coogler CE. The effect of Tai Chi Quan and computerized balance training on postural stability in older subjects. *Phys Ther.* 1997; 77(4):371–384.

46. Wolf SL, Coogler C, Xu T. Exploring the basis for Tai Chi Chuan as a therapeutic exercise approach. *Arch Phys Med Rehabil.* 1997; 79:886–892.

47. Bottomley JM. The use of Tai Chi as a movement modality in orthopaedics. *Ortho Phys Ther Clin No Amer.* 2000; 9(3):361–373.

48. Karni A, Bertini G. Learning perceptual skills: Behavioral probes into adult cortical plasticity. *Curr Opin Neurobiol.* 1997; 7(4):530–535.

49. Gomez-Beldarrain M, Garcia-Monco JC, Rubio B, Pascual-Leone A. Effect of focal cerebellar lesions on procedural learning in the serial reaction time task. *Exp Brain Res.* 1998; 120(1):25–30.

50. Westwater H, McDowall J, Siegert R, Mossman S, Abernethy D. Implicit learning in Parkinson's disease: Evidence from a verbal version of the serial reaction time task. *J Clin Exp Neuropsychol.* 1998; 20(3):413–418.

51. Behrman AL, Cauraugh JH, Light KE. Practice as an intervention to improve speeded motor performance and motor learning in Parkinson's disease. *J Neurol Sci.* 2000; 174(2):127–136.

52. Gabrieli JD, Stebbins GT, Singh J, Willingham DB, Goetz CG. Intact mirror-tracing and impaired rotary-pursuit skill learning in patients with Huntington's disease: Evidence for dissociable memory systems in skill learning. *Neuropsychology.* 1997; 11(2):272–281.

53. Poon L, Rubin D, Wilson B. *Everyday Cognition and Memory.* Hillsdale, NJ: Lawrence Erlbaum; 1986.

54. Poon L, Walsh-Sweeney L, Fozard J: Memory skill training for the elderly: Salient issues on the use of imagery mnemonics. In: Poon L, ed. *New Directions in Memory and Aging: Proceedings of the George A Talland Memorial Conference.* Hillsdale, NJ: Lawrence Erlbaum; 1980.

55. Yesavage JA. Imagery pretraining and memory training in the elderly. *Gerontology.* 1983; 29:271–275.

56. Yesavage JA, Rose T. The effects of a face-name mnemonic in young, middle aged, and elderly adults. *Exp Aging Res.* 1984; 10:55–57.

57. Zarit SH, Zarit J, Reever K. Memory training or severe memory loss: Effects of senile dementia. *Gerontologist.* 1982; 22:373–377.

58. Wilson B, Moffat N. *Clinical Management of Memory Problems.* Rockville, MD: Aspen Publishers; 1984.

59. McKitrick LA, Friedman LF, Brooks JO III, Pearman A, Kraemer HC, Yesavage JA. Predicting response of older adults to mnemonic training: Who will benefit? *Int Psychogeriatr.* 1999; 11(3):289–300.

60. Chasseigne G, Mullet E, Stewart TR. Aging and multiple cue probability learning: The case of inverse relationships. *Acta Psychol (Amst).* 1997; 97(3): 235–252.

61. McGeorge P, Crawford JR, Kelly SW. The relationship between psychometric intelligence and learning in an explicit and an implicit task. *J Exp Psychol Learn Mem Cogn*. 1997; 23(1):239–245.

62. Whitman N. Learning and teaching styles: Implications for teachers of family medicine. *Fam Med*. 1996; 28(5):321–325.

63. Wilkniss SM, Jones MG, Korol DL, Gold PE, Manning CA. Age-related differences in an ecologically based study of route learning. *Psychol Aging*. 1997; 12(2):372–375.

64. Schaie KW. Cognitive development in aging. In: Obler LK, Alpert M, eds. *Language and Communication in the Elderly*. Lexington, MA: Heath; 1980.

65. Kenney RA. *Physiology of Aging*. Chicago: Year Book Medical Publishers; 1982.

66. Cristarella MC. Visual functions of the elderly. *Am J Occup Ther*. 1987; 31:432–440.

67. Gladstone VS. Hearing loss in the elderly. *Phys & Occup Ther Geriatr*. 1992; 2:5–20.

68. Feldman HS, Lopez MA. *Developmental Psychology for the Health Care Professions: Adulthood and Aging*. Boulder CO: Westview Press; 1982: 2.

69. Okun MA. Implications of geropsychological research for the instruction of older adults. *Adult Education*. 1987; 27:139–155.

70. Rabbitt P. Changes in problem solving ability in old age. In: Birren JE, Schaie KW, eds. *Handbook of the Psychology of Aging*. New York: Van Nostrand Reinhold; 1987: 606–625.

71. Botwinick J. *Aging and Behavior*. 3rd ed. New York: Springer; 1983.

72. Siegler IC, Costa PT Jr. Health behavior relationships. In: Birren JE, Schaie KW, eds. *Handbook of the Psychology of Aging*. 2nd ed. Van Nostrand Reinhold, New York; 1985.

73. Kaplan E. Psychological factors and ischemic heart disease mortality: a focal role for perceived health.

Paper presented at the annual meeting of the American Psychological Association, Washington, DC; 1982.

74. Mossey JM, Shapiro E. Self-rated health: A predictor of mortality among the elderly. *Am J Pub Health*. 1982; 72:800–808.

75. Rosillo RA, Fagel ML. Correlation of psychologic variables and progress in physical therapy: I. Degree of disability and denial of illness. *Arch Phys Med Rehabil*. 1970; 51:227–232.

76. Stoedefalke KG. Motivating and sustaining the older adult in an exercise program. *Top Geriatr Rehab*. 1985; 1:78–83.

77. Nader IM. Level of aspiration and performance of chronic psychiatric patients on a simple motor task. *Percept Mot Skills*. 1985; 60:767–771.

78. Prohaska T, Pontiam IA, Teitleman J. Age differences in attributions to causality: Implications for intellection assessment. *Exp Aging Res*. 1984; 10: 111–117.

79. Eisdorfer L. Arousal and performance: experiments in verbal learning and a tentative theory. In: Talland GA, ed. *Human Aging and Behavior*. New York: Academic Press: 1968.

80. Weinberg R, Bruya L, Jackson A. The effects of goal proximity and goal specificity on endurance performance. *J Soc Psychol*. 1985; 7:296–301.

81. Mento A, Steele RP, Karren RJ. A metaanalytic study of the effects of goal setting on task performance: 1966–1984. *Organ Behav Hum Decis Process*. 1987; 39:52–58.

82. King DA, Cox C, Lyness JM, Conwell Y, Caine ED. Quantitative and qualitative differences in verbal learning performance of elderly depressives and healthy controls. *J Int Neuropsychol Soc*. 1998; 4(2): 115–126.

19

Administration of Geriatric Services

Pearls

- The components of administration are finance and budgeting, policies and procedures, legal concerns, employee relations, and marketing.

- Budgeting is defined as providing a monetary sketch of the department or clinic, and a realistic budget is essential to the financial well-being of the business.

- Need, advantages, disadvantages, and cost are all important considerations when purchasing equipment.

- An organizational plan is a visual chart of the administrative hierarchy.

- The plaintiff has a case if the plaintiff can show actual harm resulted from an action, or if the therapist practiced below local or national standards.

- Equipment should be calibrated annually, and more sophisticated equipment should have precautions and directions posted.

- Marketing is identifying services to be offered and promoting, pricing, and distributing these services to the patients.

INTRODUCTION

As the role of the geriatric rehabilitation therapist continues to evolve, the development of excellent clinical skills skills will be needed in administering care in nursing homes, hospitals, rehabilitation centers, outpatient clinics, and home health agencies. Therapists will be asked to provide administrative advisement and supervision for professional, as well as adjunct, staff.

It is imperative, therefore, that rehabilitation therapists become aware of all aspects of administration. This chapter has two goals: first, to familiarize therapists with administrative terms and concepts; and second, to serve as a reference for therapists working in a rehabilitation facility or a physical or occupational therapy department.

DESCRIPTION OF ADMINISTRATION

Administration is an extremely complex term. It involves not only paperwork for developing a policy and procedure manual, finance, and budgeting but also developing guidelines for effectively managing and motivating people. For the purposes of this chapter, administration will be divided into five areas:

1. Finance and budgeting;
2. Policies and procedures;
3. Legal concerns;
4. Employee relations;
5. Marketing.

The needs of administration vary by position. For example, if the therapist is a staff therapist, his or her administrative needs may be minimal. This therapist may be asked to fill out documentation forms, send in billing slips, and play a very limited role in managing employees. On the other hand, if a therapist is in charge of an entire department, he or she may need to develop human resource information, such as employee handbooks, compliance manuals, billing procedures, documentation procedures, or finance and budget procedures, as well as equipment use forms and marketing strategies. Therefore, the best approach to acquiring an understanding of administrative needs is to gain an understanding of the information in each of the five major areas listed.

FINANCING AND BUDGETING

Financing and budgeting can be defined as a monetary sketch of the needs and plans of a department in any setting. If a therapist works in an outpatient facility, for example, items that must be budgeted are rental of space, equipment, staff time, and ancillary staff (such as receptionists or aides), as well as laundry and other line items. Based on the number of patients that will be seen, the anticipated income, and the costs, the therapist must establish a workable budget for the amount of money dispersed versus the amount of incoming money.

A realistic budget is essential to the financial well-being of a physical or occupational therapy business. No matter how effective the treatment and how dedicated the staff, the hard reality is that if income does not exceed expenditures, the business will fail. Descriptions of the nuances of finance and budget can be gleaned from any elementary course in business, but the difficult part is applying the practices to an actual business.

Figure 19.1 is a notational example of a budget for a medium-sized (gross annual income between $500,000 and $1,000,000) physical therapy business, adapting data from an actual practice in a large metropolitan area. While the specifics are dependent on a wide range of variables, the rough order of magnitude of the percentages spent on various services should be a useful guide.

Figure 19.1 illustrates several points. First and foremost, a profit *must* be made to ensure the long-term viability of the practice. Next, the income comes from services delivered, and expenses should be made only for those items that contribute to earning that income. Budgets should also be living documents. No matter how well planned a budget is, actual income and expenses will vary, and the budget should be modified accordingly during the year.

The financial health of the business should be checked at least once a month. This is a useful time period, since it coincides with the normal cycle of bank statements, as well as payments by insurers and other health care agencies.

In a nursing home setting, therapists who are planning and working in a department will use a similar type of budget and have similar types of concerns. Figures 19.2A and 19.2B give examples of a financial report and budget for a nursing home.

ORGANIZING AND PLANNING FOR STAFF, EQUIPMENT, AND SUPPLIES

Equipment and supplies can be broken up into the equipment and supplies needed by the department versus the equipment and supplies needed for the patient. With respect to departmental equipment, therapists specializing in geriatrics must assess whether or not their equipment will provide a return on investment.

For example, if one were to purchase an expensive piece of exercise equipment, would this in fact provide enough revenue to justify the expense? When writing requests for equipment or in looking for equipment for self-purchase, the therapist should keep in mind these variables: need, advantages, disadvantages, and cost. Therapists, for example, can purchase parallel bars, and these bars provide needed standing support for gait, balance, and posture work. The advantage of parallel bars is that there is a well-documented history of use in the clinical setting. The main disadvantages are that they are expensive and space-consuming. Access to a sturdy railing might be an alternative. In this type of setting, the railing also can be used for gait training.

A department can be sparse, with hooks on the wall for attachment of exercise bands to be used in progressive resistance exercises, or it can be more high technology, with isokinetic equipment and high-tech balance machines. However, this level of sophistication is not always necessary. Table 19.1 presents a listing of the minimum equipment necessary for a nursing home, as well as a more comprehensive listing for a high-tech facility.

Another important category of equipment and supplies is durable medical equipment. To administer efficiently what a facility needs of this type of equipment, therapists must develop policies and procedures to monitor rental, purchase, and resale of the equipment. Therapists in the administrative capacity must develop procedures for purchase or rental of equipment for patient use based on the type of equipment that the patient needs.

Table 19.2 provides a sample of procedural record dispersement of medical supplies in a nursing home facility. This policy and procedure can be modified slightly to be used in an outpatient and hospital setting as well.

DEVELOPING GOALS, PHILOSOPHY, AND ORGANIZATIONAL PLANS

Before developing an outpatient or nursing home department, therapists should carefully review their expected goals and plan accordingly. What is the mission statement of the department? In other words, what are the goals and what kind of plan is one going to use to attain these goals in this setting? In an existing setting, the organizational goals and plans should be reviewed periodically to see that they correspond to the current structure of the practice.

Organizational Goals

Reviewing an organization's goals and objectives will provide the therapist with an idea of the direction in which the practice is or should be moving. Is the practice providing standard care to a small community, moving toward high-quality care in the current area, or expanding into a larger area, or both? Therapists must determine if these

Sample Budget for a Medium Sized Outpatient Physical Therapy Practice.

INCOME

Fees & Services	$745,000
Sales - Equipment	5,000
Total Income	$750,000

EXPENSES

Direct Expenses

Salaries: Owners/officers	$200,000
Salaries: Other employees	230,000
Medical supplies	30,000
Payroll taxes	30,000
Total Direct Expenses	490,000
Gross Profit (Loss)	260,000

Operating Expenses

Accounting	9,000
Advertising	2,000
Annual Report	100
Bank service charges	100
Business meals	4,000
Cleaning	1,000
Contributions	2,000
Data processing	1,000
State income tax (@10%)	5,000
Credit card discount	4,000
Delivery expenses	400
Depreciation	15,000
Dues and subscriptions	1,000
Entertainment	3,000
Education and seminars	2,000
Gifts	2,000
Insurance	24,000
Interest expenses	1,000
Legal fees	4,000
Licenses and permits	500
Miscellaneous expenses	1,200
Office expenses	3,000
Office supplies	6,000
Parking	2,000
Postage	3,000
Printing and stationery	5,000
Publications and books	1,000
Rent	84,000
Repairs and maintenance	2,000
Taxes, personal property	1,500
Tax, sales	200
Telephone	7,000
Travel	5,000
Temporary Help	5,000
Utilities	3,000
Total Operating Expenses	210,000
Income before taxes	50,000
Federal income tax	7,500
NET INCOME	$42,500

Figure 19.1   Sample Budget for Medium Sized Outpatient Practice.

Sample SNF Rehab Budget: Small Unit

	Physical Therapy	Occupational Therapy	Speech Therapy	Total Therapy
Charges	157,000	154,000	28,000	339,000
Expenses	84,000	88,000	14,000	186,000
Overhead	71,000	52,000	8,000	131,000
Gross Margin	2,000	14,000	6,000	22,000
Nonbillable	3,000	2,000	2,000	7,000
Adjust to Cost	2,000	14,000	6,000	22,000
Net Loss	(3,000)	(2,000)	(2,000)	(7,000)

ASSUMPTIONS/NOTES

1. 134 bed facility

2. Medicare average daily census = 7.5 beds or 5.7% of total census

3. Therapy unit staffing

	FTEs
Physical therapist	1.00
Physical therapy aide	1.00
Occupational therapist	1.00
Certified occupational therapy assistant	1.00
Speech language pathologist	0.25
Director of rehab (MD)	0.05

4. Square footage

	SQ. FEET
Physical therapy	644
Occupational therapy	50
Speech therapy	0
Total facility	23,677

5. Facility general & administrative expenses = $490,000/year

6. Rehab services payor mix:

	Mix (%)
Medicare - Part A	60
Medicare - Part B	37
Private/other	2
Welfare	1

7. Loss is due to nonbillable services to welfare patients and services under all-inclusive insurance contracts (where services are covered in the per-diem rate).

Figure 19.2A   Sample SNF Rehabilitation Budget: Small Unit. (Reprinted with permission from Kurtz, H. Medical and Rehabilitation Specialists.)

Sample SNF Rehab Budget: Large Unit

	Physical Therapy	Occupational Therapy	Speech Therapy	Total Therapy
Charges	802,000	268,000	258,000	1,328,000
Expenses	490,000	102,000	66,000	658,000
Overhead	254,000	58,000	32,000	344,000
Gross Margin	58,000	108,000	160,000	326,000
Nonbillable	45,000	50,000	46,000	141,000
Adjust to Cost	55,000	87,000	181,000	273,000
Net Loss	(42,000)	(29,000)	(17,000)	(88,000)

ASSUMPTIONS/NOTES

1. 118 bed facility

2. Medicare average daily census = 15.5 beds or 14% of total census

3. Therapy unit staffing

	FTEs
Physical therapist	5.75
Physical therapist assistant	4.00
Physical therapy aide	1.16
Occupational therapist	2.16
Certified occupational therapy assistant	1.00
Occupational therapy assistant	1.00
Speech language pathologist	1.58
Director of rehab (MD)	0.25

4. Square footage

	SQ. FEET
Physical therapy	2,071
Occupational therapy	496
Speech therapy	134
Total facility	32,584

5. Facility general & administrative expenses = $480,000/year

6. Rehab services payor mix:

	Mix (%)
Medicare - Part A	81
Medicare - Part B	8
Private/other	11
Welfare	0

7. Loss is due to nonbillable services to welfare patients and services under all-inclusive insurance contracts (where services are covered in the per-diem rate).

Figure 19.2B   Sample SNF Rehabilitation Budget: Large Unit. (Reprinted with permission from Kurtz, H. Medical and Rehabilitation Specialists.)

TABLE 19.1 Minimum and Maximum Equipment Lists for PT Departments

Basic Equipment Needs	Maximum Equipment Needs
Exercise mat	List A plus
Treatment table (plinth)	Cybex
Mirror(s)	Kinetron
Stairs	UBE
Complete set cuff weights: 1/2 to 10 lb	Fitron
Parallel bars or sturdy railings	Balance Master
Restorator or bike	KAT
Hot pack (Hydrocollator)	Tekdyne
Wall pulleys	Pro-Stretch
Assortment of ambulation aids:	Complete Theraband Line
Walkers, pick-up, 2 wheel, 4 wheel canes, single point, quad, hemicrutches	Zelex
Swiss ball	Hip Machine
	Fitter

Additional Recommended Equipment

Multimode electrical stimulator

Ultrasound

Tilt table

Whirlpool

TABLE 19.2 Sample Policy and Procedure for Equipment Purchase/Rental

Short-term rental may be appropriate if there is an occasional need for equipment. If the facility routinely uses the equipment on patients, it would be considered part of the departmental costs and would not be billable as medical supply. All equipment must be ordered by the patient's physician and billed under Part A Medicare Claims.

Examples of billable rental equipment:

1. CPM (constant passive motion machines): Used for total joint replacements.

2. Reclining wheelchairs: Used for patients allowed only minimal hip flexion.

3. Transcutaneous Electrical Neuro Stimulation units.

4. Bucks traction unit for lower extremity fractures.

goals agree with their own goals for the future. Does the therapist want to stay in a small practice, working a regular schedule, and doing the best possible job with available resources? Or is the therapist trying to expand the practice, get involved in a larger company, or both? In trying to focus on these issues, it is important to clarify the individual therapist's goals as they relate to the organizational goals of the practice.

Table 19.3 provides a sample mission statement and philosophy statement. Therapists in a supervisory role should use the type of guidelines suggested in Table 19.3 to develop their own personal philosophy, taking into consideration not only current goals but also expected goals for the next five to ten years.

TABLE 19.3 Sample Mission Statement and Philosophy Statement

Mission Statement

Our mission is to provide the highest quality rehabilitation services that:

- Meet and maximize each resident's individual needs.
- Promote the quality of life of each resident entrusted to our care.
- Use highly trained rehabilitation professionals.
- Integrate an interdisciplinary approach toward the rehabilitative potential of each resident.

Philosophy of Resident Care

- Our goal in rehabilitation services is to provide the highest quality of service to each individual resident who needs assistance in returning to his or her maximal functional abilities.
- The rehabilitation therapist at the facility plays a vital role in the operation of the skilled nursing facility, not only by being involved with the residents currently receiving therapy, but also by providing input for all residents in the facility through staff education and consultation, attendance at key meetings within the facility, routine therapy programs, and involvement in RNA programs.
- Each resident has some potential for rehabilitation, however small. It is the responsibility of the health care team to evaluate the medical, physical, and psychosocial needs of each resident. From this assessment, a health care plan is designed that encourages maximum functional independence and above all promotes the well-being and quality of life of each resident.

Reprinted with permission for Therapy Management Innovations, Inc.

Organizational Plan

The organizational plan is a visual chart of the administrative hierarchy of the department, facility, or entire company. It is a charting of the various employees' positions in relation to others (Figure 19.3). This can be done on a small scale (e.g., a one- to two person department) or on a larger scale (e.g., a company of 1000).

This can be very useful for getting an idea of how a company's hierarchy operates, how a person fits into the practice, or how a setting will change if a new person is hired. For example, an administrator can simply add the new employee to the chart in various places to see how it affects the chain of command.

LEGAL CONSTRAINTS

Legal ramifications are extremely important for therapists in both administrative and practicing capacities. Therapists must be certain that they have taken adequate measures to provide an optimal and legally safe environment for their patients.

A major concern of therapists is being sued for malpractice or negligence. The remainder of this section provides information to assist in understanding the legal climate and prepares the geriatric therapist for some common scenarios that may occur.

The malpractice scenario is as follows: the plaintiff, who is the person suing, tries to provide evidence that, through a failure to meet accepted standards, a patient has been injured. The defendant, or the person being sued, tries to show that quality care was given. Therefore, it is imperative that the therapist constantly complies with regulations and safety practices. The safety practices of the clinic should be outlined in the policy and procedure manual, and the therapist must constantly document that safety measures are in place. Legal documentation, separate from the documentation used for the purposes of reimbursement, is therefore essential. When sued, health professionals must be able to show that they provided care equal to or exceeded by the national, as well as the local, standard. If called to appear in court, local practitioners who can attest to local practices, or national experts who can testify on the differences between local and national standards, may be useful.

If a patient receives minimal or nonspecific harm because of treatment, a suit would be improper. Therapists can be sued only because actual harm resulted from treatment. For example, if a patient states that the therapist did not diagnose a particular problem, but the therapist did not prevent the patient from obtaining an adequate diagnosis, there is no fault. However, if, because of an inadequately maintained piece of equipment, a patient is injured, the therapist is at fault.

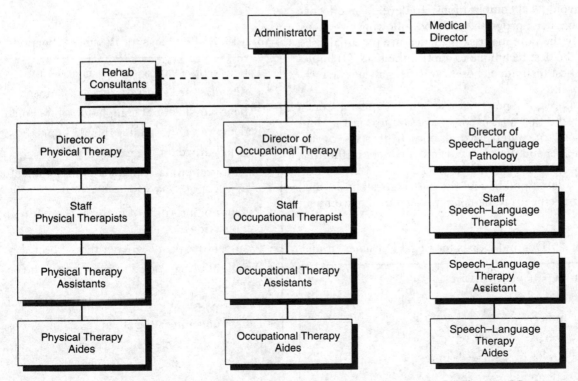

Figure 19.3   Sample Organizational Chart. (Reprinted with permission from Therapy Management Innovations, Inc.)

Additionally, liability for injury must be based on proximate cause. That is, the therapist's wrongful conduct must have actually caused the problem. For example, if the therapist walks the patient through a puddle of water, and the patient slips and falls, injuring the coccyx, that is considered proximate cause, and the therapist may be sued for unsafe practice and negligence. For the therapist in a supervisory capacity, as well as in a clinical capacity, it is advisable to use a systematic approach in writing notes, to ensure the therapist is legally covered.[1,2] The best system for this is the FACT System,[3] which stands for factual, accurate, complete, and timely. The FACT System states that therapists should write down factual comments, what they see, hear, smell, and feel, not what they suppose or assume. They should be accurate: never document for someone else and never ask other therapists to document for you. Be complete. Do not leave any blank spaces, because the attorney will allude to the possibility that space was left to be filled in at a later date.

Finally, be timely. Try to write your notes on time. If a late entry is necessary, do not write it in the margins; note that it was a late entry. If a late entry follows other entries and it is dated, it will look as though it were filled in after the fact in a methodical fashion. This reflects a better organized chart compared to squeezing notes in the margins. Do not erase errors; run a line through them and initial the correction. Table 19.4 provides additional dos and don'ts to help in legal documentation.

Finally, from an administrative advisory standpoint, therapists should keep in mind a risk management program to avoid legal complications. To develop an effective risk management program, take the following five steps: (1) identify the potential risks; (2) measure potential risks; (3) select the best technique to control the risks; (4) implement the best technique chosen; and (5) evaluate the technique chosen.

For example, if a potential risk is water spilling from a whirlpool, the therapist needs to assess if it is just a minimal amount of water leaking out. If it stays in the whirlpool area and does not move to a patient traffic area, there may not be a significant risk. If, however, the drip results in a large puddle and the patients walk in it, then some measure needs to be taken to keep the environment

safe. To drain the excess water, a pump may need to be installed in the floor, or a therapist or aide should be assigned the task of water control and clean up in the hydrotherapy unit. If either measure is used, it should be monitored to see if it is, in fact, solving the problem. If it is, it should be continued; if not, the risk assessment/management should be repeated until the situation is rectified. Some additional red flags that may indicate the liabilities of a lawsuit and of which therapists should be aware are listed in Table 19.5.[4]

Another area of legal concern for rehabilitation therapists is the malfunction or misuse of equipment. Unlike other specialties in medicine, equipment can play a large role in the legal ramifications of the physical therapy department. Therefore, therapists should be particularly aware of the following areas.

All equipment should be checked and calibrated annually or more periodically, if deemed necessary. The current certification should be clearly displayed on each piece of equipment as well as the last time that the equipment was checked. Finally, the procedure for the checking of equipment should be listed in the policy and procedure manual.

See CD for the policy and procedure manual.

Even simple equipment may pose a problem. For example, thermometers used in hot pack warmers, paraffin machines, and whirlpools may become dysfunctional.

TABLE 19.4   Dos and Don'ts for Legal Documentation

- Do put in patient's behavior.
- Don't get personal.
- Do use quotes.
- Don't advertise incident reports.
- Don't use charts to settle disputes.
- Do be neat and legible.
- Don't try to keep secrets.

TABLE 19.5   Red Flags for Possible Litigation

- Patient refuses or leaves treatment.
- Patient has cardiac arrest during treatment.
- Patient sees doctor at completion of treatment.
- Patient goes to hospital within 72 hours.
- Patient burned during treatment.
- Patient isn't properly prepared or equipment fails.
- Patient falls during visit.
- Patient not informed of his or her condition or complications.
- Postoperative pain is greater than expected.
- Patient not encouraged to call doctor if he or she has a problem.
- Patient wait is longer than 15 minutes.
- Patient uncomfortable about sexual questions.
- Patient given unclear instructions.
- Therapist unfriendly or discourteous.
- Patient feels therapist didn't spend enough time with him or her.

Temperature in these pieces of equipment should be checked monthly with a second thermometer to see if, in fact, they are correct. Hot pack covers showing bald spots and other warning signs should be replaced immediately.

Safety regulations should be posted on all pieces of equipment that require sophisticated techniques (e.g., Cybex equipment or balance machines). All timers and call bells should be checked daily, and footstools should be eliminated if they have worn pads. Wheelchairs and stretchers should be checked to make certain that locks, straps, and belts are in proper working order. Calibration of all equipment should be done annually.

The best idea for assessing safety is to have someone examine the department weekly, as though he or she were an insurance or safety inspector or a skeptical patient, keeping an eye out for hazards.

The final step of any legal administrative program is being prepared to go to court or to be deposed. Table 19.6 presents some useful hints for being an outstanding expert witness, being deposed, or being cross-examined.[4b-4d]

The following is a list of the most frequent reasons why therapists are sued, according to the APTA *Risk Management* manual:[4a]

1. Failure to perform a physical therapy diagnosis;
2. Failure to refer;
3. Failure to properly treat;

TABLE 19.6 Hints for Expert Witness

- Be sure you understand the question.
- Answer directly and simply.
- Don't volunteer information.
- Do not guess.
- Don't be too proud to admit the limits of your expertise.
- Take time to think before you answer.
- Do your homework.
- Speak clearly.
- Say yes or no; don't just shake your head.
- Always complete your answer.
- Don't let the opposing counsel cut you off.
- Be polite but firm, not cocky.
- Stop instantly when the judge interrupts you.
- Never lose your temper or argue with the attorney.
- When in court, talk directly to the members of the jury.
- Explain your answers in layperson's terms for the jury.
- Dress professionally and conservatively.

4. Failure to monitor the patient;
5. Failure to maintain equipment or equipment failure;
6. Failure to follow doctor's orders.

Improper practice by the therapist may lead to patient injury. Some common causes for patient injury are:[5-8]

1. Being improperly treated with heat or electric equipment;
2. Incorrectly performing exercises with various types of equipment;
3. Improper manipulation;
4. A slip and fall accident;
5. Improper range of motion testing.

HUMAN RESOURCES: EMPLOYEE RELATIONS

Human resources (HR) encompasses policies and procedures for employee orientation, benefits, and other programs. Providing proper supervision is another important part of HR issues. Many books have been written on how to supervise employees successfully. One of the easiest and most succinct books on supervision is *The One Minute Manager*.[9] The text, which takes about one minute to read, states that it takes one minute to acknowledge an employee's positive attributes and only one minute to reprimand an employee when necessary.

A good supervisor is one that is aware of employee needs and acknowledges good as well as inadequate performances. In addition, a good supervisor gives immediate feedback to the employee frequently.[10]

Employee orientation, quality assurance, in-services, and meeting attendance and orientations for aides are all areas that will require policy development as well as managerial expertise. Providing detailed information on this subject is beyond the scope of this text.

MARKETING

The final area to be covered in this chapter is marketing. Marketing is often a foreign concept for rehabilitation professionals. Frequently, marketing is thought of as selling, which it is not. Marketing is the process of identifying services to be offered and then promoting, pricing, and distributing these services to the patients.[10,11]

For example, before opening a rehabilitation therapy department that will provide geriatric care in the Los Angeles suburbs, it is imperative to research the composition of the population in the area to see if it will support the practice. This background information can be developed by reviewing Chamber of Commerce data, performing interviews with citizens, conducting random sampling by telephone or a mail survey, and general information gathering. Once a need has been identified, decisions can be made on pricing and promoting the service.

It is not easy to open a practice. Studies of demographics, compensation, and other factors must be thoroughly examined before a new practice can be opened. It is essential to develop a fair scheme for charging, to prepare a schedule that meets the needs of the community, to establish the most centrally located site for the services, and to make sure that the site is accessible to all clients.

The next step is to promote the service. Let people know that the service is available, show how it differs from other services in the area, and try to expose people to information about the clinic. This can be done in a number of ways, ranging from sending out letters or making telephone calls to preparing seminars or just advertising by word of mouth.

Targeting marketing efforts is very important. In many areas, therapists are dependent on physicians for referrals. Thus, marketing may need to be targeted at physicians. In other areas, targeting patients who may want physical therapy but cannot get physician orders may be the best approach.

Marketing can be divided into two categories: external and internal. External marketing has already been described and it involves letting people from the outside know about the practice's services. Internal marketing focuses on the inner workings of the facility and how the efficiency and high quality of the services provided encourages patients to return or refer others to the clinic. Good questions to assess internal marketing efforts are: (1) Is the staff courteous? (2) Is a visit to the clinic a pleasant experience? (3) Are patients provided with information about the facility? (4) Does the staff know what the goals of the clinic are and act with these in mind?

Internal marketing strategies are discussed widely in the literature and although providing more detail is beyond the scope of this section, additional references are available.[11-16] Table 19.7 provides a simple and succinct marketing strategy handout for therapists, discusses professional level marketing and community level marketing, and gives examples of how to implement these strategies.

TABLE 19.7   Marketing Strategy

Rehabilitation departments frequently succeed or fail due to their ability to plan and implement ongoing marketing programs to showcase rehabilitation services. Marketing concepts must be kept in mind at all times and not only during low volume periods. The following is an example of marketing techniques that each therapist is encouraged to develop relative to their facility and specialized programs.

Community Level

- Volunteer to an organization, such as Spinal Cord Club, Multiple Sclerosis, Muscular Dystrophy, Breast Cancer, homeless shelter.
- Advertise facility based community service programs, such as "Caring for the Stroke Patient at Home." Could be for families in the facility as well as on a local community level.
  - Organize a posture screening in a mall or senior center
  - Teach a special exercise class at a retirement center.
  - Develop educational activities for osteoporosis month (May).
- Presentations to Special Interest Groups.
  - Service clubs.
  - Elderly groups.
  - Community business groups.

Professional Level

- Doctor visits
  - Initial introduction to new physicians.
  - Introduce new programs or equipment in the rehabilitation department.
  - Discuss continuing education courses.
  - When getting started, you may want to discuss postoperative protocols (i.e., for THR, TKR to determine general approach to weight bearing, exercise).
  - Accompany patients on follow-up physician visits.
  - Send typed discharge summaries frequently.

TABLE 19.7 Marketing Strategy (Continued)

Professional Level

- Acute Care Rehabilitation Visits
  - ▪ Introduce yourself to all staff.
  - ▪ If new to area, may ask for information on local APTA chapter, TENS distributors, recommendations on good medical supply companies.
  - ▪ Tour the facility.
  - ▪ Ask for input on skilled nursing facility (SNF), rehabilitation needs in the community
- Discharge planners
  - ▪ Administrator, director of nursing, and rehabilitation professional make a good team to visit hospital discharge planners.
  - ▪ Leave brochures and business cards when available.
  - ▪ Send discharge planners typed discharge summaries on those patients they referred to you as soon as possible.
- Attend local continuing educational courses, especially those sponsored by your referring hospitals.
- Attend local professional meetings (e.g., APTA, AOTA state chapters).

Facility Level

- Admission meetings: attendance by the rehabilitation therapist is mandatory.
- Inservices to Nursing Staff and other disciplines for staff development, body mechanics, range of motion, positions, and teach rehabilitation approach.
- Form teams (e.g., wound care team, fall screening and prevention, etc.)
- Rehabilitation Conferences: used to teach rehabilitation approach to other disciplines.
- Consult with activities director to help coordinate an exercise class.

References

1. American Physical Therapy Association. Guide to physical therapist practice: Guidelines for physical therapy documentation. *Phys Ther.* 1997; 77(11): 1634–1636.
2. Lewis C. Avoid claim denials with better documentation. *ADVANCE for Phys Ther.* December 3, 2001.
3. Lewis C. *Documentation and Functional Assessment: A Home Study.* Rockville, MD: Great Seminars and Books, 2004.
4a. American Physical Therapy Association. *Risk Management.* Alexandria, VA: APTA; 1990.
4b. Klee C. Neurolitigation: A perspective on the elements of expert testimony for extending the Daubert challenge. *NeuroRehabilitation.* 2001; 16(2): 79–85.
4c. Michael, J. Expert witnessing brings nursing expertise into the legal arena. *Nurs Manage.* 2002; 33(3): 23–24.
4d. Murphy, J. Expert witnesses at trial: Where are the ethics? *Georgetown Journal of Legal Ethics.* 2001; 14: 217–239.
5. Morgan MG, Florig HK, DeKay ML, et al. Categorizing risks for risk ranking. *Risk Anal.* February 2000; 20(1):49–58.
6. Schraeder C, Britt T, Shelton P. Integrated risk assessment and feedback reporting for clinical decision making in a Medicare risk plan. *J Ambulatory Care Manag.* October 2000; 23(4):40–47.
7. Raven J, Rix P. Managing the unmanageable: Risk assessment and risk management in contemporary professional practice. *J Nurs Manag.* July 1999; 7(4): 201–206.
8. Michael JE, Summers CH. Establishing or enhancing your risk management program. Part II: The key elements of an effective risk management program. *Home Care Manag.* November–December 1997; 1(2): 10–13.
9. Blanchard K, Spencer J. *The One Minute Manager.* New York: Berkley Books; 1982.
10. Solomon R. *Clinical Practice Management.* Gaithersburg, MD: Aspen Publishers; 1991.

11. MacCracken L. *Market-Driven Strategy: An Executive's Guide to Health Care's Integrated Environment.* Chicago: American Hospital Publishing; 1997.

12. Kotler P, Clarke R. *Marketing for Health Care Organizations.* Upper Saddle River, NJ: Prentice Hall; 1987: 244.

13. Husted S, Varble D, Lowry J. *Principles of Modern Marketing.* Boston: Allyn and Bacon; 1997: 237.

14. Scott J, Warshaw M, Taylor J. *Introduction to Marketing Management.* 5th ed. Homewood, IL: Irwin Publishers; 1985: 11–12.

15. *Journal of Health Care Marketing.* American Marketing Association. 250 S. Wacker Drive, Chicago, IL 60606.

16. *Journal of Medical Practice Management.* Williams and Wilkins, 428 E. Preston Street, Baltimore, MD 21202.

20

Consultation and Research

Pearls

- The primary reasons for consultation services in geriatrics are patient care, professional education, public relations, screening, and quality assurance.
- The benefits of geriatric consultation are:
  1. Decreased length of hospitalization and responsible use of expensive health care resources.
  2. Increased use of rehabilitative services and identification of new diagnoses.
  3. Improved patient care.
  4. Greater access to educational resources.
- Rehabilitation therapists may serve as consultants in nursing homes, senior centers, hospitals, rehabilitation centers, fitness centers, industrial settings, as well as home care. The consultant's role will change in each setting.

- The steps in a successful consultation process are needs assessment, query, proposal, negotiation, implementation, and evaluation.
- The most important phase of the consultation process is the evaluation or outcome phase. This step can be as simple as checking patient satisfaction or as sophisticated as statistical analysis of postprogram scores.
- The major problems in aging research are sampling, subject recruitment, and design constraints.
- Evidence-based practice is crucial for the optimal care of older patients. Many components make up evidence-based care.

Introduction

The consultant role is not new to physical or occupational therapy, because rehabilitation professionals serve as consultants to other health care team members in daily treatment delivery. The therapist's role as a consultant is, however, new in the realm of geriatrics. Most literature on the subject of the consultant in geriatrics has been published in only the last twenty years.

Literature on geriatric consultation states several reasons for its development.[1a] These reasons include patient care, professional education, public relations screening, and quality assurance. The major reasons for requesting geriatric consultation were medical management, discharge planning, evaluation and management of dementia, and failure to thrive.[1b] According to another early study, the major reasons for requesting consultation were geriatric evaluation (28%), assessing rehabilitation potential (27%), and mental status evaluation (3%).[2]

Several benefits of geriatric consultation have been enumerated in the literature. These benefits are

1. Decreased length of hospitalization;[3a]
2. Increased use of rehabilitation services;[3b]
3. Improved patient care;[4]
4. Decreased use of expensive health care resources;[5]
5. Increased identification of new diagnoses;[6]
6. Provides a source of education.[7]

The negative aspects of geriatric consultation are:

1. Conflicts may arise among the disciplines when there is a "turf" battle over the overall management of the patient.
2. Geriatric consultation can be time consuming.
3. This type of consultation can also be costly.[7]

The final introductory point on geriatric consultation is efficacy. The general literature reveals no definitive conclusions as to the efficacy of consultation. The literature is fraught with complications about the type of patient classically referred to a medical geriatric consultant. First, the frailer patients are more frequently referred and are more difficult to manage. Second, the recommendations of the consultant are often only partially followed.[8,9,10] Even with the controversy in geriatric consultation, the potential benefit to the older person in different treatment settings outweighs the negative aspects cited. In addition in this chapter the benefits and pitfalls of geriatric research will be examined as it relates to the use of evidence-based practice in any setting.

SETTINGS FOR CONSULTING

Nursing Homes

The variety of settings available to the rehabilitation consultant in geriatrics is limited only by the therapist's imagination, but the major areas of consultation are nursing homes, home care, community senior centers, hospitals, rehabilitation centers, outpatient clinics, and industrial settings.

In the nursing home, a therapist can work as a staff therapist and receive a regular salary with all the benefits, or he or she can contract. Contract basis in the nursing home can take many forms, the most common of which are the hourly, per patient, or direct bill. In the hourly arrangement, the therapist charges the nursing home for any hours spent in the facility with the majority of time being spent in direct patient care. In addition, the therapist may set up restorative programs, provide in-service education, conduct screenings, and assist in quality assurance. The therapist is simply reimbursed on a time-spent basis.

The per patient arrangement reimburses the therapist based on how many patients are seen. This can be a flat figure per patient or based on a percentage of charges. The percentage method can be further broken down into the percentage of charges billed and the percentage of charges received. It is obvious that it is more advantageous to the therapist to contract on a percentage-billed basis, while the nursing home would prefer to use the percentage received. The pros of the first situation are that the therapist does not have to wait for the money and is not dependent on the nursing home's filing ability. In addition, the therapist does not risk a denied claim. The therapist who contracts on a percentage basis has several options in providing non-patient-care services: they can be included as part of the package on a gratis basis; the therapist can be reimbursed on a hourly basis for any time spent in presentation and preparation; or a flat fee can be assessed on a weekly, monthly, or yearly basis for these extra services.

The final, most common method of consulting in a nursing home with direct patient care as the major emphasis is direct billing of the patient. In this situation the therapist offers to treat any appropriate patients and to bill the respective insurance company. This form of consultation is riskier and more inundated with paperwork than the previously mentioned methods; however, it can prove to be the most lucrative.

For specific information on inpatient and outpatient contracting, see CD.

Home Care

Consultation in home care is identical to the situation already described when the consultant subcontracts with an agency. In this situation the therapist can be salaried, hourly, or per patient. In an even more independent situation, a therapist can hang up a shingle and treat patients in the home. The therapist will direct bill the patient and/or the insurance company.

Senior Centers

Senior centers and retirement homes provide a creative way of consulting in the geriatric realm, and therapists can serve in several capacities. For example, they can conduct environmental assessments, develop and teach exercise classes, or provide screening programs. The financial arrangements for these types of programs can be quite varied. The consultant can offer the facility a menu of these activities with a cost-per-activity charge. Another alternative is an hourly arrangement to provide whatever services are needed. The consultant can also directly charge the participants. For example, a consultant may charge each exercise class of 10 participants, $5 per session, or $20 for four sessions. The consultant may also want to provide some of the services for free as a public relations effort for future programs.

Hospitals, Rehabilitation Centers, and Outpatient Clinics

Hospital consulting is a new area of physical and occupational therapy; therefore, the therapist seeking hospital privileges is a relatively new and controversial topic.

The consultant in the hospital, rehabilitation center, and outpatient clinic can always contract to provide direct patient care on an hourly, per patient, or direct bill basis. He or she can also act to provide special assessment for older patients, which may take the form of a screening, such as an osteoporosis, balance, or foot evaluation. The consultant may also be called in to provide expert advice on how to improve the outcomes of therapy or to perform functional assessment specific for older persons (see

Chapter 10 for functional assessment tools). In addition to providing these services in the hospital, rehabilitation, and outpatient settings, the consultant can provide continuing education and screening programs to the public, as well as quality assurance expertise. The financial arrangement for this could take the form of an hourly contract, fee for service, or flat fee contract.

Industrial Settings

With increasing life expectancy, many elderly individuals choose to remain active in employment settings. In fact, many industrial entities actively recruit the older worker. As a result, industrial rehabilitation for an older population is an excellent platform for the consulting therapist. The consultant in a work-related setting can contract to do screening, functional capacity testing, ergonomic assessments and modifications, conditioning programs, and educational programs on health and wellness related topics for the older worker. Instruction in proper body mechanics for lifting and other repetitious activities can be implemented to prevent injury.

In all of these settings, the geriatric consultant may be asked to design a program where none has existed previously. This will require the consultant to create policy and procedure manuals, employee handbooks, and billing procedures and forms. In the opinion of the authors of this book, the best approach to this type of arrangement is to develop an hourly contract. A flat fee contract can also be used; however, this does not give the consultant the freedom to spend time on unforeseen complications that may arise in the process of designing a program.

IDENTIFYING CONSULTANT ACTIVITIES

Screening Programs

Screening programs are one of the major activities of the geriatric consultant. They can be conducted in any of the settings listed as well as in a public setting (e.g., shopping malls).

The CD has an example of a screening program for the community and an example of a screening mechanism for an institutional setting.

Direct Patient Care

Therapists can provide part-time or full-time direct patient care as another type of activity, and it can be very creative. In many situations the rehabilitation therapist conducts the initial evaluations and discharge evaluation, and the therapist assistant provides the hands-on treatment under the supervision of the physical therapist. Some therapists set up classes for providing care to similar

patients in the hospital, nursing home, or community setting. The options for care in this setting are limitless. Nevertheless, the important components of this type of consulting are appropriate evaluation, progressive treatment strategies, and comprehensive discharge planning. Throughout this process, the therapist must provide appropriate documentation.

Quality Assurance and Chart Review

Rehabilitation therapists can also act in a consultative capacity to provide quality assurance and chart review assistance. To provide this type of service the therapist should consult several references in this area. References[11-27] are particularly useful for information on quality assurance in the area of geriatrics. Several groups exist across the country that provide this type of service. However, if it can be done in-house or locally for less money and inconvenience, then the therapist is providing a worthwhile consultant service.

THE CONSULTATION PROCESS

To execute a successful consultation program a methodical and reproducible process should be followed. The steps in this process are:

1. Needs assessment;
2. Query;
3. Proposal;
4. Negotiation;
5. Implementation;
6. Evaluation.

A needs assessment can be conducted simply or through a very sophisticated process. In its simplest form, a needs assessment is conducted either by asking people if they think a program would be beneficial or by observing the site. Increasing in sophistication, a needs assessment would be a random phone survey, a written survey to a specific audience, or tapping the data from a community or facility survey.

The query portion of the process entails asking detailed questions to assist in the design of the program. For example, if a posture screening program is to be developed, questions about the time of day, acceptable waiting time, price, expectations, and people and facilities available would be useful (Figure 20.1).

A proposal can be simple or sophisticated. A simple proposal would be a telephone call to the general manager of a community mall, with a discussion that included information on the therapist's background. If space is available, the therapist should ask what the appropriate times are, about the available manpower, and about additional

---

Sample Query

Your group has expressed an interest in a low back exercise class. To design the class to meet your needs, please take a few moments to fill out the questions below.

1. What time of day is good for you?
2. Is five dollars per class acceptable?
3. What do you expect from this class?
4. How often would you like to come to the class?

Figure 20.1   Sample query for design of a program.

expense requirements. A letter restating the terms can follow this up.

The negotiation step of the consultation process entails discussing the therapist's needs with the facility. In this process, the therapist must come into the meeting with both an optimal situation and the minimal acceptable situation. Begin the negotiation by describing the optimal situation, and then ask the representative(s) from the facility about their optimal scenario. If the two match, both will be very happy. If the responses are completely opposite, then ask what their minimal acceptable situation is. If this situation is vastly different than the minimal criteria the therapist has established prior to this meeting, then he or she should graciously leave.

The implementation of the consulting process can be divided into four phases: long-term planning, short-term planning, execution, and continuation. Long-term planning begins from the moment the negotiation ends and the contract is signed and lasts until the day before the project begins. Activities to be accomplished during this phase are the design or completion of any administrative forms. For example, if a therapist consults to provide an exercise class, in the long-term phase he or she will need to develop medical releases and get them filled out before the class begins (Figures 20.2 and 20.3). Participant evaluation forms will be needed as well as handouts and contracts, and the class will need to be advertised. The final aspect of the long-term implementation is preparing the exercise class. In preparing for the first class, an introduction must be designed for the therapist and a way of meeting the class's participants must also be designed. Then a format for the class must be developed. Finally, the class should be practiced several times so the therapist is comfortable teaching it.

For marketing protocols, see CD.

In the short-term phase of implementation (one to two days before the class) areas to plan for are environmental and advertising. Environmentally, check the room one

more time before the class. Is there enough room? Is the temperature correct? Is the music system appropriate and do the tapes work on the equipment? Do you have tapes and do you feel comfortable working the equipment? The therapist is also part of the environment. What are you going to wear? There are several considerations here. First, you need to look professional, and yet you need to move around to teach an exercise class. Tailored slacks and a professional blouse will work. Second, the colors should be in the optimal appreciation range for the older person; that is, the reds, oranges, and golds.

The final aspect of the short-term implementation phase is intense advertising. In the last 24 to 48 hours, advertisements can be repeated for one more time. Flyers can be used to attract potential participants.

The execution phase is teaching the class. Do a last-minute check of the environment. Check to be sure the temperature and lighting are correct and that water is close by. Check to be sure the handouts are ready and that the music is working. At the very last minute, check to be sure that you are relaxed and comfortable.

The continuation phase is composed of what it takes to continue the consulting activity. In the preceding example, the continuation phase is relatively simple, but in a contracted physical therapy department, it can be much more difficult. For example, in the department setting the consultant is frequently confronted with patient load fluctuations and staff shortages. These types of problems constantly plague these settings and should be planned for in the continuation. Returning to the example of the continuation phase in the exercise classes, activities to enhance this phase are developing new handouts, programs, equipment usage, musical background, and continuing advertisement. In addition, frequent reevaluations of the class participants, using the initial evaluation to show progress, can help to motivate individuals to continue in an exercise program.

The final phase of the consultant process is the evaluation phase, which can be accomplished simply or in a more sophisticated fashion. In the simplest form, evaluation can be done by asking the recipients if they like the

Implementation Phase

	EXERCISE CLASSES	SETTING UP	PHYSICAL THERAPY DEPT.
Long-term	Medical releases Evaluation forms Contracts with individual Handouts Sign-in sheet Advertise		
Short-term	Check space Get equipment Get music Appropriate clothes Advertise		
Execution	Check water Check temperature Check music Check handouts Check lights		
Continuation	New handouts Reevalutate forms New equipment/music Advertise		

Figure 20.2 Implementation of the consulting process divided into long-term planning, short-term planning, execution, and continuation phases.

services. This can be done by spontaneous feedback or by a formal questionnaire (Figure 20.4).

In the hospital or nursing home setting, the recipients of the service are not the only consumers. Nurses and referring doctors should also receive questionnaires on the services. Evaluations can be done periodically or at set intervals (e.g., every six months), and they can also be used to assess outcomes.

Outcomes can be broken down into two broad categories. The first is patient or recipient outcomes. In the example of the exercise class, comparing initial and follow-up data can easily assess the participant outcome. The same is true for direct service consulting. Patient initial evaluation and subsequent evaluation comparison can show outcomes. The second outcome variable of overall institutional benefits is much more elusive and difficult to assess. The simplest way of assessing this variable is to choose one outcome. For example, in the direct service area, you may want to compare the number of falls prior to implementation of your rehabilitation program and after.

RESEARCH AND AGING

The last portion of this chapter will be dedicated to aging research and evidence-based practice. The issues in aging rsearch and the components of evidence-based practice as it applies and can be used in the everyday practice of geriatric rehabilitation will be discussed.

Problems with Aging Research

The problems with aging research are quite numerous, ranging from sampling and subject recruitment to cross-sectional design. In the area of sampling, the article by Wayne and associates[28] shows that people in cross-sectional samples tend to have longer nursing home stays, as well as less social support and more behavioral and functional problems than persons in the admissions sample, who tend to have shorter stays and more acute medical problems. Therefore, looking at a cross-sectional sample

Implementation Phases—Long-Term

NURSING HOME	HOSPITAL
Long-term	
Short-term	
Execution	
Continuation	

Figure 20.3   Long-term program planning during implementation phases by a consultant.

could skew the results of research findings. When conducting research in a nursing home, it is imperative to look at the samples chosen to control for the particular and cultural problems already listed.[28]

In the area of subject recruitment, several variables must be considered for the elderly. For example, older persons experience decreased mobility. Therefore, a study requiring mobility, such as the ability to drive a car or use public transportation to get to the test site, may eliminate participants from the study. To generalize the abilities of the subjects recruited is also difficult. For example, the majority of the elderly do not live in nursing homes. Therefore, to assume that they are a representative sample of all older people would be erroneous. In addition, when recruiting subjects from various settings, you may disrupt the normal functioning of the person's day and therefore make it difficult to generalize the results of the study.[29]

Gerontological researchers have been painfully aware of the effects of variability in subjects of aging research. Nelson and Dannifer,[30] however, present compelling information to the geriatric researcher to attend to the diversity and analyze the homogeneity of variance on control for aging research methodology. Their work showed an increase in variability with age up to 65%, which was more pronounced in longitudinal versus cross-sectional studies.[30]

Andrews[31] makes a very strong point for controlling cultural variables in aging research; points out that attitudinal, religious, social, and behavioral influences can affect many outcome measures commonly explored by rehabilitation researchers; and cites numerous examples, one of which is nutrition.[31] A person's religious background, for

example, can strongly influence a person's nutritional intake. This may affect rehabilitation variables, such as the ability to walk, independence, or need for assistance from others. These attitudinal, religious, and social variables should be controlled for when doing rehabilitation research to be sure to check for the effects of the study.[31]

In aging research, methodology can significantly impact research outcomes. Research designs can vary from cross-sectional to longitudinal. In cross-sectional research, all variables are measured at one point in time. Longitudinal research looks at an extended period of time and variables are measured over years. The benefits of cross-sectional studies are the short-term commitment and minimal financial implications. However, the ability to attribute differences between groups to variables of age is very difficult, and this particular study design does not take into consideration other confounding variables. For example, cohort differences can influence demographic variables. People who lived during the Depression developed a specific sense for understanding how to function in the economy when the availability of money was lowered. Therefore, as a group they have a different understanding of functioning. This shared experience is a cohort effect, which is difficult to figure out when using cross-sectional studies.[32]

Longitudinal studies, on the other hand, take a much longer amount of time and can be impractical in terms of time and money involved. In a longitudinal study, for example, a therapist may choose to examine patients/clients at age 20 to check for arthritis of the knee and follow them until they reach 90 years of age. This requires 70 years of study and is, therefore, impractical. Another

Patient Satisfaction Survey

The following is a survey that Crescent City Physical Therapy sends to patients within 30 days of their discharge date. What we hope to accomplish is to determine if we are meeting your needs and expectations. Crescent City Physical Therapy cares about what you think. We want to offer you the highest quality of patient care. So, please take a brief moment and complete this short survey, and return it in the stamped, self-addressed envelope. Thank You!!

1. The treatment you received from your physical therapist was?

   ☐ Excellent   ☐ Average   ☐ Poor   ☐ No response

2. The treatment you received from your physical therapy aid was?

   ☐ Excellent   ☐ Average   ☐ Poor   ☐ No response

3. The service you received from the front desk when you first set up an appointment was?

   ☐ Excellent   ☐ Average   ☐ Poor   ☐ No response

4. The service you received at the front desk when checking in for your appointment was?

   ☐ Excellent   ☐ Average   ☐ Poor   ☐ No response

5. The service you received at the front desk when setting up a return appointment was?

   ☐ Excellent   ☐ Average   ☐ Poor   ☐ No response

6. The manner or promptness in which billing the responsible party (insurance company, attorney, workman's compensation, or private pay) was?

   ☐ Excellent   ☐ Average   ☐ Poor   ☐ No response

7. Was the manner in which statements were sent easily understood?

   ☐ Excellent   ☐ Average   ☐ Poor   ☐ No response

8. The manner in which the Crescent City Physical Therapy office handled your telephone calls was?
   ☐ Excellent   ☐ Average   ☐ Poor   ☐ No response

Figure 20.4   Patient Satisfaction Survey. (Reprinted with permission from Cresent City Physical Therapy & Sports Rehabilitation Services, Inc.)

problem with longitudinal studies in the area of aging research is the discrimination of socialization. How, for example, can a therapist determine if the variables are actually age related or are activity related? Has a patient/client's medication or periods of rest or nutrition or depression affected the outcomes of the study, or can the findings truly be associated with the aging process?

Schale[33] proposes a cross-sectional and time-sequential analysis to differentiate the presence of cohort and age differences. He also suggests that this type of research can minimize problems of longitudinal methodologies. His method is called the cohort sequential method[33] and controls for historical events by following two or more cohorts over different age and time ranges. For example, a 20-year-old group, a 50-year-old group, and a 70-year-old group may be followed for 10 years to look at the effects of arthritis of the knee. Schale believes this method decreases the time involved in doing aging research and controls for the cohort differences. It does, however, give some longitudinal perspective to the research as to the aging process.[33]

Another problem with aging research can result from the use of the survey used. It is well known that some older persons have problems with vision, hearing, and mentation that may affect the extent to which they are able to respond to the survey instrument. The older person may also be more fearful of test taking, and therefore it may be more difficult to obtain informed consent from older populations.[34] Finally, the degree to which physical or cognitive impairments affect the older population may require special explanations and modifications of methods employed for research participation.[35,36]

Evidence-Based Practice

All of this research and scientific inquiry brings us back to the main purpose: improved patient care. This can be done through evidence-based practice. Evidence-based practice is purposefully making decisions using the most current and best scientific evidence available for each individual patient. The practitioner must use his or her professional judgment in integrating the best available evidence with individual clinical expertise.[37] This means that the practitioner must look at all the variables previously discussed plus the type and quality of the research[38]

Level of evidence is extremely important in determining the effectiveness of therapeutic interventions.[39] There are five levels of evidence. Level one is the highest level of evidence and equates to randomized control trials (RCT) that are large enough to have small false negatives or positives.[40] The second level is composed of smaller randomized trials that either show trends but may have the risk of false positives or show no impressive findings, but have the risk of false negatives. The third level is nonrandomized studies. The fourth level is formal comparison with historic controls. The fifth and final level is case series design.

Once the practitioner has looked at the study design other considerations are also important. The PEDro criteria developed by physical therapists in Australia have given us a point rating system to assess additional characteristics to ensure that the study is strong.[41] In a study that is a randomized controlled study, the outcomes would not be as strong if some of the characteristics of the study were not adhered to, such as intention to treat analysis. For example, a presenter told of a study of physical therapy for patients with total knee replacements. Half of the group received instruction in home care and half received daily physical therapy. Two weeks into the program the physician running the study switched three subjects who were doing very poorly in the home exercise group with three subjects who were doing the best in the daily physical therapy group and continued the study. Could comparisons really be made? Fortunately this study was never published. However, this factor called intention to treat analysis was not adhered to and significantly weakened the study even though it was an RCT.[42] This illustrates the importance of examining studies using the eleven points of Pedro listed below.[41]

PEDro Scale

1. Eligibility criteria were specified in the study.
2. Subjects were randomly allocated to groups.
3. Allocation was concealed.
4. The groups were similar at baseline regarding the most important prognostic indicators.
5. There was blinding of all subjects.
6. There was blinding of all therapists who administered the therapy.
7. There was blinding of all assessors who did the measurements.
8. Measurements of at least one key outcome were obtained from more than 85% of the subjects initially allocated to groups.
9. All subjects for whom outcome measurements were available received the treatment or control condition as allocated; or where this was not the case, data for at least one key outcome were analyzed by "intention to treat."
10. The results of between-group statistical comparisons are reported for at least one key outcome.
11. The study provides both point measurements and measurements of variability for at least one key outcome.

Clinicians in the area of geriatrics must become familiar with ways of using evidence in daily practice. Many organizations have developed research agendas to address common yet unanswered questions in the area of treatment efficacy.[43,44] Clinicians as well must question current care and look ahead to the future for better ways of providing care in all settings.

References

1a. Enguidanos SM, Gibbs NE, Simmons WJ, Savoni KJ, et al. Kaiser Permanente Community Partners Project: Improving geriatric management practices. *J Am Geriatr Soc.* 2003; 51:710–714.

1b. Duthie EH, Gambert SR. Geriatrics consultation implication for teaching and clinical care. *Gerontol Geriatr Edu.* 1983; 4:59.

2. Burley L, Currie C, Smith R, et al. Contribution from geriatric medicine within acute medical wards. *Brit Med J.* 1979; 2:90.

3a. Hogan DB, Fox RA, Badley BWD, et al. Effects of a geriatric consultation service on management of patients in an acute care hospital. *Can Med Assoc J.* 1987; 136:713.

3b. Studenski S, Perera S, Wallace D, Chandler JM, Duncan PW, et al. Physical performance measures in the clinical setting. *J Am Geriatr Soc.* 2003; 51: 314–322.

4. VanSwearingen JM, Brach JS. Making geriatric assessment work: Selecting useful measures. *Phys Ther.* 2001; 81(6).

5. Barker WH, Williams TF, Zimmer JG, et al. Geriatric consultation team. *J Am Geriatr Soc.* 1985; 33: 422.

6. Lichtenstein H, Winograd CH. Geriatric consultation: A functional approach. *J Am Geriatr Soc.* 1984; 32:356.

7. Lee T, Pappus EM, Goldman L. Impact of interphysician communication on the effectiveness of medical consultation. *Am J Med.* 1983; 74:105.

8. Katz P, Dube D, Calkins E, et al. Use of a structured functional assessment format in a geriatric consultation service. *J Am Geriatr Soc.* 1985; 33:681.

9. Campion EW, Jette AM, Beckman B. An interdisciplinary geriatric consultation service: A controlled trial. *J Am Geriatr Soc.* 1983; 31:792.

10. Lewis C. How to handle upcoming guidelines. *PT Bull.* June 27, 1990; 18–19.

11. Borden LP. Patient education and the quality assurance process. *QRB.* 1985; 11(4):123–127.

12. Chauhan L, Hutchings D, LePoer K. Quality assurance manual in PT services. *Clin Manage Phys Ther.* 1986; 6(5):28–31.

13. Filingliim CT, Deschler MJ. Quality control circles. *Clin Manage Phys Ther.* 1985; 5(5):42–43.

14. Gaynor L. Quality assurance quarterly screening review. *Clin Manage Phys Ther.* 1985; 5(5):38–41.

15. Glendinning M. Quality assurance in physiotherapy. *Austin Clin Rev.* November 1981; 1(3):22.

16. Goocle DH, Jamieson HD, Warrington DM. Quality assurance in physiotherapy. *Laser NZ J Physiother.* April 1984; 12(l):27–28.

17. Quality assurance. *Hosp Peer Rev.* March 1980; 5(3): 29–40.

18. Lewis C. *Health Promotion and Exercise for Older Persons.* Rockville, MD: Great Seminars and Books; 2005.

19. Coleman EA. Falling through the cracks: Challenges and opportunities for improving transitional care for persons with continuous complex care needs. *J Am Geriatr Soc.* 2003; 51:549–555.

20. Bogardus ST, Richardson E, Maciejewski PK, et al. Evaluation of a guided protocol for quality improvement in identifying common geriatric problems. *J Am Geriatr Soc.* 2002; 50:328–335.

21. Saltvedt I, Opdahl Mo ES, Fayers P, Kaasa S, Sletvold O. Reduced mortality in treating acutely sick, frail older patients in a geriatric evaluation and management unit. A prospective randomized trial. *J Am Geriatr Soc.* 2002; 50:792–798.

22. Coleman EA, Boult CB. Improving the quality of transitional care for persons with complex care needs. *J Am Geriatr Soc.* 2003; 51:556–557.

23. Home care enhances important outcomes using OASIS and structured quality improvement. *J Am Geriatr Soc.* 2002; 50:1456–1457.

24. Saliba D, Schnelle JF. Indicators of the quality of nursing home residential care. *J Am Geriatr Soc.* 2002; 50:1421–1430.

25. Berlowitz DR, Christiansen CL, Branderis GH, et al. Profiling nursing homes using Bayesian hierarchical modeling. *J Am Geriatr Soc.* 2002; 50: 1126–1130.

26. Landon BE, Normand ST, Blumenthal D, Daley J. Physician clinical performance assessment. Prospects and barriers. *J Am Geriatr Soc.* 2003; 200(9).

27. Cefalu CA. Adhering to inpatient geriatric consultation recommendations. *J Fam Pract.* 1996; 42(3): 259–263.

28. Wayne S, Rhyne RL, Thompson RF, et al. Sampling issues in nursing home research. *J Am Geriatr Soc.* 1991; 39(3):308–311.

29. Kelly P, Kroemer K. Anthropometry of the elderly: Status and recommendations. *Human Factors.* October 1990; 32(5):571–595.

30. Nelson E, Dannifer D. Aged heterogeneity: Fact or fiction? The fate of diversity in gerontological research. *Gerontologist.* 1992; 32(1):17–23.

31. Andrews G. Cross-cultural studies—An important development in aging research. *J Am Geriatr Soc.* 1989; 37(5):483–485.

32. Lewis, C. *Documentation and Functional Assessment.* Rockville, MD: Great Seminars and Books; 2003.

33. Schale KW. Quasi-experimental research designs in the psychology of aging. In: Britton SE, Schale KW, eds. *Handbook of the Psychology of Aging.* New York: Van Nostrand Rheinhold; 1985: 39.

34. Rayman I, Bloom S. Survey research as a tool for studying problems in the elderly. In: Kent B, Butler RN, eds. *Aging: Human Aging Research—Concepts and Techniques.* Vol. 34. New York: Raven Press; 1988: 51–76.

35. Mattson D. *Statistics Difficult Concepts; Understandable Explanations.* Oak Park, IL: Bolzchazy-Carducco Publishers; 1986.

36. Kinney LaPier TL, Donovan C. Statistical case scenarios in geriatric physical therapy research. *Geri-Notes.* 2000; 7(1):11–17.

37. Cormack JC. Evidence based practice . . . What is it and how do i do it? *J Orthop Sports Phys Ther.* March–April 1995; 74(2):163–170.

38. Fritz JM, Wainner RS. Examining diagnostic tests: An evidence-based perspective. *Phys Ther.* 2001; 81 (9):1546–1564.

39. Ioannidis JPA, Haidich A-B, Pappa M, Pantazis N, Kokori SI, Tektonidou MG, Contopoulos-Ioannidis DG, Lau J. Comparison of evidence of treatment effects in randomized and non-randomized studies. *JAMA.* 2001; 286(7):821–830.

40. Balk EM, Bonis PAL, Moskowitz H, Schmid CH, Ioannidis JPA, Wang C, Lau J. Correlation of quality measures with estimates of treatment effect in meta-analyses of randomized controlled trials. *JAMA.* 2002; 287(22):2973–2982.

41. Burgio LD, Fischer SE, Phillips LL, Allen RS. Establishing treatment implementation in clinical research. *Alz Care Quart.* July–September 2003; 4(3): 204–215.

42. McHorney CA. Ten recommendations for advancing patient-centered outcomes measurement for older persons. *Ann Intern Med.* 2003; 139:403–409.

43. Czaja SJ, Schulz R. Does the treatment make a real difference? The measurement of clinical significance. *Alz Care Quar.* 2003; 4(3):229–240.

44. American Physical Therapy Association. Clinical research agenda for physical therapy. *Phys Ther.* 2000; 80(5):499–513.

Index

Impregnated gauze, 403
Inactivity. *See* Activity and inactivity
Inappropriate prescribing practices, 140, 141–142
Incontinence
    fecal, 92, 93
    urinary, 91–92, 93, 416
    whirlpool for wound healing, 399
    wound evaluation, 373
    wound prevention and healing, 365, 371, 400
Infection
    diabetic ulcers, 391, 392
    wounds, 370, 378
Inflammation
    evolutionary theory of aging, 20
    secretory leukocyte protease inhibitor, 404
    ultrasound for wound healing, 399
    vasculitic ulcers, 394
    wound healing, 365, 367, 369f
Information organization, 477
Information presentation, 477–478
Information processing, 469–470
Informed consent, 451, 458–459
Institutionalization, 47, 55, 56
Insulin, 43
Insulin-like growth factor-1 (IGF-1), 23
Integumentary conditions, defined, 365–366. *See also* Skin; Wounds
Intelligence
    changes in late life, 52–53
    measuring, 472–474, 473f
Intensity of exercise, 343, 356, 357
Interface pressure, 401
Intermittent claudication
    arterial ulcers, 385
    peripheral vascular disease, 72, 73, 74, 75
Internal motivation, 431, 443, 444t
Interviews
    functional assessment, 211t
    patient evaluations, 183, 184
Intracardiac defibrillators, 358, 359
Intrinsic mutagenesis, theory of, 20–21, 25
Iodine
    nutritional deficiency, 110t
    recommended daily allowance, 114t
    supplements and natural sources, 122t
Iron
    nutritional deficiency, 110t
    recommended daily allowance, 114t
    supplements and natural sources, 122t
Ischemic heart disease, 70, 74
Isokenetic program, 325

J
JAMCO (judgment, affect, memory, cognition, and orientation) mnemonic for chronic brain syndrome, 61–62
Jeltrate mold technique, 377, 378f
Joints, 67, 79–80, 87–88
Judgment, 61
Jung's theory of development, 48

K
Kegel exercises, 92
Kidneys. *See* Renal disorders; Renal system
Kinesthesia, 31, 40, 42
Knee Society Knee Score, 265–266

Knees
    evaluation and treatment, 265–266, 268–269, 270
    exercises, 270
    extension torque, 200, 200t
    pathology of, 235, 236f
Knoll Assessment Scale, 392
Kyphosis, 229

L
Labyrinthitis, 84
Laryngectomy, 437t, 439t
Laxatives, 117
Learning
    age-related changes, 459, 467–468
    associative learning, 468–469
    changes in late life, 52–53
    contextual learning, 470
    covert strategies, 478–479
    defined, 467
    ethical issues, 459
    information organization, 477
    information presentation, 477–478
    information processing, 469–470
    intelligence, 472–474, 473f
    memory, 470–471, 471f, 472f
    motor learning, 474–475
    problem solving, 471–472
    rate of presentation, 477
    task choice, 477
    teaching in the therapeutic setting, 476–479
    teaching strategies for the elderly, 475
Legal issues, 489–491, 490t, 491t
Leukemia, 96
Levinson's seasons of adulthood, 51
Levodopa (L-dopa)
    bioavailability, 133, 134
    scheduling, 149
    side effects, 282
Lidocaine, 134
Life expectancy
    aging world population, trends in, 12–13
    U.S. aging population, 11
Life span
    caloric restriction theory of aging, 21
    maximum, as species characteristic, 19
    telomeres and aging, 24
Lipid peroxidation, 21
Lipodermatosclerosis, defined, 373
Lipofuscin
    central nervous system, 37
    free radical theory of aging, 21
Listening, 442, 442t
Litigation, risk for, 489–491, 490t
Liver
    metabolism of drugs, 135
    nutritional status, 106, 107t
Living arrangements, for aging population, 9–10
Living skin equivalents, 403
Living wills, 451, 459–460
Loneliness, 55, 56f
Losses, multiple, coping with, 58, 59, 60
Low-level functional treadmill walking test, 355
Low-level functional walking test, 355
Low-vision rehabilitation, 90

Low-voltage direct current, 398, 399
Lower extremity ulcers
    arterial, 365, 383–384t, 385–386
    diabetic, 383–384t, 389–392, 390f
    patient assessment, 365, 378, 382
    pressure, 365–392–394, 383–384t
    vasculitic, 383–384t, 394
    venous, 365, 383–384t, 386–388, 387f
Lucidity, mental, 458
Lumbar stenosis
    evaluation and treatment, 250, 251–253
    spinal pathology of the elderly, 229

M
Macular degeneration, 89, 93
Magnesium
    nutritional deficiency, 110t
    recommended daily allowance, 114t
    supplements and natural sources, 122t
Malnutrition
    immune function, 108
    wound healing, 371
Managed care, 451–452
Manganese, 122t
Manipulative techniques, 229
Marital status, 9, 10f
Marketing, 483, 491–492, 492–493t
Maslow's hierarchy of needs, 48–49, 55, 56f
Master's 2-step exercise, 354
Maximal oxygen consumption (VO$_2$), 347–348, 360
McGill-Melzak Pain Questionnaire, 185
Meals on Wheels, 123
Medical history, 184, 186t
Medicare
    foot problems, 418
    as managed care, 452
Medicare Shoe Demonstration Project, 418
Medicated elastic wraps, 388
Medication profile, 146–147
Medications. *See also* Pharmacology; specific classes of medications; specific medications
    combination drug therapy, 129, 130–131
    drug administration routes, 132
    drug clearance, 136
    drug excretion, 129, 133f, 136
    drug interactions, 141, 143–144
    drug regimen monitoring, 146–147
    duration of action, 137
    exercise, 343, 359
    hepatic system, 43
    nutrition, effects on, 105, 115–117, 118–119t
    over-the-counter, 416
    reactions to, 129, 132
    use and misuse, screening for, 415–416
    wound care, 402
    wound healing, effect on, 370–371
Memory
    chronic brain syndrome, 61
    cognitive changes in late life, 52, 52t
    intelligence, 474
    learning, 467, 468, 470–471, 471f, 472f
    teaching in the therapeutic setting, 478
    training, 475
Ménière's disease, 84
Mental status, assessment of, 191–193, 192f, 194f, 195f, 197

Pusher syndrome
   gait disturbances, 308
   stroke, 298, 302

Q
Qi Gong, 229
Quality assurance, 497
Quality of life, 452
Quinine, 142

R
Radial head fractures, 232
Radiation
   burns, 395
   somatic mutation theory of aging, 22
Range of motion
   musculoskeletal parameters, 201t, 202,
      202f, 203t, 204t
   Parkinson's disease, 290t, 291
Reaction stage of wound healing, 365, 367,
   369f
Recall stage of memory, 471
Recent memory, 471
Receptor alterations, 129, 138–140
Reciprocity, principle of, 50
Red blood cells, 36, 37
Redundant DNA theory of aging, 22, 26
REEDCO Posture Score Sheet, 202–203,
   205f
Refusal of treatment
   cardiopulmonary resuscitation, 461
   patients' rights, 457
Regeneration stage of wound healing, 365,
   367, 369f
Registration stage of memory, 471
Rehabilitation, principles and practices of
   activity *versus* inactivity, 159–161, 160t
   adapting the environment, 155, 175, 177
   assistive devices, 169
   caregivers, functional abilities of, 158
   disability, defined, 156
   disability demographics of the elderly,
      155, 156–157, 157f
   drug regimen monitoring, 146–147
   exercise, prescribed level of, 169–170
   exercise programming, 163–164,
      165–168t
   falls, 155, 172–175, 176f, 178
   frailty, 155, 157–158
   functional assessment of the elderly, 158
   geriatric rehabilitation, principles of,
      155, 158–162, 160t
   health awareness and beliefs, 163
   optimal health, 155, 161–162
   pain management, 164, 168–169
   purpose of, 155–156, 158–159
   rehabilitative measures, 162–170,
      165–168t
   restraints, 155, 170–172, 170t, 171t
   specific medication considerations, 129,
      148–149
   variability of the elderly, 155, 159
Rehabilitation centers, 496–497
Relative body weight, 109
Relaxation training, 77
Remodeling stage of wound healing, 365,
   367, 369f
Remote memory, 471

Renal disorders
   acute and chronic renal failure, 94, 98
   combination drug therapy, 131
   nutritional problems, 107t
   osteomalacia, 226
   renal disease, 93–94
Renal system
   age-related changes, 43–44
   excretion of drugs, 136
Research
   evidence-based practice, 502–503
   problems with aging research, 499–500,
      502
Resistance bands and cuff weight program,
   325
Resistance exercise
   cardiovascular pathology, 71
   depression, 54
Resistive lung disease, 75–76, 87
Resources, allocation of, 453–454
Respiratory system. *See* Cardiopulmonary
      system; Pulmonary system
Restraints, physical and chemical
   benefits and risks, 170t
   ethical issues, 462–463
   geriatric use, 155, 170–172
   side rails, 171, 171t
Retention stage of memory, 471
Retrieval stage of memory, 467, 471, 471f
Reverting postmitotic cells, 19
Rheumatoid arthritis
   evaluation and treatment, 248, 250
   orthopaedic considerations, 228–229, 228t
   pathological manifestations of aging, 67,
      79–80, 88
   spinal pathology of the elderly, 230
   wrists and hands, 232
Rheumatoid Arthritis Pain Scale, 249
Rheumatoid Hand and Functional Disabil-
      ity Scale, 260–261
Rigidity, muscular, 285, 286t, 290t
Risk management, 490
Rivermead ADL scale, 302f, 303f
Romberg's test, 314
Rotator cuff pathology, 231

S
Safety. *See also* Falls; Restraints
   assessing for, 417
   environment, adapting, 155, 175, 177
   rehabilitation department, 490–491
Sarcopenia, defined, 35–36
Schenkman's approach to treatment for
      Parkinson's disease, 285, 291
Screening programs
   cancer, 413–414
   cardiovascular disease, 413
   dementia, 416
   diabetes mellitus, 414
   foot problems, 418–424, 419–423f, 425f,
      426f, 427f
   geriatric consultation activities, 497
   health habits, 414–416
   health problems of the elderly, 411
   high-risk populations, 412–413
   osteoporosis, 414
   prevention, advantages of, 409–410
   prevention types, 410–411

primary prevention, 410, 412, 417–418
   psychological problems, 416
   safety, 417
   secondary prevention tests, 413
   sensory deficits, 416
   special considerations, 424
   urinary incontinence, 416
Seborrhea, 287t
Secondary prevention
   community-based screening programs,
      412
   prevention, types of, 410–411
   screening tests, 413
Secretory leukocyte protease inhibitor, 404
Sedatives, 370, 371
Selenium, 114t, 123t
Self-appraisal of health
   mortality, 163
   teaching in the therapeutic setting, 478
Self-care
   Parkinson's disease, 287t
   teaching in the therapeutic setting, 477
Self-Care Guidelines: Recommended Foot
      Care, 426f
Self-determination, 452
Self-Evaluation of Life Function question-
      naire, 412
Self-medication, 129, 131
Self-paced learning, 476
Semipermeable foam dressings, 403
Semmes-Weinstein monofilaments, 356
Senile purpura, 39
Senior centers, 496
Sensorineural hearing loss, 40, 431, 432
Sensory changes. *See also* Hearing; Vestibu-
      lar system; Vision
   debridement for wound healing, 400
   deficit screening, 416
   hearing, 40, 41–42, 431–434, 432t, 433f,
      434t, 435t
   immobilization, 159
   proprioception/kinesthesia, 31, 40, 42,
      312
   taste and smell, 40, 42, 434
   temperature, protective, and vibration,
      356
   touch, 39, 41, 89, 434
   vestibular system, 40, 42
   vision, 39–40, 41, 434
Sensory integration techniques, 164
Shoes
   balance and falls, 317
   foot problems, 237
   Medicare coverage, 418
Short-term (immediate) memory, 471
Shoulder Pain and Disability Index, 258
Shoulders
   evaluation and treatment, 258–259
   hemiplegia with stroke, 308
   orthopaedic considerations, 230–232
   range of motion, 202, 203t, 204t
Side rails, bed, 171, 171t
Silver sulfadiazine, 391
Single platform step test, 354
Sinus tracts of wounds, 376–377, 377f
Skeletal system. *See* Musculoskeletal system
Skin. *See also* Wounds
   age-related changes, 39, 41